Edited by
Timo Jäger, Oliver Koch, and Leopold Flohé

Trypanosomatid Diseases

Titles of the Series "Drug Discovery in Infectious Diseases"

Selzer, P. M. (ed.)

Antiparasitic and Antibacterial Drug Discovery

From Molecular Targets to Drug Candidates

2009

ISBN: 978-3-527-32327-2

Becker, K. (ed.)

Apicomplexan Parasites

Molecular Approaches toward Targeted Drug Development

2011

ISBN: 978-3-527-32731-7

Conor R. Caffrey (ed.)

Parasitic Helminths

Targets, Screens, Drugs and Vaccines

2012

ISBN 978-3-527-33059-1

Forthcoming Topics of the Series

• Protein Phosphorylation in Parasites: Novel Targets for Antiparasitic Intervention

Related Titles

Lucius, R., Loos-Frank, B., Grencis, R. K., Striepen, B., Poulin, R. (eds.)

The Biology of Parasites

2014

ISBN: 978-3-527-32848-2

Lamb, T.

Immunity to Parasitic Infections

2013

ISBN: 978-0-470-97247-2

Zajac, A. M., Conboy, G. A. (eds.)

Veterinary Clinical Parasitology

2012

ISBN: 978-0-8138-2053-8

Scott, I., Sutherland, I.

Gastrointestinal Nematodes of Sheep and Cattle

Biology and Control

2009

ISBN: 978-1-4051-8582-0

Edited by Timo Jäger, Oliver Koch, and Leopold Flohé

Trypanosomatid Diseases

Molecular Routes to Drug Discovery

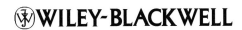

The Editors

Volume Editors:

Dr. Timo Jäger
German Centre for Infection Research
Inhoffenstraße 7
38124 Braunschweig
Germany
timo.jaeger@dzif.de

Dr. Oliver Koch
TU Dortmund University
Faculty of Chemistry
Otto-Hahn-Straße 6
44227 Dortmund
Germany
Oliver.Koch@tu-dortmund.de

Prof. Dr. med. Dr. h.c. Leopold Flohé
Otto-von-Guericke-Univeristät
Department of Chemistry
Universitätsplatz 2
39106 Magdeburg
Germany
l.flohe@t-online.de

Series Editor:

Prof. Dr. Paul M. Selzer
MSD Animal Health Innovation GmbH
Zur Propstei
55270 Schwabenheim
Germany
Paul.Selzer@msd.de

Cover Legend

The cover depicts the three-dimensional structure of a trypanothione synthetase model containing ATP, glutathione, and glutathionylspermidine in the active site. The protein is shown in ribbon representation. Glutathionylsperimidine, ATP, and glutathione are depicted in ball-and-stick representation. Two magnesium ions are shown as green spheres. The structure visualization was prepared by R. Marhöfer, MSD Animal Health Innovation GmbH, Schwabenheim, Germany on the basis of a structural model, kindly provided by O. Koch *et al.*, Chapter 23. The inset shows an artificially colored scanning electron microscope image of *Trypanosoma brucei* (blue) surrounded by erythrocytes (red discs) and a single leukocyte (yellow sphere). The original scanning electron microscope image was kindly provided by M. Duszenko, University of Tübingen, Germany.

Library of Congress Card No.: applied for

British Library Cataloguing-in-Publication Data
A catalogue record for this book is available from the British Library.

Bibliographic information published by the Deutsche Nationalbibliothek
The Deutsche Nationalbibliothek lists this publication in the Deutsche Nationalbibliografie; detailed bibliographic data are available on the Internet at http://dnb.d-nb.de.

© 2013 Wiley-VCH Verlag GmbH & Co. KGaA, Boschstr. 12, 69469 Weinheim, Germany

Wiley-Blackwell is an imprint of John Wiley & Sons, formed by the merger of Wiley's global Scientific, Technical, and Medical business with Blackwell Publishing.

Composition   Thomson Digital, Noida, India
Printing and Binding   betz-druck GmbH, Darmstadt
Cover Design   Adam-Design, Weinheim

Print ISBN: 978-3-527-33255-7
ePDF ISBN: 978-3-527-67039-0
epub ISBN: 978-3-527-67040-6
mobi ISBN: 978-3-527-67041-3
oBook ISBN: 978-3-527-67038-3

Printed in the Federal Republic of Germany
Printed on acid-free paper

Contents

Foreword *IX*

Acknowledgment *XV*

Preface *XVII*

List of Contributors *XIX*

Part One Disease Burden, Current Treatments, Medical Needs, and Strategic Approaches *1*

1 **Visceral Leishmaniasis – Current Treatments and Needs** *3*
*Poonam Salotra, Ruchi Singh, and Karin Seifert**

2 **Chemotherapy of Leishmaniasis: A Veterinary Perspective** *17*
*María Jesús Corral-Caridad and José María Alunda**

3 **Pharmacological Metabolomics in Trypanosomes** *37*
*Darren J. Creek, Isabel M. Vincent, and Michael P. Barrett**

4 **Drug Design and Screening by *In Silico* Approaches** *57*
*Mattia Mori and Maurizio Botta**

5 **Computational Approaches and Collaborative Drug Discovery for Trypanosomal Diseases** *81*
Sean Ekins and Barry A. Bunin*

Part Two Metabolic Peculiarities in the Trypanosomatid Family Guiding Drug Discovery *103*

6 **Interaction of *Leishmania* Parasites with Host Cells and its Functional Consequences** *105*
*Uta Schurigt, Anita Masic, and Heidrun Moll**

7 Function of Glycosomes in the Metabolism of Trypanosomatid Parasites and the Promise of Glycosomal Proteins as Drug Targets *121*
Melisa Gualdrón-López, Paul A.M. Michels, Wilfredo Quiñones, Ana J. Cáceres, Luisana Avilán, and Juan-Luis Concepción*

8 Glyoxalase Enzymes in Trypanosomatids *153*
*Marta Sousa Silva, António E.N. Ferreira, Ricardo Gomes, Ana M. Tomás, Ana Ponces Freire, and Carlos Cordeiro**

9 Trypanothione-Based Redox Metabolism of Trypanosomatids *167*
Marcelo A. Comini and Leopold Flohé*

10 Thiol Peroxidases of Trypanosomatids *201*
Helena Castro and Ana M. Tomás*

11 Peroxynitrite as a Cytotoxic Effector Against *Trypanosoma cruzi*: Oxidative Killing and Antioxidant Resistance Mechanisms *215*
*Madia Trujillo, María Noel Alvarez, Lucía Piacenza, Martín Hugo, Gonzalo Peluffo, and Rafael Radi**

12 Selenoproteome of Kinetoplastids *237*
*Alexei V. Lobanov and Vadim N. Gladyshev**

13 Replication Machinery of Kinetoplast DNA *243*
*Rachel Bezalel-Buch, Nurit Yaffe, and Joseph Shlomai**

14 Life and Death of *Trypanosoma brucei*: New Perspectives for Drug Development *261*
*Torsten Barth, Jasmin Stein, Stefan Mogk, Caroline Schönfeld, Bruno K. Kubata, and Michael Duszenko**

Part Three Validation and Selection of Drug Targets in Kinetoplasts *279*

15 Rational Selection of Anti-Microbial Drug Targets: Unique or Conserved? *281*
*Boris Rodenko and Harry P. de Koning**

16 Drug Targets in Trypanosomal and Leishmanial Pentose Phosphate Pathway *297*
Marcelo A. Comini, Cecilia Ortíz, and Juan José Cazzulo*

17 GDP-Mannose: A Key Point for Target Identification and Drug Design in Kinetoplastids *315*
Sébastien Pomel and Philippe M. Loiseau*

18 Transporters in Anti-Parasitic Drug Development and Resistance   *335*
Vincent Delespaux and Harry P. de Koning*

19 Peptidases in Autophagy are Therapeutic Targets for Leishmaniasis   *351*
Roderick A.M. Williams*

20 Proteases of *Trypanosoma brucei*   *365*
Dietmar Steverding*

Part Four   Examples of Target-Based Approaches and Compounds Under Consideration   *383*

21 Screening Approaches Towards Trypanothione Reductase   *385*
Mathias Beig, Frank Oellien, R. Luise Krauth-Siegel, and Paul M. Selzer*

22 Redox-Active Agents in Reactions Involving the Trypanothione/Trypanothione Reductase-based System to Fight Kinetoplastidal Parasites   *405*
Thibault Gendron, Don Antoine Lanfranchi, and Elisabeth Davioud-Charvet*

23 Inhibition of Trypanothione Synthetase as a Therapeutic Concept   *429*
Oliver Koch*, Timo Jäger, Leopold Flohé, and Paul M. Selzer

24 Targeting the Trypanosomatidic Enzymes Pteridine Reductase and Dihydrofolate Reductase   *445*
Stefania Ferrari, Valeria Losasso, Puneet Saxena, and Maria Paola Costi*

25 Contribution to New Therapies for Chagas Disease   *473*
Patricia S. Doyle* and Juan C. Engel

26 Ergosterol Biosynthesis for the Specific Treatment of Chagas Disease: From Basic Science to Clinical Trials   *489*
Julio A. Urbina*

27 New Developments in the Treatment of Late-Stage Human African Trypanosomiasis   *515*
Cyrus J. Bacchi, Robert T. Jacobs, and Nigel Yarlett*

Index   *531*

Foreword
Drug Discovery for Neglected Diseases –
Past and Present and Future

The kinetoplastid diseases – sleeping sickness, the leishmaniases, and Chagas disease – are "neglected diseases of poverty," afflicting millions of people and collectively responsible for over 100 000 deaths per annum. No vaccines are available and current insect vector control methods and other public health measures are insufficient to eliminate them. The currently available drug therapies are far from satisfactory due to issues such as poor efficacy, toxicity, the need for hospitalization, the requirement for prolonged parenteral treatment, and high cost. This book is a timely attempt to address some of these unmet medical needs.

It is somewhat ironic that, at the beginning of the twentieth century, many of the ground-breaking developments in drug discovery were driven by economic and colonial expansion in Africa and Asia. The African trypanosome in particular was an early model for experimental chemotherapy along two main lines of investigation: synthetic dyes, and organic arsenicals and antimonials (for further details, see reviews by Williamson [1] and Steverding [2]). Indeed, the first synthetic compound to cure an infectious disease in an animal model was the dye, Trypan red (Ehrlich, 1904), which was a forerunner of suramin (1916–1920), the first effective trypanocidal drug for human African trypanosomiasis (HAT). The demonstration by Thomas and Breinl in 1905 of the trypanocidal activity in mice of atoxyl (*p*-aminophenylarsonic acid) formed the basis of Ehrlich's pioneering work on organic arsenicals that culminated in the development of arsphenamine (606, Salvarsan) for the treatment of syphilis (Ehrlich and Hata, 1910) and tryparsamide for the treatment of HAT (Jacobs and Heidelberger, 1919). Tryparsamide, which caused blindness in 10–20% of patients, was finally replaced by melarsoprol (Friedheim, 1949). Trivalent antimony, in the form of tartar emetic, was shown to be trypanocidal in mice (Plimmer and Thompson, 1908), but lacked efficacy in humans. However, potassium antimony tartrate was found to have some activity in the treatment of leishmaniasis (Vianna, 1912) and was the forerunner of the pentavalent antimonial drugs, sodium stibogluconate (Pentostam®) and meglumine antimonate (Glucantime®), both introduced in the 1940s. Along with the diamidine, pentamidine (1937), all of these drugs are still in use today.

From the 1950s, subsequent drug treatments have largely been discovered by serendipity through repurposing of existing drugs used for other indications. The nitrofuran, nifurtimox, and the nitroimidazole, benznidazole, used for the treatment of Chagas disease arose from research into nitro-compounds as antibacterial agents. Amphotericin B, isolated in 1953, was originally developed for the treatment of systemic mycoses, but later found use in the treatment of visceral leishmaniasis in the 1990s as the expensive, but highly efficacious liposomal formulation (AmBisome®) or as the cheaper, but more toxic amphotericin B deoxycholate. Both formulations were included in the World Health Organization's Essential Medicines List in 2009. The off-patent aminoglycoside, paromomycin, originally developed as an oral treatment for intestinal infections in the 1960s, finally gained approval as paromomycin intramuscular injection for the treatment of visceral leishmaniasis in India in 2006. Two anticancer agents, the phospholipid analog, miltefosine, registered as the first oral treatment for visceral leishmaniasis in India in 2002, and eflornithine (now in combination with oral nifurtimox as nifurtimox–eflornithine combination therapy (NECT), 2009) for the treatment of HAT caused by *Trypanosoma brucei gambiense* complete the woefully inadequate treatment options for these diseases. Notably, none of these newer developments have completely displaced their forerunners that were developed prior to the 1950s.

After nearly a century of research, only 10 novel chemical entities for three diseases is a singularly unimpressive output by the pharmaceutical industry. The reason for this lamentable performance is not hard to find. Poor economic return on investment by pharma is a major factor, since these are diseases of poverty. The thalidomide disaster of the late 1950s kick-started regulatory demands for greater patient safety resulting in ever-increasing development costs. Blockbuster drugs were "in;" smaller, less profitable markets were "out." Ninety percent of research and development was aimed at 10% of the world's unmet medical need – the so-called "10–90 gap." The drive for greater efficiency and profitability through mergers and acquisitions resulted in the loss of parasitology expertise in most pharma companies. Medicinal chemists were seduced by combinatorial chemistry without due regard for chemical space and drug-likeness. Miniaturization of chemical synthesis restricted the use of animal disease models and shifted emphasis towards target screening. Intellectual property rights were increasingly used as an obstructive, rather than an enabling tool.

At the end of the twentieth century, the situation had become so dire that a radical new approach was required. One of the most encouraging developments was the founding of "public–private partnerships" (PPPs), such as the Drugs for Neglected Diseases *initiative* (DNDi) and Medicines for Malaria Venture (MMV) – non-profit organizations who strive to forge drug discovery partnerships between multiple academic, biotech, and pharma partners with funding from the governmental and charitable sector [3]. PPPs were initially met with much skepticism, but by 2005, an analysis by Mary Moran and colleagues concluded that PPPs were responsible for three-quarters of an expanded research and development portfolio for neglected diseases [4]. Another important development was the publication of annotated genomes for *T. brucei*, *L. major*, and *T. cruzi* in 2005 [5–7]. As Barry Bloom optimistically prophesized 10 years earlier "Sequencing bacterial and parasitic pathogens . . . could buy the sequence of every virulence determinant, every protein antigen and every drug target . . . for all time" [8]. Certainly, pathogen genomes are proving to be a valuable resource for target discovery, but without a deeper understanding of parasite biology the full potential of these genomes will not be realized. About the same time as genome sequencing was getting underway, C.C. Wang threw down the gauntlet that academics needed genetic evidence of essentiality to justify their claims of the therapeutic potential of their research field [9]. This dogma has now been refined and extended to include chemical evidence of druggability, driven by a defined therapeutic product profile [10]. These challenges have encouraged some academics to move out of their traditional comfort zones to fill the early-stage drug discovery gap in translational medicine not adequately covered by the PPPs [11]. The concept of "one gene, one target, one drug" has been very much at the forefront of current academic (and industry) thinking, with structure-based design an important adjunct in this strategy. Thus, it is timely that much of this book is devoted to the identification of metabolic peculiarities in the kinetoplastids that can be chemically and genetically validated as drug targets.

However, what of the future? Experience in industry and in academia suggests that the rate of validation of new targets is failing to keep pace with the rate of attrition of currently validated targets. Despite initial promise, the target-based approach has yielded disappointing results in anti-bacterial discovery in pharma [12] and lessons need to be learned from this if we are to avoid making the same mistakes. Rapid and robust methods of genetic target validation are still needed for parasites causing visceral leishmaniasis and Chagas disease, and we need a better understanding of basic biology to understand why targets fail. Certainly, not all targets are equal from a medicinal chemistry point of view. Greater attention needs to be paid to drug likeness [13] and ligand efficiency [14] for lead selection. Screening of fragment libraries using biophysical methods should help to weed out "undruggable" targets without recourse to expensive high-throughput screens [15]. From a pharmacology perspective, cytocidal activity is much preferable to cytostatic, so biologists should address this question early in discovery. Likewise, the potential ease for resistance arising as a result of point mutations in a single-target strategy should be a research priority for biologists. Systems biology suggests that exquisitely selective, single-target compounds may exhibit lower than desired clinical efficacy compared with multitarget drugs due to the robustness of biological networks [16]. Thus, polypharmacology (network pharmacology) is undergoing a resurgence of interest. Given the paucity of validated druggable targets, phenotypic screening is undergoing a revival aided by access to large compound collections held by pharma and the development of suitable miniaturized whole-parasite screens and mammalian counter-screens. This approach has the advantage of addressing the key druggability issues of cell permeability, desirable cytocidal activity, and a suitable parasite–host selectivity window. Phenotypic screening can also identify compounds hitting non-protein targets (e.g., amphotericin B) or compounds that act as prodrugs (e.g., nitroimidazoles). However, the future challenge will be to identify the often complex mode(s) of action of such phenotypic hits (target deconvolution), and to use modern technologies to improve the potency and selectivity of these molecules [17]. Finally, we should ask ourselves whether our compound collections are too "clean" in terms of chemical reactivity. After all, arsenicals, antimonials, nitro-drugs, and eflornithine all undergo reaction with one or more targets, and about one-quarter of all drugs that inhibit enzymes are essentially irreversible reactions [18].

I believe that there is every cause for optimism in the battle against neglected diseases. As long as "donor fatigue" does not set in, and industry continues to engage in a positive and productive manner with academia, future prospects look better than at any time in history. However, we should all remember the dictum by Sir James Black "to first purge your project of wishful thinking" if we are to succeed!

Dundee, UK

Alan Fairlamb

References

1 Williamson, J. (1970) Review of chemotherapeutic and chemoprophylactic agents, in *The African Trypanosomiases* (ed. H.W. Mulligan), Allen & Unwin, London, pp. 125–221.

2 Steverding, D. (2010) The development of drugs for treatment of sleeping sickness: a historical review. *Parasit. Vectors*, **3**, e15.

3 Matter, A.. and Keller, T. H. (2008) Impact of non-profit organizations on drug discovery: opportunities, gaps, solutions. *Drug Discov. Today*, **13**, 347–352.

4 Moran, M., Ropars, A.-L., Guzman, J., Diaz, J., and Garrison, C. (2005) *The New Landscape of Neglected Disease Drug Development*, The Wellcome Trust, London, pp. 1–99.

5 Berriman, M., Ghedin, E., Hertz-Fowler, C., Blandin, G., Renauld, H., Bartholomeu, D.C., Lennard, N.J., Caler, E., Hamlin, N.E., Haas, B., Bohme, U., Hannick, L., Aslett, M.A., Shallom, J., Marcello, L., Hou, L., Wickstead, B., Alsmark, U.C., Arrowsmith, C., Atkin, R.J., Barron, A.J., Bringaud, F., Brooks, K., Carrington, M., Cherevach, I., Chillingworth, T.J., Churcher, C., Clark, L.N., Corton, C.H., Cronin, A., Davies, R. M., Doggett, J., Djikeng, A., Feldblyum, T., Field, M.C., Fraser, A., Goodhead, I., Hance, Z., Harper, D., Harris, B.R., Hauser, H., Hostetler, J., Ivens, A., Jagels, K., Johnson, D., Johnson, J., Jones, K., Kerhornou, A.X., Koo, H., Larke, N., Landfear, S., Larkin, C., Leech, V., Line, A., Lord, A., MacLeod, A., Mooney, P.J., Moule, S., Martin, D.M., Morgan, G.W., Mungall, K., Norbertczak, H., Ormond, D., Pai, G., Peacock, C.S., Peterson, J., Quail, M.A., Rabbinowitsch, E., Rajandream, M.A., Reitter, C., Salzberg, S.L., Sanders, M., Schobel, S., Sharp, S., Simmonds, M., Simpson, A.J., Tallon, L., Turner, C.M., Tait, A., Tivey, A.R., Van Aken, S., Walker, D., Wanless, D., Wang, S., White, B., White, O., Whitehead, S., Woodward, J., Wortman, J., Adams, M.D., Embley, T.M., Gull, K., Ullu, E., Barry, J. D., Fairlamb, A.H., Opperdoes, F., Barrell, B.G., Donelson, J.E., Hall, N., Fraser, C.M., Melville, S.E., and El Sayed, N. M. (2005) The genome of the African trypanosome *Trypanosoma brucei*. *Science*, **309**, 416–422.

6 Ivens, A.C., Peacock, C.S., Worthey, E.A., Murphy, L., Aggarwal, G., Berriman, M., Sisk, E., Rajandream, M.A., Adlem, E., Aert, R., Anupama, A., Apostolou, Z., Attipoe, P., Bason, N., Bauser, C., Beck, A., Beverley, S.M., Bianchettin, G., Borzym, K., Bothe, G., Bruschi, C.V., Collins, M., Cadag, E., Ciarloni, L., Clayton, C., Coulson, R.M., Cronin, A., Cruz, A.K., Davies, R.M., De Gaudenzi, J., Dobson, D.E., Duesterhoeft, A., Fazelina, G., Fosker, N., Frasch, A.C., Fraser, A., Fuchs, M., Gabel, C., Goble, A., Goffeau, A., Harris, D., Hertz-Fowler, C., Hilbert, H., Horn, D., Huang, Y., Klages, S., Knights, A., Kube, M., Larke, N., Litvin, L., Lord, A., Louie, T., Marra, M., Masuy, D., Matthews, K., Michaeli, S., Mottram, J.C., Muller-Auer, S., Munden, H., Nelson, S., Norbertczak, H.,

Oliver, K., O'neil, S., Pentony, M., Pohl, T.M., Price, C., Purnelle, B., Quail, M.A., Rabbinowitsch, E., Reinhardt, R., Rieger, M., Rinta, J., Robben, J., Robertson, L., Ruiz, J.C., Rutter, S., Saunders, D., Schafer, M., Schein, J., Schwartz, D.C., Seeger, K., Seyler, A., Sharp, S., Shin, H., Sivam, D., Squares, R., Squares, S., Tosato, V., Vogt, C., Volckaert, G., Wambutt, R., Warren, T., Wedler, H., Woodward, J., Zhou, S., Zimmermann, W., Smith, D.F., Blackwell, J.M., Stuart, K. D., Barrell, B., and Myler, P.J. (2005) The genome of the kinetoplastid parasite, *Leishmania major. Science*, **309**, 436–442.

7 El-Sayed, N.M., Myler, P.J., Bartholomeu, D.C., Nilsson, D., Aggarwal, G., Tran, A. N., Ghedin, E., Worthey, E.A., Delcher, A. L., Blandin, G., Westenberger, S.J., Caler, E., Cerqueira, G.C., Branche, C., Haas, B., Anupama, A., Arner, E., Aslund, L., Attipoe, P., Bontempi, E., Bringaud, F., Burton, P., Cadag, E., Campbell, D.A., Carrington, M., Crabtree, J., Darban, H., da Silveira, J.F., de Jong, P., Edwards, K., Englund, P.T., Fazelina, G., Feldblyum, T., Ferella, M., Frasch, A.C., Gull, K., Horn, D., Hou, L.H., Huang, Y.T., Kindlund, E., Ktingbeil, M., Kluge, S., Koo, H., Lacerda, D., Levin, M.J., Lorenzi, H., Louie, T., Machado, C.R., McCulloch, R., McKenna, A., Mizuno, Y., Mottram, J.C., Nelson, S., Ochaya, S., Osoegawa, K., Pai, G., Parsons, M., Pentony, M., Pettersson, U., Pop, M., Ramirez, J.L., Rinta, J., Robertson, L., Salzberg, S.L., Sanchez, D. O., Seyler, A., Sharma, R., Shetty, J., Simpson, A.J., Sisk, E., Tammi, M.T., Tarteton, R., Teixeira, S., Van Aken, S., Vogt, C., Ward, P.N., Wickstead, B., Wortman, J., White, O., Fraser, C.M., Stuart, K.D., and Andersson, B. (2005) The genome sequence of *Trypanosoma cruzi*, etiologic agent of Chagas disease. *Science*, **309**, 409–415.

8 Bloom, B.R. (1995) Genome sequences – a microbial minimalist. *Nature*, **378**, 236.

9 Wang, C.C. (1997) Validating targets for antiparasite chemotherapy. *Parasitology*, **114**, S31–S44.

10 Wyatt, P.G., Gilbert, I.H., Read, K.D., and Fairlamb, A.H. (2011) Target validation: linking target and chemical properties to desired product profile. *Curr. Top. Med. Chem.*, **11**, 1275–1283.

11 Renslo, A.R. and McKerrow, J.H. (2006) Drug discovery and development for neglected parasitic diseases. *Nat. Chem. Biol.*, **2**, 701–710.

12 Payne, D.J., Gwynn, M.N., Holmes, D.J., and Pompliano, D.L. (2007) Drugs for bad bugs: confronting the challenges of antibacterial discovery. *Nat. Rev. Drug Discov.*, **6**, 29–40.

13 Lipinski, C.A., Lombardo, F., Dominy, B. W., and Feeney, P.J. (1997) Experimental and computational approaches to estimate solubility and permeability in drug discovery and development settings. *Adv. Drug Deliv. Rev.*, **23**, 3–25.

14 Hopkins, A.L., Groom, C.R., and Alex, A. (2004) Ligand efficiency: a useful metric for lead selection. *Drug Discov. Today*, **9**, 430–431.

15 Edfeldt, F.N.B., Folmer, R.H.A., and Breeze, A.L. (2011) Fragment screening to predict druggability (ligandability) and lead discovery success. *Drug Discov. Today*, **16**, 284–287.

16 Hopkins, A.L. (2008) Network pharmacology: the next paradigm in drug discovery. *Nat. Chem. Biol.*, **4**, 682–690.

17 Cong, F., Cheung, A.K., and Huang, S.M. A. (2012) Chemical genetics-based target identification in drug discovery. *Ann. Rev. Pharmacol. Toxicol.*, **52**, 57–78.

18 Robertson, J.G. (2005) Mechanistic basis of enzyme-targeted drugs. *Biochemistry*, **44**, 5561–5571.

Acknowledgment

This publication is supported by COST.

COST – the acronym for European Cooperation in Science and Technology – is the oldest and widest European intergovernmental network for cooperation in research. Established by the Ministerial Conference in November 1971, COST is presently used by the scientific communities of 36 European countries to cooperate in common research projects supported by national funds.

The funds provided by COST – less than 1% of the total value of the projects – support the COST cooperation networks (COST Actions) through which, with EUR 30 million per year, more than 30 000 European scientists are involved in research having a total value which exceeds EUR 2 billion per year. This is the financial worth of the European added value which COST achieves.

A "bottom-up approach" (the initiative of launching a COST Action comes from the European scientists themselves), "à la carte participation" (only countries interested in the Action participate), "equality of access" (participation is open also to the scientific communities of countries not belonging to the European Union), and "flexible structure" (easy implementation and light management of the research initiatives) are the main characteristics of COST.

As precursor of advanced multidisciplinary research COST has a very important role for the realization of the European Research Area (ERA) anticipating and complementing the activities of the Framework Programmes, constituting a "bridge" towards the scientific communities of emerging countries, increasing the mobility of researchers across Europe, and fostering the establishment of "Networks of Excellence" in many key scientific domains such as: Biomedicine and Molecular Biosciences; Food and Agriculture; Forests, their Products and Services; Materials, Physical, and Nanosciences; Chemistry and Molecular Sciences and Technologies; Earth System Science and Environmental Management; Information and Communication Technologies; Transport and Urban Development; Individuals, Societies, Cultures, and Health. It covers basic and more applied research and also addresses issues of a prenormative nature or of societal importance.

Web: http://www.cost.eu

Legal Notice by COST Office

Preface

Infections caused by parasites of the trypanosomatid family are considered to belong to the most neglected diseases. They comprise the African sleeping sickness (*Trypanosoma brucei rhodesiense, T. brucei gambiense*), the Chagas' disease in Latin America (*T. cruzi*), the black fever or Kala-Azar (*Leishmania donovani*) and other forms of Leishmaniasis (various *Leishmania* species). They affect about 30 million of people and account for half a million of fatalities per year. Trypanosomatids also cause substantial economic losses by affecting life stock (*T. brucei brucei, T. congolense, T. evansi*). Available treatments of the diseases are unsatisfactory in terms of safety and efficacy. Industrial commitments to meet the therapeutic needs remain limited because of unfavourable economic perspectives for drugs acting on diseases that prevail in countries with poor socio-economic conditions. In fact, currently used drugs are overwhelmingly those developed many decades ago when the 'Western World' had still to be concerned about the health of administrators and soldiers in their tropical colonies.

The present book originates from an interdisciplinary network of academic and industrial researchers devoted to the development of "new drugs for neglected diseases". The initiative was sponsored by the European Union (COST Action CM0801) and in the beginnings was largely restricted to Europe. Over the four years of its operation, however, the exchange of experience and cooperative projects expanded far beyond its geographical basis, particularly by integrating countries in Latin America, Africa and Asia where the diseases are endemic. The progress achieved by this network is reflected in many of the contributions to the book. The editors, however, took care not just to present a 'progress report' but the state-of-the-art in the entire field of drug discovery for trypanosomatid diseases, as reviewed by leading scientists from all over the world. It is hoped that the compiled knowledge will become instrumental to shorten the time from basic discoveries to the urgently needed new drugs for the neglected diseases.

The editor's heartfelt thanks go to the contributing authors for their excellent work, to the series editor Paul M. Selzer for his constructive advice, and to the COST Office in Brussels for financial support.

Braunschweig, Ingelheim, Potsdam, Germany
March 2013

Timo Jäger
Oliver Koch
Leopold Flohé

List of Contributors

José María Alunda[*]
Universidad Complutense
Department of Animal Health
Faculty of Veterinary Medicine
Avenida Puerta de Hierro s/n
28040 Madrid
Spain
jmalunda@ucm.es

María Noel Alvarez
Departamento de Bioquímica and
Center for Free Radical and
Biomedical Research
Facultad de Medicina
Universidad de la República
Avenida General Flores 2125
11800 Montevideo
Uruguay

Luisana Avilán
Universidad de los Andes
Laboratorio de Fisiología
Facultad de Ciencias
La Hechicera
Av. Alberto Carnevalli
Mérida 5101
Venezuela

Cyrus J. Bacchi
Pace University
The Haskins Laboratories
41 Park Row
New York, NY 10038
USA

Michael P. Barrett[*]
University of Glasgow
Wellcome Trust Centre for Molecular
Parasitology
Institute of Infection, Immunity and
Inflammation
College of Medical, Veterinary and
Life Sciences
120 University Place
Glasgow G12 8TA
UK
michael.barrett@glasgow.ac.uk

Torsten Barth
Eberhard Karls Universität Tübingen
Interfakultäres Institut für
Biochemie
Hoppe-Seyler-Strasse 4
72076 Tübingen
Germany
torsten.barth@uni-tuebingen.de

Mathias Beig
MSD Animal Health Innovation
GmbH
Zur Propstei
55270 Schwabenheim
Germany

[*]Corresponding Author

Rachel Bezalel-Buch
The Hebrew University-Hadassah
Medical School
Department of Microbiology and
Molecular Genetics
Kuvin Center for the Study of
Infectious and Tropical Diseases
Institute for Medical Research
Israel–Canada
PO Box 12272
Jerusalem 91120
Israel

Maurizio Botta*
University of Siena
Faculty of Pharmacy
Via Aldo Moro 2
53100 Siena
Italy
botta.maurizio@gmail.com

Barry A. Bunin
Collaborative Drug Discovery, Inc.
1633 Bayshore Highway Suite 342
Burlingame, CA 94010
USA

Ana J. Cáceres
Universidad de los Andes
Laboratorio de Enzimología de
Parásitos
Facultad de Ciencias
La Hechicera
Av. Alberto Carnevalli
Mérida 5101
Venezuela

Helena Castro*
Universidade do Porto
Instituto de Biologia Molecular e
Celular
Rua do Campo Alegre 823
4150-180 Porto
Portugal
hcastro@ibmc.up.pt

Juan José Cazzulo
Universidad Nacional General San
Martín/CONICET
Instituto de Investigaciones
Biotecnológicas (IIB/INTECH)
Campus Miguelete
Avenida 25 de Mayo y Francia
1650 San Martín
Buenos Aires
Argentina
jcazzulo@iibintech.com.ar

Marcelo A. Comini*
Institut Pasteur de Montevideo
Group Redox Biology of
Trypanosomes
Mataojo 2020
11400 Montevideo
Uruguay
mcomini@pasteur.edu.uy

Juan-Luis Concepción
Universidad de los Andes
Laboratorio de Enzimología de
Parásitos
Facultad de Ciencias
La Hechicera
Av. Alberto Carnevalli
Mérida 5101
Venezuela

Carlos Cordeiro*
Universidade de Lisboa
Faculdade de Ciências
Departamento de Química e
Bioquímica
Centro de Química e Bioquímica
Edifício C8 Campo Grande
1749-016 Lisboa
Portugal
cacordeiro@fc.ul.pt

María Jesús Corral-Caridad
Universidad Complutense
Department of Animal Health
Faculty of Veterinary Medicine
Avenida Puerta de Hierro s/n
28040 Madrid
Spain
mariajco@ucm.es

Maria Paola Costi*
University of Modena and Reggio
Emilia
Department of Life Science
Via Campi 183
41125 Modena
Italy
mariapaola.costi@unimore.it

Darren J. Creek
University of Glasgow
Wellcome Trust Centre for Molecular
Parasitology
Institute of Infection, Immunity and
Inflammation
College of Medical, Veterinary and
Life Sciences
120 University Place
Glasgow G12 8TA
UK

and

University of Melbourne
Department of Biochemistry and
Molecular Biology
Bio21 Molecular Science and
Biotechnology Institute
Flemington Road
Parkville
Victoria 3010
Australia

Elisabeth Davioud-Charvet*
UMR CNRS 7509
European School of Chemistry,
Polymers and Materials (ECPM)
Bioorganic and Medicinal Chemistry
25 rue Becquerel
67087 Strasbourg Cedex 2
France
elisabeth.davioud@unistra.fr

Harry P. de Koning*
University of Glasgow
Institute of Infection
Immunity and Inflammation
College of Medical
Veterinary and Life Sciences
120 University Place
Glasgow G12 8TA
UK
Harry.de-Koning@glasgow.ac.uk

Vincent Delespaux
Institute of Tropical Medicine
Antwerpen
Department of Biomedical Sciences
Nationalestraat 155
2000 Antwerp
Belgium

Patricia S. Doyle*
University of California
San Francisco
Department of Pathology and Sandler
Center for Drug Discovery
1700 4th Street 508
San Francisco, CA 94158-2330
USA
patricia.doyle.engel@gmail.com

Michael Duszenko*
Eberhard Karls Universität Tübingen
Interfakultäres Institut für
Biochemie
Hoppe-Seyler-Strasse 4
72076 Tübingen
Germany
michael.duszenko@uni-tuebingen.de

Sean Ekins*
Collaborative Drug Discovery, Inc.
1633 Bayshore Highway Suite 342
Burlingame, CA 94010
USA
sekins@collaborativedrug.com

and

Collaborations in Chemistry
5616 Hilltop Needmore Road
Fuquay Varina, NC 27526
USA

and

University of Maryland
Department of Pharmaceutical
Sciences
20 North Pine Street
Baltimore, MD 21201
USA

and

University of Medicine & Dentistry of
New Jersey (UMDNJ)
Robert Wood Johnson Medical
School
Department of Pharmacology
675 Hoes lane
Piscataway, NJ 08854
USA

Juan C. Engel
University of California
San Francisco
Department of Pathology and Sandler
Center for Drug Discovery
1700 4th Street 508
San Francisco, CA 94158-2330
USA
juan.engel@ucsd.edu

Alan Fairlamb*
Division of Biological Chemistry &
Drug Discovery
College of Life Sciences
University of Dundee
Dundee DD1 5EH
UK
a.h.fairlamb@dundee.ac.uk

Stefania Ferrari
University of Modena and Reggio
Emilia
Department of Life Science
Via Campi 183
41125 Modena
Italy

António E.N. Ferreira
Universidade de Lisboa
Faculdade de Ciências
Departamento de Química e
Bioquímica
Centro de Química e Bioquímica
Edifício C8 Campo Grande
1749-016 Lisboa
Portugal

Leopold Flohé
Otto-von-Guericke-Universität
Magdeburg
Chemisches Institut
Universitätsplatz 2
39106 Magdeburg
Germany

Thibault Gendron
UMR CNRS 7509
European School of Chemistry,
Polymers and Materials (ECPM)
Bioorganic and Medicinal Chemistry
25 rue Becquerel
67087 Strasbourg Cedex 2
France

Vadim N. Gladyshev*
Harvard Medical School
Division of Genetics
Department of Medicine
Brigham and Women's Hospital
75 Francis Street
Boston, MA 02115
USA
vgladyshev@rics.bwh.harvard.edu

Ricardo Gomes
Universidade de Lisboa
Faculdade de Ciências
Departamento de Química e
Bioquímica
Centro de Química e Bioquímica
Edifício C8 Campo Grande
1749-016 Lisboa
Portugal

Melisa Gualdrón-López
Université catholique de Louvain
Research Unit for Tropical Diseases
de Duve Institute
Avenue Hippocrate 74
La Hechicera
Av. Alberto Carnevalli
1200 Brussels
Belgium

Martín Hugo
Departamento de Bioquímica and
Center for Free Radical and
Biomedical Research
Facultad de Medicina
Universidad de la República
Avenida General Flores 2125
11800 Montevideo
Uruguay

Robert T. Jacobs
Scynexis, Inc.
PO Box 12878
Research Triangle Park
NC 27709-2878
USA

Timo Jäger
German Centre for Infection
Research (DZIF)
Inhoffenstraße 7
38124 Braunschweig
Germany
timo.jaeger@dzif.de

Oliver Koch*
Junior Research Group Leader
"Medicinal Chemistry"
Chemical Biology – Faculty
of Chemistry
Technische Universität Dortmund
Otto-Hahn-Straße 6
44227 Dortmund
Oliver.Koch@tu-dortmund.de

R. Luise Krauth-Siegel
Heidelberg University
Biochemistry Center
Im Neuenheimer Feld 328
69120 Heidelberg
Germany

Bruno K. Kubata
Research for Health Africa & Pharma
Innovation
AU/NEPAD Agency Regional Office
in Nairobi
C/o the AU/Inter African Bureau for
Animal Resources
P.O. BOX 13601-00800
Kenya
brunokubata@yahoo.com

Don Antoine Lanfranchi
UMR CNRS 7509
European School of Chemistry,
Polymers and Materials (ECPM)
Bioorganic and Medicinal Chemistry
25 rue Becquerel
67087 Strasbourg Cedex 2
France

Alexei V. Lobanov
Harvard Medical School
Division of Genetics
Department of Medicine
Brigham and Women's Hospital
75 Francis Street
Boston, MA 02115
USA

Philippe M. Loiseau
Université Paris-Sud 11
Faculté de Pharmacie
UMR 8076 CNRS
Chimiothérapie Antiparasitaire
5 rue Jean-Baptiste Clément
92290 Châtenay-Malabry
France

Valeria Losasso
University of Modena and
Reggio Emilia
Department of Life Science
Via Campi 183
41125 Modena
Italy

and

Scientific Computing Department,
Science and Technology Facilities
Council
Daresbury Laboratory
Keckwick Lane
Warrington WA4 4AD
UK

Anita Masic
University of Würzburg
Institute for Molecular Infection
Biology
Josef-Schneider-Strasse 2/D15
97080 Würzburg
Germany

Paul A.M. Michels*
Université catholique de Louvain
Research Unit for Tropical Diseases
de Duve Institute
Avenue Hippocrate 74
1200 Brussels
Belgium
paul.michels@uclouvain.be

Stefan Mogk
Eberhard Karls Universität Tübingen
Interfakultäres Institut für
Biochemie
Hoppe-Seyler-Strasse 4
72076 Tübingen
Germany
labor@virtualmogk.de

Heidrun Moll*
University of Würzburg
Institute for Molecular Infection
Biology
Josef-Schneider-Strasse 2/D15
97080 Würzburg
Germany
heidrun.moll@uni-wuerzburg.de

Mattia Mori
University of Siena
Faculty of Pharmacy
Via Aldo Moro 2
53100 Siena
Italy

Frank Oellien
MSD Animal Health Innovation
GmbH
Zur Propstei
55270 Schwabenheim
Germany

Cecilia Ortíz
Institut Pasteur de Montevideo
Group Redox Biology of
Trypanosomes
Mataojo 2020
11400 Montevideo
Uruguay
cortiz@pasteur.edu.uy

Gonzalo Peluffo
Departamento de Bioquímica and
Center for Free Radical and
Biomedical Research
Facultad de Medicina
Universidad de la República
Avenida General Flores 2125
11800 Montevideo
Uruguay

Lucía Piacenza
Departamento de Bioquímica and
Center for Free Radical and
Biomedical Research
Facultad de Medicina
Universidad de la República
Avenida General Flores 2125
11800 Montevideo
Uruguay

Sébastien Pomel*
Université Paris-Sud 11
Faculté de Pharmacie
UMR 8076 CNRS
Chimiothérapie Antiparasitaire
5 rue Jean-Baptiste Clément
92290 Châtenay-Malabry
France
sebastien.pomel@u-psud.fr

Ana Ponces Freire
Universidade de Lisboa
Faculdade de Ciências
Departamento de Química e
Bioquímica
Centro de Química e Bioquímica
Edifício C8 Campo Grande
1749-016 Lisboa
Portugal

Wilfredo Quiñones
Universidad de los Andes
Laboratorio de Enzimología de
Parásitos
Facultad de Ciencias
La Hechicera
Av. Alberto Carnevalli
Mérida 5101
Venezuela

Rafael Radi*
Departamento de Bioquímica and
Center for Free Radical and
Biomedical Research
Facultad de Medicina
Universidad de la República
Avenida General Flores 2125
11800 Montevideo
Uruguay
rradi@fmed.edu.uy

Boris Rodenko
University of Glasgow
Institute of Infection, Immunity and
Inflammation
College of Medical, Veterinary and
Life Sciences
120 University Place
Glasgow G12 8TA
boris.rodenko@glasgow.ac.uk

and

The Netherlands Cancer Institute
Department of Chemical Biology
Division of Cell Biology
Plesmanlaan 121
1066 CX Amsterdam
The Netherlands

Poonam Salotra
National Institute of Pathology
(ICMR)
Safdarjung Hospital Campus
Post Box 4909
New Delhi 110029
India

Puneet Saxena
University of Modena and Reggio
Emilia
Department of Life Science
Via Campi 183
41125 Modena
Italy

Caroline Schönfeld
Eberhard Karls Universität Tübingen
Interfakultäres Institut für
Biochemie
Hoppe-Seyler-Strasse 4
72076 Tübingen
Germany
caroline.schoenfeld@uni-tuebingen.de

Uta Schurigt
University of Würzburg
Institute for Molecular Infection
Biology
Josef-Schneider-Strasse 2/D15
97080 Würzburg
Germany

Karin Seifert*
London School of Hygiene & Tropical
Medicine
Faculty of Infectious and Tropical
Diseases
Keppel Street
London WC1E 7HT
UK
karin.seifert@lshtm.ac.uk

Paul M. Selzer*
MSD Animal Health Innovation
GmbH
Zur Propstei
55270 Schwabenheim
Germany
paul.selzer@msd.de

and

University of Tübingen
Interfaculty Institute of Biochemistry
Hoppe-Seyler-Strasse 4
72076 Tübingen
Germany

and

University of Glasgow
Institute of Infection, Immunity and
Inflammation
120 University Place
Glasgow G12 8TA
UK

Joseph Shlomai*
The Hebrew University-Hadassah
Medical School
Department of Microbiology and
Molecular Genetics
Kuvin Center for the Study of
Infectious and Tropical Diseases
Institute for Medical Research
Israel–Canada
PO Box 12272
Jerusalem 91120
Israel
josephs@ekdm.huji.ac.il

Ruchi Singh
National Institute of Pathology
(ICMR)
Safdarjung Hospital Campus
Post Box 4909
New Delhi 110029
India

Marta Sousa Silva
Universidade de Lisboa
Faculdade de Ciências
Departamento de Química e
Bioquímica
Centro de Química e Bioquímica
Edifício C8 Campo Grande
1749-016 Lisboa
Portugal

Jasmin Stein
Eberhard Karls Universität Tübingen
Interfakultäres Institut für
Biochemie
Hoppe-Seyler-Strasse 4
72076 Tübingen
Germany
Jasmin_Stein@gmx.de

Dietmar Steverding*
University of East Anglia
BioMedical Research Centre
Norwich Medical School
Norwich Research Park
Norwich NR4 7TJ
UK
dsteverding@hotmail.com

Ana M. Tomás
Universidade do Porto
Instituto de Biologia Molecular e
Celular
Rua do Campo Alegre 823
4150-180 Porto
Portugal

and

Universidade do Porto
Instituto de Ciências Biomédicas
Abel Salazar
Rua de Jorge Viterbo Ferreira 228
4050-313 Porto
Portugal

and

Faculdade de Ciências
Departamento de Química e
Bioquímica
Centro de Química e Bioquímica
Edifício C8 Campo Grande
1749-016 Lisboa
Portugal

Madia Trujillo
Departamento de Bioquímica and
Center for Free Radical and
Biomedical Research
Facultad de Medicina
Universidad de la República
Avenida General Flores 2125
11800 Montevideo
Uruguay

Julio A. Urbina*
Instituto Venezolano de
Investigaciones Científicas
Centro de Biofisica y Bioquimica
Apartado 21827
Caracas 1020A
Venezuela

and

200 Lakeside Drive No. 503
Oakland, CA 94612-3503
United States
jurbina@mac.com

Isabel M. Vincent
University of Glasgow
Wellcome Trust Centre for Molecular
Parasitology
Institute of Infection, Immunity and
Inflammation
College of Medical, Veterinary and
Life Sciences
120 University Place
Glasgow G12 8TA
UK

and

Université Laval
Centre de Recherche en Infectiologie
du CHUL
2705 Boulevard Laurier
Québec G1V 4G2
Canada

Roderick A.M. Williams*
University of Strathclyde
Strathclyde Institute for Pharmacy
and Biological Sciences
161 Cathedral Street
Glasgow G4 0RE
UK
roderick.williams@strath.ac.uk

and

University of the West of Scotland
School of Science
High Street
Paisley PA1 2BE
UK
roderick.williams@uws.ac.uk

Nurit Yaffe
The Hebrew University-Hadassah
Medical School
Department of Microbiology and
Molecular Genetics
Kuvin Center for the Study of
Infectious and Tropical Diseases
Institute for Medical Research
Israel–Canada
PO Box 12272
Jerusalem 91120
Israel

Nigel Yarlett*
Pace University
The Haskins Laboratories and
Chemistry and Physical Sciences
41 Park Row
New York, NY 10038
USA
nyarlett@pace.edu

Part One
Disease Burden, Current Treatments, Medical Needs,
and Strategic Approaches

Trypanosomatid Diseases: Molecular Routes to Drug Discovery, First edition. Edited by T. Jäger, O. Koch, and L. Flohé.
© 2013 Wiley-VCH Verlag GmbH & Co. KGaA. Published 2013 by Wiley-VCH Verlag GmbH & Co. KGaA.

1
Visceral Leishmaniasis – Current Treatments and Needs

*Poonam Salotra, Ruchi Singh, and Karin Seifert**

Abstract

The last decade has seen significant advances in the treatment of visceral leishmaniasis. Two new drugs (miltefosine and paromomycin) have been registered for the treatment of visceral leishmaniasis since 2002. Multidrug treatments have been investigated in systematic clinical studies and are now recommended as a new treatment approach for visceral leishmaniasis. However, the range of available drugs is still limited. Regional differences in response rates to anti-leishmanial available drugs as well as treatment of post-kala-azar dermal leishmaniasis, a complication of visceral leishmaniasis, are examples of the continued need for improved treatments for visceral leishmaniasis. In this chapter we discuss current treatments for visceral leishmaniasis and needs for drug discovery and development and translation to the clinic.

Introduction

Visceral leishmaniasis belongs to the group of neglected tropical diseases (NTDs), a group of chronic parasitic and related bacterial and viral infections that promote poverty [1]. Visceral leishmaniasis is caused by different species of the intracellular protozoan parasite *Leishmania*; predominantly by *L. donovani* in Asia and Africa, *L. infantum* in Europe and Latin America, and to a lesser extent in Africa [1–4]. Parasites, promastigotes as the insect stage, are transmitted by the bite of female phlebotomine sandflies to mammalian hosts [5]. Transmission can be zoonotic (transmission from animal to vector to human) or anthroponotic (transmission from human to vector to human). Inside the host the parasites invade monocytes and macrophages of the mononuclear phagocyte system and transform to the mammalian stage, intracellular amastigotes, which survive and multiply within host cell phagolysosomes. Parasite dissemination occurs through lymphatic and vascular systems. Clinical features of established visceral leishmaniasis include fever, abdominal pain, weight loss, splenomegaly, hepatomegaly, and lymphadenopathy [6]. It should be noted that infection can remain subclinical or develop into clinical disease. The latter displays fatality rates of 100% if untreated. Risk factors to develop

* Corresponding Author

Trypanosomatid Diseases: Molecular Routes to Drug Discovery, First edition. Edited by T. Jäger, O. Koch, and L. Flohé.

clinical disease include malnutrition and immune suppression, and are often linked to the overarching factor of poverty [7–9]. Visceral leishmaniasis is also an important infection associated with HIV/AIDS [10].

Major geographical areas affected are South Asia, which carries around 60% of cases worldwide [1], East Africa [4], North Africa and the Middle East [11], Latin America [2], and Southern Europe [3]. There are an estimated 50 000 new visceral leishmaniasis cases and 59 000 deaths per year [12]. However, under-reporting, misdiagnosis, and forced human migration obscure the establishment of exact numbers [4,6,12]. Importantly 90% of cases occur in only six countries: India, Bangladesh, Sudan, Brazil, Nepal, and Ethiopia [13].

Post-kala-azar dermal leishmaniasis (PKDL) is a complication of visceral leishmaniasis characterized by a spectrum of skin lesions following a visceral leishmaniasis episode mainly in areas where *L. donovani* is endemic. Reported incidence and time of onset of PKDL vary between countries; from 50 to 60% of cured visceral leishmaniasis cases within weeks to few months in Sudan to 5–10% generally after 2–4 years in India. There are sporadic reports of PKDL cases with no previous recorded history of visceral leishmaniasis. PKDL lesions contain parasites and are seen as an important reservoir for transmission [14].

In the following sections we will address (i) treatment options for visceral leishmaniasis and geographical differences in treatment response (see the "Current Anti-Leishmanial Drugs and Treatment Options for Visceral Leishmaniasis" section), and (ii) pathology, immunopathology, and treatment options for PKDL (see the "PKDL" section).

Current Anti-Leishmanial Drugs and Treatment Options for Visceral Leishmaniasis

Available Drugs

Pentavalent antimonials (sodium stibogluconate (SSG), generic sodium antimony gluconate, and meglumine antimoniate depending on country and region) have been the standard drugs for the last 60 years. Due to high rates of clinical unresponsiveness their use has been largely abandoned in Bihar state, India [15], but they continue to be used in other endemic areas [16,17]. SSG is still used to a wide extent in Africa, where limited availability of other drugs persists. Toxicity, lot-to-lot variations and need for hospitalization are severe limitations of antimonial treatment [16]. The polyene antibiotic amphotericin B is highly effective. It is used as amphotericin B deoxycholate, which suffers from toxicity [16], and as a liposomal formulation (AmBisome®) approved for the treatment of visceral leishmaniasis [18]. Notably, liposomal amphotericin B is the safest and most effective drug available [19]. Recently, a preferential pricing agreement for developing countries has reduced the cost of liposomal amphotericin B from US$200 to 20 per 50 mg vial [20]. Following this agreement a single infusion of liposomal amphotericin B at a dose of 10 mg/kg body weight was shown to be non-inferior and less expensive than treatment with conventional amphotericin B deoxycholate [21]. A single infusion of 10 mg/kg liposomal amphotericin B is now recommended as first-line treatment for anthroponotic visceral leishmaniasis in the Indian subcontinent [22] and one component in recently trialed short-course multidrug treatment regimes [23,24]. Sadly, despite the price reduction, cost is still an inhibiting factor for use of liposomal amphotericin B in some endemic areas. Another limitation is temperature stability as temperatures above 25 °C and below 0 °C can alter liposome characteristics, and impact on drug efficacy and toxicity [19]. Miltefosine, an alkylphosphocholine, was the first oral anti-leishmanial drug registered for visceral leishmaniasis in India in 2002 following clinical trials with 94% cure rates [25]. It is used as a potential tool in the visceral leishmaniasis elimination program in India, Bangladesh, and Nepal [16,17]. The gastrointestinal tract is the main target organ for side-effects [26] and gastrointestinal symptoms were recognized as the most common adverse effect in clinical trials [27]. The major limitation of miltefosine is its contraindication in pregnancy, and mandatory contraception for women in child-bearing age for the duration of therapy and 2–3 months beyond. This restriction is based on a teratogenic effect seen in one species (rat) in preclinical studies and the pharmacokinetic profile of miltefosine [26]. Paromomycin, an aminoglycoside antibiotic, is the latest drug registered for visceral leishmaniasis in India in 2006. Non-inferiority of paromomycin to amphotericin B was shown in a phase III trial in India [28]. Safety and efficacy of both miltefosine [27] and paromomycin [29] were confirmed in phase IV studies in an outpatient setting.

Current drugs and treatment regimes are summarized in Table 1.1.

New Treatment Regimes

Treatment courses for visceral leishmaniasis have been long (3–4 weeks) with a negative impact on compliance and cost. Experimental resistance to the new drugs, miltefosine [30–33] and paromomycin [34,35], was easily generated in the laboratory. Antimony-resistant Indian visceral leishmaniasis parasites show increased tolerance to miltefosine and amphotericin B, but not to paromomycin [36,37]. In addition, miltefosine has a long terminal half-life and concerns have been raised about the emergence of resistance when used as monotherapy [38]. Drug combinations and multidrug treatment regimes are in practice for infectious diseases such as malaria and tuberculosis. The rational for use of combination chemotherapy or multidrug treatments is reduction of treatment duration and total drug doses (resulting in decreased toxicity, higher compliance, and less burden on health systems), and delay of emergence of resistance (and hence an increase of a drug's lifespan) [39,40].

Multidrug treatments against visceral leishmaniasis have been trialed earlier on smaller scales with a limited number of drugs available. Examples are SSG plus paromomycin in Sudan (which became standard treatment used by Médecins Sans Frontières) and India [41,42], and SSG plus allopurinol in Kenya [43] in the 1990s and 1980s. With the registration of new drugs and the efficacy of single-dose treatment of liposomal amphotericin B, multidrug treatment regimes became a real possibility for systematic use in visceral leishmaniasis. Non-overlapping drug toxicities and

Table 1.1 Current drugs for visceral leishmaniasis and treatment regimes in Europe, Middle East, Latin America, South Asia, and East Africa.

Drug	Dosage	Regimen and clinical efficacy			Limitations
		South Asia: visceral leishmaniasis due to L. donovani	East Africa: visceral leishmaniasis due to L. donovani	Europe, Middle East, and Latin America: visceral leishmaniasis due to L. infantum	
SSG	20 mg/kg intramuscular/intravenous injection	30 d; effective in Bangladesh, Nepal, and Indian states of Jharkhand, West Bengal, and Uttar Pradesh	30 d; effective and first-line treatment; >95% cure rate	28 d; effective >95% cure rate	Liver and cardiac toxicity; widespread resistance in Indian state of Bihar
Amphotericin B deoxycholate	0.75–1 mg/kg slow infusion	Daily or alternate days infusion 15–20 d, total dose 15 mg/kg; 99% cure rate in India	Daily or alternate days infusion 15–20 d, total dose 15 mg/kg; 97% cure rate in Uganda	Daily or alternate days infusion 20–30 d, total dose 2–3 g effective, but not used	Renal and cardiac toxicity
Liposomal amphotericin B	3–5 mg/kg infusion in 5% dextrose	Daily infusion given over 3–5 d; total dose 15 mg/kg; >90% cure rate; single-dose infusion of 10 mg/kg recommended as first line, 95% cure rate	Daily infusion given over 6–10 d; total dose 30 mg/kg; 88% cure rate in Sudan. 93% in Ethiopia; single-dose infusion drug trials ongoing	Daily infusion given over 3–6 d; total dose 18–24 mg/kg; >95% cure rate and recommended as first-line drug	Significantly less toxic than Amphotericin B, but highly expensive, temperature stability
Miltefosine	2–11 yr: 2.5 mg/kg; >12 yr and <25 kg: 50 mg daily; 25–50 kg: 50 mg b.i.d.; >50 kg: 50 mg thrice orally	28 d; used as first line in Indian control program in Bihar, 94% cure rate; 85% cure rate in Bangladesh	28 d; 90% cure rate in Ethiopia	Not used so far for primary visceral leishmaniasis, recommended as an alternative drug for relapse treatment in visceral leishmaniasis–HIV coinfection	Potential teratogenicity implicates cautionary use in women of child-bearing age; gastrointestinal side-effects; to ensure compliance DOTS (directly observed treatment strategy) should be used
Paromomycin	15 mg/kg daily intramuscular injection	21 d; 93–95% cure rate	At 20 mg/kg/day for 21 d; 85% cure rate; used in combination with SSG at recommended doses for 17 d with 93% cure rate	Not used so far	

matching half-lives are important considerations in the design of drug combinations [44] as is the relationship between drug concentrations, drug resistance, and tolerance [45]. These questions have been explored in the field of anti-malarial drug combinations. The issues related to drug combinations for visceral leishmaniasis have recently been summarized [39]. Importantly, there are no drugs available for fixed-dose combinations for visceral leishmaniasis and the arsenal of drugs to chose from for coadministration or sequential administration is still limited. Hence, experimental studies [46] and clinical trials [23,24,47,48] are focused on coadministration of available drugs in a pragmatic approach. This approach in visceral leishmaniasis is not yet fully guided by a pharmacological or biological evidence base since our understanding of the pharmacokinetic/pharmacodynamic profiles of visceral leishmaniasis drugs, combination treatment regimes, and evolution of drug resistance in the field is still limited. Based on the different modes of action of current anti-leishmanial drugs [49,50] mutual protection against resistance may be achieved, but ultimately (experimental) proof-of-concept and integrated pharmacokinetic/pharmacodynamic studies are still to be carried out. The need for increased knowledge of parasite biology and pharmacology has been voiced [39]. Assessment of pharmacodynamic properties of three treatment arms (single-dose liposomal amphotericin B plus SSG, single-dose liposomal amphotericin B plus miltefosine, and miltefosine alone), pharmacokinetic properties of miltefosine alone and in combination with liposomal amphotericin B, and subsequent modeling of pharmacokinetic/pharmacodynamic relationships for miltefosine are planned for a phase II study for treatment of visceral leishmaniasis in East Africa [47]. This integrated approach will provide highly valuable information. The significant advantage that multidrug treatment regimens in visceral leishmaniasis have shown so far over monotherapy is reduction of treatment duration, cost, and frequency of adverse events [23]. This treatment approach is expected to be the strategy for visceral leishmaniasis in the future.

Recent clinical trials have been reviewed and summarized elsewhere [39,40]. Further information on ongoing trials may be found at www.dndi.org and www.clinicaltrials.gov.

Another combination approach discussed for PKDL [51] and HIV coinfected individuals is the combination of an immunotherapy or therapeutic vaccine with drug treatment. One rational for this approach is to decrease the parasite burden with an effective (preferentially fast killing) drug used at low dose or as a short-course treatment and boost the effector immune response with an immunostimulatory agent [52]. This approach has been tried with first-generation vaccines, recombinant proteins, adjuvant, and cytokines, but lacked availability of defined products suitable for registration. With defined vaccines and immunotherapies currently in development this approach is set to gain future attention.

Regional Differences in Clinical Drug Efficacy

Regional differences in clinical drug efficacy have been reported between and within countries. The most recent example is the finding for paromomycin in East Africa. A dose of 15 mg/kg/day paromomycin sulfate for 21 days was efficacious in a phase III trial in India with a 94.6% cure rate, but gave an unacceptable low overall cure rate of 63.8% in East African countries [8]. The pharmacological and/or biological basis, patient or parasite factor, for this difference still needs to be established. Differences in treatment response to liposomal amphotericin B between Indian, Kenyan, and Brazilian patients have also been reported earlier in a phase II study [53]. A recent report addressed the question of differences in visceral leishmaniasis patient (demographic and nutritional) profiles in Brazil, East Africa, and South Asia [9], highlighting potential requirements of distinct strategies between geographical settings. These may be based on differences at the level of parasite, host or parasite host interactions.

PKDL

Pathology and Immunopathology of PKDL

PKDL, predominantly observed in the Indian subcontinent and East Africa, is a dermal manifestation in a fraction of treated visceral leishmaniasis patients caused by *L. donovani* [54]. Sporadic cases of PKDL have been reported due to *L. infantum*, especially in HIV–visceral leishmaniasis coinfection [55]. The clinical spectrum of disease ranges from hypopigmented macular lesions to infiltrated plaques to the chronic and most aggravated nodular form. Most patients present with a combination of lesions described as polymorphic form [54,56,57].

Dermal infiltration of lymphocytes, macrophages, and plasma cells in varying proportion is observed in granuloma of Indian PKDL in contrast to Sudanese PKDL, where plasma cells are virtually absent [54,57,58]. The parasites are mainly present in the superficial epidermis, and easily detected in nodular lesion compared to macular and papular lesions [59]. Neuritis in small cutaneous nerves indicating peripheral nerve involvement, mucosal lesions with destructive complication in oronasal regions, and ocular lesions have been described in Sudanese PKDL, but appear rare in Indian PKDL with a sole report of neuritis [54,57,60].

Immunosuppression, reactivation of residual parasite, or reinfection in a viscerally immune person is thought to be the underlying mechanism in the development of PKDL [54,58,61]. Mechanisms of parasite persistence in the host are not yet well established. However, increasing evidence indicates the involvement of host as well as parasite factors.

Predominantly, CD8$^+$ T cells are observed in dermal lesions as well as in lymph nodes of Indian PKDL, unlike in Sudanese PKDL patients where a preponderance of CD4$^+$ T cells is observed [57,62]. Increased production of interleukin (IL)-10 by keratinocytes and high levels of IL-10 in plasma and peripheral blood mononuclear cell cultures as well as elevated C-reactive proteins predicted the development of PKDL in Sudan [57]. Persistence of parasites in Indian PKDL despite high interferon (IFN)-γ and tumor necrosis factor (TNF)-α expression has been accounted to the presence of counteracting cytokines and minimal expression of IFN-γ receptor 1, and the TNF receptors TNFR1 and R2 [63,64]. Ample evidence is available to conclude that an IL-10-rich milieu promotes *Leishmania* parasite persistence and reactivation in skin.

In the Sudanese population, PKDL susceptibility has been associated with polymorphism observed at promoter regions of IFN-γ receptor 1 and IL-10 genes. However, confirmatory experimental analysis to demonstrate a regulatory role of this polymorphism is awaited [65,66]. Such studies are yet to be performed in Indian PKDL.

In addition to immunological mechanisms, *Leishmania* genetic determinants also contribute to alterations of the host–parasite equilibrium in favor of the parasite, resulting in the persistence in the human host for up to 20 years in Indian PKDL. It is well established that parasites isolated from visceral leishmaniasis and PKDL patients are essentially the same [67], although polymorphism is observed at the 28S rRNA locus and β-tubulin locus [68,69]. Transient changes such as preferential expression of surface proteases in parasites isolated from PKDL lesions are suggestive of altered interaction with macrophages and may be responsible for the predilection of parasite to the dermis [69].

Current Treatment Options for PKDL

Treating PKDL patients is an important aspect of visceral leishmaniasis control programs as PKDL patients are deemed as the major reservoir in anthroponotic transmission settings. High incidence of refractoriness to antimony has been attributed to anthroponotic transmission via PKDL in India [70]. Three to four times longer treatment regimens than for visceral leishmaniasis, increasing antimony resistance, and poor patient compliance pose major challenges for treatment of PKDL. In Sudan, most of the PKDL patients self heal, and only severe and chronic patients are treated, while in Indian PKDL treatment is always required. In India, SSG is extensively used at a dose of 20 mg/kg/day for 120 days with cure rates of 64–92% [57,71]. As an alternative, various drugs including allopurinol, ketoconazole, and rifampicin alone or in combination with pentavalent antimonials have been tried in Indian PKDL with variable cure rates [72]. Amphotericin B and miltefosine, the frontline drugs for visceral leishmaniasis, have potential benefits for PKDL patients. Amphotericin B deoxycholate at a dose of 1 mg/kg/day by infusion for 60–80 doses over a period of 120 days was found 100% effective [73]. Miltefosine at a dose of 100 mg/day in divided doses for 12 weeks has been found effective in Indian PKDL [74]. However, a shorter regimen of 150 mg/day in three doses for 60 days was also found curative and advocated in patients capable of tolerating gastrointestinal symptoms caused by the drug [75].

Non-healing Sudanese PKDL patients with severe lesions are best treated with SSG at a dose of 20 mg/kg/day for 30 days, which may be prolonged to 2–3 months if necessary [57]. Liposomal amphotericin B at 2.5 mg/kg/day by infusion for 20 days has been effective with a cure rate of 83% without side-effects in Sudan [76]. Novel immunochemotherapy using alum-precipitated autoclaved *L. major* (Alum/ALM) vaccine plus Bacille Calmette-Guerin (BCG) and SSG was found safe and effective with a cure rate of 87% by day 60 in Sudanese PKDL [77].

However, systematic studies on larger sets of patients to evaluate drugs for treatment of PKDL are urgently needed to accomplish improved, effective, and shortened treatments.

Open Questions and Needs

Without doubt real progress has been made in the treatment of visceral leishmaniasis over the last decade. However, this progress was also driven by the repurposing of drugs initially developed for other indications and pragmatic approaches. A new chemical entity (NCE) dedicated to visceral leishmaniasis has yet to be identified along with candidates for fixed-dose combinations. Screening campaigns over the last 5 years have focused on high-throughput and high-content screening formats, yet the complexity of the *Leishmania* parasite and its lifestyle do not make it an easy candidate for this approach. Consideration has to be given to crucial aspects of parasite biology in order to identify compounds that hold potential to progress into treatments for visceral leishmaniasis [78]. There is also a strong need for refined models and approaches for preclinical candidate selection, optimal drug use, and dosing regimes with inclusion of pharmacokinetic/pharmacodynamic relationships in anti-leishmanial drug development.

Understanding of pathogenesis, host factors, host–parasite interactions, and regional differences in clinical treatment response require continued research efforts and are crucial to design optimal treatments for visceral leishmaniasis and PKDL. Lastly, the importance of access to treatment has to be emphasized for the effort of all disciplines involved in the drug discovery and development process to yield long-lasting fruits. Poor access to care for leishmaniasis remains a major barrier to control. Factors that determine access to drugs (drug affordability, drug availability, forecasting, distribution and storage, drug quality, drug legislation and pharmacovigilance, user-friendliness, etc.) have recently been reviewed and the importance of a concerted effort by all stakeholders emphasized [13].

Promising directions and strategies have been set and are ongoing. Now research efforts have to continue to support further progress in treatment of visceral leishmaniasis and PKDL.

References

1 Lobo, D.A., Velayudhan, R., Chatterjee, P., Kohli, H., and Hotez, P.J. (2011) The neglected tropical diseases of India and South Asia: review of their prevalence, distribution, and control or elimination. *PLoS Negl. Trop. Dis.*, **5**, e1222.

2 Hotez, P.J., Bottazzi, M.E., Franco-Paredes, C., Ault, S.K., and Periago, M.R. (2008) The neglected tropical diseases of Latin America and the Caribbean: a review of disease burden and distribution and a roadmap for control and elimination. *PLoS Negl. Trop. Dis.*, **2**, e300.

3 Hotez, P.J. and Gurwith, M. (2011) Europe's neglected infections of poverty. *Int. J. Infect. Dis.*, **15**, e611–e619.

4 Hotez, P.J. and Kamath, A. (2009) Neglected tropical diseases in sub-Saharan

Africa: review of their prevalence, distribution, and disease burden. *PLoS Negl. Trop. Dis.*, **3**, e412.

5 Bates, P.A. (2007) Transmission of *Leishmania* metacyclic promastigotes by phlebotomine sand flies. *Int. J. Parasitol.*, **37**, 1097–1106.

6 Chappuis, F., Sundar, S., Hailu, A., Ghalib, H., Rijal, S., Peeling, R.W., Alvar, J., and Boelaert, M. (2007) Visceral leishmaniasis: what are the needs for diagnosis, treatment and control? *Nat. Rev. Microbiol.*, **5**, 873–882.

7 Bern, C., Courtenay, O., and Alvar, J. (2010) Of cattle, sand flies and men: a systematic review of risk factor analyses for South Asian visceral leishmaniasis and implications for elimination. *PLoS Negl. Trop. Dis.*, **4**, e599.

8 Hailu, A., Musa, A., Wasunna, M., Balasegaram, M., Yifru, S., Mengistu, G., Hurissa, Z., Hailu, W., Weldegebreal, T., Tesfaye, S., Makonnen, E., Khalil, E., Ahmed, O., Fadlalla, A., El-Hassan, A., Raheem, M., Mueller, M., Koummuki, Y., Rashid, J., Mbui, J., Mucee, G., Njoroge, S., Manduku, V., Musibi, A., Mutuma, G., Kirui, F., Lodenyo, H., Mutea, D., Kirigi, G., Edwards, T., Smith, P., Muthami, L., Royce, C., Ellis, S., Alobo, M., Omollo, R., Kesusu, J., Owiti, R., and Kinuthia, J. (2010) Geographical variation in the response of visceral leishmaniasis to paromomycin in East Africa: a multicentre, open-label, randomized trial. *PLoS Negl. Trop. Dis.*, **4**, e709.

9 Harhay, M.O., Olliaro, P.L., Vaillant, M., Chappuis, F., Lima, M.A., Ritmeijer, K., Costa, C.H., Costa, D.L., Rijal, S., Sundar, S., and Balasegaram, M. (2011) Who is a typical patient with visceral leishmaniasis? Characterizing the demographic and nutritional profile of patients in Brazil, East Africa, and South Asia. *Am. J. Trop. Med. Hyg.*, **84**, 543–550.

10 Alvar, J., Aparicio, P., Aseffa, A., Den Boer, M., Canavate, C., Dedet, J.P., Gradoni, L., Ter Horst, R., Lopez-Velez, R., and Moreno, J. (2008) The relationship between leishmaniasis and AIDS: the second 10 years. *Clin. Microbiol. Rev.*, **21**, 334–359.

11 Hotez, P.J., Savioli, L., and Fenwick, A. (2012) Neglected tropical diseases of the middle East and north Africa: review of

their prevalence, distribution, and opportunities for control. *PLoS Negl. Trop. Dis.*, **6**, e1475.

12 Desjeux, P. (2004) Leishmaniasis: current situation and new perspectives. *Comp. Immunol. Microbiol. Infect. Dis.*, **27**, 305–318.

13 den Boer, M., Argaw, D., Jannin, J., and Alvar, J. (2011) Leishmaniasis impact and treatment access. *Clin. Microbiol. Infect.*, **17**, 1471–1477.

14 Uranw, S., Ostyn, B., Rijal, A., Devkota, S., Khanal, B., Menten, J., Boelaert, M., and Rijal, S. (2011) Post-kala-azar dermal leishmaniasis in Nepal: a retrospective cohort study (2000–2010). *PLoS Negl. Trop. Dis.*, **5**, e1433.

15 Sundar, S., More, D.K., Singh, M.K., Singh, V.P., Sharma, S., Makharia, A., Kumar, P. C., and Murray, H.W. (2000) Failure of pentavalent antimony in visceral leishmaniasis in India: report from the center of the Indian epidemic. *Clin. Infect. Dis.*, **31**, 1104–1107.

16 Alvar, J., Croft, S., and Olliaro, P. (2006) Chemotherapy in the treatment and control of leishmaniasis. *Adv. Parasitol.*, **61**, 223–274.

17 Croft, S.L. and Olliaro., P. (2011) Leishmaniasis chemotherapy – challenges and opportunities. *Clin. Microbiol. Infect.*, **17**, 1478–1483.

18 Meyerhoff, A. (1999) U.S. Food and Drug Administration approval of AmBisome (liposomal amphotericin B) for treatment of visceral leishmaniasis. *Clin. Infect. Dis.*, **28**, 42–48, discussion 49–51.

19 Bern, C., Adler-Moore, J., Berenguer, J., Boelaert, M., den Boer, M., Davidson, R.N., Figueras, C., Gradoni, L., Kafetzis, D.A., Ritmeijer, K., Rosenthal, E., Royce, C., Russo, R., Sundar, S., and Alvar, J. (2006) Liposomal amphotericin B for the treatment of visceral leishmaniasis. *Clin. Infect. Dis.*, **43**, 917–924.

20 Olliaro, P., Darley, S., Laxminarayan, R., and Sundar, S. (2009) Cost-effectiveness projections of single and combination therapies for visceral leishmaniasis in Bihar, India. *Trop. Med. Int. Health*, **14**, 918–925.

21 Sundar, S., Chakravarty, J., Agarwal, D., Rai, M., and Murray, H.W. (2010) Single-

dose liposomal amphotericin B for visceral leishmaniasis in India. *N. Engl. J. Med.*, **362**, 504–512.

22 Matlashewski, G., Arana, B., Kroeger, A., Battacharya, S., Sundar, S., Das, P., Sinha, P.K., Rijal, S., Mondal, D., Zilberstein, D., and Alvar, J. (2011) Visceral leishmaniasis: elimination with existing interventions. *Lancet Infect. Dis.*, **11**, 322–325.

23 Sundar, S., Sinha, P.K., Rai, M., Verma, D. K., Nawin, K., Alam, S., Chakravarty, J., Vaillant, M., Verma, N., Pandey, K., Kumari, P., Lal, C.S., Arora, R., Sharma, B., Ellis, S., Strub-Wourgaft, N., Balasegaram, M., Olliaro, P., Das, P., and Modabber, F. (2011) Comparison of short-course multidrug treatment with standard therapy for visceral leishmaniasis in India: an open-label, non-inferiority, randomised controlled trial. *Lancet*, **377**, 477–486.

24 Sundar, S., Sinha, P.K., Verma, D.K., Kumar, N., Alam, S., Pandey, K., Kumari, P., Ravidas, V., Chakravarty, J., Verma, N., Berman, J., Ghalib, H., and Arana, B. (2011) Ambisome plus miltefosine for Indian patients with kala-azar. *Trans. R. Soc. Trop. Med. Hyg.*, **105**, 115–117.

25 Sundar, S., Jha, T.K., Thakur, C.P., Engel, J., Sindermann, H., Fischer, C., Junge, K., Bryceson, A., and Berman, J. (2002) Oral miltefosine for Indian visceral leishmaniasis. *N. Engl. J. Med.*, **347**, 1739–1746.

26 Sindermann, H. and Engel, J. (2006) Development of miltefosine as an oral treatment for leishmaniasis. *Trans. R. Soc. Trop. Med. Hyg.*, **100** (Suppl. 1), S17–S20.

27 Bhattacharya, S.K., Sinha, P.K., Sundar, S., Thakur, C.P., Jha, T.K., Pandey, K., Das, V. R., Kumar, N., Lal, C., Verma, N., Singh, V. P., Ranjan, A., Verma, R.B., Anders, G., Sindermann, H., and Ganguly, N.K. (2007) Phase 4 trial of miltefosine for the treatment of Indian visceral leishmaniasis. *J. Infect. Dis.*, **196**, 591–598.

28 Sundar, S., Jha, T.K., Thakur, C.P., Sinha, P.K., and Bhattacharya, S.K. (2007) Injectable paromomycin for visceral leishmaniasis in India. *N. Engl. J. Med.*, **356**, 2571–2581.

29 Sinha, P.K., Jha, T.K., Thakur, C.P., Nath, D., Mukherjee, S., Aditya, A.K., and Sundar, S. (2011) Phase 4

pharmacovigilance trial of paromomycin injection for the treatment of visceral leishmaniasis in India. *J. Trop. Med.*, **2011**, 645203.

30 Perez-Victoria, F.J., Gamarro, F., Ouellette, M., and Castanys, S. (2003) Functional cloning of the miltefosine transporter. A novel P-type phospholipid translocase from *Leishmania* involved in drug resistance. *J. Biol. Chem.*, **278**, 49965–49971.

31 Perez-Victoria, F.J., Sanchez-Canete, M.P., Castanys, S., and Gamarro, F. (2006) Phospholipid translocation and miltefosine potency require both *L. donovani* miltefosine transporter and the new protein LdRos3 in *Leishmania* parasites. *J. Biol. Chem.*, **281**, 23766–23775.

32 Seifert, K., Matu, S., Javier Perez-Victoria, F., Castanys, S., Gamarro, F., and Croft, S. L. (2003) Characterisation of *Leishmania donovani* promastigotes resistant to hexadecylphosphocholine (miltefosine). *Int. J. Antimicrob. Agents*, **22**, 380–387.

33 Seifert, K., Perez-Victoria, F.J., Stettler, M., Sanchez-Canete, M.P., Castanys, S., Gamarro, F., and Croft, S.L. (2007) Inactivation of the miltefosine transporter, LdMT, causes miltefosine resistance that is conferred to the amastigote stage of *Leishmania donovani* and persists *in vivo*. *Int. J. Antimicrob. Agents*, **30**, 229–235.

34 Jhingran, A., Chawla, B., Saxena, S., Barrett, M.P., and Madhubala, R. (2009) Paromomycin: uptake and resistance in *Leishmania donovani*. *Mol. Biochem. Parasitol.*, **164**, 111–117.

35 Maarouf, M., Adeline, M.T., Solignac, M., Vautrin, D., and Robert-Gero, M. (1998) Development and characterization of paromomycin-resistant *Leishmania donovani* promastigotes. *Parasite*, **5**, 167–173.

36 Kulshrestha, A., Singh, R., Kumar, D., Negi, N.S., and Salotra, P. (2011) Antimony-resistant clinical isolates of *Leishmania donovani* are susceptible to paromomycin and sitamaquine. *Antimicrob. Agents Chemother.*, **55**, 2916–2921.

37 Kumar, D., Kulshrestha, A., Singh, R., and Salotra, P. (2009) *In vitro* susceptibility of field isolates of *Leishmania donovani* to miltefosine and amphotericin B:

correlation with sodium antimony gluconate susceptibility and implications for treatment in areas of endemicity. *Antimicrob. Agents Chemother.*, **53**, 835–838.

38 Bryceson, A. (2001) A policy for leishmaniasis with respect to the prevention and control of drug resistance. *Trop. Med. Int. Health*, **6**, 928–934.

39 Olliaro, P.L. (2010) Drug combinations for visceral leishmaniasis. *Curr. Opin. Infect. Dis.*, **23**, 595–602.

40 van Griensven, J., Balasegaram, M., Meheus, F., Alvar, J., Lynen, L., and Boelaert, M. (2010) Combination therapy for visceral leishmaniasis. *Lancet Infect. Dis.*, **10**, 184–194.

41 Seaman, J., Pryce, D., Sondorp, H.E., Moody, A., Bryceson, A.D., and Davidson, R.N. (1993) Epidemic visceral leishmaniasis in Sudan: a randomized trial of aminosidine plus sodium stibogluconate versus sodium stibogluconate alone. *J. Infect. Dis.*, **168**, 715–720.

42 Thakur, C.P., Olliaro, P., Gothoskar, S., Bhowmick, S., Choudhury, B.K., Prasad, S., Kumar, M., and Verma, B.B. (1992) Treatment of visceral leishmaniasis (kala-azar) with aminosidine (= paromomycin)–antimonial combinations, a pilot study in Bihar, India. *Trans. R. Soc. Trop. Med. Hyg.*, **86**, 615–616.

43 Chunge, C.N., Gachihi, G., Muigai, R., Wasunna, K., Rashid, J.R., Chulay, J.D., Anabwani, G., Oster, C.N., and Bryceson, A.D. (1985) Visceral leishmaniasis unresponsive to antimonial drugs. III. Successful treatment using a combination of sodium stibogluconate plus allopurinol. *Trans. R. Soc. Trop. Med. Hyg.*, **79**, 715–718.

44 Kremsner, P.G. and Krishna, S. (2004) Antimalarial combinations. *Lancet*, **364**, 285–294.

45 Hastings, I.M. and Watkins, W.M. (2006) Tolerance is the key to understanding antimalarial drug resistance. *Trends Parasitol.*, **22**, 71–77.

46 Seifert, K. and Croft, S.L. (2006) *In vitro* and *in vivo* interactions between miltefosine and other antileishmanial drugs. *Antimicrob Agents Chemother.*, **50**, 73–79.

47 Omollo, R., Alexander, N., Edwards, T., Khalil, E.A., Younis, B.M., Abuzaid, A.A., Wasunna, M., Njoroge, N., Kinoti, D., Kirigi, G., Dorlo, T.P., Ellis, S., Balasegaram, M., and Musa, A.M. (2011) Safety and efficacy of miltefosine alone and in combination with sodium stibogluconate and liposomal amphotericin B for the treatment of primary visceral leishmaniasis in East Africa: study protocol for a randomized controlled trial. *Trials*, **12**, 166.

48 Sundar, S., Rai, M., Chakravarty, J., Agarwal, D., Agrawal, N., Vaillant, M., Olliaro, P., and Murray, H.W. (2008) New treatment approach in indian visceral leishmaniasis: single-dose liposomal amphotericin B followed by short-course oral miltefosine. *Clin. Infect. Dis.*, **47**, 1000–1006

49 Croft, S.L., Sundar, S., and Fairlamb, A.H. (2006) Drug resistance in leishmaniasis. *Clin. Microbiol. Rev.*, **19**, 111–126.

50 Seifert, K. (2011) Structures, targets and recent approaches in anti-leishmanial drug discovery and development. *Open Med. Chem. J.*, **5**, 31–39.

51 Ghalib, H. and Modabber, F. (2007) Consultation meeting on the development of therapeutic vaccines for post kala azar dermal leishmaniasis. *Kinetoplastid Biol. Dis.*, **6**, 7.

52 Musa, A.M., Noazin, S., Khalil, E.A., and Modabber, F. (2010) Immunological stimulation for the treatment of leishmaniasis: a modality worthy of serious consideration. *Trans. R. Soc. Trop. Med. Hyg.*, **104**, 1–2.

53 Berman, J.D., Badaro, R., Thakur, C.P., Wasunna, K.M., Behbehani, K., Davidson, R., Kuzoe, F., Pang, L., Weerasuriya, K., and Bryceson, A.D. (1998) Efficacy and safety of liposomal amphotericin B (AmBisome) for visceral leishmaniasis in endemic developing countries. *Bull. World Health Organ.*, **76**, 25–32.

54 Ramesh, V. (2007) Post-kala-azar dermal leishmaniasis with visceral leishmaniasis, or a rare presentation of visceral leishmaniasis with extensive skin manifestations. *Int. J. Dermatol.*, **46**, 1326.

55 Stark, D., Pett, S., Marriott, D., and Harkness, J. (2006) Post-kala-azar dermal leishmaniasis due to *Leishmania infantum* in a human immunodeficiency virus type

1-infected patient. *J. Clin. Microbiol.*, **44**, 1178–1180.

56 Ramesh, V. and Mukherjee, A. (1995) Post-kala-azar dermal leishmaniasis. *Int. J. Dermatol.*, **34**, 85–91.

57 Zijlstra, E.E., Musa, A.M., Khalil, E.A., el-Hassan, I.M., and el-Hassan, A.M. (2003) Post-kala-azar dermal leishmaniasis. *Lancet Infect. Dis.*, **3**, 87–98.

58 Mukherjee, A., Ramesh, V., and Misra, R.S. (1993) Post-kala-azar dermal leishmaniasis: a light and electron microscopic study of 18 cases. *J. Cutan. Pathol.*, **20**, 320–325.

59 Beena, K.R., Ramesh, V., and Mukherjee, A. (2003) Identification of parasite antigen, correlation of parasite density and inflammation in skin lesions of post kala-azar dermal leishmaniasis. *J. Cutan. Pathol.*, **30**, 616–620.

60 Khandpur, S., Ramam, M., Sharma, V.K., Salotra, P., Singh, M.K., and Malhotra, A. (2004) Nerve involvement in Indian post kala-azar dermal leishmaniasis. *Acta Derm. Venereol.*, **84**, 245–246.

61 el Hassan, A.M., Ghalib, H.W., Zijlstra, E.E., Eltoum, I.A., Satti, M., Ali, M.S., and Ali, H.M. (1992) Post kala-azar dermal leishmaniasis in the Sudan: clinical features, pathology and treatment. *Trans. R. Soc. Trop. Med. Hyg.*, **86**, 245–248.

62 Rathi, S.K., Pandhi, R.K., Chopra, P., and Khanna, N. (2005) Lesional T-cell subset in post-kala-azar dermal leishmaniasis. *Int. J. Dermatol.*, **44**, 12–13.

63 Ansari, N.A., Katara, G.K., Ramesh, V., and Salotra, P. (2008) Evidence for involvement of TNFR1 and TIMPs in pathogenesis of post-kala-azar dermal leishmaniasis. *Clin. Exp. Immunol.*, **154**, 391–398.

64 Ansari, N.A., Ramesh, V., and Salotra, P. (2006) Interferon (IFN)-gamma, tumor necrosis factor-alpha, interleukin-6, and IFN-gamma receptor 1 are the major immunological determinants associated with post-kala azar dermal leishmaniasis. *J. Infect. Dis.*, **194**, 958–965.

65 Farouk, S., Salih, M.A., Musa, A.M., Blackwell, J.M., Miller, E.N., Khalil, E.A., Elhassan, A.M., Ibrahim, M.E., and Mohamed, H.S. (2010) Interleukin 10 gene polymorphisms and development of post kala-azar dermal leishmaniasis in a selected Sudanese population. *Public Health Genom.*, **13**, 362–367.

66 Salih, M.A., Ibrahim, M.E., Blackwell, J.M., Miller, E.N., Khalil, E.A., ElHassan, A.M., Musa, A.M., and Mohamed, H.S. (2007) IFNG and IFNGR1 gene polymorphisms and susceptibility to post-kala-azar dermal leishmaniasis in Sudan. *Genes Immun.*, **8**, 75–78.

67 Alam, M.Z., Kuhls, K., Schweynoch, C., Sundar, S., Rijal, S., Shamsuzzaman, A.K., Raju, B.V., Salotra, P., Dujardin, J.C., and Schonian, G. (2009) Multilocus microsatellite typing (MLMT) reveals genetic homogeneity of *Leishmania donovani* strains in the Indian subcontinent. *Infect. Genet. Evol.*, **9**, 24–31.

68 Dey, A. and Singh, S. (2007) Genetic heterogeneity among visceral and post-Kala-Azar dermal leishmaniasis strains from eastern India. *Infect. Genet. Evol.*, **7**, 219–222.

69 Salotra, P., Duncan, R.C., Singh, R., Subba Raju, B.V., Sreenivas, G., and Nakhasi, H. L. (2006) Upregulation of surface proteins in *Leishmania donovani* isolated from patients of post kala-azar dermal leishmaniasis. *Microbes Infect.*, **8**, 637–644.

70 Singh, R., Kumar, D., Ramesh, V., Negi, N. S., Singh, S., and Salotra, P. (2006) Visceral leishmaniasis, or kala azar (KA): high incidence of refractoriness to antimony is contributed by anthroponotic transmission via post-KA dermal leishmaniasis. *J. Infect. Dis.*, **194**, 302–306.

71 Thakur, C.P. and Kumar, K. (1990) Efficacy of prolonged therapy with stibogluconate in post kala-azar dermal leishmaniasis. *Indian J. Med. Res.*, **91**, 144–148.

72 Ramesh, V., Kumar, J., Kumar, D., and Salotra, P. (2010) A retrospective study of intravenous sodium stibogluconate alone and in combinations with allopurinol, rifampicin, and an immunomodulator in the treatment of Indian post-kala-azar dermal leishmaniasis. *Indian J. Dermatol. Venereol. Leprol.*, **76**, 138–144.

73 Thakur, C.P., Narain, S., Kumar, N., Hassan, S.M., Jha, D.K., and Kumar, A. (1997) Amphotericin B is superior to sodium antimony gluconate in the treatment of Indian post-kala-azar dermal leishmaniasis. *Ann. Trop. Med. Parasitol.*, **91**, 611–616.

74 Sundar, S., Kumar, K., Chakravarty, J., Agrawal, D., Agrawal, S., Chhabra, A., and Singh, V. (2006) Cure of antimony-unresponsive Indian post-kala-azar dermal leishmaniasis with oral miltefosine. *Trans. R. Soc. Trop. Med. Hyg.*, **100**, 698–700.

75 Ramesh, V., Katara, G.K., Verma, S., and Salotra, P. (2011) Miltefosine as an effective choice in the treatment of post-kala-azar dermal leishmaniasis. *Br. J. Dermatol.*, **165**, 411–414.

76 Musa, A.M., Khalil, E.A., Mahgoub, F.A., Hamad, S., Elkadaru, A.M., and El Hassan, A.M. (2005) Efficacy of liposomal amphotericin B (AmBisome) in the treatment of persistent post-kala-azar dermal leishmaniasis (PKDL). *Ann. Trop. Med. Parasitol.*, **99**, 563–569.

77 Musa, A.M., Khalil, E.A., Mahgoub, F.A., Elgawi, S.H., Modabber, F., Elkadaru, A.E., Aboud, M.H., Noazin, S., Ghalib, H.W., and El-Hassan, A.M. (2008) Immunochemotherapy of persistent post-kala-azar dermal leishmaniasis: a novel approach to treatment. *Trans. R. Soc. Trop. Med. Hyg.*, **102**, 58–63.

78 De Muylder, G., Ang, K.K., Chen, S., Arkin, M.R., Engel, J.C., and McKerrow, J.H. (2011) A screen against *Leishmania* intracellular amastigotes: comparison to a promastigote screen and identification of a host cell-specific hit. *PLoS Negl. Trop. Dis.*, **5**, e1253.

2
Chemotherapy of Leishmaniasis: A Veterinary Perspective

*María Jesús Corral-Caridad and José María Alunda**

Abstract

Leishmania species cause a variety of in part fatal diseases in man and animals, the prominent veterinary manifestation being canine leishmaniasis caused by *L. infantum* (syn. *L. chagasi*), which also causes visceral leishmaniasis in humans. Canine leishmaniasis is common in the Mediterranean basin, Central and South America, the Middle East, and China, and the infected dogs, depending on the spread of transmitting vectors, represent a permanent threat to human health as reservoir of the parasite. The status of leishmaniasis treatment, as well as recent progress, is reviewed with special emphasis on canine leishmaniasis, and the problems arising from *L. infantum* being both a zoonotic and anthroponotic parasite. In essence, treatment of canine leishmaniasis relies on the same drugs used for human leishmaniasis (i.e., pentavalent antimonials, amphotericin, paromomycin and miltefosine with or without drug delivery systems). Despite demonstrated clinical efficacy, none of these drugs reliably achieves a parasitological cure in dogs, which implies the risk of relapses, spread of the disease within the dog population, human infection, and development of drug resistance. A critical evaluation of the present therapeutic scenario reveals that more efficacious, safer, and affordable drugs are required to solve the veterinary and public health problems resulting from the infections by *L. infantum* and *Leishmania* species in general.

Introduction

Status of the Chemotherapy of Leishmaniasis

More than 25 medications have been approved for use in *Leishmania* infections. This large number constitutes evidence of the shortcomings of present-day antileishmanial chemotherapy. Different chapters of this book stress the difficulties of satisfactory treatment of Leishmaniasis: limited efficacy of some compounds, high toxicity and severe side-effects of others, lack of socioeconomic conditions allowing the administration of the drugs in remote regions, variability in the

---

* Corresponding Author

Trypanosomatid Diseases: Molecular Routes to Drug Discovery, First edition. Edited by T. Jäger, O. Koch, and L. Flohé.

sensitivity of different *Leishmania* species and isolates, or the reported appearance of isolates resistant to the drugs most commonly used (pentavalent antimonials) [1,2]. Moreover, first-line drugs against these infections have a high price [3], making them simply unaffordable under the economic conditions in many areas of the world. Therefore, it is not surprising that research efforts are carried out all over the world to develop new treatments for leishmaniasis. Up to now, attempts at rational therapy – parasite target-oriented compounds – have yielded only limited success, and the deep knowledge of the physiology and molecular biology of *Leishmania* has not yet fostered the development of new drugs. The compounds used in both human medicine and veterinary clinics or those under clinical study are actually more a consequence of incidental findings than of focused research [4]. In 2004, the World Health Organization TDR, the Special Programme for Research and Training in Tropical Diseases, identified liposomal amphotericin B, miltefosine, and paromomycin as the most promising anti-*Leishmania* compounds (http://www.who.int/tdr/diseases/leish). However, none of these compounds is new. Amphotericin B has been employed as an efficacious treatment of leishmaniasis for decades, besides its antifungal properties; miltefosine (hexadecylphosphocholine) was originally developed as an anti-neoplasic agent; the aminoglycoside antibiotic paromomycin (aminosidine) has been used as anti-microbial since the 1960s. Presently, these three drugs and the pentavalent antimonials still constitute the chemotherapeutic agents of reference for the treatment of leishmaniasis. Miltefosine has been shown to have efficacy comparable to that of amphotericin B deoxycholate and has been proposed as an alternative chemotherapy in India [3]. This compound has a strong limitation due to its long half-life (greater than 120 h) in combination with teratogenic properties. This precludes its use during reproductive life, unless a contraception method is applied. Also, its high accessibility, oral administration potentially without medical supervision, and long half-life facilitate rapid appearance of resistance. In fact, under laboratory conditions, it is relatively easy to select resistant clonal lines of *L. donovani*.

Paromomycin is a low-cost compound, classified as an "orphan drug" (US Food and Drug Administration/European Medicines Agency) by the Institute for One World Health (www.iowh.com), after a long time of being used as an anti-microbial. Short-time administration, efficacy, and low toxicity make it a potential first-line drug against leishmaniasis. However, induction of resistance in *L. donovani* [5] suggests that resistant isolates might appear if the drug is used in monotherapy. Amphotericin B is highly efficacious against *Leishmania* (particularly *L. donovani* and *L. infantum*). No resistant isolates have been reported even after prolonged therapy in humans coinfected with HIV and *L. infantum* [6], although some resistant lines of *L. donovani* and *L. mexicana* have been obtained *in vitro* under pharmacological pressure [7,8]. This compound has two major shortcomings: high cost and high toxicity of the free compound as deoxycholate. Introduction of a liposomal formulation (AmBisome®), approved in both the United States and Europe, reduced the toxicity problems. However, the costs of treatment with AmBisome or the colloidal (Amphocil®) or lipidic (Abelcet®) formulations are unaffordable in low-income areas.

Chemotherapy of Canine Leishmaniasis

Canine Leishmaniasis by *L. infantum* (=*L. chagasi*)

Animal leishmaniases, particularly those from domestic animals, present a double interest: animals infected with zoonotic *Leishmania* species are potential reservoirs for human infections and are equally important from a strictly veterinary perspective. Most *Leishmania* species causing disease in humans have a zoonotic nature and even for those considered exclusively or predominantly anthroponotic (*L. donovani* and *L. tropica*) some potential animal reservoirs have been reported [9]. On the other hand, infections of dogs by *L. infantum*, apart from their role in the epidemiology of human infections, are a first-order pathology in veterinary clinics in some parts of the world. Thus, the transmission pattern of human and animal leishmaniases in endemic areas, in particular that of *L. infantum*, is more complex than previously thought [10]. In any case, the control of animal leishmaniasis (clinical recovery, infectivity for sandflies) is considered a critical issue when trying to reduce the prevalence and incidence of human leishmaniases.

Infections by *L. infantum* in dogs are mainly present in the Mediterranean basin, Central and South America, the Middle East, and China. Moreover, apparently autochthonous infection is occasionally diagnosed in North America (United States and Canada) and Central Europe. Presence of the infection is related to the distribution of sandfly vectors. Other transmission mechanisms (i.e., direct dog to dog, vertical, ticks as mechanical vectors) have been reported to occur, although their epidemiological role is probably negligible as compared to the vectorial one. Prevalence of canine infection is variable, even within an endemic region, with areas of low infection pressure close to hotspots. Many studies, particularly those carried out in the Mediterranean, support these findings. However, a comparison between many of these epidemiological studies is hardly feasible, since different diagnostic methods (direct observation, indirect fluorescent antibody test (IFAT), enzyme-linked immunosorbent assay, polymerase chain reaction (PCR)) of variable sensitivity and specificity have been employed. Moreover, they include surveys carried out in different years and comparable sampling methods are not guaranteed. Generally speaking, a prevalence of *L. infantum* between 5 and 7% of the total canine population of the Mediterranean area would be a reasonable estimate.

Canine leishmaniasis is a chronic disease with incubation periods (i.e., the time between inoculation and the appearance of clinical signs) varying from 2 to several months. Pathogenesis is related to the multiplication of the parasite within cells of the mononuclear phagocytic system. Therefore, splenomegaly and generalized lymphadenomegaly are commonly found. The clinical picture comprises irregular fever, cachexy and muscle atrophy, epistaxis, uveitis, blepharitis, keratoconjunctivitis, onychogryphosis, dermatitis with or without alopecia, ulcerations, vomiting, diarrhea, polyuria and polydypsia, nose hyperkeratosis, and, eventually, renal failure by glomerulonephritis and tubulointerstitial nephritis. The outcome of the disease is related to the general status of the animal, immune response elicited by

Leishmania, balance of $CD4^+/CD8^+$ T-cells, presence of inter-current infections, and, possibly, differential virulence of *Leishmania* isolates. Therefore, the clinical course of canine leishmaniasis is highly variable from one animal to another; some infections are subclinical (so-called "cryptic infections"), whereas in other cases the infection is not self-limiting and is fatal unless treated.

Chemotherapy of Canine Leishmaniasis

Chemotherapy of infected animals, particularly in the Mediterranean, includes the use of the same compounds employed in the treatment of the human infection [11,12]. A large body of information has been obtained by veterinary practitioners, especially with pentavalent antimonials and combinations, along their clinical practice. However, this experience has hardly been published and the treatment conditions were mostly not controlled, thus failing to meet statistical standards and rendering the data difficult to interpret. The drugs most frequently employed are pentavalent antimonials, particularly meglumine antimoniate, administered as monotherapy or in combination, amphotericin B, miltefosine, and paromomycin [13–15]. The latter drugs have been found to be less efficacious than "traditional" drugs and tend to be used in combination with antimonials. The variability of treatment schedules (number of doses, total dose administered, administration route, duration of treatment), sometimes contradictory results (i.e., with AmBisome and others), or the use of different systems of post-treatment monitoring have demanded standardized treatment protocols. Generally speaking, however, none of the available drugs reliably clears the *Leishmania* infection; treatment provokes clinical improvement or clinical cure of infected dogs, but relapses are the rule as a consequence of parasites surviving in the host [16,17]. The prognosis of the animals subjected to anti-leishmanial treatment is highly unpredictable and probably depends on the initial physiological status of the infected dogs, particularly renal function, degree of disease, presence of inter-current infections, and other features [18,19]. It has been stated that affected dogs treated with meglumine antimoniate followed by a subsequent treatment at the time of recurrences have a 75% probability of living an additional 4 years [16]. All therapeutic regimens established for canine leishmaniasis must be accompanied by supportive therapy, appropriate diet, and a monitoring system during chemotherapy (clinical and hematological parameters, biochemical profile, serum protein levels, liver, and, particularly, renal functionality markers and anti-*Leishmania* antibody levels) [15]. In short, thus, there is not only a need for effective treatment schedules with the available chemotherapeutic agents and for adequate surveillance, but also for the discovery of new drugs.

Pentavalent Antimonials

Pentavalent antimonials (Sb(V)) have been available since 1920 and in the form of stibogluconate since 1945 [20]. Pentavalent antimonials, administered by the parenteral route, are the classical drugs for visceral leishmaniasis and the drugs of choice to treat canine leishmaniasis. There are two marketed formulations, N-methylglucamine (meglumine) antimoniate (Glucantime[®]) containing 85 mg Sb(V)/ml, and sodium stibogluconate (SSG; Pentostam[®]) with 100 mg of Sb(V)/ml [21]. In spite of the use of antimonials against *Leishmania* for over 50 years, their mechanism of action is far from clear. Leishmanicidal activity of antimonials has been related to the selective inhibition of enzymes required for energy metabolism (glycolysis and Krebs cycle) and fatty acids oxidation [22,23]. However, Sb(III) killed promastigotes of *L. mexicana in vitro*, while they were unaffected by Sb(V), and neither antimonial inhibited hexokinase, phosphofructo-kinase, pyruvate kinase, malate dehydrogenase, or phosphoenolpyruvate carboxy-kinase [24]. Comparable results were obtained in *L. tropica* promastigotes without any noticeable effect of glucantime on the activity of hexokinase and phosphofruc-tokinase [25]. Another possible mechanism of action of antimonials is the inhibition of type I DNA topoisomerase [26], but no relationship has been found by Walker and Saravia [27] between leishmanicidal activity of Sb(III) and inhibition of topoisomer-ase I in *L. donovani*. In addition, it has been shown that Sb(III) interferes with trypanothione metabolism by two different mechanisms: rapid efflux of intracellular trypanothione and glutathione, and inhibition of trypanothione reductase [28]. Most of this experimental work has been carried out under *in vitro* or *ex vivo* conditions and in some cases with promastigotes. Therefore, in the infected host other mechanisms could still be involved.

Both Pentostam and, especially, Glucantime are usually employed in the control of canine leishmaniasis, particularly in the Mediterranean, and, on occasion, they have been recommended to prevent the development of the disease in asympto-matic infected dogs. This presymptomatic treatment could, in addition, induce an important reduction of the available parasites for sandflies [29,30], thus dimin-ishing the risk of transmission for other dogs or humans.

The use of antimonials is restricted by the side-effects, mainly nephrotoxicity [23,31]. However, toxicity of antimonials is a controversial issue, since the apparent toxicity disappears when the doses are applied more separatedly [32]. Actually, antimonials have a short-half life (21, 42, and 122 min after intravenous, intra-muscular, and subcutaneous administration, respectively), and are quickly eliminated by urine and do not accumulate; after 6–9 h, 80–95% of meglumine antimoniate is eliminated through the kidneys [33]. The renal toxicity after administration of the antimonial reported in some studies is due possibly to previous kidney damage caused by intraglomerular deposition of circulating immunocomplexes inducing glomeru-lonephritis [34,35]. Oliva *et al.* [18] concluded that no scientific evidence is presently available that supports a genuine nephrotoxicity of antimonials in dogs.

Other side-effects observed after administration include painful local swellings at the site of the injection, gastrointestinal disturbances, locomotor problems, joint stiffness, anorexia, and fatigue [16,23,36]. Apathy has been observed during the first days post-treatment [17].

Certain studies reported that a variable amount of Sb(III), the most active and toxic form of the antimonials, could be present in the marketed preparations and this could partially explain the toxicity of the drug [21]. Sb(V) has been suggested to act as a pro-drug, being converted to the more active anti-leishmanial and toxic Sb(III) form in the host. However, this link between toxicity for the host and anti-leishmanial activity of Sb(III) forms has been challenged, since only a marginal effect on *Leishmania* of the residual Sb(III) in pentavalent antimonial drugs administered could be observed *in vivo* [37].

Meglumine antimoniate induces a rapid improvement of the clinical condition of the infected dogs, temporary recovery of cell-mediated immune response [38], and a differential IgG1/IgG2 pattern up to 5–12 months post-treatment [39]. This is observed in 75–90% of the animals treated. However, parasitological cure of the dogs is not achieved and relapses are the rule in about 75% of the cases 6–8 months post-treatment [40–42]. As observed in human leishmaniasis, the presence of resistant strains of *L. infantum* to meglumine antimoniate in dogs has sporadically been reported [40,43]; this resistance development could be related to inappropriate under-dosage of the drug.

As mentioned, treatment schedules in canine leishmaniasis are variable and this holds also true for meglumine antimoniate dosing. Doses from 40 to 75 mg/kg, twice a day for 4 weeks or 75–100 mg/kg/day administered by subcutaneous injection are currently employed [16,19,33,36,44]. Separation of daily doses is recommended on the basis of the pharmacokinetic properties to sustain tissue levels. Treatments are supposed to be repeated after relapses and a prolonged treatment (2–3 additional weeks) could be used if no improvement of the animals is observed. Meglumine antimoniate is used as monotherapy, although practitioners favor its combination with allopurinol and to a lesser extent with miltefosine (see below). The most frequent treatment schedule used by veterinary clinicians is meglumine antimoniate (100 mg/kg/day for 4 weeks) plus allopurinol (10 mg/kg *per os*, twice a day, 6–12 months). Dogs treated with the combination show a prolonged period of clinical remission [36]. Comparable results have been obtained in naturally infected dogs with *L. infantum* treated with the combination of allopurinol (15 mg/kg *per os* twice a day until clinical improvement, followed by allopurinol plus SSG, 30 mg/kg/day, subcutaneously for 1 month, followed by allopurinol at the same dose up to 8 months) [45].

Adverse effects of the combination are those of the drugs administered in monotherapy. In spite of the scarce evidence of toxicity associated with meglumine antimoniate, some drug delivery systems, particularly liposomes, have been employed. These formulations have shown promising results as they retain the leishmanicidal ability of this compound and reduce its potential toxicity [46]. Despite this success, Schettini *et al.* [47] observed that treatment with liposomal forms could not provoke the complete elimination of parasites either. Other formulations of SSG in non-ionic surfactant vesicles have been tested on rodent models (mouse and hamster) and dogs. In all cases, the encapsulated forms increased efficacy with lower toxicity when compared to the free form [48].

Allopurinol

Allopurinol is an analog of purine (hypoxanthine) that was first used against leishmaniasis in the 1980s. Its mechanism of action is based on the inhibition of enzymes of purine metabolism such as xanthine oxidase. In *Leishmania*, but not in mammals, this compound is also metabolized to various nucleosides and nucleotides that exert toxicity via incorporation into RNA [49,50]. Allopurinol does not usually generate side-effects and thus is recommended in individuals with chronic nephritis due to leishmaniasis [51] or locations where first-choice drugs are not available. However, it has been shown that this leishmaniostatic compound alone cannot completely eliminate the parasites from the human body [18,52,53] and does not prevent infection of healthy individuals [54]. In spite of this limitation it has been used in canine leishmaniasis both in monotherapy or combined with antimonials. Doses are variable, ranging from 5 to 30 mg/kg every 12 h *per os*. The treatment should be maintained for at least 6 months [16,18]. The most frequently used dose is 10 mg/kg twice a day [19,52]. Side-effects are not common, but hepatic and renal function must be monitored during prolonged treatment since xanthinuria and xanthine urolithiasis can occur, particularly in dogs with hepatic disease [55]. A moderate clinical improvement of the animals treated with allopurinol has been described [52,56] and 20 mg/kg/day, 1 week every month, of this compound was effective in maintaining clinical remission in naturally infected dogs. Moreover, allopurinol has been reported to ameliorate renal function, preventing deterioration of the glomerular filtration rate in infected dogs with proteinuria, provided that there is no renal insufficiency [51]. Since parasitological cure is not achieved [53], relapses appear once the administration of allopurinol is interrupted [52,57]. The comparatively poor efficacy of allopurinol monotherapy demands combination with antimonials or miltefosine, except for cases with severe renal injury [19].

Alkylphosphocholine (Miltefosine)

Hexadecylphosphocholine or miltefosine was originally developed as an anti-neoplasic by its ability to induce apoptosis selectively in tumor cells. Some derivatives of alkyllysophospholipids such as miltefosine, edelfosine, or ilmofosine have anti-leishmanial activity (in promastigotes and amastigotes) [58,59]. Miltefosine was able to reduce by 89% the parasite burden in spleen and liver of mice experimentally infected with *L. infantum* [60]. It has been used against human visceral leishmaniasis (Impavido®) and a veterinary formulation to treat dog leishmaniasis (Milteforan®) is available. Apart from its anti-leishmanial activity, the compound has immunostimulating properties by activating T cells and macrophages with an increase of NO production [23]. No major acute toxic effects of miltefosine have been described in humans or dogs [61] apart from vomiting and diarrhea. Treatment of naturally infected dogs with *L. infantum* using 2 mg/kg/day miltefosine for 28 consecutive days yielded clinical improvement of the animals, recovery of pre-treatment hematologic abnormalities (50%) and seronegativity (IFAT test) in about 50% of pretrial seropositive dogs [62]. Comparable results were obtained by Mateo *et al.* [63] using the same treatment schedule.

Combination of miltefosine with allopurinol (2 mg/kg/day, oral administration miltefosine plus 10 mg allopurinol/kg/day *per os*) for 30 days, followed by treatment with allopurinol alone for 1 year, induced a rapid improvement of the clinical condition of severely affected dogs (1 week after starting the treatment) and recovery of normal renal function after 2 weeks [64]. Impressive clinical improvement with progressive reduction of *L. infantum* burden in lymph node aspirates and increase of interferon-γ was observed even during an extended follow-up period after various miltefosine-based treatment regimens, but again parasitological clearance of the animals was not achieved, as evidenced by PCR 24 months after treatment [65].

The main limitation of miltefosine is the induction of fetal malformations, which limits its use to non-fertile individuals or those under anti-conceptional treatment [66]. Moreover, the potential of this compound to generate resistant *Leishmania* under field conditions is high. The ability of miltefosine-exposed *Leishmania* to overexpress a transporter protein expelling the drug from the parasite, the long half-life (greater than 120 h) of the compound, and the prolonged treatment required, often associated with subtherapeutic drug levels, favor rapid emergence of resistance [67]. Moreover, oral administration of miltefosine, a logistic advantage to treat human leishmaniasis in remote regions even with poor sanitary standards, implies a lack of control of resistance development. Similar considerations can be made in a veterinary scenario.

Amphotericin B

Amphotericin B is a polyene macrolide antibiotic obtained from the fermentation of the fungus *Streptomyces nodosus*. Its leishmanicidal capacity was discovered in the 1960s. The compound was mainly used as an anti-fungal, especially for the treatment of systemic mycoses. Its mechanism of action has been related to the ability to bind to ergosterol in membranes of *Leishmania*, which results in cell death due to loss of ions [68]. This primary mechanism of action could explain why clinically significant resistance to amphotericin B is so rare [69]. Amphotericin B is marketed in a colloidal suspension of amphotericin B deoxycholate to be administered parenterally. A large number of studies have shown the leishmanicidal efficacy of this compound, although toxicity restricts its general use. Toxicity for mammals has been attributed to the similarity between ergosterol from the *Leishmania* membranes and cholesterol, the major sterol in mammalian cells, causing non-specific binding and thereby altering potassium permeability. Amphotericin B affinity for sterols, and therefore toxicity, depends on its state of aggregation: the monomeric form of amphotericin B does not interact with ergosterol, whereas its affinity increases with aggregation [70]. Moreover, the sterol composition of the membrane also influences the selectivity of amphotericin B for ergosterol [71], which could contribute to differential sensitivity of *Leishmania* species to amphotericin B.

Amphotericin B has been employed in human medicine as a second-choice drug against leishmaniasis, but its use, particularly as liposomal formulation, is increasing due to the emerging resistance to antimonials [2,21,23]. Dogs naturally infected with *L. infantum* have been treated with different dosage regimens of amphotericin B (between 1 and 2–5 mg/kg, twice per week, slow intravenous infusion in normal saline followed by 10 ml/kg mannitol 20%). All animals receiving a total dose beyond 10 mg/kg were apparently cured after treatment and 14 out of 17 were PCR-negative [72]. With the same emulsion all dogs were clinically cured and 5 months post-treatment only 38% of the dogs were positive by PCR [73].

Use of Drug Delivery Systems for Amphotericin B

The main side-effect of amphotericin B associated to the treatment of canine leishmaniasis is nephrotoxicity caused by renal vasoconstriction and possibly by its direct action on renal epithelial cells [23]. Many drug delivery systems of the compound have been developed to reduce its adverse effects in the mammalian host. The most successful vehicles have been liposomes, maintaining the leishmanicidal properties of amphotericin B and reducing its toxicity. The rationale of this approach is to target the large-size amphotericin B-charged liposomes in the bloodstream to the mononuclear phagocytic system. Thus, the leishmanicidal drug reaches the actual intracellular location where *Leishmania* amastigotes multiply. In turn, the amphotericin B thus trapped can no longer interact with mammalian sterols and accordingly the toxicity for the host is substantially lowered. Preparations of lower toxicity of amphotericin B would make this compound an almost ideal treatment of visceral leishmaniasis in humans [74].

A number of formulations of amphotericin B are currently available [75]. The one most commonly used is AmBisome, a formulation of amphotericin B in sonicated liposomes. Another liposomal preparation (Fungisome®), developed in India in 2003, indeed yielded most promising results in kala-azar patients (100% cure after 1 month and 90% sustained cure 6 months after treatment) with doses of 10 mg/kg (twice 5 mg/kg) [76]. Non-liposomal drug delivery systems of amphotericin B in clinical use are Amphocil, a colloidal dispersion of amphotericin B in cholesterol, and Abelcet, a lipid complex, which was the first lipid formulation of amphotericin B that was approved by the US Food and Drug Administration for the treatment of fungal infections [4,77–79]. Some of these amphotericin B formulations have also been used to treat canine leishmaniasis. Treatment with amphotericin B induces a rapid clinical cure, although in dogs the improvement is followed by relapses [18]. In addition to some public health considerations (see below), its high cost makes the use of liposomal amphotericin B for canine leishmaniasis not generally feasible.

Over recent years alternative drug delivery systems of amphotericin B of lower cost and higher stability (i.e., niosomes, nanodisks, polymers conjugates, micro/nanopolymeric particles) have been tested against leishmaniasis. Nanospheres of poly(ε-caprolactone) with amphotericin B have been employed *in vitro* against *L. donovani* amastigotes [80]. These nanospheres, coated with poloxamer 188, have also been utilized to treat fungal infections [81]. Amphotericin B conjugated with arabinogalactan [82] and phospholipid bilaminar complexes and apolipoprotein [83] displayed low toxicity and high leishmanicidal activity in mice infected with *L. major*. Using a polysaccharide matrix with anionic lipids, amphotericin B retained the leishmanicidal activity against *L. donovani* infections and was substantially less toxic in a mouse model [84]. Similarly, lecithin micro-emulsions [85,86] or nanospheres of egg albumin [87] had lower toxicity than the free antibiotic. Also, superaggregated amphotericin B, obtained by heat treatment, has a reduced toxicity [88,89]. Human albumin microspheres containing amphotericin B have been tested *in vitro* and *in vivo* models (hamster) of *L. infantum* infection. This low-cost drug delivery system showed a reduced toxicity (10-fold) when compared to amphotericin B deoxycholate and similar leishmanicidal properties [90–92]. Pilot experiments carried out with dogs naturally infected with *L. infantum* yielded inconsistent results, although a clinical improvement of the animals treated was observed (unpublished results). The use of drug delivery systems against *Leishmania* has been critically reviewed [93].

It has often been stated that the use of amphotericin B for the treatment of canine leishmaniasis is not recommended, since parasite clearance is not achieved and resistance development appears possible [11,18,74]. However, its mechanism of action does not likely favor resistance [69] and no resistant strains of *L. infantum*, despite the long history of amphotericin B use in human medicine, have ever been identified in humans [6] or dogs (unpublished results). This observation is indeed surprising, since amphotericin B was, and still is, the preferred treatment for systemic fungal infections in humans and domestic animals including dogs, and frequent exposure of *L. infantum* to this antibiotic must be rated as more than likely over the 50 years since its introduction.

Aminosidine (Paromomycin), Pentamidine, and Other Compounds

Aminosidine is an aminoglycoside antibiotic produced by *Streptomyces* spp. The compound shows both anti-bacterial and anti-parasitic activity [23]. Parenterally administered, aminosidine reduced the parasite burden in a model infection of *L. infantum* in mice, although the efficacy was lower than that obtained with antimonials. Treatment of dogs naturally infected with *L. infantum* with this antibiotic significantly reduced the antibody titers in the animals [94]. Aminosidine is not likely suited for monotherapy given the relapses observed 50–100 days after treatment with a dose of 20 mg/kg/day and the casualties associated with higher doses (80 mg/kg/day) [13]. A combined therapy of aminosidine and antimonials appears more realistic, since interference between these anti-leishmanial agents has not been observed and renal function was not altered after treatment of healthy Beagle dogs [95]. Oliva *et al.* [18] suggest a combination of aminosidine (5 mg/kg, subcutaneous, daily for 3 weeks) plus 60 mg meglumine antimoniate, intramuscular, twice a day for 4 weeks. Also in mice models of infection, the combination of antimonials and aminosidine proved to be more efficacious than the individual drugs, but still the parasites persisted in liver and spleen and toxicity was not abrogated [96].

Pentamidine isethionate is an aromatic diamidine used to treat pneumonia caused by *Pneumocystis carinii* and also has anti-leishmanial properties. A formulation for parenteral use (Pentacarinat®) is available. A closely related compound, pentamidine dimetasulfonate (Lomidine®), is also marketed [4,23]. The action mechanism of pentamidines is believed to comprise induction of conformational changes in DNA, inhibition of polyamine metabolism, and interference with purine metabolism [97–99]. In canine leishmaniasis, an apparently complete clinical and immunologic recovery has been observed after pentamidine treatment [100], but relapses occur. Associated side-effects are irritation at the injection site, vomiting, tachycardia, and hypotension [23]. As with other anti-leishmanial compounds, various drug delivery systems have been investigated (nanospheres of polylactic acid and polymethacrylate containing pentamidine) and the results obtained in mouse models of *L. infantum* infections showed a significant increase of efficacy when compared to the free compound [101,102].

A number of anti-fungal azoles (ketoconazole, metronidazole, and fluconazole) have also been investigated for activity against *Leishmania* because of the similarity between fungal and *Leishmania* membranes [1]. In canine leishmaniasis, however, their efficacy was lower than that of Sb(V) antimonials [23,103].

Exploration of New Anti-Leishmanial Drugs

No ideal drug to control leishmaniasis, human or canine, is presently available. The search for novel, safe, affordable and effective chemotherapeutic agents to control this infection has followed different strategies. The anti-leishmanial activity of compounds with anti-proliferative (i.e., anti-neoplasic, anti-protozoal and anti-bacterial) or anti-fungal properties is being explored. In this context, tamoxifen, a triphenyl-ethylene derivative with anti-neoplasic and anti-fungal activity, was shown to have anti-leishmanial efficacy *in vitro* (*L. braziliensis* and *L. infantum*) and proved to be effective (95–98% reduction in spleen parasite burden) in a hamster model of *L. infantum* infection at a dose of 20 mg/kg/day for 15 days administered intraperitoneally [104].

Based on the observation that lactation protects against experimental leishmaniasis in hamsters [105], domperidone (EV-4820), a dopamine D2 receptor antagonist stimulating prolactin production, was tested in dogs naturally infected with *L. infantum*. Oral administration of domperidone (1 mg/kg/twice a day for 1 month) was effective in controlling and reducing clinical signs and improved cellular responses [106]. Unfortunately, neither parasite burden of the animals nor their infection status was determined.

Naphthoquinones showed anti-leishmanial activity *in vitro* [107]. However, the screening tests were carried out with promastigotes and the predictive value of data obtained with this extracellular stage of the parasite is considered to be low. Accordingly, buparvaquone, 2-[*trans*(4-*t*-butylcyclohexyl)-methyl]-3-hydroxy-1,4-naphthoquinone, which is active against *Theileria* and marketed for veterinary use (Butalex®), showed good anti-leishmanial activity against amastigotes *in vitro*, but limited success in a murine model of *L. donovani* infection (62% reduction of parasite burden in liver) [108]. In dogs naturally infected with *L. infantum* four doses of 5 mg/kg live weight over 12 days only caused minor clinical improvements and no parasitological cure or halting of disease progression [14].

One of the most favored approaches to new treatments for leishmaniasis is the exploration of natural products extracted from plants. For example, some alkaloids showed activity on both promastigotes and amastigotes of *Leishmania* [109], and some betulin derivatives are able to inhibit by 50% the multiplication of intracellular amastigotes *in vitro* at low micromolar concentrations [110]. Cystatins, natural inhibitors of cysteine proteases, induce the production of NO by macrophages and therefore reduce the multiplication of amastigotes in peritoneal macrophages *ex vivo*, and can control the infection in mouse infections by *L. donovani* [111,112]. Recombinant barley cystatins showed *in vitro* activity against amastigotes of the two major causative agents of visceral leishmaniasis, *L. donovani* and *L. infantum*, in the micromolar range (IC$_{90}$ about 4.8 μM) [113]. The potential of many natural products to control leishmaniasis, human and canine, has recently been reviewed [114]. Such information, together with target-based drug design, provides reasonable chances to develop new drugs for leishmaniasis in the forthcoming years.

Concluding Remarks

Currently available control systems of dog leishmaniasis include the use of repellents, immunoprophylaxis, dog culling, and chemotherapy. Recently marketed vaccines have some shortcomings, including their price, need for annual revaccination, and absence of total protection of vaccinated animals. From a public health point of view, reduction of infection levels in infected reservoirs to lower transmission rates to the human population by sandflies is the objective. However, euthanasia of infected dogs is ethically not acceptable, not commonly accepted by owners, and the results obtained are inconsistent and hardly promise a solution for the problem [10]. Therefore, even in endemic areas where human and dog populations are exposed to *L. infantum*, chemotherapy is a need. Present chemotherapeutic control of dog leishmaniasis is far from ideal, and for the most part, being realistic, the same drugs are used for human and canine leishmaniasis in the endemic areas. Scientific evidence of the potential risks associated with this therapeutic practice is urgently needed.

Acknowledgments

M.J.C. has a PhD fellowship from the Spanish Ministry of Science and Innovation. This contribution was carried out under the umbrella of the COST Action CM0801. J.M.A. gratefully acknowledges financial support by grant from CYCYT (AGL2009-13009).

References

1 Croft, S.L. and Coombs, G.H. (2003) Leishmaniasis – current chemotherapy and recent advances in the search for novel drugs. *Trends Parasitol.*, **19**, 502–508.

2 Croft, S.L., Sundar, S., and Fairlamb, A.H. (2006) Drug resistance in leishmaniasis. *Clin. Microbiol. Rev.*, **19**, 111–126.

3 Sundar, S. and Chatterjee, M. (2006) Visceral leishmaniasis – current therapeutic modalities. *Indian J. Med. Res.*, **123**, 345–352.

4 Guerin, P.J., Olliaro, P., Sundar, S., Boelaert, M., Croft, S.L., Desjeux, P., Wasunna, M.K., and Bryceson, A.D.M. (2002) Visceral leishmaniasis: current status of control, diagnosis, and treatment, and a proposed research and development agenda. *Lancet Infect. Dis.*, **2**, 494–501.

5 Maarouf, M., Adeline, M.T., Solignac, M., Vautrin, D., and Robert-Gero, M. (1998) Development and characterization of paromomycin-resistant *Leishmania donovani* promastigotes. *Parasite*, **5**, 167–173.

6 Durand, R., Paul, M., Pratlong, F., Rivollet, D., Dubreuil-Lemaire, M.L., Houin, R., Astier, A., and Deniau, M. (1998) *Leishmania infantum*: lack of parasite resistance to amphotericin B in a clinically resistant visceral leishmaniasis. *Antimicrob. Agents Chemother.*, **42**, 2141–2143.

7 Espuelas, S., Legrand, P., Loiseau, P.M., Bories, C., Barratt, C., and Irache, J.M. (2000) *In vitro* reversion of amphotericin B resistance in *Leishmania donovani* by poloxamer 188. *Antimicrob. Agents Chemother.*, **44**, 2190–2192.

8 Al-Mohammed, H.I., Chance, M.L., and Bates, P.A. (2005) Production and characterization of stable amphotericin-resistant amastigotes and promastigotes of *Leishmania mexicana*. *Antimicrob. Agents Chemother.*, **49**, 3274–3280.

9 Gramiccia, M. and Gradoni, L. (2005) The current status of zoonotic leishmaniases and approaches to disease control. *Int. J. Parasitol.*, **35**, 1169–1180.

10 Costa, C.H.N. (2011) How effective is dog culling in controlling zoonotic visceral leishmaniasis? A critical evaluation of the science, politics and ethics behind this public health policy. *Rev. Soc. Bras. Med. Trop.*, **44**, 232–242.

11 Oliva, G., Manzillo, V.F., and Pagano, A. (2004) Canine leishmaniasis: evolution of the chemotherapeutic protocols. *Parassitologia*, **46**, 231–234.

12 Noli, C. and Auxilia, S.T. (2005) Treatment of canine Old World visceral leishmaniasis: a systematic review. *Vet. Dermatol.*, **16**, 213–232.

13 Vexenat, J.A., Croft, S.L., Campos, J.H.F., and Miles, M.A. (1998) Failure of buparvaquone (Butalex) in the treatment of canine visceral leishmaniosis. *Vet. Parasitol.*, **77**, 71–73.

14 Vexenat, J.A., Olliaro, P.L., De Castro, J.A. F., Cavalcante, R., Campos, J.H.F., Tavares, J.P., and Miles, M.A. (1998) Clinical recovery and limited cure in canine visceral Leishmaniasis treated with aminosidine (paromomycin). *Am. J. Trop. Med. Hyg.*, **58**, 448–453.

15 Vulpiani, M.P., Iannetti, L., Paganico, D., Iannino, F., and Ferri, N. (2011) Methods of control of the *Leishmania infantum* dog reservoir: state of the art. *Vet. Med. Int.*, **2011**, ID 215964.

16 Noli, C. (1999) Canine leishmaniasis. *Waltham Focus*, **9**, 16–24.

17 Ferrer, L. and Roura, X. (2012) Tratamiento de la leishmaniosis canina. *Argos*, August 2012, noticia 6787.

18 Oliva, G., Roura, X., Crotti, A., Maroli, M., Castagnaro, M., Gradoni, L., Lubas, G., Paltrinieri, S., Zatelli, A., and Zini, E. (2010) Guidelines for treatment of leishmaniasis in dogs. *J. Am. Vet. Med. Assoc.*, **236**, 1192–1198.

19 Solano-Gallego, L., Miró, G., Koutinas, A., Cardoso, L., Pennisi, M.G., Ferrer, L., Bourdeau, P., Oliva, G., and Baneth, G. (2011) LeishVet guidelines for the practical management of canine leishmaniosis. *Parasit. Vectors*, **4**, 86.

20 Ramos, J.M. and Segovia, M. (1997) Estado actual del tratamiento farmacológico de la leishmaniasis. *Rev. Española Quimioter.*, **10**, 26–35.

21 Croft, S.L. and Yardley, V. (2002) Chemotherapy of leishmaniasis. *Curr. Pharm. Des.*, **8**, 319–342.

22 Berman, J.D., Waddell, D., and Hanson, B.D. (1985) Biochemical mechanisms of the antileishmanial activity of sodium stibogluconate. *Antimicrob. Agents Chemother.*, **27**, 916–920.

23 Baneth, G. and Shaw, S.E. (2002) Chemotherapy of canine leishmaniosis. *Vet. Parasitol.*, **106**, 315–324.

24 Mottram, J.C. and Coombs, G.H. (1985) *Leishmania mexicana* – enzyme activities of amastigotes and promastigotes and their inhibition by antimonials and arsenicals. *Exp. Parasitol.*, **59**, 151–160.

25 Foulquie, M.R., Louassini, M., Castanys, S., Gamarro, F., Benitz, R., and Adroher, F.J. (1999) Different catalytic activities of hexokinase and phosphofructokinase in wild type and Glucantime-resistant *Leishmania* promastigotes appears not causatively related to resistance. *Eur. J. Protistol.*, **35**, 338–341.

26 Chakraborty, A.K. and Majumder, H.K. (1988) Mode of action of pentavalent antimonials-specific inhibition of type-I DNA topoisomerase of *Leishmania donovani. Biochem. Biophys. Res. Commun.*, **152**, 605–611.

27 Walker, J. and Saravia, N.G. (2004) Inhibition of *Leishmania donovani* promastigote DNA topoisomerase I and human monocyte DNA topoisomerases I and II by antimonial drugs and classical antitopoisomerase agents. *J. Parasitol.*, **90**, 1155–1162.

28 Wyllie, S., Cunningham, M.L., and Fairlamb, A.H. (2004) Dual action of antimonial drugs on thiol redox metabolism in the human pathogen *Leishmania donovani. J. Biol. Chem.*, **279**, 39925–39932.

29 Gradoni, L., Maroli, M., Gramiccia, M., and Mancianti, F. (1987) *Leishmania infantum* infection rates in *Phlebotomus perniciosus* fed on naturally infected dogs under antimonial treatment. *Med. Vet. Entomol.*, **1**, 339–342.

30 Mancianti, F., Gramiccia, M., Gradoni, L., and Pieri, S. (1988) Studies on canine leishmaniasis control.1. Evolution of infection of different clinical forms of canine leishmaniasis following antimonial treatment. *Trans. R. Soc. Trop. Med. Hyg.*, **82**, 566–567.

31 Veiga, J.P.R., Khanam, R., Rosa, T.T., Junqueira, L.F., Brant, P.C., Raick, A.N., Friedman, H., and Marsden, P.D. (1990) Pentavalent antimonial nephrotoxicity in

the rat. *Rev. Inst. Med. Trop. Sao. Paulo*, **32**, 304–309.

32 Valladares, J.E., Riera, C., Alberola, J., Gállego, M., Portús, M., Cristofol, C., Franquelo, C., and Arboix, M. (1998) Pharmacokinetics of meglumine antimoniate after administration of a multiple dose in dogs experimentally infected with *Leishmania infantum. Vet. Parasitol.*, **75**, 33–40.

33 Tassi, P., Ormas, P., Madonna, M., Carli, S., Belloli, C., Denatale, G., Ceci, L., and Marcotrigiano, G.O. (1994) Pharmacokinetics of *N*-methylglucamine antimoniate after intravenous, intramuscular and subcutaneous administration in the dog. *Res. Vet. Sci.*, **56**, 144–150.

34 Mancianti, F., Poli, A., and Bionda, A. (1989) Analysis of renal immune deposits in canine leishmaniasis. Preliminary results. *Parassitologia*, **31**, 213–230.

35 Poli, A., Abramo, F., Mancianti, F., Nigro, M., Pieri, S., and Bionda, A. (1991) Renal involvement in canine leishmaniasis. A light microscopic, immunohistochemical and electron microscopic study. *Nephron*, **57**, 444–452.

36 Denerolle, P. and Bourdoiseau, G. (1999) Combination allopurinol and antimony treatment versus antimony alone and allopurinol alone in the treatment of canine leishmaniasis (96 cases). *J. Vet. Intern. Med.*, **13**, 413–415.

37 Dzamitika, S.A., Falcao, C.A.B., de Oliveira, F.B., Marbeuf, C., Garnier-Suillerot, A., Demicheli, C., Rossi-Bergmann, B., and Frezard, F. (2006) Role of residual Sb(III) in meglumine antimoniate cytotoxicity and MRP1-mediated resistance. *Chem. Biol. Interact.*, **160**, 217–224.

38 Bourdoiseau, G., Bonnefont, C., Hoareau, E., Boehringer, C., Stolle, T., and Chabanne, L. (1997) Specific IgG1 and IgG2 antibody and lymphocyte subset levels in naturally *Leishmania infantum*-infected treated and untreated dogs. *Vet. Immunol. Immunopathol.*, **59**, 21–30.

39 Fernández-Pérez, F.J., Gómez-Muñoz, T., Méndez, S., and Alunda, J.M. (2003) *Leishmania*-specific lymphoproliferative responses and IgG1/IgG2

immunodetection patterns by Western blot in asymptomatic, symptomatic and treated dogs. *Acta Trop.*, **86**, 83–91.

40 Gramiccia, M., Gradoni, L., and Orsini, S. (1992) Decreased sensitivity to meglumine antimoniate (Glucantime) of *Leishmania infantum* isolated from dogs after several courses of drug treatment. *Ann. Trop. Med. Parasitol.*, **86**, 613–620.

41 Slappendel, R.J. and Teske, E. (1997) The effect of intravenous or subcutaneous administration of meglumine antimonate Glucantime® in dogs with leishmaniasis. A randomized clinical trial. *Vet. Quart.*, **19**, 10–13.

42 Ikeda-Garcia, F.A., Lopes, R.S., Marques, F.J., Felix de Lima, V.M., Morinishi, C.K., Bonello, F.L., Zanette, M.F., Venturoli Perrio, S.H., and Feitosa, M.M. (2007) Clinical and parasitological evaluation of dogs naturally infected by *Leishmania (Leishmania) chagasi* submitted to treatment with meglumine antimoniate. *Vet. Parasitol.*, **143**, 254–259.

43 Carrió, J. and Portús, M. (2002) *In vitro* susceptibility to pentavalent antimony in *Leishmania infantum* strains is not modified during *in vitro* or *in vivo* passages but is modified after host treatment with meglumine antimoniate. *BMC Pharmacol.*, **2**, 11.

44 Manna, L., Reale, S., Vitale, F., Picillo, E., Pavone, L.M., and Gravino, A.E. (2008) Real-time PCR assay in *Leishmania*-infected dogs treated with meglumine antimoniate and allopurinol. *Vet. J.*, **177**, 279–282.

45 Pasa, S., Toz, S.O., Voyvoda, H., and Ozbel, Y. (2005) Clinical and serological follow-up in dogs with visceral leishmaniosis treated with allopurinol and sodium stibogluconate. *Vet. Parasitol.*, **128**, 243–249.

46 Valladares, J.E., Riera, C., González-Ensenyat, P., Díez-Cascón, A., Ramos, G., Solano-Gallego, L., Gállego, M., Portús, M., Arboix, M., and Alberola, J. (2001) Long term improvement in the treatment of canine leishmaniosis using an antimony liposomal formulation. *Vet. Parasitol.*, **97**, 15–21.

47 Schettini, D.A., Val, A.P.C., Souza, L.F., Demicheli, C., Rocha, O.G.F., Melo, M.N.,

Michalick, M.S.M., and Frezard, F. (2005) Pharmacokinetic and parasitological evaluation of the bone marrow of dogs with visceral leishmaniasis submitted to multiple dose treatment with liposome-encapsulated meglumine antimoniate. *Braz. J. Med. Biol. Res.*, **38**, 1879–1883.

48 Nieto, J., Alvar, J., Mullen, A.B., Carter, K. C., Rodríguez, C., San Andrés, M.I., San Andrés, M.D., Baillie, A.J., and González, F. (2003) Pharmacokinetics, toxicities, and efficacies of sodium stibogluconate formulations after intravenous administration in animals. *Antimicrob. Agents Chemother.*, **47**, 2781–2787.

49 Nelson, D.J., Bugge, C.J.L., Elion, G.B., Berens, R.L., and Marr, J.J. (1979) Metabolism of pyrazolo (3,4-D) pyrimidines in *Leishmania braziliensis* and *Leishmania donovani* – allopurinol, oxipurinol and 4-aminopyrazolo (3,4-D) pyrimidine. *J. Biol. Chem.*, **254**, 3959–3964.

50 Nelson, D.J., Lafon, S.W., Tuttle, J.V., Miller, W.H., Miller, R.L., Krenitsky, T.A., and Elion, G.B. (1979) Allopurinol ribonucleoside as an antileishmanial agent. Biological effects, metabolism, and enzymatic phosphorylation. *J. Biol. Chem.*, **254**, 1544–1549.

51 Plevraki, K., Koutinas, A.F., Kaldrymidou, H., Roumpies, N., Papazoglou, L.G., Saridomichelakis, M.N., Savvas, I., and Leondides, L. (2006) Effects of allopurinol treatment on the progression of chronic nephritis in canine leishmaniosis (*Leishmania infantum*). *J. Vet. Intern. Med.*, **20**, 228–233.

52 Cavaliero, T., Arnold, P., Mathis, A., Glaus, T., Hofmann-Lehmann, R., and Deplazes, P. (1999) Clinical, serologic, and parasitologic follow-up after long-term allopurinol therapy of dogs naturally infected with *Leishmania infantum. J. Vet. Intern. Med.*, **13**, 330–334.

53 Koutinas, A.F., Saridomichelakis, M.N., Mylonakis, M.E., Leontides, L., Polizopoulou, Z., Billinis, C., Argyriadis, D., Diakou, N., and Papadopoulos, O. (2001) A randomised, blinded, placebo-controlled clinical trial with allopurinol in canine leishmaniosis. *Vet. Parasitol.*, **98**, 247–261.

54 Saridomichelakis, M.N., Mylonakis, M.E., Leontides, L.S., Billinis, C., Koutinas, A. F., Galatos, A.D., Gouletsou, P., Diakou, A., and Kontos, V.I. (2005) Periodic administration of allopurinol is not effective for the prevention of canine leishmaniosis (*Leishmania infantum*) in the endemic areas. *Vet. Parasitol.*, **130**, 199–205.

55 Ling, G.V., Ruby, A.L., Harrold, D.R., and Johnson, D.L. (1991) Xanthine containing urinary calculi in dogs given allopurinol. *J. Am. Vet. Med. Assoc.*, **198**, 1935–1940.

56 Vercammen, F., Fernández-Pérez, F.J., del Amo, C., and Alunda, J.M. (2002) Follow-up of *Leishmania infantum* naturally infected dogs treated with allopurinol: immunofluorescence antibody test, ELISA and Western blot. *Acta Trop.*, **84**, 175–181.

57 Ginel, P.J., Lucena, R., Lopez, R., and Molleda, J.M. (1998) Use of allopurinol for maintenance of remission in dogs with leishmaniasis. *J. Small Anim. Pract.*, **39**, 271–274.

58 Escobar, P., Matu, S., Marques, C., and Croft, S.L. (2002) Sensitivities of *Leishmania* species to hexadecylphosphocholine (miltefosine), ET-18-OCH3 (edelfosine) and amphotericin B. *Acta Trop.*, **81**, 151–157.

59 Azzouz, S., Maache, M., García, R.G., and Osuna, A. (2005) Leishmanicidal activity of edelfosine, miltefosine and ilmofosine. *Basic Clin. Pharmacol. Toxicol.*, **96**, 60–65.

60 Le Fichoux, Y., Rousseau, D., Ferrua, B., Ruette, S., Lelievre, A., Grousson, D., and Kubar, J. (1998) Short- and long-term efficacy of hexadecylphosphocholine against established *Leishmania infantum* infection in BALB/c mice. *Antimicrob. Agents Chemother.*, **42**, 654–658.

61 Olliaro, P.L., Ridley, R.G., Engel, J., Sindermann, H., and Bryceson, A.D.M. (2003) Miltefosine in visceral leishmaniasis. *Lancet Infect. Dis.*, **3**, 70–70.

62 Woerly, V., Maynard, L., Sanquer, A., and Eun, H.-M. (2009) Clinical efficacy and tolerance of miltefosine in the treatment of canine leishmaniosis. *Parasitol. Res.*, **105**, 463–469.

63 Mateo, M., Maynard, L., Vischer, C., Bianciardi, P., and Miró, G. (2009)

Comparative study on the short term efficacy and adverse effects of miltefosine and meglumine antimoniate in dogs with natural leishmaniosis. *Parasitol. Res.*, **105**, 155–162.

64 Manna, L., Viola, E., Pavone, L., Staiano, N., and Gravino, A. (2005) Leishmanicidal activity of miltefosine in acute renal failure of naturally infected dogs, Worldleish3, Palermo-Terrasini, Sicily, p. 165.

65 Andrade, H.M., Toledo, V.P.C.P., Pinheiro, M.B., Guimaraes, T.M.P.D., Oliveira, N.C., Castro, J.A., Silva, R.N., Amorim, A.C., Brandao, R.M.S.S., Yoko, M., Silva, A.S., Dumont, K., Ribeiro, M.L. Jr., Bartchewsky, W., and Monte, S.J.H. (2011) Evaluation of miltefosine for the treatment of dogs naturally infected with *L. infantum* (=*L. chagasi*) in Brazil. *Vet. Parasitol.*, **181**, 83–90.

66 Sindermann, H. and Engel, J. (2006) Development of miltefosine as an oral treatment for leishmaniasis. *Trans. R. Soc. Trop. Med. Hyg.*, **100**, S17–S20.

67 Pérez-Victoria, F.J., Sánchez-Cañete, M. P., Seifert, K., Croft, S.L., Sundar, S., Castanys, S., and Gamarro, F. (2006) Mechanisms of experimental resistance of *Leishmania* to miltefosine: implications for clinical use. *Drug Resist. Update*, **9**, 26–39.

68 Ramos, H., Valdivieso, E., Gamargo, M., Dagger, F., and Cohen, B.E. (1996) Amphotericin B kills unicellular leishmanias by forming aqueous pores permeable to small cations and anions. *J. Membr. Biol.*, **152**, 65–75.

69 Gray, K.C., Palacios, D.S., Dailey, I., Endo, M.M., Uno, B.E., Wilcock, B.C., and Burke, M.D. (2012) Amphotericin primarily kills yeast by simply binding ergosterol. *Proc. Natl. Acad. Sci. USA*, **109**, 2234–2239.

70 Gruda, I. and Dussault, N. (1988) Effect of the aggregation state of amphotericin B on its interaction with ergosterol. *Biochem. Cell Biol.*, **66**, 177–183.

71 Barwicz, J. and Tancrede, P. (1997) The effect of aggregation state of amphotericin-B on its interactions with cholesterol- or ergosterol-containing phosphatidylcholine monolayers. *Chem. Phys. Lipids*, **85**, 145–155.

72 Lamothe, J. (2001) Activity of amphotericin B in lipid emulsion in the initial treatment of canine leishmaniasis. *J. Small Anim. Pract.*, **42**, 170–175.

73 Cortadellas, O. (2003) Initial and long-term efficacy of a lipid emulsion of amphotericin B deoxycholate in the management of canine leishmaniasis. *J. Vet. Intern. Med.*, **17**, 808–812.

74 Alvar, J., Croft, S., and Olliaro, P. (2006) Chemotherapy in the treatment and control of leishmaniasis. *Adv. Parasitol.*, **61**, 223–274.

75 Sundar, S. and Chakravarty, J. (2010) Liposomal amphotericin B and leishmaniasis: dose and response. *J. Global Infect. Dis.*, **2**, 159–166.

76 Mondal, S., Bhattacharya, P., Rahaman, M., Ali, N., and Goswami, R.P. (2010) A curative immune profile one week after treatment of Indian Kala-Azar patients predicts success with a short-course liposomal amphotericin B therapy. *PLoS Negl. Trop. Dis.*, **4**, 1–8.

77 Berman, J.D., Ksionski, G., Chapman, W. L., Waits, V.B., and Hanson, W.L. (1992) Activity of amphotericin-B cholesterol dispersion (Amphocil) in experimental visceral leishmaniasis. *Antimicrob. Agents Chemother.*, **36**, 1978–1980.

78 Berman, J.D. (1999) US Food and Drug Administration approval of AmBisome (liposomal amphotericin B) for treatment of visceral leishmaniasis – Editorial response. *Clin. Infect. Dis.*, **28**, 49–51.

79 Robinson, R.F. and Nahata, M.C. (1999) A comparative review of conventional and lipid formulations of amphotericin B. *J. Clin. Pharm. Ther.*, **24**, 249–257.

80 Espuelas, M.S., Legrand, P., Loiseau, P. M., Bories, C., Barratt, G., and Irache, J. M. (2002) *In vitro* antileishmanial activity of amphotericin B loaded in poly(epsilon-caprolactone) nanospheres. *J. Drug Target*, **10**, 593–599.

81 Espuelas, M.S., Legrand, P., Campanero, M.A., Appel, M., Cheron, M., Gamazo, C., Barratt, G., and Irache, J.M. (2003) Polymeric carriers for amphotericin B: *in vitro* activity, toxicity and therapeutic efficacy against systemic candidiasis in neutropenic mice. *J. Antimicrob. Chemother.*, **52**, 419–427.

82 Golenser, J., Frankenburg, S., Ehrenfreund, T., and Domb, A.J. (1999) Efficacious treatment of experimental leishmaniasis with amphotericin B-arabinogalactan water-soluble derivatives. *Antimicrob. Agents Chemother.*, **43**, 2209–2214.

83 Nelson, K.G., Bishop, J.V., Ryan, R.O., and Titus, R. (2006) Nanodisk-associated amphotericin B clears *Leishmania major* cutaneous infection in susceptible BALB/c mice. *Antimicrob. Agents Chemother.*, **50**, 1238–1244.

84 Loiseau, P.M., Imbertie, L., Bories, C., Betbeder, D., and De Miguel, I. (2002) Design and antileishmanial activity of amphotericin B-loaded stable ionic amphiphile biovector formulations. *Antimicrob. Agents Chemother.*, **46**, 1597–1601.

85 Moreno, M., Frutos, P., and Ballesteros, M.P. (2001) Lyophilized lecithin based oil–water microemulsions as a new and low toxic delivery system for amphotericin B. *Pharm. Res.*, **18**, 344–351.

86 Brime, B., Frutos, P., Bringas, P., Nieto, A., Ballesteros, M.P., and Frutos, G. (2003) Comparative pharmacokinetics and safety of a novel lyophilized amphotericin B lecithin-based oil–water microemulsion and amphotericin B deoxycholate in animal models. *J. Antimicrob. Chemother.*, **52**, 103–109.

87 Santhi, K., Dhanaraj, S.A., Rajendran, S. D., Raja, K., Ponnusankar, S., and Suresh, B. (1999) Nonliposomal approach – a study of preparation of egg albumin nanospheres containing amphotericin-B. *Drug Dev. Ind. Pharm.*, **25**, 547–551.

88 Petit, C., Yardley, V., Gaboriau, F., Bolard, J., and Croft, S.L. (1999) Activity of a heat-induced reformulation of amphotericin B deoxycholate (Fungizone) against *Leishmania donovani*. *Antimicrob. Agents Chemother.*, **43**, 390–392.

89 Bau, P., Bolard, J., and Dupouy-Camet, J. (2003) Heated amphotericin to treat leishmaniasis. *Lancet Infect. Dis.*, **3**, 188–188.

90 Dea-Ayuela, M.A., Rama-Íñiguez, S., Sánchez-Brunete, J.A., Torrado, J.J., Alunda, J.M., and Bolás-Fernández, F. (2004) Anti-leishmanial activity of a new

formulation of amphotericin B. *Trop. Med. Int. Health*, **9**, 981–990.

91 Sánchez-Brunete, J.A., Dea, M.A., Rama, S., Bolás, F., Alunda, J.M., Torrado-Santiago, S., and Torrado, H.H. (2004) Amphotericin B molecular organization as an essential factor to improve activity/toxicity ratio in the treatment of visceral leishmaniasis. *J. Drug Target.*, **12**, 453–460.

92 Ordóñez-Gutiérrez, L., Espada-Fernández, R., Dea-Ayuela, M.A., Torrado, J.J., Bolás-Fernández, F., and Alunda, J.M. (2007) *In vitro* effect of new formulations of amphotericin B on amastigote and promastigote forms of *Leishmania infantum*. *Int. J. Antimicrob. Agents*, **30**, 325–329.

93 Romero, E.L. and Morilla, M.J. (2008) Drug delivery systems against leishmaniasis? Still an open question. *Expert Opin. Drug. Del.*, **5**, 805–823.

94 Poli, A., Sozzi, S., Guidi, G., Bandinelli, P., and Mancianti, F. (1997) Comparison of aminosidine (paromomycin) and sodium stibogluconate for treatment of canine leishmaniasis. *Vet. Parasitol.*, **71**, 263–271.

95 Belloli, C., Crescenzo, G., Carli, S., Zaghini, A., Mengozzi, G., Bertini, S., and Ormas, P. (1999) Disposition of antimony and aminosidine combination after multiple subcutaneous injections in dogs. *Vet. J.*, **157**, 315–321.

96 Gangneux, J.P., Sulahian, A., Garin, Y.J. F., and Derouin, F. (1997) Efficacy of aminosidine administered alone or in combination with meglumine antimoniate for the treatment of experimental visceral leishmaniasis caused by *Leishmania infantum*. *J. Antimicrob. Chemother.*, **40**, 287–289.

97 Nguewa, P.A., Fuertes, M.A., Cepeda, V., Iborra, S., Carrión, J., Valladares, B., Alonso, C., and Pérez, J.M. (2005) Pentamidine is an antiparasitic and apoptotic drug that selectively modifies ubiquitin. *Chem. Biodivers.*, **2**, 1387–1400.

98 Calonge, M., Johnson, R., Balaña Fouce, R., and Ordóñez, D. (1996) Effects of cationic diamidines on polyamine content and uptake on *Leishmania infantum* in in

vitro cultures. *Biochem. Pharmacol.*, **52**, 835–841.

99 Johnson, R., Cubría, J.C., Reguera, R.M., Balaña-Fouce, R., and Ordóñez, D. (1998) Interaction of cationic diamidines with *Leishmania infantum* DNA. *Biol. Chem.*, **379**, 925–930.

100 Rhalem, A., Sahibi, H., Lasri, S., and Jaffe, C.L. (1999) Analysis of immune responses in dogs with canine visceral leishmaniasis before, and after, drug treatment. *Vet. Immunol. Immunopathol.*, **71**, 69–76.

101 Durand, R., Paul, M., Rivollet, D., Fessi, H., Houin, R., Astier, A., and Deniau, M. (1997) Activity of pentamidine-loaded poly-(D,L-lactide) nanoparticles against *Leishmania infantum* in a murine model. *Parasite*, **4**, 331–336.

102 Durand, R., Paul, M., Rivollet, D., Houin, R., Astier, A., and Deniau, M. (1997) Activity of pentamidine-loaded methacrylate nanoparticles against *Leishmania infantum* in a mouse model. *Int. J. Parasitol.*, **27**, 1361–1367.

103 Pennisi, M.G., De Majo, M., Masucci, M., Britti, D., Vitale, F., and Del Maso, R. (2005) Efficacy of the treatment of dogs with leishmaniosis with a combination of metronidazole and spiramycin. *Vet. Rec.*, **156**, 346–349.

104 Miguel, D.C., Zauli-Nascimento, R.C., Yokoyama-Yasunaka, J.K.U., Katz, S., Barbieri, C.L., and Uliana, S.R.B. (2009) Tamoxifen as a potential antileishmanial agent: efficacy in the treatment of *Leishmania braziliensis* and *Leishmania chagasi* infections. *J. Antimicrob. Chemother.*, **63**, 365–368.

105 Gómez-Ochoa, P., Gascón, F.M., Lucientes, J., Larraga, V., and Castillo, J.A. (2003) Lactating females Syrian hamster (*Mesocricetus auratus*) show protection against experimental *Leishmania infantum* infection. *Vet. Parasitol.*, **116**, 61–64.

106 Gómez-Ochoa, P., Castillo, J.A., Gascón, M., Zárate, J.J., Álvarez, F., and Couto, C. G. (2009) Use of domperidone in the treatment of canine visceral leishmaniasis: a clinical trial. *Vet. J.*, **179**, 259–263.

107 Kayser, O., Kiderlen, A.F., Laatsch, H., and Croft, S.L. (2000) *In vitro*

leishmanicidal activity of monomeric and dimeric naphthoquinones. *Acta Trop.*, **77**, 307–314.

108 Croft, S.L., Hogg, J., Gutteridge, W.E., Hudson, A.T., and Randall, A.W. (1992) The activity of hydroxynaphthoquinones against *Leishmania donovani. J. Antimicrob. Chemother.*, **30**, 827–832.

109 Di Giorgio, C., Delmas, F., Ollivier, E., Elias, R., Balansard, G., and Timon-David, P. (2004) *In vitro* activity of the beta-carboline alkaloids harmane, harmine, and harmaline toward parasites of the species *Leishmania infantum. Exp. Parasitol.*, **106**, 67–74.

110 Wert, L., Alakurtti, S., Corral, M.J., Sánchez-Fortún, S., Yli-Kauhaluoma, J., and Alunda, J.M. (2011) Toxicity of betulin derivatives and *in vitro* effect on promastigotes and amastigotes of *Leishmania infantum* and *L. donovani. J. Antibiot.*, **64**, 475–481.

111 Das, L., Datta, N., Bandyopadhyay, S., and Das, P.K. (2001) Successful therapy of lethal murine visceral leishmaniasis with cystatin involves up-regulation of nitric oxide and a favorable T cell response. *J. Immunol.*, **166**, 4020–4028.

112 Mukherjee, S., Ukil, A., and Das, P.K. (2007) Immunomodulatory peptide from cystatin, a natural cysteine protease inhibitor, against leishmaniasis as a model macrophage disease. *Antimicrob. Agents Chemother.*, **51**, 1700–1707.

113 Ordóñez-Gutiérrez, L., Martínez, M., Rubio-Somoza, I., Díaz, I., Méndez, S., and Alunda, J.M. (2009) *Leishmania infantum*: antiproliferative effect of recombinant plant cystatins on promastigotes and intracellular amastigotes estimated by direct counting and real-time PCR. *Exp. Parasitol.*, **123**, 341–346.

114 Shukla, A.K., Singh, B.K., Patra, S., and Dubey, V.K. (2010) Rational approaches for drug designing against leishmaniasis. *Appl. Biochem. Biotechnol.*, **160**, 2208–2218.

3
Pharmacological Metabolomics in Trypanosomes

Darren J. Creek, Isabel M. Vincent, and Michael P. Barrett[*]

Abstract

Many drugs act by perturbing aspects of cellular metabolism. Human African trypanosomiasis can be treated with five drugs, depending on the causative subspecies and the stage of the disease. For only one drug, eflornithine (difluoromethylornithine), has a mode of action been ascertained – it inhibits ornithine decarboxylase, a key enzyme in polyamine biosynthesis. Modes of action remain unknown for the other drugs, which include the organic arsenical melarsoprol, the naphthalene suramin, the diamidine pentamidine, and the nitrofuran nifurtimox, although it has recently been shown that nifurtimox acts following its metabolism to a reactive trinitrile derivative. Metabolomics aims to quantify all low-molecular-weight chemicals within a given system. Metabolomic techniques have recently been developed and applied to trypanosomes, and might be expected to reveal how drugs perturb metabolism. Here, we review methods to study the trypanosome's metabolome and discuss the current knowledge with respect to the effects of anti-trypanosomal drugs on parasite metabolism.

Introduction

Human African trypanosomiasis (HAT) is caused by *Trypanosoma brucei* subspecies [1]. The disease has two defined stages. In stage 1, which follows transmission of the parasites by the tsetse fly vector, trypanosomes replicate in the hemolymphatic system, causing relatively non-specific symptoms, including general malaise, fever, and headache [1]. In stage 2, parasites have entered the central nervous system (CNS) and their presence induces various neurological sequelae, including psychological changes and disruptions to sleep/wake patterns after which the common name of "sleeping sickness" is derived [2].

In Central and West Africa the subspecies *T. b. gambiense* causes a chronic form of HAT taking around 2 years before CNS infection, followed by progressive neurological deterioration during stage 2 disease, then death [1,2]. In Eastern and Southern Africa, *T. b. rhodesiense* causes an acute disease and is fatal within months.

---

[*] Corresponding Author

Trypanosomatid Diseases: Molecular Routes to Drug Discovery, First edition. Edited by T. Jäger, O. Koch, and L. Flohé.
© 2013 Wiley-VCH Verlag GmbH & Co. KGaA. Published 2013 by Wiley-VCH Verlag GmbH & Co. KGaA.

Trypanosomes escape immunological destruction using a process of antigenic variation [3], which renders vaccination an unlikely proposition for HAT. Chemotherapy remains pre-eminent, although tsetse fly control can also be an effective means of intervention [1]. A decade of sustained and enhanced intervention has led to HAT prevalence declining with fewer than 7000 cases reported in 2010 [4].

However, the history of trypanosomiasis control has seen previous declines preceding resurgence, owing to the cessation of intervention programs perceived as uneconomical for a low-prevalence disease [5].

Until recently, investigations into the mode of action of trypanocidal drugs have depended upon testing inhibition of predicted enzyme targets. In the case of eflornithine, a specific inhibitor of ornithine decarboxylase, several studies confirmed this mode of action [2,6]. For other drugs, however, which were introduced empirically based on their ability to kill trypanosomes, modes of action have remained elusive [2]. The new methodologies collectively referred to as "metabolomics" now offer the means to determine how drugs perturb trypanosome metabolism in a hypothesis-free, untargeted fashion. Here, we review the published literature on the application of metabolomics technology to trypanosomes and also on what is known about actions of anti-trypanosomal drugs on metabolism.

Metabolomics – New Technologies Applied to Trypanosomes

The relative homogeneity of the chemical building blocks of nucleic acids and proteins, respectively, has enabled rapid development of generic techniques to enable the analysis of these biological constituents making genomics, transcriptomics, and proteomics relatively mature technologies. Metabolomics, the measurement of the low-molecular-weight constituents of biosystems, has been hampered by the chemical diversity and broad concentration range of different metabolites. No individual analytical platform is capable of measuring all metabolites simultaneously. However, variations on the nuclear magnetic resonance (NMR) and mass spectrometry (MS) themes have, in recent years, allowed increasing coverage of the metabolome [7–12], and these techniques are now being applied with increasing intensity to the study of trypanosomes and also drug action.

Sample Preparation

Sample preparation is critical in metabolomics. Levels of many metabolites can change profoundly in response to external stimuli (including dramatic perturbations involved in harvesting cells for metabolite extraction). Various controls to report on deviations not related to the specific biological question addressed by an experiment are vital. Rapid quenching [13] to capture the metabolome as close to its physiological state as possible is desirable. In some microbes, including yeast, tough cell walls make them extremely robust and cells in suspension can be applied directly to solvents such as methanol at temperatures as low as $-80\,°C$. Metabolism ceases instantaneously and the cells can be washed free of medium prior to metabolite extraction [14]. Unfortunately, trypanosomes lyse under such conditions. Another way to rapidly stop metabolism and separate trypanosomes from their medium has been to use a rapid filtration method followed by hypotonic lysis and extraction in aqueous solvent [15]. Although suitable for *T. brucei* procyclic forms, the method causes on-filter lysis of bloodstream forms. Metabolites can be collected by application of trypanosome suspensions directly to organic solvents including hot ethanol [16] and cold chloroform/methanol/water [17]. However, medium carries over many abundant metabolites that can swamp their intracellular counterparts. Moreover, high cell numbers are needed to provide detectable quantities of most metabolites (5×10^7 to 10^9 trypanosomes [17–19]). This "direct-squirt" method remains useful in obtaining rapid flux measurements in systems where heavy isotope precursors are followed and hence not subject to interference from extracellular metabolites (provided controls on medium at different time points are included). A rapid chilling method, where flasks of cells are cooled to 0 °C, without freezing, in a dry-ice ethanol bath before centrifugation for removal of medium was developed for analyzing polar metabolites in *Leishmania* [17–19] and is currently the method of choice in detecting changes in steady-state intracellular metabolite levels by liquid chromatography (LC)-MS in trypanosomes [20]. Metabolite extraction from quenched cell pellets is generally achieved by addition of organic solvents, such as 80% ethanol or chloroform/methanol/water (1 : 3 : 1) followed by vigorous mixing and centrifugation to remove insoluble material. Rapid enzyme inactivation and cellular disruption may be improved by using higher temperatures (80 °C) [16]. However, generally extractions should be performed below 4 °C to minimize the degradation of metabolites [19]. Samples should be stored, preferably under argon to minimize oxidation, at −80 °C prior to analysis, or may be dried by evaporation and reconstituted prior to analysis with solvents appropriate for the analytical platform (MS or NMR).

NMR-Based Metabolomics

NMR has been used for broad untargeted metabolite profiling for many years, and its reproducibility, simple sample preparation, and ability to provide absolute quantification offer some advantages [21,22]. The spin properties of atomic nuclei are detected by NMR, and in metabolite analysis ^1H, ^{13}C, and ^{31}P signals can be used to report on the structure and abundance of metabolites. NMR is capable of detecting only the most abundant metabolites in a given sample, which limits the approach, although it has been used successfully in unraveling the metabolic pathways operative in procyclic trypanosomes [23–28], and in detecting metabolic changes in blood and urine of trypanosome infected mice [29,30].

NMR studies on glucose metabolism in bloodstream trypanosomes under anaerobic conditions [31,32] showed that glycerol and pyruvate were major end-products of glycolysis. However, significant amounts of alanine were also detected. Alanine is produced from pyruvate using alanine aminotransferase, which has subsequently been shown to be essential to bloodstream-form as well as procyclic trypanosomes [33], possibly contributing to pyruvate removal if its efflux rate cannot match production [34]. ^{31}P-NMR was also used to quantify the main phosphorylated metabolites in various trypanosomatids including *T. brucei* [35]. Bringaud's systematic application of NMR to characterize secreted metabolites from procyclic trypanosomes, modified using the reverse genetic approaches, has identified roles for numerous genes [23–28]. MS-based approaches have now also been applied to determine steady state levels of metabolites in various procyclic mutants [15]. ^{13}C-NMR was also used effectively to analyze an aconitase mutant cell line, revealing that most succinate in trypanosomes is not generated within the tricarboxylic acid (TCA) cycle [36]. Proline metabolism by procyclic *T. brucei* was also probed [15,37] and shifts in metabolism noted depending on whether parasites were grown on glucose or proline as their main carbon source. [^{13}C]proline is converted into succinate if glucose is present in medium but to alanine if glucose is absent [15].

^{1}H-NMR applied to *T. brucei* infection in mouse urine and plasma [29] showed progressive changes to the plasma metabolome from day 1 postinfection whilst urine was clearly distinguishable in infected mice from day 7. Elevated lactate was detected in both plasma and urine of infected animals. Urine also showed increases in the branched chain amino acid metabolites 3-methyl-2-oxovalerate and 2-oxoisovalerate, and D-3-hydroxybutyrate while the branched chain amino acids leucine, isoleucine and valine themselves were diminished in plasma. Diminished quantities of hippurate were also reported in urine along with increases in trimethylamine and 4-hydroxyphenylacetic acid. In mixed infections [30] some strain-specific changes were apparent in highly parasitized rodents. The very low parasitemias that accompany *T. b. gambiense* infection in man mean that careful studies should be performed to determine whether metabolic biomarkers can also be found that diagnose human disease.

MS-Based Metabolomics

MS approaches are generally of greater sensitivity than NMR [38]. Chromatographic separation methods (including gas chromatography (GC)), high-performance liquid chromatography (HPLC), ultra-performance liquid chromatography (UPLC), or capillary electrophoresis (CE) improve the technique as they separate metabolites prior to entry into the MS. Chromatography decreases problems with ion suppression (where highly ionizable chemical species can outcompete others in acquiring a charge during the ionization process), can distinguish multiple isomeric metabolites, and also provides key information on metabolite structure from the chromatographic behavior. GC-electron impact ionization (EI)-MS and LC-electrospray ionization (ESI)-MS are the most commonly used approaches in contemporary metabolomics research [38] and both approaches have been applied to the study of *T. brucei*.

GC-MS-Based Metabolomics
GC-MS is the best method to study inherently volatile metabolites and can also detect other compounds made volatile by chemical derivatization. Capillary GC can reproducibly separate hundreds of metabolites in complex biological mixtures by

phase partitioning between a carrier gas phase and the liquid phase on the inner surface of the column. Eluted metabolites are then ionized (usually by EI) and detected using a quadrupole mass spectrometer [38]. Chemical ionization (CI) can also be used as a "softer" alternative to EI and (quadrupole) time-of-flight (TOF) or high-resolution Fourier transform ion cyclotron resonance (FT-ICR) mass spectrometers have improved identification. GC-MS has been popular in metabolomics due to its capacity to detect many intermediates in central carbon metabolism (e.g., organic acids, sugar phosphates, lipids, and amino acids), and highly reproducible GC retention time and EI-generated mass spectra. Complex sample processing protocols, including the need for derivatization, and a failure to detect many polar metabolites, however, are limitations to its use. GC-MS is currently being applied to great effect in pioneering metabolomics analysis in *Leishmania* parasites [17,18,39]. In *T. brucei* GC-MS was used to identify changes to hosts (rodents) infected with trypanosomes. *T. b. gambiense* was shown to metabolize tryptophan, tyrosine, and phenylalanine to indole 3-pyruvic acid, 4-hydroxphenylpyruvic acid, and phenylpyruvic acid, respectively [40–42], and *T. brucei gambiense*-infected rodents also secreted abnormal quantities of catabolites of these aromatic amino acids [43–46].

GC-MS was also used to show that host-derived cholesterol is the predominant sterol (96% of the total sterol content) in bloodstream forms while procyclic forms have other sterols such as ergosta-5,7,25(27)-trienol [47] as a major proportion of the total sterol content. It is likely that GC-MS will be used increasingly in the analysis of *T. brucei* as metabolomic technologies become more accessible and more groups exploit their capabilities.

LC-MS-Based Metabolomics

LC separates chemicals based primarily on their lipophilicity and/or charge. Reversed-phase LC combined with MS is particularly suited to lipophilic metabolites. However, polar or charged metabolites are generally not retained on reversed-phase columns, making this approach unsuitable for separation of many polar cellular metabolites. Hydrophilic interaction chromatography (HILIC) is now preferentially used in many LC-MS-based metabolomics analyses [48,49]. ESI in positive mode (usually adding protons to metabolites) or negative mode (removing protons) in the ionization source is the most common way to generate ions. Ideally samples should be analyzed in both modes to detect as many metabolites as possible [49]. The Exactive Orbitrap (Thermo) in "switching mode" alternates between positive and negative mode thus yielding data in both modes from a single sample injection [49]. A confounding problem in LC-MS arises from the variable effect of ion suppression by coeluting metabolites, salts, or other chemicals in the ionization source, which is highly dependent on the matrix under study. It is possible to provide quantification, however, by spiking of samples with internal standards that can be obtained from, for example, *Escherichia coli* extracts in which all metabolites are labeled with ^{13}C. Metabolites of interest can then be compared to the heavy isotope spike whose quantity in the *E. coli* extract can be calculated by titration against authentic, pure standards [50].

Ultra-high mass accuracy MS has revolutionized metabolomics. TOF detectors offer high mass accuracy and have been successfully deployed in metabolomic studies, but FT-ICR and Orbitrap mass spectrometers offer the best results in terms of mass accuracy (below 1 ppm) and resolution (above 100 000) allowing assignment of a putative molecular formula to each observed mass for many metabolites of interest [7].

Triple-quadrupole mass spectrometers have also found great utility in LC-MS approaches where the multiple reaction monitoring (MRM) approaches involve fragmentation of selected analytes, allowing identification of metabolite-specific fragments. The MRM approach is highly sensitive, but limited by the fact that it can only identify metabolites for which fragmentation patterns have been predetermined and thus cannot be used for untargeted metabolomics. Nevertheless, some detailed analyses of metabolism in *T. brucei* procyclic forms have shown its utility [15,51].

Targeted LC-MS approaches have been used successfully to track sugar nucleotide incorporation into glycoconjugates in trypanosomatids [52]. In a first untargeted LC-MS study, FT-ICR-MS was used to probe the metabolome of bloodstream forms of *T. brucei* [53]. Although the number of metabolites identified was not great, this study also introduced a method where metabolites identified on accurate mass can be linked to others based on the exact mass of known metabolic transformations, allowing the development of *ab initio* metabolic networks. This type of approach may prove useful in pharmacological metabolomics to facilitate the discovery of novel drug metabolites or adducts. ZIC®-HILIC chromatography, coupled to Orbitrap MS, has become a powerful way to obtain data from trypanosome samples [49]. The first untargeted metabolomic analysis of procyclic forms of *T. brucei* focused on parasites grown in either glucose- or proline-rich medium [16]. Significant changes were found in several metabolites including the precursor substrates and key metabolites of central carbon metabolism and proline catabolism consistent with those predicted using NMR analysis of end-products in various mutants [23–28].

Considerable advances have also been made in the lipidomic analysis of *T. brucei* using LC-MS approaches (reviewed in [54–56]). Phosphatidylethanolamine and phosphatidylcholine glycerolipids are abundant, while phosphatidylinositol, phosphatidylserine, and cardiolipin are relatively minor species. Ether-linked lipids are found relatively abundantly in both forms and sphingolipids are abundant too. Major changes to lipid metabolism appear to correlate to a number of major events in *T. brucei*, including differentiation and drug assault [54–56].

Data Analysis

Hundreds, or even thousands, of metabolites can now be identified simultaneously. However, the analytical runs that identify these metabolites are also polluted by tens of thousands of peaks that do not represent true metabolites (including contaminating species from solvents, buffers, plasticware, tubing within machines, and also a multitude of fragments, adducts, multicharged species, isotopomers, and clusters derived from all chemicals within the samples). It is crucial to distinguish true metabolites from the artifacts. In GC-MS, many common metabolites can be identified based on relatively comprehensive databases that offer specific information on retention time and EI fragmentation patterns (http://www.sisweb.com/software/ms/nist.htm). Assigning metabolite identifications from LC-MS analyses based on exact mass alone, however, often results in false-positive identifications [57]. For *T. brucei*, the Scottish Metabolomics Facility has focused largely on exact mass data from an Orbitrap mass spectrometer. A variety of filters using mzMatch [58] select and annotate the most reproducible peaks representing metabolites. Prefiltered datasets are then further filtered and represented using the Ideom software package – a Microsoft Excel-based application that allows for advanced data analysis in a user-friendly interface [59]. Caution is still needed in interpreting data and ideally any metabolites that emerge as biologically significant in a given experiment should be verified with authentic standards, using comparative chromatography and tandem MS (MS/MS or MS^n), although mass and retention times of common metabolite standards and prior knowledge of the presence (or not) of a metabolites in trypanosomes can offer reliable identification of some metabolites [60].

The *T. brucei* genome [61] (and comparisons to the other TriTryps genomes, e.g., *Leishmania major* and *T. cruzi*) has enabled generation of a predicted metabolome at the Kyoto Encyclopedia of Genes and Genomes (KEGG) [62]. The MetaCyc family of databases [63] offers an alternative community-based representation of genome-predicted metabolomes. A clearly annotated version of the *Leishmania* metabolome has been assembled under LeishCyc [64] (http://leishcyc.bio21.unimelb.edu.au/). Automated reconstruction of the *T. brucei* metabolome (TrypanoCyc) has also been constructed [65], and is currently being improved with links to the TriTryp genome projects at the GeneDB [66] and TritrypDB [67] databases. Pathos (http://motif.gla.ac.uk/Pathos/index.html) [68] is an interactive web application that allows direct representation of identified metabolites and their relative abundance in the KEGG environment. MetExplore [69] (http://metexplore.toulouse.inra.fr/metexplore/index.php) has also been used extensively to analyze trypanosome metabolomics datasets in network-based representations that allows gap filling between detected metabolites in related metabolic pathways [70].

Stoichiometry-based models of metabolism have been built for many organisms, including *T. cruzi* [71] and *L. major* [72]. A model of *T. brucei* metabolism is currently being built. Such stoichiometric models have been helpful in identifying choke points; reactions that are the single route to production or consumption of key metabolites in the network that often represent potentially good drug targets, if choke point enzymes are druggable according to pharmacological criteria [73].

One of the most advanced fine-grained, dynamic models of metabolism, based on a series of ordinary differential equations reporting kinetic parameters of enzymes, has been produced for glycolysis in the bloodstream-form African trypanosome [74–76], which occurs within the glycosome, a membrane bound organelle, related to peroxisomes [77,78]. The pentose phosphate pathway has recently been added to the glycolytic model [79] and NADPH offers the potential to link glycolysis to the main redox active pathway in trypanosomes via the N^1,N^8-bis(glutathionyl) spermidine adduct, termed trypanothione. Measurements of protein and RNA abundance, as achieved for phosphoglycerate kinase [80], are also being put together with an ultimate aim of a full mathematical description of trypanosome metabolism or "the silicon trypanosome" [81,82].

Metabolic Affects of Trypanocidal Drugs

An area of natural interest is metabolomic analysis of modes of action of trypanocidal drugs. Current drugs for HAT all suffer drawbacks, including toxicity, parenteral administration, and restricted efficacy [2]. For *T. b. gambiense*, pentamidine is used for stage 1 disease while eflornithine or a nifurtimox–eflornithine combination therapy (NECT) is used preferentially for stage 2. For *T. b. rhodesiense*, suramin is preferred for stage 1 and melarsoprol is the only option for stage 2 disease [1,2]. Modes of action have not been ascertained for most drugs, although eflornithine acts as an inhibitor of polyamine biosynthesis through its inactivation of the enzyme ornithine decarboxylase.

Pentamidine

Pentamidine has been used for over 60 years to treat stage 1 *T. b. gambiense* disease [1,2]. *In vitro* trypanocidal potency (IC$_{50}$) is of the order of 1–10 nM in a typical 3-day drug sensitivity assay [83]. Pentamidine is concentrated to high (millimolar) levels by trypanosomes using the P2 amino-purine permease and other transporters that include a high-affinity pentamidine transporter (HAPT1) and a low-affinity pentamidine transporter (LAPT1) [84]. How it actually kills trypanosomes is not certain [85,86], although diamidines bind to DNA and mitochondrial dysfunction has been associated with diamidine treatment. Pentamidine binds avidly to DNA and accumulates within the mitochondrion, leading to a disintegration of the kinetoplast. However, *Trypanosoma evansi* strains that are lacking a kinetoplast are only a few fold less sensitive to diamidines than kinetoplast containing *T. brucei*, indicating other modes of action [87].

Electrostatic interactions also mediate dicationic pentamidine binding to numerous enzymes. In one study, mice infected with trypanosomes were treated with pentamidine and the parasites then analyzed using a targeted metabolite profiling approach. The basic amino acids lysine and arginine were increased in concentration by 13- and 2.5-fold, respectively [88]. Pentamidine has been speculated to interfere with polyamine function in cells and the drug is a potent inhibitor of *S*-adenosylmethionine decarboxylase (SAMDC) when assayed in a purified form [89]. However, trypanosomes purified from pentamidine-treated mice showed no perturbations in polyamine abundance. Moreover, gene knockouts of SAMDC in *Leishmania* yielded no change in sensitivity to pentamidine [90]. Studies in the related protist *Crithidia fasiculata* revealed inhibition of nucleic acid, protein, and phospholipid synthesis, suggesting that numerous biosynthetic enzymes are implicated in pentamidine action [91]. Untargeted metabolomic analysis will enable direct testing of the various proposals already made on metabolic actions for pentamidine and also reveal if unexpected changes to metabolism might accompany treatment with the drug.

The advent of other postgenomic technologies in addition to metabolomics is also reporting on modes of action and mechanisms of resistance to drugs. Exploitation of the RNA interference (RNAi) pathway operative in *T. brucei* [92], for example, has enabled a comprehensive search for all genes whose loss of function can lead to diminished drug sensitivity and this, in turn, can point to modes of action [93–95]. Transformation of trypanosomes with a library of DNA fragments permitting inducible downregulation of genes by RNAi, followed by selection in drugs, allowed identification of multiple genes whose loss of function can cause resistance. This so-called RITSeq approach [95], applied to selection with pentamidine, has yielded several key observations. It has long been known that loss of the P2 adenosine transporter contributes to pentamidine resistance. The RITSeq screen also yielded an aquaglyceroporin (AQP2) [95] that might represent one of the other transporters involved in uptake whose loss relates to resistance [84] (or else regulate that second transporter). A proton ATPase was also identified, although genes encoding specific metabolic enzymes were not apparent, which might relate to the drug's activity associating principally with disruption to nucleic acid metabolism.

Suramin

Suramin is a large (molecular weight 1297) polysulfonated naphthalene derivative that was originally derived from a group of trypanocidal dyes including Trypan blue in 1916. It is administered through five slow intravenous injections of 20 mg/kg every 3–7 days for 28 days [2]. Side-effects include nausea, rashes, and circulatory problems. The *in vitro* inhibitory concentrations (50%) for suramin are in the low nanomolar range [2] and *in vivo* activity is enhanced by the long half-life (44–92 days). This large polyanionic molecule is highly plasma protein bound (99.7%) and cannot cross the blood–brain barrier (BBB), and so is ineffective for stage 2 CNS disease, although it does increase the concentration of eflornithine entering the CNS in mice [96]. Suramin was proposed to enter trypanosomes by endocytosis [97]. Low-density lipoprotein was proposed as a possible carrier [98], although this was shown not to be the case [99]. The RITSeq approach has indicated that ISG75 is the ligand that binds suramin [95]. Those experiments revealed several components of the endocytic vesicular cascade as being lost in selection of drug resistance [95]. Interestingly, downregulation of several enzymes involved in polyamine biosynthesis and *N*-acetylglucosamine biosynthesis also yielded a positive impact on growth for *T. brucei* [95]. Polyamines have recently been shown to play a role in vesicular trafficking in mammalian cells [100] so such a role is also likely in trypanosomes and *N*-acetylglucosamine loss might also perturb endocytosis.

Even with the RITSeq breakthroughs, the mode of action of suramin remains unknown. Numerous theories have sought to explain how the drug exerts its effects.

Targeted analysis of glucose, oxygen, glycerol, and pyruvate levels suggested the trypanocidal activity resulted from inhibition of glycolysis, which could be explained by specific inhibition of numerous glycolytic enzymes in cell-free assays [101]. In *Onchocerca* spp., an inhibition of dihydrofolate reductase (DHFR) (the inhibition was 35 times more efficient on the parasite enzyme than on the mammalian enzyme) was noted [102,103]. Folate metabolism in trypanosomes has been subject to a relatively elegant targeted metabolite profiling study [104], but no evidence of suramin impact is apparent. Inhibition of thymidine kinase has also been reported, suggesting disruption of nucleotide synthesis underlies the mode of suramin action [105], but proven modes of action remain unknown.

Melarsoprol

Melarsoprol, a melaminophenyl-based organic arsenical, is extraordinarily toxic with many patients taking the drug suffering a reactive encephalopathy that frequently kills. A 3.6% solution in propylene glycol is administered, generally now over a 10-day course that superseded earlier long-term interrupted regimens. Melarsoprol converts rapidly to an active metabolite melarsen oxide *in vivo*, which shows a mean elimination half-life of 3.9 h [106]. Cyclodextrin-based formulations [107] enable oral uptake of melarsoprol in mice [108] and it is hoped that this could ameliorate some of the toxic effects associated with the drug.

Rapid uptake via the P2 (*Tb*AT1) aminopurine transporter and at least one other carrier (probably the HAPT1 transporter [109]) contributes to the selective activity of the drug and loss of transport relates to resistance [110]. The *Tb*AT1 and the aquaglyceroporin gene found in the pentamidine screen also emerged in the RITSeq melarsoprol screen [95]. Roles for several protein kinases and reduced expression of both trypanothione synthase and trypanothione reductase pointed to the previously identified melarsen oxide–trypanothione conjugate (MelT) [111] as contributing to toxicity to the parasites. This, however, is the opposite of the situation in *Leishmania* treated with the related heavy metal (antimony), where overexpression of enzymes (ornithine decarboxylase and γ-glutamylcysteine synthetase) [112] relates to resistance via production of excess trypanothione to bind the toxic heavy metal.

The mode of action of melarsoprol remains to be definitively elucidated. Dithiols are structurally important for many proteins and are also key residues in many enzyme active sites, which explains the large number of metabolic enzymes that are inhibited by melarsoprol and related arsenicals. Melarsoprol inhibition of several trypanosomal glycolytic enzymes has been demonstrated, including glycerol 3-phosphate dehydrogenase [113], 6-phosphogluconate dehydrogenase [114], pyruvate kinase [115], glucose 6-phosphate dehydrogenase, malic dehydrogenase, and hexokinase [116], although cell death precedes significant inhibition of glycolysis and ATP levels are not significantly decreased at the time of cell lysis [117]. The application of metabolomics to pharmacological evaluation will require great care to distinguish specific drug-induced metabolic changes from non-specific changes associated with cell death.

Trypanothione, an essential dithiol antioxidant molecule in trypanosomes, binds to melarsoprol and has been proposed as the molecular target [111]. Accumulation of the melarsen–trypanothione adduct (MelT) may be responsible for increasing the intracellular concentration of melarsen, but trypanothione levels are not significantly depleted by melarsoprol. Although trypanothione reductase is inhibited by melarsoprol (and by MelT) *in vitro*, parasites with altered expression of this enzyme did not show altered sensitivity to melarsen oxide [118]. One suggestion is that trypanothione sequestration of melarsoprol may be a protective mechanism [119] although the RITSeq data [95] was more consistent with MelT toxicity. Lipoic acid and lipoamide have been proposed as alternative targets, due to formation of drug-dithiol adducts that are 500-fold more stable than MelT [120].

Trivalent arsenicals have also been studied for their action against leukemia cell lines, demonstrating induction of apoptosis. Proteomic analysis of As_2O_3-treated cells revealed changes to levels of more than 50 proteins, including a number of enzymes [121]. Whilst the modes of action of melarsoprol and As_2O_3 are not identical, it is assumed that multiple biochemical changes will also be associated with melarsoprol action.

Eflornithine

Eflornithine (D,L-difluoromethyl ornithine (DFMO)) is an analog of the amino acid ornithine and inhibits the polyamine biosynthetic enzyme ornithine decarboxylase (ODC). The drug is active against the *T. b. gambiense* trypanosome subspecies, but less active against the related *T. b rhodesiense*. The usual treatment regimen involves intravenous infusions of 100 mg/kg body weight at 6-h intervals (i.e. 400 mg/kg/day) for 14 days. This intensive dosage schedule is necessary, because the compound is only weakly active against *T. brucei* bloodstream stages when compared to the other licensed drugs (IC_{50} values of 20–40 µM rather than the low nanomolar range) and *in vivo* activity depends upon an additional contribution from the host immune system [122].

Eflornithine's target in trypanosomes has been confirmed by HPLC-based analyses that show decreases in putrescine (the direct product of ODC) and other polyamines, spermidine and trypanothione, and increases in ornithine (the direct substrate of ODC) and adenosylmethionine levels after 48 h of treatment in rats [123,124]. The knockout of the gene could only be obtained *in vitro* if using putrescine-supplemented medium to bypass the lesion in the polyamine pathway [125]. An RNAi knockdown of ODC expression was also achieved, which mimicked the effects of eflornithine treatment and could be rescued with exogenous putrescine, but not spermidine [126]. In a first global metabolomics approach using the HILIC-Orbitrap approach to the determination of drug action, eflornithine was shown to induce the expected changes to ornithine and polyamine levels (and also revealed unexpected acetylated derivatives) as the most significant drug-induced perturbations [127]. A lack of off-target effects observed during sublethal drug exposure suggested that additional metabolic alterations only become apparent subsequent to the onset of membrane lysis and cell death.

The specificity of the drug against trypanosomes may relate to the enzyme target being far less rapidly turned over in trypanosomes than in mammalian cells, hence ODC inactivation leads to long-term loss of polyamine biosynthesis in *T. b. gambiense* trypanosomes while enzyme activity is continuously replenished in mammals. In bloodstream forms of the parasite, the drug enters the cell via a transporter-mediated process and recent evidence points to loss of a particular amino acid transporter, *Tb*AAT6, as underlying eflornithine resistance [93,94,128]. This transporter was shown to be lost during selection of resistance to eflornithine and sensitivity to eflornithine was restored when the gene was reintroduced to the resistant trypanosome's genome [128]. Interestingly the RITSeq approach identified *Tb*AAT6 as the only gene whose knockdown related to improved survival in eflornithine [95].

NECT

Recently it was recommended that eflornithine be given with nifurtimox in a combination therapy (NECT) [129] where eflornithine is given by intravenous infusion at 200 mg/kg every 12 h for 7 days (rather than 100 mg/kg every 6 h for 14 days as in monotherapy), in addition to 15 mg/kg nifurtimox orally every day for 10 days.

A rationale behind the combination was that eflornithine leads to depletion of spermidine, a key component of the trypanosome-specific redox active metabolite trypanothione (N^1,N^8-bis(glutathionyl)spermidine). Since nifurtimox was proposed to generate reactive oxygen species, a synergistic effect with eflornithine in redox-sensitive parasites could be inferred [130,131].

Curiously, eflornithine and nifurtimox are not synergistic in *in vitro* assays [127], possibly because nifurtimox's mode of action involves reduction by an unusual type I nitroreductase in *T. brucei* [132] followed by further metabolism to a highly reactive nitrile derivative [133], which may react with macromolecules by acting as a Michael acceptor [133]. In addition to the nitroreductase itself, the RITSeq approach yielded a flavokinase implicated in the synthesis of FMN, the cofactor of the nitroreductase enzyme [95]. Downregulation of proteins of the ubiquinol biosynthetic pathway also yielded improved viability in nifurtimox, pointing to a physiological role for the nitroreductase in the ubiquinol reduction pathway. The recent untargeted metabolomic analyses provide evidence for this theory with increases in nucleotides and nucleobases suggestive of DNA and RNA breakdown after nifurtimox treatment *in vitro* [127]. Of note too is that metabolomic changes with eflornithine and nifurtimox are additive rather than synergistic.

Conclusion

The biochemical investigation of drug mechanisms has long interested parasitologists, and previous studies have supported numerous hypotheses regarding the mechanisms responsible for the trypanocidal activity of existing drugs. Recent advances in metabolomics technology provide a new tool to investigate the metabolic impact of each drug from an untargeted (hypothesis-free) perspective, and a recent proof-of-concept study has revealed the mode of action of eflornithine and confirmed a metabolic activation of nifurtimox [127]. Knowledge of the mechanisms of existing drugs will support optimal utilization of these drugs by consideration of potential resistance mechanisms, drug interactions, adverse effects, and contraindications. Perhaps more importantly, elucidation of the mode of action of existing drugs will allow rational design of new compounds that retain optimal trypanocidal activity, but overcome the existing drawbacks with respect to pharmacokinetics and toxicity (an approach recently demonstrated for peroxide antimalarials based on the action of artemisinin [134]).

The potential role of metabolomics in pharmacology extends beyond the investigations of drug mechanisms described here, including biomarker discovery, which has enormous potential for diagnostic applications and monitoring of treatment response. Metabolomics may also provide improved methods for detection of drug toxicity and understanding of the mechanisms responsible for host toxicity and adverse effects.

Acknowledgments

M.P.B. thanks the Biotechnology and Biological Sciences Research Council (BBSRC) for funding the Systryp project as part of the BBSRC-ANR Systems Biology initiative and the *"insilico tryp"* project as part of the SysMO initiative. D.C. is an Australian National Health and Medical Research Council Training Fellow. I.V. was funded by the BBSRC and Pfizer as a Case student.

References

1 Brun, R., Blum, J., Chappuis, F., and Burri, C. (2010) Human African trypanosomiasis. *Lancet*, **375**, 148–159.

2 Barrett, M.P., Boykin, D.W., Brun, R., and Tidwell, R.R. (2007) Human African trypanosomiasis: pharmacological re-engagement with a neglected disease. *Br. J. Pharmacol.*, **152**, 1155–1171.

3 Stockdale, C., Swiderski, M.R., Barry, J.D., and McCulloch, R. (2008) Antigenic variation in *Trypanosoma brucei*: joining the DOTs. *PLoS Biol.*, **6**, e185.

4 Simarro, P.P., Franco, J., Diarra, A., Postigo, J.A., and Jannin, J. (2012) Update on field use of the available drugs for the chemotherapy of human African trypanosomiasis. *Parasitology*, **6**, 1–5.

5 Steverding, D. (2008) The history of African trypanosomiasis. *Parasit. Vectors*, **12**, 3.

6 Burri, C. and Brun, R. (2003) Eflornithine for the treatment of human African trypanosomiasis. *Parasitol. Res.*, **90**, S49–52.

7 Breitling, R., Vitkup, D., and Barrett, M.P. (2008) New surveyor tools for charting microbial metabolic maps. *Nat. Rev. Microbiol.*, **6**, 156–161.

8 Weckwerth, W. (2010) Metabolomics: an integral technique in systems biology. *Bioanalysis*, **2**, 829–836.

9 van der Werf, M.J., Jellema, R.H., and Hankemeier, T. (2005) Microbial metabolomics: replacing trial-and-error by

the unbiased selection and ranking of targets. *J. Ind. Microbiol. Biotechnol.*, **32**, 234–252.

10 Dunn, W.B., Broadhurst, D.I., Atherton, H.J., Goodacre, R., and Griffin, J.L. (2010) Systems level studies of mammalian metabolomes: the roles of mass spectrometry and nuclear magnetic resonance spectroscopy. *Chem. Soc. Rev.*, **40**, 387–426.

11 Saito, N., Ohashi, Y., Soga, T., and Tomita, M. (2010) Unveiling cellular biochemical reactions via metabolomics-driven approaches. *Curr. Opin. Microbiol.*, **13**, 358–362.

12 Kafsack, B.F. and Llinas, M. (2010) Eating at the table of another: metabolomics of host–parasite interactions. *Cell Host Microbe*, **7**, 90–99.

13 van Gulik, W.M. (2010) Fast sampling for quantitative microbial metabolomics. *Curr. Opin. Biotechnol.*, **21**, 27–34.

14 de Koning, W. and van Dam, K. (1992) A method for the determination of changes of glycolytic metabolites in yeast on a subsecond time scale using extraction at neutral pH. *Anal. Biochem.*, **204**, 118–123.

15 Ebikeme, C., Hubert, J., Biran, M., Gouspillou, G., Morand, P., Plazolles, N., Guegan, F. *et al.* (2010) Ablation of succinate production from glucose metabolism in the procyclic trypanosomes induces metabolic switches to the glycerol 3-phosphate/dihydroxyacetone phosphate shuttle and to proline metabolism. *J. Biol. Chem.*, **285**, 32312–32324.

16 Kamleh, A., Barrett, M.P., Wildridge, D., Burchmore, R.J.S., Scheltema, R.A., and Watson, D.G. (2008) Metabolomic profiling using Orbitrap Fourier transform mass spectrometry with hydrophilic interaction chromatography: a method with wide applicability to analysis of biomolecules. *Rapid Commun. Mass Spectrom.*, **22**, 1912–1918.

17 Saunders, E.C., De Souza, D.P., Naderer, T., Sernee, M.F., Ralton, J.E., Doyle, M.A., Macrae, J.I. *et al.* (2010) Central carbon metabolism of *Leishmania* parasites. *Parasitology*, **137**, 1303–1313.

18 Saunders, E.C., Ng, W.W., Chamber, J.M., Ng, M., Naderer, T., Kroemer, J.O., Likic, V.A., and McConville, M.J. (2011)

Isotopomer profiling of *Leishmania mexicana* promastigotes reveals important roles for succinate fermentation and aspartate uptake in TCA cycle anaplerosis, glutamate synthesis and growth. *J. Biol. Chem.*, **286**, 27706–27717.

19 t'Kindt, R., Jankevics, A., Scheltema, R., Zheng, L., Watson, D., Dujardin, J.-C., Breitling, R. *et al.* (2010) Towards an unbiased metabolic profiling of protozoan parasites: optimisation of a *Leishmania* sampling protocol for HILIC-Orbitrap analysis. *Anal. Bioanal. Chem.*, **398**, 59–2069.

20 Creek, D.J., Anderson, J., McConville, M. J., and Barrett, M.P. (2012) Metabolomic analysis of trypanosomatid protozoa. *Mol. Biochem. Parasitol.*, **181**, 73–84.

21 Fan, T.W. and Lane, A.N. (2011) NMR-based stable isotope resolved metabolomics in systems biochemistry. *J. Biomol. NMR*, **49**, 267–280.

22 Beckonert, O., Keun, H.C., Ebbels, T.M. D., Bundy, J., Holmes, E., Lindon, J.C., and Nicholson, J.K. (2007) Metabolic profiling, metabolomic and metabonomic procedures for NMR spectroscopy of urine, plasma, serum and tissue extracts. *Nat. Protocols*, **2**, 2692–2703.

23 Coustou, V., Biran, M., Breton, M., Guegan, F., Riviere, L., Plazolles, N., Nolan, D. *et al.* (2008) Glucose-induced remodeling of intermediary and energy metabolism in procyclic *Trypanosoma brucei*. *J. Biol. Chem.*, **283**, 16342–16354.

24 Coustou, V., Besteiro, S., Biran, M., Diolez, P., Bouchaud, V., Voisin, P., Michels, P.A. *et al.* (2003) ATP generation in the *Trypanosoma brucei* procyclic form: cytosolic substrate level is essential, but not oxidative phosphorylation. *J. Biol. Chem.*, **278**, 49625–49635.

25 Coustou, V., Besteiro, S., Riviere, L., Biran, M., Biteau, N., Franconi, J.M., Boshart, M. *et al.* (2005) A mitochondrial NADH-dependent fumarate reductase involved in the production of succinate excreted by procyclic *Trypanosoma brucei*. *J. Biol. Chem.*, **280**, 16559–16570.

26 Coustou, V., Biran, M., Besteiro, S., Riviere, L., Baltz, T., Franconi, J.M., and Bringaud, F. (2006) Fumarate is an essential intermediary metabolite

produced by the procyclic *Trypanosoma brucei*. *J. Biol. Chem.*, **281**, 26832–26846.

27 Besteiro, S., Biran, M., Biteau, N., Coustou, V., Baltz, T., Canioni, P., and Bringaud, F. (2002) Succinate secreted by *Trypanosoma brucei* is produced by a novel and unique glycosomal enzyme, NADH-dependent fumarate reductase. *J. Biol. Chem.*, **277**, 38001–38012.

28 Riviere, L., Moreau, P., Allmann, S., Hahn, M., Biran, M., Plazolles, N., Franconi, J.M. *et al.* (2009) Acetate produced in the mitochondrion is the essential precursor for lipid biosynthesis in procyclic trypanosomes. *Proc. Natl. Acad. Sci. USA*, **106**, 12694–12699.

29 Wang, Y., Utzinger, J.R., Saric, J., Li, J.V., Burckhardt, J., Dirnhofer, S., Nicholson, J. K. *et al.* (2008) Global metabolic responses of mice to *Trypanosoma brucei brucei* infection. *Proc. Natl. Acad. Sci. USA*, **105**, 6127–6132.

30 Li, J.V., Saric, J., Wang, Y., Utzinger, J., Holmes, E., and Balmer, O. (2011) Metabonomic investigation of single and multiple strain *Trypanosoma brucei brucei* infections. *Am. J. Trop. Med. Hyg.*, **84**, 91–98.

31 Mackenzie, N.E., Hall, J.E., Flynn, I.W., and Scott, A.I. (1983) ^{13}C nuclear magnetic resonance studies of anaerobic glycolysis in *Trypanosoma brucei* spp. *Biosci. Rep.*, **3**, 141–151.

32 Mackenzie, N.E., Hall, J.E., Seed, J.R., and Scott, A.I. (1982) Carbon-13 nuclear-magnetic-resonance studies of glucose catabolism by *Trypanosoma brucei gambiense*. *Eur. J. Biochem.*, **121**, 657–661.

33 Spitznagel, D., Ebikeme, C., Biran, M., Nic a' Bhaird, N., Bringaud, F., Henehan, G.T., and Nolan, D.P. (2009) Alanine aminotransferase of *Trypanosoma brucei* – a key role in proline metabolism in procyclic life forms. *FEBS J.*, **276**, 7187–7199.

34 Achcar, F., Kerkhoven, E.J., Bakker, B.M., Barrett, M.P., and Breitling, R. (2012) Dynamic modelling under uncertainty: the case of *Trypanosoma brucei* energy metabolism. *PLoS Comput. Biol.*, **8**, e1002352.

35 Moreno, B., Urbina, J.A., Oldfield, E., Bailey, B.N., Rodrigues, C.O., and Docampo, R. (2000) ^{31}P NMR spectroscopy of *Trypanosoma brucei*, *Trypanosoma cruzi*, and *Leishmania major*. Evidence for high levels of condensed inorganic phosphates. *J. Biol. Chem.*, **275**, 28356–28362.

36 van Weelden, S.W., Fast, B., Vogt, A., van der Meer, P., Saas, J., van Hellemond, J.J., Tielens, A.G. *et al.* (2003) Procyclic *Trypanosoma brucei* do not use Krebs cycle activity for energy generation. *J. Biol. Chem.*, **278**, 12854–12863.

37 Lamour, N., Riviere, L., Coustou, V., Coombs, G.H., Barrett, M.P., and Bringaud, F. (2005) Proline metabolism in procyclic *Trypanosoma brucei* is down-regulated in the presence of glucose. *J. Biol. Chem.*, **280**, 11902–11910.

38 Lenz, E.M. and Wilson, I.D. (2006) Analytical strategies in metabonomics. *J. Proteome. Res.*, **6**, 443–458.

39 De Souza, D.P., Saunders, E.C., McConville, M.J., and Likic, V.A. (2006) Progressive peak clustering in GC-MS Metabolomic experiments applied to *Leishmania* parasites. *Bioinformatics*, **22**, 1391–1396.

40 Stibbs, H.H. and Seed, J.R. (1975) Further studies on the metabolism of tryptophan in *Trypanosoma brucei gambiense*: cofactors, inhibitors, and end-products. *Experientia*, **31**, 274–278.

41 Stibbs, H.H. and Seed, J.R. (1975) Metabolism of tyrosine and phenylalanine in *Trypanosoma brucei gambiense*. *Int. J. Biochem.*, **6**, 197–203.

42 Hall, J.E., Dahm, K.H., and Seed, J.R. (1981) Quantification of tryptophan catabolites from *Trypanosoma brucei gambiense in vitro*. *Comp. Biochem. Physiol. B*, **68**, 521–526.

43 Hall, J.E. and Seed, J.R. (1981) Quantitation of aromatic amino acid catabolites in urine of mice acutely infected with *Trypanosoma brucei gambiense*. *Comp. Biochem. Physiol. B*, **69**, 791–796.

44 Hall, J.E. and Seed, J.R. (1984) Increased urinary excretion of aromatic amino acid catabolites by Microtus montanus chronically infected with *Trypanosoma brucei gambiense*. *Comp. Biochem. Physiol. B*, **77**, 755–760.

45 Hall, J.E., Seed, J.R., and Sechelski, J.B. (1985) Multiple alpha-keto aciduria in *Microtus montanus* chronically infected with *Trypanosoma brucei gambiense. Comp. Biochem. Physiol. B*, **82**, 73–78.

46 Newport, G.R., Page, C.R., Ashman, P.U., Stibbs, H.H., and Seed, J.R. (1977) Alteration of free serum amino acids in voles infected with *Trypanosoma brucei gambiense. J. Parasitol.*, **63**, 15–24.

47 Zhou, W., Cross, G.A., and Nes, W.D. (2007) Cholesterol import fails to prevent catalyst-based inhibition of ergosterol synthesis and cell proliferation of *Trypanosoma brucei. J. Lipid. Res.*, **48**, 665–673.

48 Lu, W., Bennett, B.D., and Rabinowitz, J.D. (2008) Analytical strategies for LC-MS-based targeted metabolomics. *J. Chromatogr. B*, **871**, 236–242.

49 Watson, D.G. (2010) The potential of mass spectrometry for the global profiling of parasite metabolomes. *Parasitology*, **137**, 1409–1423.

50 Kiefer, P., Portais, J.C., and Vorholt, J.A. (2008) Quantitative metabolome analysis using liquid chromatography-high-resolution mass spectrometry. *Anal. Biochem.*, **382**, 94–100.

51 Stoffel, S.A., Alibu, V.P., Hubert, J., Ebikeme, C., Portais, J.C., Bringaud, F., Schweingruber, M.E. *et al.* (2011) Transketolase in *Trypanosoma brucei. Mol. Biochem. Parasitol.*, **179**, 1–7.

52 Turnock, D.C. and Ferguson, M.A. (2007) Sugar nucleotide pools of *Trypanosoma brucei, Trypanosoma cruzi*, and *Leishmania major. Eukaryot. Cell*, **6**, 1450–1463.

53 Breitling, R., Ritchie, S., Goodenowe, D., Stewart, M.L., and Barrett, M.P. (2006) *Ab initio* prediction of metabolic networks using Fourier transform mass spectrometry data. *Metabolomics*, **2**, 155–164.

54 Serricchio, M. and Bütikofer, P. (2011) *Trypanosoma brucei*: a model microorganism to study eukaryotic phospholipid biosynthesis. *FEBS J.*, **278**, 1035–1046.

55 Smith, T.K. and Bütikofer, P. (2010) Lipid metabolism in *Trypanosoma brucei. Mol. Biochem. Parasitol.*, **172**, 66–79.

56 Richmond, G.S., Gibellini, F., Young, S.A., Major, L., Denton, H., Lilley, A., and Smith, T.K. (2010) Lipidomic analysis of bloodstream and procyclic form *Trypanosoma brucei. Parasitology*, **137**, 1357–1392.

57 Scheltema, R., Decuypere, S., Dujardin, J., Watson, D., Jansen, R., and Breitling, R. (2009) Simple data-reduction method for high-resolution LCMS data in metabolomics. *Bioanalysis*, **1**, 1551–1557.

58 Scheltema, R.A., Jankevics, A., Jansen, R.C., Swertz, M.A., and Breitling, R. (2011) PeakML/mzMatch: a file format, Java library, R library, and tool-chain for mass spectrometry data analysis. *Anal. Chem.*, **83**, 2786–2793.

59 Creek, D.J., Jankevics, A., Burgess, K.E., Breitling, R., and Barrett, M.P. (2012) IDEOM: an Excel interface for analysis of LC-MS based metabolomics data. *Bioinformatics*, **28**, 1048–1049.

60 Creek, D.J., Jankevics, A., Breitling, R., Watson, D.G., Barrett, M.P., and Burgess, K.E. (2011) Toward global metabolomics analysis with hydrophilic interaction liquid chromatography-mass spectrometry: improved metabolite identification by retention time prediction. *Anal. Chem.*, **83**, 8703–8710.

61 Berriman, M., Ghedin, E., Hertz-Fowler, C., Blandin, G., Renauld, H., Bartholomeu, D.C., Lennard, N.J. *et al.* (2005) The genome of the African trypanosome *Trypanosoma brucei. Science*, **309**, 416–422.

62 Kanehisa, M., Goto, S., Furumichi, M., Tanabe, M., and Hirakawa, M. (2010) KEGG for representation and analysis of molecular networks involving diseases and drugs. *Nucleic Acids Res.*, **38**, D355–D360.

63 Caspi, R., Altman, T., Dale, J.M., Dreher, K., Fulcher, C.A., Gilham, F., Kaipa, P. *et al.* (2010) The MetaCyc database of metabolic pathways and enzymes and the BioCyc collection of pathway/genome databases. *Nucleic Acids Res.*, **38**, D473–D479.

64 Doyle, M.A., MacRae, J.I., De Souza, D.P., Saunders, E.C., McConville, M.J., and Likic, V.A. (2009) LeishCyc: a biochemical pathways database for *Leishmania major. BMC Syst. Biol.*, **3**, 57.

65 Chukualim, B., Peters, N., Fowler, C., and Berriman, M. (2008) TrypanoCyc – a

metabolic pathway database for
Trypanosoma brucei. BMC Bioinformatics,
9, P5.

66 Logan-Klumpler, F.J., De Silva, N.,
Boehme, U., Rogers, M.B., Velarde, G.,
McQuillan, J.A., Carver, T. *et al.* (2012)
GeneDB–an annotation database
for pathogens. *Nucleic Acids Res.*, **40**,
D98–108.

67 Aslett, M., Aurrecoechea, C., Berriman,
M., Brestelli, J., Brunk, B.P., Carrington,
M., Depledge, D.P. *et al.* (2010)
TriTrypDB: a functional genomic resource
for the Trypanosomatidae. *Nucleic Acids
Res.*, **38**, D457–D462.

68 Leader, D.P., Burgess, K., Creek, D., and
Barrett, M.P. (2011) Pathos: a web facility
that uses metabolic maps to display
experimental changes in metabolites
identified by mass spectrometry. *Rapid
Commun. Mass Spectrom.*, **25**,
3422–3426.

69 Cottret, L., Wildridge, D., Vinson, F.,
Barrett, M.P., Charles, H., Sagot, M.F.,
and Jourdan, F. (2010) MetExplore: a web
server to link metabolomic experiments
and genome-scale metabolic networks.
Nucleic Acids Res., **38** (Suppl.),
W132–W137.

70 Jourdan, F., Cottret, L., Huc, L.,
Wildridge, D., Scheltema, R., Hillenweck,
A., Barrett, M.P. *et al.* (2010) Use of
reconstituted metabolic networks to assist
in metabolomic data visualization and
mining. *Metabolomics*, **6**, 312–321.

71 Roberts, S.B., Robichaux, J.L., Chavali, A.
K., Manque, P.A., Lee, V., Lara, A.M.,
Papin, P.A. *et al.* (2009) Proteomic and
network analysis characterize stage-
specific metabolism in *Trypanosoma cruzi.*
BMC Syst. Biol., **3**, 52.

72 Chavali, A.K., Whittemore, J.D., Eddy, J.
A., Williams, K.T., and Papin, J.A. (2008)
Systems analysis of metabolism in the
pathogenic trypanosomatid *Leishmania
major. Mol. Syst. Biol.*, **4**, 177.

73 Magariños, M.P., Carmona, S.J.,
Crowther, G.J., Ralph, S.A., Roos, D.S.,
Shanmugam, D., Van Voorhis, W.C., and
Agüero, F. (2012) TDR Targets: a
chemogenomics resource for
neglected diseases. *Nucleic Acids Res.*, **40**,
D1118–D1127.

74 Bakker, B.M., Michels, P.A., Opperdoes,
F.R., and Westerhoff, H.V. (1997)
Glycolysis in bloodstream form
Trypanosoma brucei can be understood in
terms of the kinetics of the glycolytic
enzymes. *J. Biol. Chem.*, **272**, 3207–3215.

75 Bakker, B.M., Mensonides, F.I., Teusink,
B., van Hoek, P., Michels, P.A., and
Westerhoff, H.V. (2000)
Compartmentation protects
trypanosomes from the dangerous design
of glycolysis. *Proc. Natl. Acad. Sci. USA*,
97, 2087–2092.

76 Haanstra, J.R., van Tuijl, A., Kessler, P.,
Reijnders, W., Michels, P.A., Westerhoff,
H.V., Parsons, M. *et al.* (2008)
Compartmentation prevents a lethal
turbo-explosion of glycolysis in
trypanosomes. *Proc. Natl. Acad. Sci. USA*,
105, 17718–17723.

77 Opperdoes, F.R. and Borst, P. (1977)
Localization of nine glycolytic enzymes in
a microbody-like organelle in
Trypanosoma brucei: the glycosome. *FEBS
Lett.*, **80**, 360–364.

78 Michels, P.A., Bringaud, F., Herman, M.,
and Hannaert, V. (2006) Metabolic
functions of glycosomes in
trypanosomatids. *Biochim. Biophys. Acta*,
1763, 1463–1477.

79 Kerkhoven, E.J. (2012) Extending a
dynamic mathematical model of
metabolism in Trypanosoma brucei PhD
thesis University of Glasgow.

80 Haanstra, J.R., Stewart, M., Luu, V.D., van
Tuijl, A., Westerhoff, H.V., Clayton, C.,
and Bakker, B.M. (2008) Control and
regulation of gene expression:
quantitative analysis of the expression of
phosphoglycerate kinase in bloodstream
form *Trypanosoma brucei. J. Biol. Chem.*,
283, 2495–2507.

81 Haanstra, J.R., Kerkhoven, E.J., van Tuijl,
A., Blits, M., Wurst, M., van Nuland, R.,
Albert, M.A. *et al.* (2011) A domino effect
in drug action: from metabolic assault
towards parasite differentiation. *Mol.
Microbiol.*, **79**, 94–108.

82 Bakker, B.M., Krauth-Siegel, R.L., Clayton,
C., Matthews, K., Girolami, M.,
Westerhoff, H.V., Michels, P.A. *et al.*
(2010) The silicon trypanosome.
Parasitology, **137**, 1333–1341.

83 Räz, B., Iten, M., Grether-Bühler, Y., Kaminsky, R., and Brun, R. (1997) The Alamar Blue assay to determine drug sensitivity of African trypanosomes (*T. b. rhodesiense* and *T. b. gambiense*) *in vitro*. *Acta Trop.*, **68**, 139–147.

84 De Koning, H.P. (2001) Uptake of pentamidine in *Trypanosoma brucei brucei* is mediated by three distinct transporters: implications for cross-resistance with arsenicals. *Mol. Pharmacol.*, **59**, 586–592.

85 Werbovetz, K. (2006) Diamidines as antitrypanosomal, antileishmanial and antimalarial agents. *Curr. Opin. Investig. Drugs*, **7**, 147–157.

86 Paine, M.F., Wang, M.Z., Generaux, C.N., Boykin, D.W., Wilson, W.D., De Koning, H.P., Olson, C.A. *et al.* (2010) Diamidines for human African trypanosomiasis. *Curr. Opin. Investig. Drugs*, **11**, 876–883.

87 Gillingwater, K., Kumar, A., Ismail, M.A., Arafa, R.K., Stephens, C.E., Boykin, D.W., Tidwell, R.R., and Brun, R. (2010) *In vitro* activity and preliminary toxicity of various diamidine compounds against *Trypanosoma evansi*. *Vet. Parasitol.*, **169**, 264–272.

88 Berger, B.J., Carter, N.S., and Fairlamb, A. H. (1993) Polyamine and pentamidine metabolism in African trypanosomes. *Acta Trop.*, **54**, 215–224.

89 Bitonti, A.J., Dumont, J.A., and McCann, P.P. (1986) Characterization of *Trypanosoma brucei brucei* S-adenosyl-L-methionine decarboxylase and its inhibition by Berenil, pentamidine and methylglyoxal bis(guanylhydrazone). *Biochem. J.*, **237**, 685–689.

90 Roberts, S.C., Scott, J., Gasteier, J.E., Jiang, Y., Brooks, B., Jardim, A., Carter, N. S. *et al.* (2002) S-adenosylmethionine decarboxylase from *Leishmania donovani*. Molecular, genetic, and biochemical characterization of null mutants and overproducers. *J. Biol. Chem.*, **277**, 5902–5909.

91 Gutteridge, W.E., McCormack, J.J., and Jaffe, J.J. (1969) Presence and properties of dihydrofolate reductases within the genus *Crithidia*. *Biochim. Biophys. Acta*, **178**, 453–458.

92 Kolev, N.G., Tschudi, C., and Ullu, E. (2011) RNA interference in protozoan parasites: achievements and challenges. *Eukaryot. Cell*, **10**, 1156–1163.

93 Schumann-Burkard, G., Jutzi, P., and Roditi, I. (2011) Genome-wide RNAi screens in bloodstream form trypanosomes identify drug transporters. *Mol. Biochem. Parasitol.*, **175**, 91–94.

94 Baker, N., Alsford, S., and Horn, D. (2011) Genome-wide RNAi screens in African trypanosomes identify the nifurtimox activator NTR and the eflornithine transporter AAT6. *Mol. Biochem. Parasitol.*, **176**, 55–57.

95 Alsford, S., Eckert, S., Baker, N., Glover, L., Sanchez-Flores, A., Leung, K.F., Turner, D.J. *et al.* (2012) High-throughput decoding of antitrypanosomal drug efficacy and resistance. *Nature*, **482**, 232–236.

96 Sanderson, L., Dogruel, M., Rodgers, J., Bradley, B., and Thomas, S.A. (2008) The blood–brain barrier significantly limits eflornithine entry into *Trypanosoma brucei* infected mouse brain. *J. Neurochem.*, **107**, 1136–1146.

97 Fairlamb, A.H. and Bowman, I.B. (1980) Uptake of the trypanocidal drug suramin by bloodstream forms of *Trypanosoma brucei* and its effect on respiration and growth rate *in vivo*. *Mol. Biochem. Parasitol.*, **1**, 315–333.

98 Vansterkenburg, E.L., Coppens, I., Wilting, J., Bos, O.J., Fischer, M.J., Janssen, L.H., and Opperdoes, F.R. (1993) The uptake of the trypanocidal drug suramin in combination with low-density lipoproteins by *Trypanosoma brucei* and its possible mode of action. *Acta Trop.*, **54**, 237–250.

99 Pal, A., Hall, B.S., and Field, M.C. (2002) Evidence for a non-LDL-mediated entry route for the trypanocidal drug suramin in *Trypanosoma brucei*. *Mol. Biochem. Parasitol.*, **122**, 217–221.

100 Kanerva, K., Mäkitie, L.T., Bäck, N., and Andersson, L.C. (2010) Ornithine decarboxylase antizyme inhibitor 2 regulates intracellular vesicle trafficking. *Exp. Cell Res.*, **316**, 1896–1906.

101 Willson, M., Callens, M., Kuntz, D.A., Perié, J., and Opperdoes, F.R. (1993) Synthesis and activity of inhibitors highly specific for glycolytic enzymes from

T. brucei. Mol. Biochem. Parasitol., **59**, 201–210.

102 Awadzi, K., Hero, M., Opoku, N.O., Addy, E.T., Büttner, D.W., and Ginger, C.D. (1995) The chemotherapy of onchocerciasis XVIII. Aspects of treatment with suramin. *Trop. Med. Parasitol.*, **46**, 19–26.

103 Jaffe, J.J., McCormack, J.J., and Meymarian, E. (1972) Comparative properties of schistosomal and filarial dihydrofolate reductases. *Biochem. Pharmacol.*, **21**, 719–731.

104 Sienkiewicz, N., Jarosławski, S., Wyllie, S., and Fairlamb, A.H. (2008) Chemical and genetic validation of dihydrofolate reductase–thymidylate synthase as a drug target in African trypanosomes. *Mol. Microbiol.*, **69**, 520–533.

105 Chello, P.L. and Jaffe, J.J. (1972) Comparative properties of trypanosomal and mammalian thymidine kinases. *Comp. Biochem. Physiol. B*, **43**, 543–562.

106 Keiser, J., Ericsson, O., and Burri, C. (2000) Investigations of the metabolites of the trypanocidal drug melarsoprol. *Clin. Pharmacol. Ther.*, **67**, 478–488.

107 Gibaud, S., Gaia, A., and Astier, A. (2002) Slow-release melarsoprol microparticles. *Int. J. Pharm.*, **243**, 161–166.

108 Rodgers, J., Jones, A., Gibaud, S., Bradley, B., McCabe, C., Barrett, M.P., Gettinby, G., and Kennedy, P.G. (2011) Melarsoprol cyclodextrin inclusion complexes as promising oral candidates for the treatment of human African trypanosomiasis. *PLoS Negl. Trop. Dis.*, **5**, e1308.

109 Bridges, D.J., Gould, M.K., Nerima, B., Mäser, P., Burchmore, R.J., and de Koning, H.P. (2007) Loss of the high-affinity pentamidine transporter is responsible for high levels of cross-resistance between arsenical and diamidine drugs in African trypanosomes. *Mol. Pharmacol.*, **71**, 1098–1108.

110 Barrett, M.P., Vincent, I.M., Burchmore, R.J., Kazibwe, A.J., and Matovu, E. (2011) Drug resistance in human African trypanosomiasis. *Future Microbiol.*, **6**, 1037–1047.

111 Fairlamb, A.H., Henderson, G.B., and Cerami, A. (1989) Trypanothione is the primary target for arsenical drugs against African trypanosomes. *Proc. Natl. Acad. Sci. USA*, **86**, 2607–2611.

112 Mukhopadhyay, R., Dey, S., Xu, N., Gage, D., Lightbody, J., Ouellette, M., and Rosen, B.P. (1996) Trypanothione overproduction and resistance to antimonials and arsenicals in *Leishmania*. *Proc. Natl. Acad. Sci. USA*, **93**, 10383–10387.

113 Denise, H. and Barrett, M.P. (2001) Uptake and mode of action of drugs used against sleeping sickness. *Biochem. Pharmacol.*, **61**, 1–5.

114 Hanau, S., Rippa, M., Bertelli, M., Dallocchio, F., and Barrett, M.P. (1996) 6-Phosphogluconate dehydrogenase from *Trypanosoma brucei*. *Eur. J. Biochem.*, **240**, 592–599.

115 Flynn, I.W. and Bowman, I.B.R. (1974) The action of trypanocidal arsenical drugs on *Trypanosoma brucei* and *Trypanosoma rhodesiense*. *Comp. Biochem. Physiol. B*, **48**, 261–273.

116 Bacchi, C.J., Ciaccio, E.I., and Koren, L.E. (1969) Effects of some antitumor agents on growth and glycolytic enzymes of the flagellate crithidia. *J. Bacteriol.*, **98**, 23–28.

117 Van Schaftingen, E., Opperdoes, F.R., and Hers, H.G. (1987) Effects of various metabolic conditions and of the trivalent arsenical melarsen oxide on the intracellular levels of fructose 2,6-bisphosphate and of glycolytic intermediates in *Trypanosoma brucei*. *Eur. J. Biochem.*, **166**, 653–661.

118 Krieger, S., Schwarz, W., Ariyanayagam, M.R., Fairlamb, A.H., Krauth-Siegel, R.L., and Clayton, C. (2000) Trypanosomes lacking trypanothione reductase are avirulent and show increased sensitivity to oxidative stress. *Mol. Microbiol.*, **35**, 542–552.

119 Cunningham, M.L., Zvelebil, M.J., and Fairlamb, A.J. (1994) Mechanism of inhibition of trypanothione reductase and glutathione reductase by trivalent organic arsenicals. *Eur. J. Biochem.*, **221**, 285–295.

120 Fairlamb, A.H., Smith, K., and Hunter, K.J. (1992) The interaction of arsenical drugs with dihydrolipoamide and dihydrolipoamide dehydrogenase from arsenical resistant and sensitive strains of *Trypanosoma brucei brucei*. *Mol. Biochem. Parasitol.*, **53**, 223–231.

121 Xiong, L. and Wang., Y. (2010) Quantitative proteomic analysis reveals the perturbation of multiple cellular pathways in HL-60 cells induced by arsenite treatment. *J. Prot. Res.*, **9**, 1129–1137.

122 Bitonti, A.J., McCann, P.P., and Sjoerdsma, A. (1986) Necessity of antibody response in the treatment of African trypanosomiasis with alpha-difluoromethylornithine. *Biochem. Pharmacol.*, **35**, 331–334.

123 Fairlamb, A.H., Henderson, G.B., Bacchi, C.J., and Cerami, A. (1987) *In vivo* effects of difluoromethylornithine on trypanothione and polyamine levels in bloodstream forms of *Trypanosoma brucei*. *Mol. Biochem. Parasitol.*, **24**, 185–191.

124 Byers, T.L., Bush, T.L., McCann, P.P., and Bitonti, A.J. (1991) Antitrypanosomal effects of polyamine biosynthesis inhibitors correlate with increases in *Trypanosoma brucei brucei* S-adenosyl-L-methionine. *Biochem. J.*, **274**, 527–533.

125 Li, F., Hua, S.B., Wang, C.C., and Gottesdiener, K.M. (1998) *Trypanosoma brucei brucei*: characterization of an ODC null bloodstream form mutant and the action of alpha-difluoromethylornithine. *Exp. Parasitol.*, **88**, 255–257.

126 Xiao, Y., McCloskey, D.E., and Phillips, M.A. (2009) RNA interference-mediated silencing of ornithine decarboxylase and spermidine synthase genes in *Trypanosoma brucei* provides insight into regulation of polyamine biosynthesis. *Eukaryot. Cell*, **8**, 747–755.

127 Vincent, I.M., Creek, D.J., Burgess, K., Woods, D.J., Burchmore, R.J.S., and Barrett, M.P. (2012) Untargeted metabolomics reveals a lack of synergy between nifurtimox and eflornithine against *Trypanosoma brucei*. *PLoS Negl. Trop. Dis.*, **6**, e1618.

128 Vincent, I.M., Creek, D., Watson, D.G., Kamleh, M.A., Woods, D.J., Wong, P.E., Burchmore, R.J. *et al.* (2010) A molecular mechanism for eflornithine resistance in African trypanosomes. *PLoS Pathog.*, **6**, e1001204.

129 Priotto, G., Kasparian, S., Mutombo, W., Ngouama, D., Ghorashian, S., Arnold, U., and Ghabri, S. (2009) Nifurtimox–eflornithine combination therapy for second-stage African *Trypanosoma brucei gambiense* trypanosomiasis: a multicentre, randomized, phase III, non-inferiority trial. *Lancet*, **374**, 56–64.

130 Docampo, R., Moreno, S.N., Stoppani, A.O., Leon, W., Cruz, F.S., Villalta, F., and Muniz, R.F. (1981) Mechanism of nifurtimox toxicity in different forms of *Trypanosoma cruzi*. *Biochem. Pharmacol.*, **30**, 1947–1951.

131 Enanga, B., Ariyanayagam, M.R., Stewart, M.L., and Barrett, M.P. (2003) Activity of megazol, a trypanocidal nitroimidazole, is associated with DNA damage. *Antimicrob. Agents Chemother.*, **47**, 3368–3370.

132 Wilkinson, S.R., Taylor, M.C., Horn, D., Kelly, J.M., and Cheeseman, I. (2008) A mechanism for cross-resistance to nifurtimox and benznidazole in trypanosomes. *Proc. Natl. Acad. Sci. USA*, **105**, 5022–5027.

133 Hall, B.S., Bot, C., and Wilkinson, S.R. (2011) Nifurtimox activation by trypanosomal type I nitroreductases generates cytotoxic nitrile metabolites. *J. Biol. Chem.*, **286**, 13088–13095.

134 Charman, S.A., Arbe-Barnes, S., Bathurst, I.C., Brun, R., Campbell, M., Charman, W.N., Chiu, F.C. *et al.* (2011) Synthetic ozonide drug candidate OZ439 offers new hope for a single-dose cure of uncomplicated malaria. *Proc. Natl. Acad. Sci. USA*, **108**, 4400–4405.

4
Drug Design and Screening by *In Silico* Approaches

*Mattia Mori and Maurizio Botta**

Abstract
Hundreds of millions of people worldwide are affected by infectious diseases caused by Kinetoplastida parasites. Especially in non-industrialized countries, these diseases represent one of the most serious health problems. Since current drugs lack efficacy, specificity, and suffer from several side-effects, there is an urgent need for novel therapeutics. In modern drug discovery, more and more relevance is given to the use of computer-aided (or *in silico*) techniques. Especially in the early phases of projects, *in silico* tools based on the knowledge of the target receptor structure (structure-based) or on the chemical structure of active small molecules (ligand-based) are routinely used for discovering and optimizing hit or lead compounds of pharmaceutical interest. Here, *in silico* approaches for discovering anti-trypanosomal compounds are described and general remarks on computer-aided methods are provided.

Introduction

Chagas disease is one of the most serious parasitic health problems with a wide extension in Latin American countries up to the United States. Other devastating diseases such as leishmaniasis and African sleeping sickness are, like Chagas, due to infection by parasitic trypanosomatids of the Kinetoplastida order. Taken together, these diseases are one of the most severe causes of human morbidity, mortality, and livestock losses, especially in non-industrialized countries [1]. Rising levels of industrialization and migration are among the major causes of the diffusion of parasites, which are principally transmitted by congenital ways, by transfusion with infected blood, or by insect vectors, the latter being the most common way of transmission in endemic countries.

At present, leishmaniasis is treated with unspecific, although effective, drugs such as paromomycin and amphotericin B, whereas only two drugs are available for the therapy of Chagas disease: nifurtimox and benznidazole. These drugs suffer from

---

* Corresponding Author

Trypanosomatid Diseases: Molecular Routes to Drug Discovery, First edition. Edited by T. Jäger, O. Koch, and L. Flohé.
© 2013 Wiley-VCH Verlag GmbH & Co. KGaA. Published 2013 by Wiley-VCH Verlag GmbH & Co. KGaA.

limited efficacy in the chronic stages of the illness and toxic effects (e.g., vomiting, allergy, neuropathy, and cardiac and renal injury) that limit their widespread use. The therapeutic options in the treatment of African sleeping sickness are similarly unsatisfactory. Therefore, there is an urgent need of more effective and less toxic drugs or drug candidates for the therapy of the diseases caused by Kinetoplastida [2].

Several drug discovery projects have been started in the last two decades, aiming at the identification of anti-trypanosomal hit or lead compounds endowed with drug-like properties. In the early phases of common drug discovery, computer-aided techniques have often been used to discover and to optimize novel hit or lead compounds of pharmaceutical interest. These methods are briefly described below as well as their application for discovering small molecules with anti-kinetoplastida activity.

Computer-Aided Drug Design: General Remarks

One of the first reports describing the use of computers for studying atomic or molecular properties dates back to 1966 when Cyrus Levinthal modeled the behavior of some small proteins in three-dimensional (3-D) space [3]. Since then, incredible steps forward have been recorded in the technical performance of hardware components and in the development of software for predicting more and more specific molecular properties with great accuracy and reliability.

At present, molecular modeling is the term that better encompasses all the types of computer simulations of molecular systems having biological or pharmaceutical relevance. For the sake of clarity, a major distinction has to be made between molecular mechanics (MM) and quantum mechanics (QM) methods. Basically, MM is based on the approximation that considers atoms as solid spheres, each characterized by the Van der Waals radius, the atomic weight, and partial charge, while the bond between atoms is treated as a spring with an equilibrium distance taken from experiments or QM simulations and with a force constant that is proportional to the bond valence. Bond and dihedral angles are similarly approximated as systems of harmonic springs. Electrons are not explicitly accounted for in MM, and atomic and molecular motions follow the laws of classic physics. MM methods are mostly used for exploring the conformational and the energetic space of large molecular systems. In contrast, in QM approaches electrons are treated explicitly and molecular properties are calculated *ab initio* starting only from the initial coordinates of the molecular system. In general, QM calculations are slower than MM, and are used for studying electronic properties of molecular systems with restricted dimensions (up to tens of atoms) and for studying reaction pathways involving electron transfer between atomic species in catalyzed or other chemical reactions.

These *in silico* tools have being widely applied to multiple fields of current research, as highlighted by the increasing numbers papers reporting on the use of computer-aided methodologies for ligand design or for predicting the behavior of biological systems. In this respect, it is interesting to note that a parallelism exists between technical progress and the increasing number of literature reports on the use of molecular modeling. This could have a dual cause. (i) Computer-aided methods are being considered as reliable tools for studying biomolecules, because theoretical results are often in very good agreement with experimental data. (ii) High-performance machines are available that render calculations computationally less expensive than a few years ago. Moreover, several user-friendly programs have been developed, thus allowing researchers with limited experience in the field to approach computer simulations.

Supercomputers and Other Technical Resources

An interesting point we want to address is the existence of many supercomputer centers around the world that provide large computational resources to researchers of both academia and industry. The world most potent supercomputer (as of December 2011) is the Japanese K computer with a performance of 8.16 petaflop/s, followed by the Chinese Tianhe-1 with a 2.57 petaflop/s performance, which is composed of 14 336 central processing units (CPUs) and 7168 graphic processing units (GPUs). Alternatively, a defined percentage of the CPU resources of several computers worldwide can be used by the so-named GRID computing technique to run calculations. Scientists can apply to these centers to obtain extensive CPU time for running simulations, while the computational setup and data analysis can be done by using the basic computer equipment that is commonly available in most laboratories. Last, but not least, one of the biggest technological improvements recorded in recent years is the use of GPUs for performing calculations. GPUs are significantly faster than classical CPUs, especially for running algorithms where processing is done in parallel. Most software for computer-aided drug design has been recently upgraded for using GPUs, providing therefore a significant reduction of the simulation time and allowing researchers to study very complex systems.

Molecular Modeling and Anti-Kinetoplastida Drug Design

Molecular modeling has been applied for discovering anti-trypanosomal hit compounds, some of which have been further optimized and tested *in vitro* and *in vivo*. When applying molecular modeling, one of two main situations is faced, depending on the availability of experimental data:

- The 3-D structure of the target receptor has not yet been solved or the target receptor itself is still unknown. Only some active compounds having a common mechanism of action or interacting with the selected target receptor have been described. In these cases, the drug design is generally done on the basis of the chemical structure of active ligands or starting from their pharmacophoric alignment. These approaches are referred to as "ligand-based."

- The 3-D structure of the target receptor has been solved by experimental methods (X-ray, nuclear magnetic resonance (NMR), electron microscopy) or the 3-D structure of a homologous protein is known. In this latter case, the structure of the target receptor can be predicted by homology modeling. Irrespective of the source of the 3-D protein structure, the drug design is carried out according to complementarity criteria between the shape and physicochemical properties of the receptor binding site and those of the small molecules. These approaches are referred to as "structure-" or "receptor-based".

The main features of these *in silico* approaches have been largely reviewed in papers and books [4–6]. Briefly, by using ligand-based methods the chemical diversity between query and results is generally poor, while it is rather easy to discover new active small molecules belonging to the same (or a similar) chemical scaffold as the reference compounds. On the other hand, structure-based approaches starting from the knowledge of the active site geometry and physico-chemical features are more suitable for identifying chemically diverse hit com-pounds by means of virtual screening. In projects aiming at the discovery and optimization of anti-kinetoplastida drug candidates, ligand-based approaches are mostly used to perform a retrospective analysis of active compounds, to identify possible structural or electronic descriptors that might correlate with biological activity, while structure-based methods have mostly been used to discover novel chemical entities with trypanocidal activity through the massive screening of large and diverse chemical libraries.

Ligand-based methods have been largely applied especially in early medicinal chemistry projects carried out before 2005, when the number of available 3-D structures of target proteins for Kinetoplastida in the Protein Data Bank (PDB) was relatively low (Figure 4.1). In parallel with the increased number of protein structures available in public repositories, a growing number of papers reporting

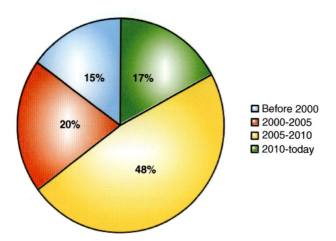

Figure 4.1 Statistics of X-ray *Trypanosoma*'s protein structures deposited on the PDB (updated in December 2011). Structures are equally divided between *T. cruzi* and *T. brucei*.

on structure-based works began appearing in the literature. In the subsequent sections we provide an overview of the use of *in silico* computational tools for discovering hit and/or lead compounds with anti-trypanosomal activity, on the basis of our own and others' experience.

Ligand-Based Approaches Against Trypanosoma Parasites

First, we want to recall the general concept that ligand-based approaches have been used in this field more frequently to perform a retrospective rationalization of biological data, rather than for performing virtual screening. Therefore, most of the results we are going to discuss in this section do not refer to a massive search of possibly active compounds in large chemical libraries or databases, but aim at understanding the nature of structural or chemical/physical determinants involved in anti-trypanosomal activity.

Although different ligand-based methods have been developed and validated, a significant contribution to anti-kinetoplastida research has been provided by the so-called TOMOCOMD approach (acronym for TOpological MOlecular COMputer Design), which is based on non-stochastic quadratic fingerprints. This method was presented in 2004 by Marrero-Ponce *et al.* [7] as a novel tool for molecular design. Since that time, the method has been successfully applied in several research projects aiming at discovering anti-helmintic, anti-trypanosomal, anti-malarial, and anti-bacterial compounds, as well as for studying nucleic acid–drug interaction. The first work describing the application of quadratic fingerprints for studying anti-trypanosomal compounds was published in 2005 by Montero-Torres [8], where the TOMOCOMD was used to develop quantitative structure–activity relationship (QSAR) or quantitative structure–property relationship (QSPR) models based on a training set of 153 bio-active compounds, 62 of which had anti-trypanosomal records and 91 had other clinical uses. Briefly, the linear discriminant analysis (LDA) was used to obtain a predictive model, which was able to correctly classify about 90% of the training set. To stress the applicability of such generated QSAR model for *in silico* anti-trypanosomal drug design, its predictive capability was assessed against a test set of 10 compounds not included in the training set. As predicted, five compounds were trypanocidal at 100 μg/ml, whereas **1** (Figure 4.2) showed more than 80% of epimastigote inhibition at 1 μg/ml. Even though none of the tested compounds was more active than the reference drug nifurtimox, this work has laid the foundations for the use of mathematical methods in classifying compounds active against the epimastigote forms of *Trypanosoma* cruzi. In a similar way, in 2006 the TOMOCOMD software was used to develop a linear classification function able to discriminate between anti-trypanosomal and inactive compounds, with a confidence of 95% [9], thus confirming the high potential of the method. Three compounds inhibited epimastigote and amastigote replication at 10 μg/ml. The hit endowed with the best compromise between anti-amastigote activity and unspecific toxicity, namely **2** (Figure 4.2), showed a suppressive activity of 60% on the peak of parasitemia *in vivo*, where the activity was normalized against that of

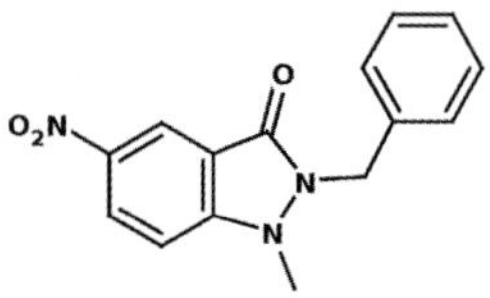

1, %AE = 82.8 at 1 µg/mL [8]

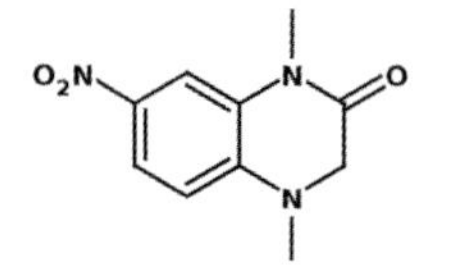

2, %AE = 72.7 at 100 µg/mL
%AA = 85.4 at 100 µg/mL [9]

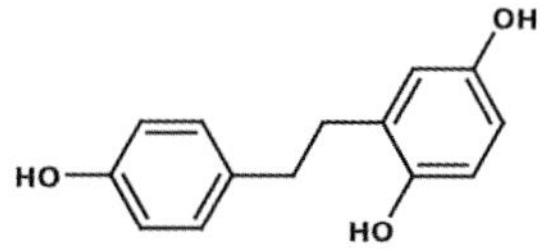

3, 14-hydroxylunularin
IC_{50} = 17.3 µM (AA)
IC_{50} = 5.8 µM (AE) [10]

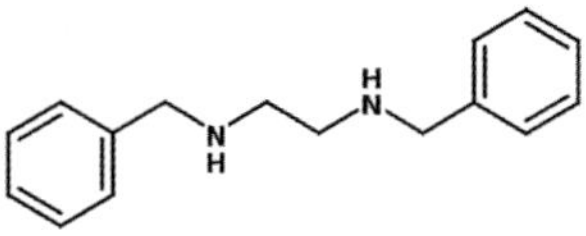

4, %AE = 78.2 at 10 µg/mL [11]

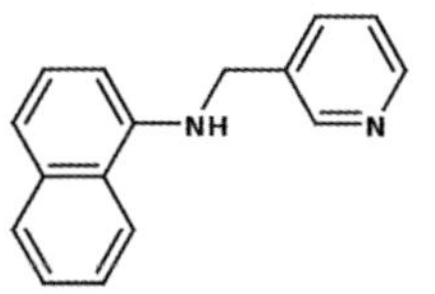

5, %AE = 81.3 at 10 µg/mL [11]

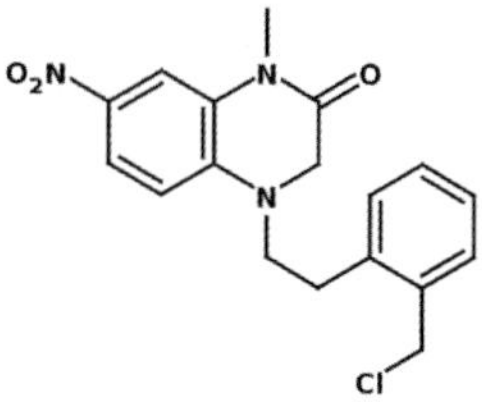

6, %AE = 65.5 at 1 µg/mL
%AA = 35.4 at 1 µg/mL [12]

Figure 4.2 Chemical structure and biological activity against *T. cruzi* of most active compounds discovered by using the *in silico* ligand-based TOMOCOMD approach. Biological activity data are expressed as the percentage of anti-epimastigote (%AE) or anti-amastigote (%AA) activity, or by the IC_{50} value.

nifurtimox. According to this initial work, the algorithm seems unable to select compounds with higher activity than the reference drug, while the classification between active and inactive works nicely. The TOMOCOMD software was also used in 2008 by Roldos *et al.* [10] to probe the activity of the natural compound 14-hydroxylunularin **3** (Figure 4.2) and some chemical derivatives, highlighting the strict correlation between *in silico* prediction and experimental structure–activity relationship (SAR) data. The reliability of this computational approach in antiparasitic drug design was further emphasized by a work published in 2010, where the QSAR model was built starting from a training set larger than those of previous reports; it comprised 440 small molecules, 143 having trypanocidal activity and 297 having different clinical use [11]. After internal and external validation, the predictive model was used to classify nine compounds with unknown activity. As predicted, compounds **4** and **5** (Figure 4.2) showed significant epimastigote inhibition at 10 µg/ml, but were less active than nifurtimox.

Finally, the issue of the lower activity of compounds classified by the TOMOCOMD with respect to nifurtimox was recently addressed by Castillo-Garit *et al.* [12], who reported on the use of *in silico* two-dimensional (2-D) bond-based linear indices and LDA for building a QSAR model capable of classifying very active trypanocidal compounds. The QSAR model was built starting from a large training set as in [11] and was used to filter a test set of 90 small molecules. Nine compounds, never described before as trypanocidal, were selected for *in vitro* studies. Five of them were active against the epimastigotes at 100 µg/ml. The best compromise between activity and unspecific cytotoxicity was represented by **6** (Figure 4.2), which belongs to the same scaffold as **2** [9]. Notably,

6 showed an epimastigote elimination activity comparable with that exerted by nifurtimox. As **6** is less toxic than nifurtimox, it could be considered as the most promising lead compound discovered *in silico* by using the TOMOCOMD software.

Apart from the TOMOCOMD software, different ligand-based approaches have been carried out, typically aiming at retrospective analyses of biological activity data rather than at virtual screening of large libraries or databases. However, *in silico* understanding of the chemical/physical determinants that correlate with bioactivity data is of key relevance for driving the rational optimization of active compounds.

One of the first research articles describing the use of *in silico* ligand-based methods in the anti-kinetoplastida field was published in 2005 by Molfetta *et al.* [13] who used QM methods at the density functional theory (DFT) level for calculating atomic and molecular properties of 25 trypanocidal quinones. SARs of quinones were investigated by calculating steric, electronic, hydrophobic, and topological descriptors, four of which were found in agreement with biological activity data. Two of them described electronic properties, namely the sum of partial charges and the energy of the highest occupied molecular orbital (HOMO), while the remaining descriptors accounted for structural features (i.e., the torsional angles and the steric hindrance of chemical substitutions). In summary, active quinones should have a particular geometry restrained by the torsion of atoms in the core region, while bulky as well as electron-poor substitutions might increase the overall trypanocidal activity. These findings were used to setup a drug design exercise, where three quinones not included in the training set were correctly classified by the predictive model. A similar approach was followed in 2008 by Gasteiger *et al.* [14], who performed QM calculations at the AM1 theory level for predicting atomic and molecular properties of a large training set, composed of 179 *N*-oxide-containing heterocycles belonging to four different scaffolds (benzimidazoles, benzofuraxans, indazoles, and benzopyrazines). This very precise and accurate computational study showed that an electrophilic center placed at 4.1–4.9 Å from the oxygen atom of the *N*-oxide moiety is crucial for anti-trypanosomal activity. Even if this feature did not correlate with all biological data available for the training set, it could be used in the rational optimization of *N*-oxide compounds. An interesting ligand-based virtual screening exercise was further published in 2006 by Prieto *et al.* for studying trypanothione reductase (TR) inhibitors [15]. Although several crystal structures of the TR were available at that time, the authors used a ligand-based method for discovering novel potential TR inhibitors. LDA was used to obtain a reliable QSAR model, starting from a training set of 58 molecules, 29 having TR inhibitory activity and 29 having other clinical uses. The predictive model was used to screen a library of more than 400 000 compounds. In total, 739 *in silico* hits were selected as promising anti-chagasic agents through TR inhibition but, to our knowledge, biological results have not yet been published. Nevertheless, this work represents a valuable example of ligand-based virtual screening.

To verify the hypothesis that the biochemical reduction of a nitro group is crucial for anti-trypanosomal activity, Paula *et al.* in 2009 applied an *in silico* ligand-based strategy to study the SAR of nifuroxazide analogs [16]. Ten trypanocidal nitroderivatives were analyzed through a validated QSAR model. Surprisingly, electronic descriptors proved not to be sufficient for explaining bioactivity data. In contrast, the lipophilicity index, which nicely correlated with biological activity data, was found as the most important descriptor in this series. A similar *in silico* strategy was also followed by Vera-Divaio *et al.* [17] for building a QSAR model based on a new series of anti-trypanosomal *N*-phenylpyrazole benzylidene-carbo-hydrazides. Also in this case electronic descriptors such as energy of HOMO or LUMO (lowest unoccupied molecular orbital) orbitals did not correlate properly with the activity trend observed *in vitro*, while structural descriptors such as the bulkiness of substituents in the *para* position to the benzylidene scaffold did. A very interesting computational work was recently published by Planche *et al.* [18] who used descriptors based on chemical fragments and topological substructural molecular design descriptors to obtain a QSAR model capable of classifying anti-trypanosomal agents only on the basis of their chemical structure. In fact, the quantitative contribution to the anti-trypanosomal activity due to chemical fragments contained in active compounds was calculated and implemented in the QSAR model. In this way, the trypanocidal activity of lead molecules could be improved by introducing some chemical fragments that are quantitatively associated with strong anti-trypanosomal activity. Alternatively, possibly active molecules could be *de novo* designed by combining several fragments with considerable positive contributions to the trypanocidal activity. This QSAR model was used to design and correctly classify 15 small molecules that showed a significant inhibitory activity against *T. cruzi*.

Finally, Muscia *et al.* [19] reported the use of computational methods for building a QSAR model capable of classifying 10 chloro-quinoline derivatives, which had been synthesized to improve the activity of the lead compound **7** (Figure 4.3). In line with the QSAR study discussed above [13], several descriptors were calculated for the training set and then correlated with biological activity data. Again, geometric properties turned out to play a more important role than electronic properties. The distance between the chloro-quinoline scaffold and a

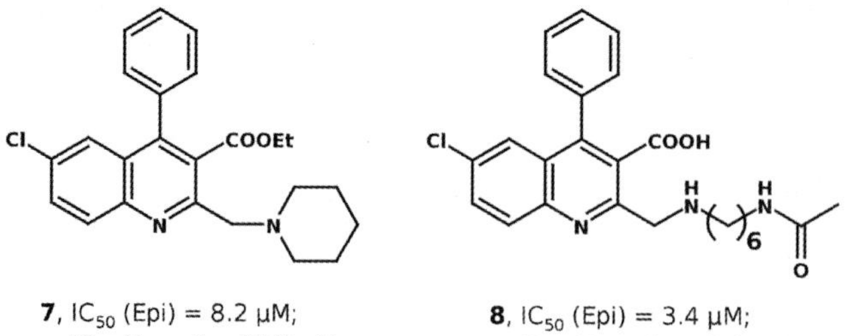

7, IC$_{50}$ (Epi) = 8.2 μM;
IC$_{50}$ (Amas) = 37.9 μM

8, IC$_{50}$ (Epi) = 3.4 μM;
IC$_{50}$ (Amas) = 12.8 μM

Figure 4.3 Chemical structure and biological activity of anti-trypanosomal compounds discovered by using the *in silico* ligand-based approach described in reference [19]. Biological activity data are presented as the IC$_{50}$ values against the epimastigote (Epi) and the amastigote (Amas) forms of *T. cruzi*.

nitrogen atom on the alkyl chain was proportional to the trypanocidal activity up to an optimum distance as in **8**, which is the most active of the series (Figure 4.3). It should be emphasized that **8** is more active than benznidazole against the epimastigote and the trypomastigote forms of the parasite (mammal stages), and has a good activity also against the amastigote form, thus being a promising lead compound for further studies.

Structure-Based Drug Design and Screening

The basic requirement for structure-based approaches is the availability of the 3-D structure of the target receptor or, at least, of a highly homologous protein. The principal source of protein structures is, undoubtedly, the freely accessible Protein Data Bank (PDB, www.pdb.org) which currently contains more than 75 000 structures (December 2011).

The philosophy of structure-based virtual screening is to apply subsequent filters for drastically reducing the dimension of compounds in the chemical space to a few hits having physicochemical properties suitable for interacting with the target receptor. Hit compounds identified by means of virtual screening must be necessarily tested *in vitro* and/or *in vivo*, but the enrichment of active compounds after experiments is, in general, significantly higher than in a random selection. Several different methods have been developed for performing virtual screening, based on the different combination of filters and algorithms. In particular, the selection of filters for setting-up a virtual screening workflow strictly depends on the nature of the chemical library and of the target protein. In Figure 4.4 we present a general virtual screening workflow, with the only aim to facilitate the understanding of literature data discussed below. Even though this

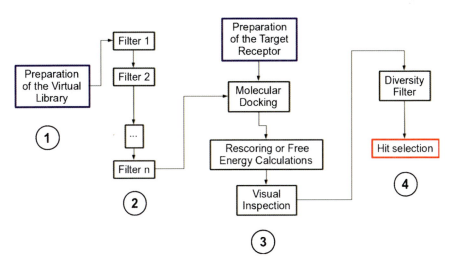

Figure 4.4 General workflow for structure-based virtual screening approaches.

workflow corresponds to our own experience and includes most of the virtual screening approaches commonly used by medicinal chemists, we are aware that different virtual screening strategies could be realized. For the sake of clarity, the workflow of Figure 4.4 has been divided into four steps.

i) Small molecules included in chemical libraries are often represented by heavy atoms connected in the 2-D space. Thus, after the addition of hydrogen atoms, the conversion to a 3-D format is generally required, alongside the conformational analysis and the selection of appropriate tautomers and ionization states for physiological conditions. From an informatics standpoint, this step might significantly increase the physical and virtual memory usage, but is essential to make the library suitable for being handled in the next steps.

ii) The subsequent application of filters aims at eliminating from the library those compounds that violate certain rules, such as Lipinski's rules for drug-like molecules, or custom rules that could be defined by the users. Some filters, for example, eliminate compounds on the basis of their ADME/Tox (absorption, distribution, metabolism, elimination, and toxicity) profile, which can be easily predicted *in silico*; some software can drive through the selection of compounds having a particular chemical scaffold (or chemical moiety) by using monodimensional fingerprints, whereas some other filters classify compounds on the basis of their pharmacophore alignment toward the coordinates of a reference active ligand in its biologically active conformation. Among the latter, LigandScout is a smart and user-friendly software that, starting from the coordinates of a protein–ligand complex, is capable of generating structure-based pharmacophore models that can be used as a 3-D query to filter chemical libraries [20]. Useful programs have also been developed by OpenEye (www.eyesopen.com) for filtering chemical libraries on the basis of the shape and chemical similarity to a reference active molecule or on the basis of the electrostatic similarity. Molecules that survive these filtrations can be studied by docking.

iii) The third step is probably the most time and computation consuming one of the workflow. Coordinates of the target receptor come most frequently from X-ray crystallography or NMR spectroscopy. However, despite the reliability of these biophysical methods, a computational refinement of experimental structures should be done to overcome intrinsic limitations, before starting a drug design study [21]. Compounds that survived previous filters are docked toward the target receptor and the interaction energy (or score) is calculated for each ligand binding pose. Docking usually represents the core process of a classic structure-based approach, and reliability of docking results depends on the type of program and docking and scoring function used. To reduce the number of possible false-positive hits selected by docking, an alternative scoring function could be used to calculate the ligand binding energy (or score). Many docking programs (e.g., GOLD or Glide) have been implemented with internal scoring functions, while external scoring functions such as the X-score and the MM-PBSA or MM-GBSA approaches for free energy calculations (Poisson–Boltzmann surface area or generalized Born surface area, respectively) may be used. These latter have been discussed in several recent works and represent a powerful tool for rescoring docking poses [22]. Finally, visual inspection of docking poses is essential to discard possible artifacts or binding poses that are away from the selected cluster of target residues.

iv) Last, but not least, the diversity filter should be applied to avoid the selection of closely related chemicals. In fact, stressing the chemical diversity of selected hits could drive toward the discovery of multiple novel scaffolds having the desired biological activity.

Hit compounds selected *in silico* need to be tested *in vitro* but, in comparison to high-throughput screening (HTS), experimental efforts after virtual screening are reduced to a few compounds having a high probability of success. Currently, virtual screening is a widely appreciated tool for drug discovery, because it is faster and cheaper than experimental methods, and often provides highly reliable results.

Virtual Screening Approaches against Trypanosome Proteins

Structures of several proteins from trypanosome parasites have been solved so far. In detail, 394 structures equally distributed between *T. cruzi* and *T. brucei* are available in the PDB, in addition to 26 still unreleased structures and 200 ligand hits, which emphasizes the growing interest in ligand–protein interactions and their implication in drug discovery. Most of these structures belong to the biochemical class of isomerases (26%), followed by a comparable amount of hydrolases (24%), oxidoreductases (23%), and transferases (18%). Structures of lyases (6%) and ligases (3%) are also available, although in a limited amount. As reported in Figure 4.5 , most of the 384 structures solved by X-ray crystallography have a resolution lower than 2.5 Å. Only 10 structures have been solved in solution by using NMR spectroscopy.

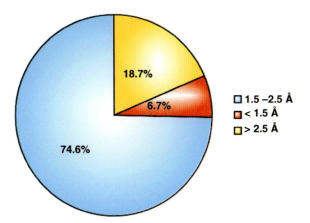

18.7%

6.7%

74.6%

☐ 1.5 –2.5 Å
◼ < 1.5 Å
☐ > 2.5 Å

Figure 4.5 Statistics on the X-ray resolution of protein structures from *T. cruzi* and *T. brucei* available in the PDB.

Starting from these statistical considerations, it should not be surprising that the number of papers describing structure-based approaches against infections by Kinetoplastida is numerically surpassing the ligand-based approaches. Moreover, in respect of the ligand-based projects discussed above, most of the structure-based approaches performed in this field aimed at discovering novel anti-trypanosomal agents through the massive *in silico* screening of large chemical libraries. In the following, virtual screening campaigns carried out against Kinetoplastida are discussed on the basis of our own and others' examples. Results are grouped by target proteins.

Cruzain is the recombinant form of cruzipaine – a major cysteine protease present in every stage of the parasite life cycle. To date, coordinates of 19 cruzain structures in complex with covalent and non-covalent inhibitors have been solved by means of X-ray crystallography, emphasizing its potential role as a drug target. A structure-based virtual screening was performed in 2008 by Malvezzi *et al.* [23] with the aim of highlighting possible pitfalls of that *in silico* approach. Thereafter, a massive virtual screening of a library of about 200 000 compounds was performed by the group of Shoichet in 2010 [24]. Although the primary aim of this work was to compare the performance of the virtual screening with that of the HTS by using the same library of compounds, five novel scaffolds for competitive inhibitors of cruzain were discovered. These active molecules (**9–13** in Figure 4.6) showed *in vitro* K_i values ranging from 65 nM to 6 μM, and their scaffolds were similarly prioritized by *in silico* docking and *in vitro* HTS. These findings highlight that, at least for the system

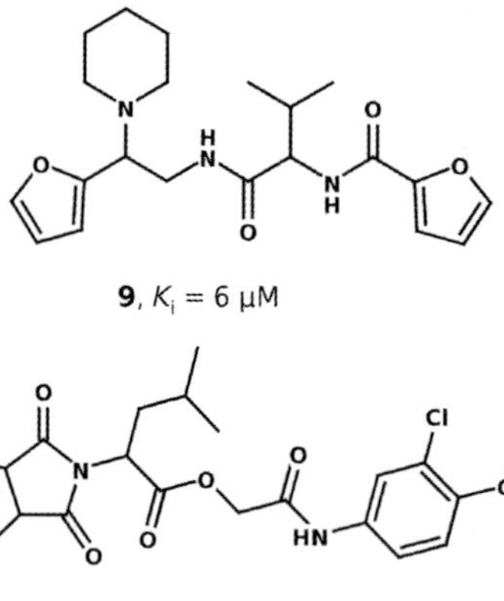

9, K_i = 6 μM

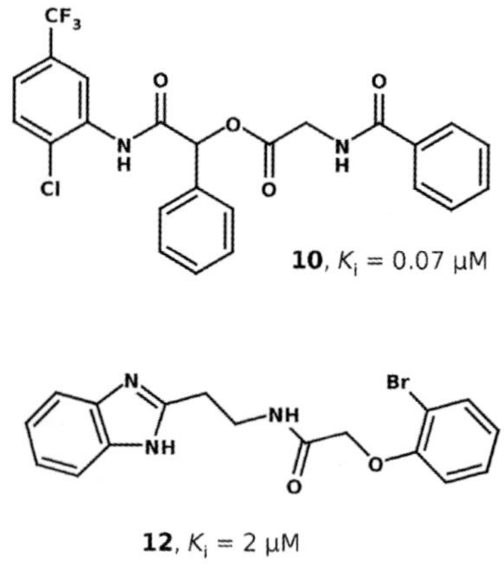

10, K_i = 0.07 μM

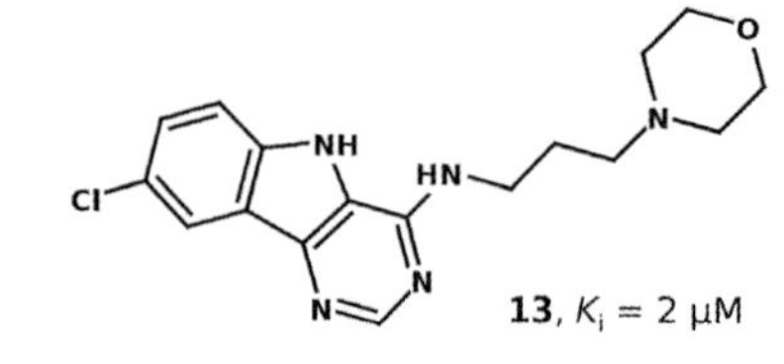

11, K_i = 0.08 μM

12, K_i = 2 μM

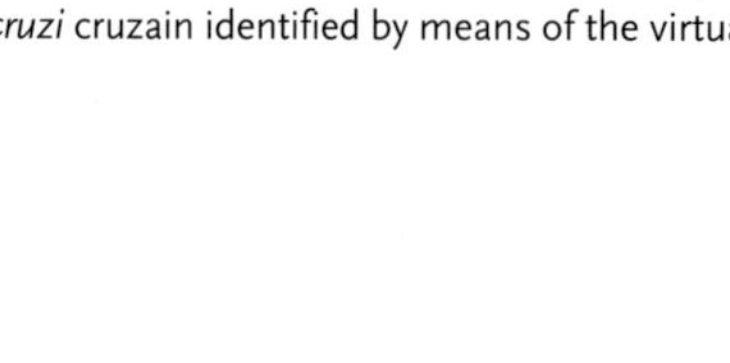

13, K_i = 2 μM

Figure 4.6 Chemical structure and inhibitory activity of the most potent competitive inhibitors of *T. cruzi* cruzain identified by means of the virtual screening according to reference [24].

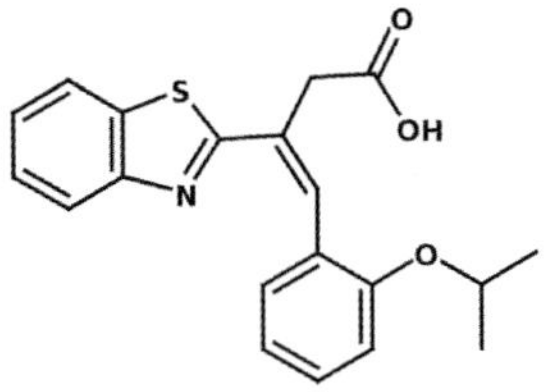

14, 92% inhibition at 1 mM; IC$_{50}$ = 0.29 mM

Figure 4.7 Chemical structure and inhibitory activity of the *TcTS* inhibitor **14** identified by means of the structure-based virtual screening approach according to reference [25].

studied, virtual screening provides similar results as experimental procedures, but with a significant gain of time and money.

The enzyme *T. cruzi trans*-sialidase (TcTS) has recently emerged as a possible target for the treatment of Chagas disease. Since several crystal structures of the enzyme in complex with small-molecule inhibitors have been solved, structure-based approaches for ligand design are facilitated. In 2009, Neres *et al.* [25] described a virtual screening exercise for discovering novel *TcTS* inhibitors. Starting from a database containing 2.5 million structures, only compounds having drug-like properties in agreement with Lipinski's Rule of Five and a negative charge were selected by subsequent application of multiple filters. Docking was then performed within the active site of the *TcTS* and, after rescoring, 1819 compounds were visually inspected. According to the diversity criteria, the 23 most diverse compounds were selected for *in vitro* fluorimetric assays and X-ray crystallography. The most active compound was **14** (Figure 4.7). However, due the weak inhibition constant observed, **14** still needs to be improved.

T. cruzi **dihydrofolate reductase (DHFR)**. Human DHFR is a validated drug target for the therapy of various diseases such as cancers or bacterial infections and could also be targeted by anti-kinetoplastida agents. Structures of the *T. cruzi* and *T. brucei* DHFR in complex with inhibitors have been solved by means of X-ray crystallography and were used by Schormann *et al.* [26] to dock known competitive DHFR inhibitors. The docking was used to align the possible bioactive conformations of these compounds within the receptor active site. Afterwards, a 3-D-QSAR model, which nicely correlated with biological activity data, was generated and used to screen about 3000 molecules taken from the ZINC database [27], sharing the 2,4-diaminopyrimidine or the 2,4-diaminopteridine scaffold. To the best of our knowledge, biological activity of hit compounds selected *in silico* has not been declared, but a follow-up of the work has recently been published by the same authors [28] who presented the synthesis and biological activity of a series of 2,4-diaminoquinazoline derivatives as potent *T. cruzi* DHFR inhibitors. Most potent compounds were **15** and **16** (Figure 4.8), which showed $K_i = 1.6$ nM and 1.3 nM, respectively, although being poorly selective against the human DHFR.

T. brucei **pteridine reductase 1 (PTR1)**. DHFR inhibitors experienced a limited efficacy against *T. brucei* and *Leishmania major*. A possible reason of this failure has been ascribed to the specificity of pteridine reductase that, in *T. brucei*, not only

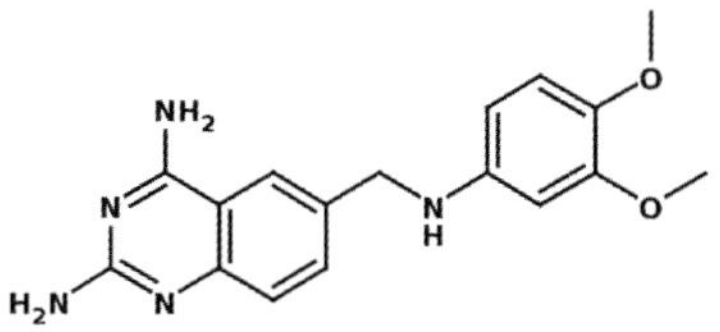

15
TcDHFR: $IC_{50} = 27.1 \pm 4.7$ nM
$K_i = 1.6 \pm 0.4$ nM
hDHFR: $IC_{50} = 85.5 \pm 11.2$ nM
$K_i = 11.8 \pm 0.8$ nM

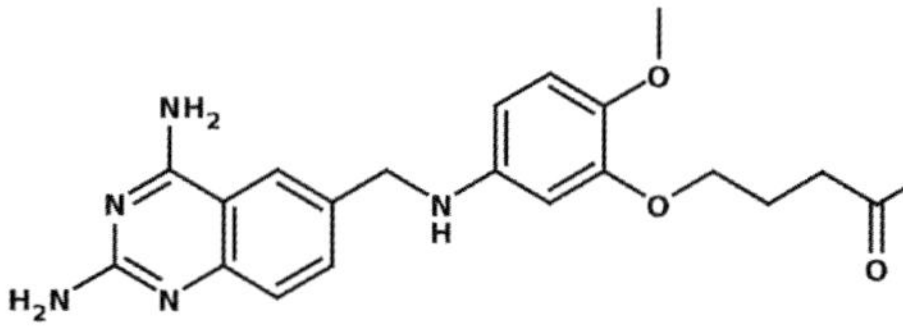

16
TcDHFR: $IC_{50} = 23.8 \pm 7.0$ nM
$K_i = 1.3 \pm 0.2$ nM
hDHFR: $IC_{50} = 68.3 \pm 5.6$ nM
$K_i = 9.6 \pm 1.5$ nM

Figure 4.8 Chemical structure and inhibitory activity of potent *T. cruzi* DHFR inhibitors. IC_{50} and K_i values are reported for both the *T. cruzi* and the human isoforms of the enzyme.

reduces its primary substrates (biopterin and dihydrobiopterin), but also dihydrofolate, thus overcoming the function of DHFR inhibitors and serving as possible resistance mechanism. PTR1 knockdown *T. brucei* also resulted in the loss of viability and virulence in cultures and animal models [29]. PTR1, thus, is a potential drug target for the treatment of African trypanosomiasis. The first *in silico* attempt to discover novel PTR1 inhibitors was done by Mpamhanga *et al.* [30] who performed the virtual screening of a custom fragment library composed of 26 084 individual entries. The docking toward the crystallographic structure of PTR1, followed by the application of some filters such as pharmacophore-like alignment and the visual inspection, led the selection of 45 compounds for *in vitro* tests. The aminobenzimidazole derivative **17** (Figure 4.9) showed PTR1 inhibition at low micromolar concentration, while its analog **18** (Figure 4.9) bearing a 3′,4′-dichlorobenzyl substituent was more active ($K_i = 0.4 \mu M$). X-ray crystallography studies on these fragments in complex with PTR1 suggested some possible chemical modification to improve ligand affinity and selectivity against DHFR. Accordingly, **19** (Figure 4.9) reached nanomolar affinity for PTR1. Furthermore, authors explored the aminobenzimidazole scaffold by means of chemical substitutions in different position [31], establishing SAR for this series and discovering **20** (Figure 4.9) as a potent and selective PTR1 inhibitor.

Trypanothione **Reductase (TR)** is the trypanothione-related protein most extensively investigated by *in silico* structure-based approaches. Starting from the late 1990s, a conspicuous number of papers describing the use of virtual screening or molecular modeling procedures in the search for TR inhibitors has been

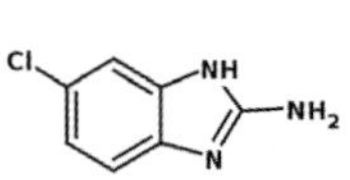

17, $K_i = 10.6$ 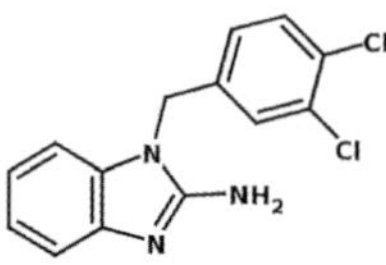   **18**, $K_i = 0.4 \mu M$ 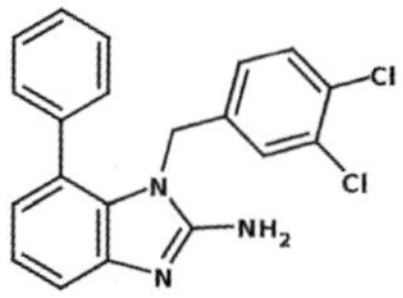   **19**, $K_i = 0.007 \mu M$ 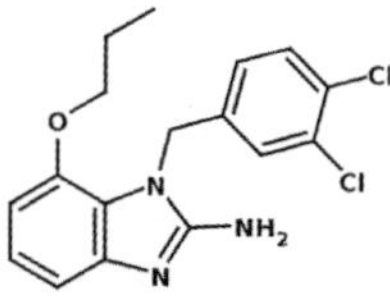   **20**, $K_i = 0.047 \mu M$

Figure 4.9 PTR1 inhibitors belonging to the aminobenzimidazole scaffold.

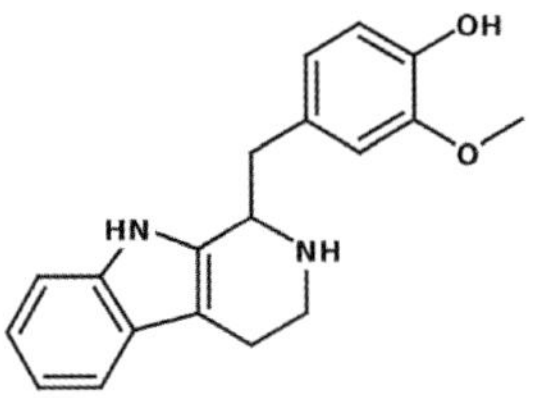

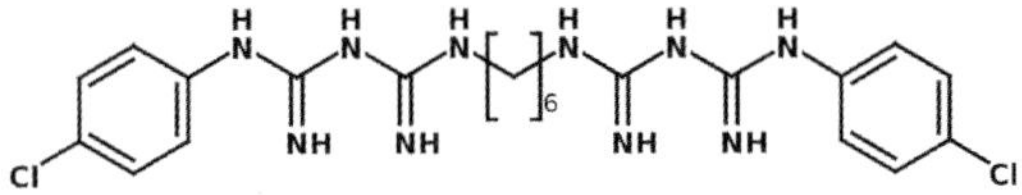

21, 27% inhibition at 57 μM [32]

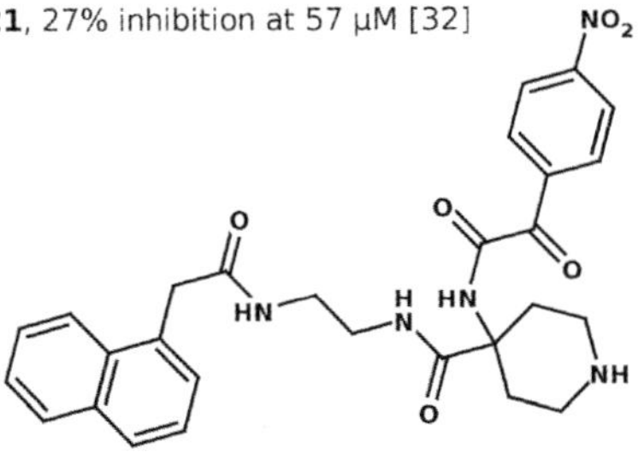

chlorexidine **23**, K_i = 2 ± 1 μM [33]

22, K_i = 6.2 ± 2 μM; K_i' = 8.2 ± 2 μM [33]

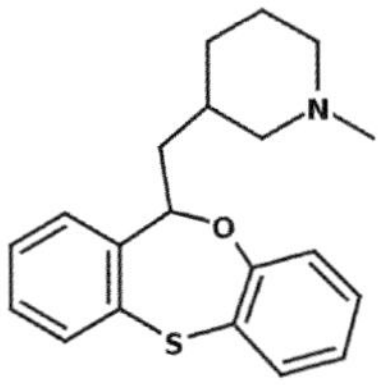

24, TcTR IC$_{50}$ = 11.5 μM
TbTR IC$_{50}$ = 14.6 μM [36]

Figure 4.10 Chemical structure and biological activity data of representative TR inhibitors obtained by *in silico* virtual screening approaches.

published. To the best of our knowledge, the first work in this field was published in 1997 by Horvath [32] who described the development of an algorithm for virtual screening against the TR enzyme. This method was used to screen a library of about 2500 small molecules. The 13 most promising and diverse virtual hits were then submitted to biological tests, and nine out of them were active. Particular attention was given to the discovery of the polycyclic compound **21** (Figure 4.10), which does not bear the linear alkylammonium moiety contained in many known TR inhibitors. Despite the great potential disclosed by this early work, it took a long time before another *in silico* screening against TR was published. In 2005, Meiering *et al.* presented a structure-based virtual screening campaign based on the application of two different docking programs, FlexX and ProPose, to screen about 1 million commercially available compounds toward the active site of the *T. cruzi* TR [33]. Upon a consensus analysis of docking results, 25 compounds were tested *in vitro*. The piperidine derivative **22** and the antimicrobial chlorexidine **23** (Figure 4.10) experienced more than 90% TR inhibition at 100 μM. These compounds exerted a different mechanism of action against TR, **22** being a mixed inhibitor and **23** a pure competitive inhibitor. The existence of multiple mechanisms for TR inhibition was also observed one year later by Vega-Teijido *et al.* [34] who combined crystallographic and molecular modeling studies to explore possible binding sites of *TR* and human glutathione reductase (hGR), indicating a possible way for gaining TR selectivity against hGR. Similar issues were also addressed by means of molecular dynamics simulations [35], while a novel virtual screening cascade was presented in 2009 by Perez-Pineiro *et al.* [36]. In detail, 1312 possible TR inhibitors were extracted from the PubChem library by using a ligand similarity filter, based on a training set of 135 known TR inhibitors. Ligands with a suitable ADME/Tox profile were then docked toward the active site of the TR by means of the AutoDock4 program, whereas the X-score function was used to rescore docking poses (i.e., by calculating the ligand binding affinity). Nineteen compounds were selected for *in vitro* tests upon visual inspection of docking poses. Ten hits were able to inhibit TR *in vitro* at concentrations lower than 100 µM. The most active compound (**24** in Figure 4.10) showed IC_{50} values of 11.5 and 14.6 µM against the *T. cruzi* and *T. brucei* isoforms of the TR, respectively. It should be emphasized that some of the active hits belong to chemical scaffolds never identified before as TR inhibitors, such as dibenzothiepine, dibenzooxathiepine, dibenzodithiepine, thiaazatetracyclo, and 2,4,6-trioxohexahydro pyrimidine, thus stressing the capability of this novel virtual screening protocol to promote the chemical diversity among active compounds.

A virtual screening protocol based on the combination of ligand similarity search and structure-based modeling has been also recently optimized by Maccari *et al.* in our own molecular modeling laboratory for discovering potent TR inhibitors [37]. First, a training set composed of 19 known TR inhibitors with micromolar and submicromolar affinity was docked toward the active site of TR by means of the FRED program. Docking poses were then refined by means of energy minimization performed by using the Szybki program. These are two very fast and accurate programs from OpenEye. Individual shape- and electrostatic-based queries were then generated on the basis of docking poses for the training set, and were used to filter the whole ASINEX database containing about 600 000 small molecules. By this filtering, 5640 unique molecules having electrostatic properties and shape similar to the training set were selected, and then docked toward TR by using both the ChemScore and the GoldScore docking functions implemented in the GOLD docking program. A consensus "rank-by-rank" analysis of docking results was done for reducing as much as possible the number of possible false positive hits. Upon visual inspection, the most promising and diverse molecules were tested *in vitro*. Interestingly, nine compounds bearing the imidazole moiety were active, showing $K_i < 27$ µM. The most active compound, namely **25** (Figure 4.11), showed a K_i of 5.7 µM. Moreover, active compounds are significantly different from known TR inhibitors included in the training set and do not present the chemical moieties most often considered crucial for TR inhibition, such as the tricyclic system or the protonated alkylamine.

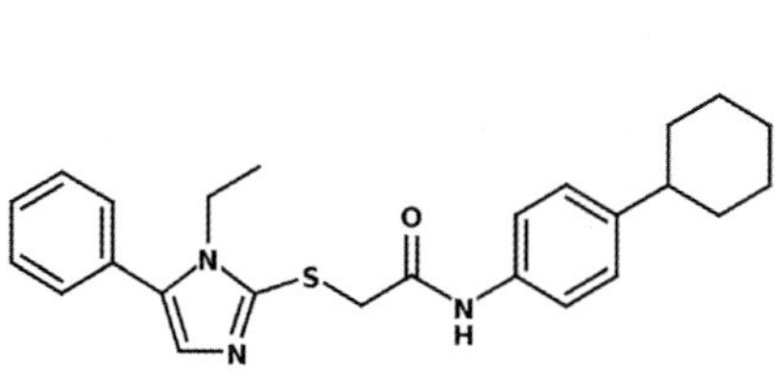

25, $K_i = 5.7 \pm 0.1$ µM

Figure 4.11 Chemical structure and inhibitory activity of the most active *T. cruzi* TR inhibitor discovered by means of the fast virtual screening approach [37].

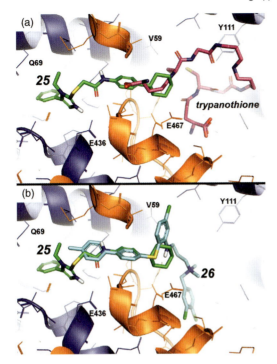

Figure 4.12 Structural alignment of (a) the docking-based binding mode of **25** and the crystallographic binding mode of trypanothione (PDB ID: 1BZL) or (b) the docking-based binding mode of the competitive inhibitor **26**. Protein coordinates and residue numbers are taken from PDB ID: 1BZL. Chain A is shown as a blue cartoon and lines, chain B as an orange cartoon and lines; organic molecules are showed as sticks; carbon atoms are colored green in **25**, magenta in trypanothione, and cyan in **26**, while the non-carbon atom color code follows the default settings of the PyMOL visualizer.

Analysis of docking-based binding mode of **25** reveals that it partially overlaps with the crystallography-based binding mode of trypanothione (Figure 4.12a) as well as with the predicted binding conformation of **26** (Figure 4.12b), which is a well-known diarylsulfide competitive inhibitor of TR included in the training set [38].

Interestingly, docking analysis also reveals that the lipophilic part of the molecule is well inserted into the initial part of the buried TR dimerization interface site, also known as the "Z site". The predicted binding mode of **25** within both active and interface sites (Figure 4.13) permits the rational growth of the ligand either toward the active site, for enhancing the competition with trypanothione, and toward the buried interface site, for enhancing the ligand affinity by performing polar as well as hydrophobic contacts with the protein.

Finally, this investigation identified novel TR inhibitors by means of a fast virtual screening protocol based on the combination of ligand similarity search and structure-based docking. These inhibitors share a common imidazole moiety and are significantly diverse from known TR inhibitors, highlighting the capability

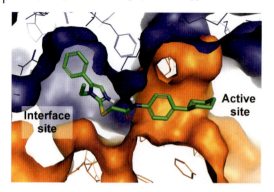

Figure 4.13 Docking-based binding mode of **25**. Surface and residues of the TR chains A and B are shown in orange and blue, respectively (PDB ID: 1BZL).

of this computational protocol to promote the chemical diversity. These active hits might represent a profitable starting point for further optimizations.

Some of the filters described in these virtual screening projects have been also used individually to perform structure-based studies. In particular, molecular docking and molecular dynamics have been widely used to study the possible binding conformation of active ligands or to align a series of compounds within the binding site of a target protein. This latter approach would be useful, for example, to build quantitative statistical models such as CoMFA/CoMSIA and 3-D-QSAR, which correlate structural features of ligands with their biological activity. Examples of speculative molecular modeling approaches have been described against several Kinetoplastida drug targets such as kinetoplast DNA [39], cruzain [40], superoxide dismutase [41], glyceraldehyde-3-phosphate dehydrogenase [42], hexokinase [43], and N-myristoltransferase [44].

In Silico Prediction of Protein Druggability

The choice of the target protein represents a crucial step in drug discovery. The ideal target should be clearly involved in pathogenesis and disease progression, and its modulation should induce a rapid regression of the disease and an improvement of patient's health without promoting toxic effects. Accordingly, the availability of a plethora of information coming from different fields is required to assess the so-called druggability of a target protein, where druggability is the term that describes the capability of a protein to interact with a small-molecule compound able to modulate its activity. Gene knockdown and knockout strategies have been widely applied to demonstrate the involvement of a protein in specific pathways and are considered the most powerful tools for the validation of possible target proteins, although they often require considerable economic efforts and experimental time, and provide little, if any, information on target druggability. With the aim of accelerating drug discovery and reducing the cost associated with target identification, *in silico* tools have therefore been developed to predict protein druggability. In this section we will provide a general overview of such methods, while for more detail we refer to original publications.

Early *in silico* strategies were based on genomic sequence similarity search, while more sophisticated algorithms have later been developed for identifying deep and, generally, lipophilic pockets on the surface of a target receptor. These latter strategies require, of course, the knowledge of the 3-D structure of the target protein and are included within structure-based methods. Most appreciated algorithms identify druggable binding pockets on the basis of shape and geometry features, as for example PocketPicker (example in Figure 4.14a) [45] and LIGSITE, which is also available as a Web server [46], or make use of the interaction energy of probe atoms

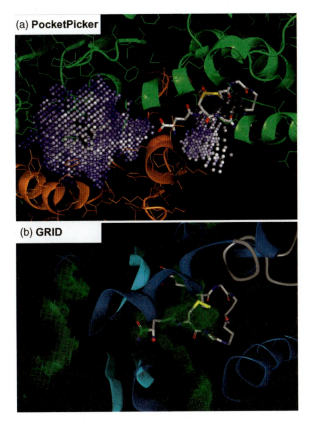

(a) **PocketPicker**

(b) **GRID**

Figure 4.14 Application of software for binding pocket prediction for TR (PDB ID: 1BZL). Trypanothione is shown as sticks. (a) Binding pockets identified by PocketPicker are filled by dots. The most probable pocket is that on the left side at the interface between TR monomers. The second possible binding pocket is found within the trypanothione binding site. (b) Binding pockets identified by GRID by using the DRY probe for hydrophobic interactions. Visualization of the interaction energy map is done with the LigandScout software. Binding pockets are shown as green meshes; the results are comparable with those obtained by PocketPicker.

toward the protein such as the widely appreciated GRID program (example in Figure 4.14b) [47].

Additional features determining protein druggability have been reported by Hadjuk *et al.* [48,49], who derived druggability indices from NMR screenings and from the physicochemical properties of known ligand binding sites. Quantitative descriptors for hydrophobicity, electrostatic properties, and shape were found to be crucial for correctly predicting protein druggability. The use of these quantitative descriptors also facilitates the direct comparison between multiple proteins. In a similar way, Sugaya and Ikeda recently developed a computational approach for discovering druggable protein–protein interactions [50] by searching for the existence of possible ligand binding sites at the protein–protein interaction interface. This approach was further implemented in 2009 by the introduction of a supervised machine learning method for studying physicochemical, structural, and ligand-related properties [51]. Recently, Crowther *et al.* presented the open-access TDRtargets.org Web resource containing multiple and diverse information of potential targets for neglected disease, including proteins from trypanosomes [52]. The target prioritization is made *in silico* and is based on whether protein properties meet criteria established for a potential drug target. Finally, FLAP (Fingerprint for Ligands And Proteins) is a new software from Molecular Discovery that might facilitate the prediction of protein druggability. Starting from GRID force field parameterization, it generates fingerprints for protein cavities that permit a rapid comparison between different protein pockets [53]. All these methods are based on the analysis of the 3-D protein structure, thus restricting the applicability only to the biological systems whose 3-D structure has been already solved or predicted by means of homology modeling. Moreover, since several factors are involved in determining the druggability of a protein, *in silico* methods have to be flanked by the experimental validation of a target. In the anti-trypanosomal field, some drug targets have been validated by chemical and/or biological methods; useful examples have been described by Bland for the case of *T. brucei* phosphodiesterases B1 and B2 [54], by Torrie and by Flohé for the trypanothione synthetase [55,56], and by Spinks for the TR [57].

References

1 Kirchhoff, L.V. (1993) American trypanosomiasis (Chagas' disease) – a tropical disease now in the united states. *N. Engl. J. Med.*, **329**, 639–644.

2 Fairlamb, A.H., Ridley, R.G., and Vial, H.J. (eds) (2003) *Drugs Against Parasitic Diseases. R&D Methodologies and Issues.* WHO/TDR, Geneva.

3 Levinthal, C. (1966) Molecular model-building by computer. *Sci. Am.*, **214**, 42–52.

4 Andricopulo, A.D. (2009) Structure- and ligand-based drug design: advances and perspectives. *Curr. Top. Med. Chem.*, **9**, 754.

5 Merz, K.M., Ringe, D., and Reynolds, C.H. (eds) (2010) *Drug Design: Structure- And Ligand-Based Approaches.* Cambridge University Press, Cambridge.

6 Marhöfer, R.J., Oellien, F., and Selzer, P.M. (2011) Drug discovery and the use of computational approaches for infectious diseases. *Future Med. Chem.*, **3**, 1011–1025.

7 Marrero Ponce, Y., Cabrera Pérez, M.A., Romero Zaldivar, V., González Díaz, H., and Torrens, F. (2004) A new topological descriptors based model for predicting intestinal epithelial transport of drugs in caco-2 cell culture. *J. Pharm. Pharm. Sci.*, **7**, 186–199.

8 Montero-Torres, A., Vega, M.C., Marrero-Ponce, Y., Rolón, M., Gómez-Barrio, A. *et al.* (2005) A novel non-stochastic quadratic fingerprints-based approach for the *in silico* discovery of new antitrypanosomal compounds. *Bioorg. Med. Chem.*, **13**, 6264–6275.

9 Vega, M.C., Montero-Torres, A., Marrero-Ponce, Y., Rolón, M., Gómez-Barrio, A. *et al.* (2006) New ligand-based approach for the discovery of antitrypanosomal compounds. *Bioorg. Med. Chem. Lett.*, **16**, 1898–1904.

10 Roldos, V., Nakayama, H., Rolón, M., Montero-Torres, A., Trucco, F. *et al.* (2008) Activity of a hydroxybibenzyl bryophyte constituent against *Leishmania* spp. and *Trypanosoma cruzi*: *in silico, in vitro* and *in vivo* activity studies. *Eur. J. Med. Chem.*, **43**, 1797–1807.

11 Castillo-Garit, J.A., Vega, M.C., Rolon, M., Marrero-Ponce, Y., Kouznetsov, V.V. *et al.* (2010) Computational discovery of novel trypanosomicidal drug-like chemicals by using bond-based non-stochastic and stochastic quadratic maps and linear discriminant analysis. *Eur. J. Pharm Sci.*, **39**, 30–36.

12 Castillo-Garit, J.A., Vega, M.C., Rolón, M., Marrero-Ponce, Y., Gómez-Barrio, A. *et al.* (2011) Ligand-based discovery of novel trypanosomicidal drug-like compounds: *in silico* identification and experimental support. *Eur. J. Med. Chem.*, **46**, 3324–3330.

13 Molfetta, F.A., Bruni, A.T., Honório, K.M., and da Silva, A.B.F. (2005) A structure–activity relationship study of quinone compounds with trypanocidal activity. *Eur. J. Med. Chem.*, **40**, 329–338.

14 Boiani, M., Cerecetto, H., Gonzalez, M., and Gasteiger, J. (2008) Modeling anti-*Trypanosoma cruzi* activity of *N*-oxide containing heterocycles. *J. Chem. Inf. Model*, **48**, 213–219.

15 Prieto, J.J., Talevi, A., and Bruno-Blanch, L.E. (2006) Application of linear discriminant analysis in the virtual screening of antichagasic drugs through trypanothione reductase inhibition. *Mol. Divers.*, **10**, 361–375.

16 Paula, F.R., Jorge, S.D., de Almeida, L.V., Pasqualoto, K.F.M., and Tavares, L.C. (2009) Molecular modeling studies and *in vitro* bioactivity evaluation of a set of novel 5-nitro-heterocyclic derivatives as anti-*T. cruzi* agents. *Bioorg. Med. Chem.*, **17**, 2673–2679.

17 Vera-Divaio, M.A.F., Freitas, A.C.C., Castro, H.C., de Albuquerque, S., Cabral, L.M. *et al.* (2009) Synthesis, antichagasic *in vitro* evaluation, cytotoxicity assays, molecular modeling and SAR/QSAR studies of a 2-phenyl-3-(1-phenyl-1H-pyrazol-4-yl)-acrylic acid benzylidene-carbohydrazide series. *Bioorg. Med. Chem.*, **17**, 295–302.

18 Planche, A.S., Scotti, M.T., Emerenciano, V.D.P., López, A.G., Pérez, E.M. *et al.* (2010) Designing novel antitrypanosomal agents from a mixed graph-theoretical substructural approach. *J. Comput. Chem.*, **31**, 882–894.

19 Muscia, G.C., Cazorla, S.I., Frank, F.M., Borosky, G.L., Buldain, G.Y. *et al.* (2011) Synthesis, trypanocidal activity and molecular modeling studies of 2-alkylaminomethylquinoline derivatives. *Eur. J. Med. Chem.*, **46**, 3696–3703.

20 Wolber, G. and Langer, T. (2005) LigandScout: 3-D pharmacophores derived from protein-bound ligands and their use as virtual screening filters. *J. Chem. Inf. Model*, **45**, 160–169.

21 Marco, E. and Gago, F. (2007) Overcoming the inadequacies or limitations of experimental structures as drug targets by using computational modeling tools and molecular dynamics simulations. *ChemMedChem*, **2**, 1388–1401.

22 Mori, M., Manetti, F., and Botta, M. (2011) Predicting the binding mode of known NCp7 inhibitors to facilitate the design of novel modulators. *J. Chem. Inf. Model.*, **51**, 446–454.

23 Malvezzi, A., de Rezende, L., Izidoro, M.A., Cezari, M.H.S., Juliano, L. *et al.* (2008) Uncovering false positives on a virtual screening search for cruzain inhibitors. *Bioorg. Med. Chem. Lett.*, **18**, 350–354.

24 Ferreira, R.S., Simeonov, A., Jadhav, A., Eidam, O., Mott, B.T. *et al.* (2010) Complementarity between a docking and a high-throughput screen in discovering new cruzain inhibitors. *J. Med. Chem.*, **53**, 4891–4905.

25 Neres, J., Brewer, M.L., Ratier, L., Botti, H., Buschiazzo, A. *et al.* (2009) Discovery of novel inhibitors of *Trypanosoma cruzi trans*-sialidase from *in silico* screening. *Bioorg. Med. Chem. Lett.*, **19**, 589–596.

26 Schormann, N., Senkovich, O., Walker, K., Wright, D.L., Anderson, A.C. *et al.* (2008) Structure-based approach to pharmacophore identification, *in silico* screening, and three-dimensional quantitative structure–activity relationship studies for inhibitors of *Trypanosoma cruzi* dihydrofolate reductase function. *Proteins*, **73**, 889–901.

27 Irwin, J.J. and Shoichet, B.K. (2005) ZINC – a free database of commercially available compounds for virtual screening. *J. Chem. Inf. Model.*, **45**, 177–182.

28 Schormann, N., Velu, S.E., Murugesan, S., Senkovich, O., Walker, K. *et al.* (2010) Synthesis and characterization of potent inhibitors of *Trypanosoma cruzi* dihydrofolate reductase. *Bioorg. Med. Chem.*, **18**, 4056–4066.

29 Sienkiewicz, N., Ong, H.B., and Fairlamb, A.H. (2010) *Trypanosoma brucei* pteridine reductase 1 is essential for survival *in vitro* and for virulence in mice. *Mol. Microbiol.*, **77**, 658–671.

30 Mpamhanga, C.P., Spinks, D., Tulloch, L.B., Shanks, E.J., Robinson, D.A. *et al.* (2009) One scaffold, three binding modes: novel and selective pteridine reductase 1 inhibitors derived from fragment hits discovered by virtual screening. *J. Med. Chem.*, **52**, 4454–4465.

31 Spinks, D., Ong, H.B., Mpamhanga, C.P., Shanks, E.J., Robinson, D.A. *et al.* (2011) Design, synthesis and biological evaluation of novel inhibitors of *Trypanosoma brucei* pteridine reductase 1. *ChemMedChem*, **6**, 302–308.

32 Horvath, D. (1997) A virtual screening approach applied to the search for trypanothione reductase inhibitors. *J. Med. Chem.*, **40**, 2412–2423.

33 Meiering, S., Inhoff, O., Mies, J., Vincek, A., Garcia, G. *et al.* (2005) Inhibitors of *Trypanosoma cruzi* trypanothione reductase revealed by virtual screening and parallel synthesis. *J. Med. Chem.*, **48**, 4793–4802.

34 Vega-Teijido, M., Caracelli, I., and Zukerman-Schpector, J. (2006) Conformational analyses and docking studies of a series of 5-nitrofuran- and 5-nitrothiophen-semicarbazone derivatives in three possible binding sites of trypanothione and glutathione reductases. *J. Mol. Graph. Model.*, **24**, 349–355.

35 Iribarne, F., Paulino, M., Aguilera, S., and Tapia, O. (2009) Assaying phenothiazine derivatives as trypanothione reductase and glutathione reductase inhibitors by theoretical docking and molecular dynamics studies. *J. Mol. Graph. Model.*, **28**, 371–381.

36 Perez-Pineiro, R., Burgos, A., Jones, D.C., Andrew, L.C., Rodriguez, H. *et al.* (2009) Development of a novel virtual screening cascade protocol to identify potential trypanothione reductase inhibitors. *J. Med. Chem.*, **52**, 1670–1680.

37 Maccari, G., Jaeger, T., Moraca, F., Biava, M., Flohé, L. *et al.* (2011) A fast virtual screening approach to identify structurally diverse inhibitors of trypanothione reductase. *Bioorg. Med. Chem. Lett.*, **21**, 5255–5258.

38 Stump, B., Eberle, C., Kaiser, M., Brun, R., Krauth-Siegel, R.L. *et al.* (2008) Diaryl sulfide-based inhibitors of trypanothione reductase: inhibition potency, revised binding mode and antiprotozoal activities. *Org. Biomol. Chem.*, **6**, 3935–3947.

39 Athri, P., Wenzler, T., Ruiz, P., Brun, R., Boykin, D.W. *et al.* (2006) 3-D QSAR on a library of heterocyclic diamidine derivatives with antiparasitic activity. *Bioorg. Med. Chem.*, **14**, 3144–3152.

40 Trossini, G.H.G., Guido, R.V.C., Oliva, G., Ferreira, E.I., and Andricopulo, A.D. (2009) Quantitative structure–activity relationships for a series of inhibitors of cruzain from *Trypanosoma cruzi*: molecular modeling, comfa and comsia studies. *J. Mol. Graph. Model.*, **28**, 3–11.

41 de Paula da Silva, C.H.T., Sanches, S.M., and Taft, C.A. (2004) A molecular modeling and QSAR study of suppressors of the growth of *Trypanosoma cruzi* epimastigotes. *J. Mol. Graph. Model.*, **23**, 89–97.

42 Guido, R.V.C., Oliva, G., Montanari, C.A., and Andricopulo, A.D. (2008) Structural basis for selective inhibition of trypanosomatid glyceraldehyde-3-phosphate dehydrogenase: molecular docking and 3D QSAR studies. *J. Chem. Inf. Model.*, **48**, 918–929.

43 Willson, M., Sanejouand, Y.H., Perie, J., Hannaert, V., and Opperdoes, F. (2002) Sequencing, modeling, and selective inhibition of *Trypanosoma brucei* hexokinase. *Chem. Biol.*, **7**, 839–847.

44 Sheng, C., Ji, H., Miao, Z., Che, X., Yao, Y., Wang, W. *et al.* (2009) Homology modeling and molecular dynamics simulation of *N*-myristoyltransferase from protozoan parasites: active site characterization and insight into rational inhibitor design. *J. Comput. Aided Mol. Des.*, **6**, 375–389.

45 Weisel, M., Proschak, E., and Schneider, G. (2007) PocketPicker: analysis of ligand binding-sites with shape descriptors. *Chem. Cent. J.*, **1**, 7–23.

46 Huang, B. and Schroeder, M. (2006) LIGSITEcsc: predicting ligand binding sites using the Connolly surface and degree of conservation. *BMC Struct. Biol.*, **6**, 19–29.

47 Goodford, P.J. (1985) A computational procedure for determining energetically favorable binding sites on biologically important macromolecules. *J. Med. Chem.*, **28**, 849–857.

48 Hajduk, P.J., Huth, J.R., and Tse, C. (2005) Predicting protein druggability. *Drug Discov. Today*, **10**, 1675–1682.

49 Hajduk, P.J., Huth, J.R., and Fesik, S.W. (2005) Druggability indices for protein targets derived from NMR-based screening data. *J. Med. Chem.*, **48**, 2518–2525.

50 Sugaya, N., Ikeda, K., Tashiro, T., Takeda, S., Otomo, J. *et al.* (2007) An integrative *in silico* approach for discovering candidates for drug-targetable protein–protein interactions in interactome data. *BMC Pharmacol.*, **7**, 10–24.

51 Sugaya, N. and Ikeda, K. (2009) Assessing the druggability of protein–protein interactions by a supervised machine-learning method. *BMC Bioinformatics*, **10**, 263–275.

52 Crowther, G.J., Shanmugam, D., Carmona, S.J., Doyle, M.A., Hertz-Fowler, C. *et al.* (2010) Identification of attractive drug targets in neglected-disease pathogens using an *in silico* approach. *PLoS Negl. Trop. Dis.*, **4**, e804.

53 Baroni, M., Cruciani, G., Sciabola, S., Perruccio, F., and Mason, J.S. (2007) A common reference framework for analyzing/comparing proteins and ligands. Fingerprints for ligands and proteins (FLAP): theory and application. *J. Chem. Inf. Model.*, **47**, 279–294.

54 Bland, N.D., Wang, C., Tallman, C., Gustafson, A.E., Wang, Z. *et al.* (2011) Pharmacological validation of *Trypanosoma brucei* phosphodiesterases B1 and B2 as druggable targets for African sleeping sickness. *J. Med. Chem.*, **54**, 8188–8194.

55 Flohé, L. (2011) The trypanothione system and the opportunities it offers to create drugs for the neglected kinetoplast diseases. *Biotechnol. Adv.*, **30**, 294–301.

56 Torrie, L.S., Wyllie, S., Spinks, D., Oza, S.L., Thompson, S. *et al.* (2009) Chemical validation of trypanothione synthetase: a potential drug target for human trypanosomiasis. *J. Biol. Chem.*, **284**, 36137–36145.

57 Spinks, D., Shanks, E.J., Cleghorn, L.A.T., McElroy, S., Jones, D. *et al.* (2009) Investigation of trypanothione reductase as a drug target in *Trypanosoma brucei*. *ChemMedChem*, **4**, 2060–2069.

5
Computational Approaches and Collaborative Drug Discovery for Trypanosomal Diseases

Sean Ekins and *Barry A. Bunin*

Abstract

Over the past decade there have been several studies that have employed high-throughput screening against *Trypanosoma brucei* or *T. cruzi* or their specific targets. Some of these datasets have been collated in the Collaborative Drug Discovery (CDD) database and made available to the community. In addition, there have been numerous computational drug discovery approaches applied to trypanosomal diseases in different laboratories. A collaborative database like CDD could bring together neglected disease and other researchers, to collaborate and share compounds and drug discovery data, which could avoid repetition and increase research efficiency. This chapter describes the CDD software and summarizes the computational drug discovery approaches used for research in trypanosomal diseases.

Introduction

Trypanosoma brucei is the causative agent behind African sleeping sickness, which is transmitted via the tsetse fly. The disease is known to have neurological symptoms and can be fatal [1]. There are currently four drugs used as treatments and these can cause frequent side-effects. *T. cruzi* is the protozoan parasite that causes Chagas disease (also known as American trypanosomiasis). To date there are two drugs marketed for this disease. These diseases, which primarily impact the African and American continents, have not received a great deal of interest from the pharmaceutical industry, and research is therefore dependent on academic and not-for-profit organizations. A recent review by McKerrow *et al.* described a listing of the laboratories doing drug discovery research for Chagas diseases [2]. One group also discussed the potential impact on drug development arising from new consortia among academic, corporate, and public partners committed to the discovery of new, effective anti-protozoan drugs [3]. There is an urgent need for new drugs due to resistance and to improve upon the toxicity profile of existing drugs.

* Corresponding Author

Trypanosomatid Diseases: Molecular Routes to Drug Discovery, First edition. Edited by T. Jäger, O. Koch, and L. Flohé.
© 2013 Wiley-VCH Verlag GmbH & Co. KGaA. Published 2013 by Wiley-VCH Verlag GmbH & Co. KGaA.

Anti-protozoan drug research reviews have focused on how advances in high-throughput screening (HTS) technologies and availability of diverse small-molecule libraries facilitate the discovery of new drug targets and new drugs that will reduce disease burdens imposed on humanity by parasitic protozoa [3]. HTS can be used with the whole organism or against specific targets. HTS by whole-cell screening resulted in 17 novel trypanocidal drugs versus *T. brucei* [4]. The same group found 55 compounds including 13 drugs with a greater than 5-fold selectivity window against high-content screening for the intracellular stage of *T. cruzi* [5] (Table 5.1). Such efforts could help rapidly find compounds for repurposing. Whole-organism screens for other organisms (e.g., hookworm [6] and schistosomiasis [7]) have also found new potential uses for US Food and Drug Administration (FDA)-approved drugs. These are in addition to some of the many examples of groups performing HTS screens with FDA compound libraries for other diseases [8,9]. Large-scale whole-cell HTS has potential issues with reconfirmation by independent laboratories. In one documented case, 23 actives were followed up and 11 failed to have activity [10]. This is not surprising, given the range of possible variations in cell growth conditions, buffers, and other assay condition variables, as well as the inherent variability and signal-to-noise ratios observed even for simply reproducing results on different days for whole-cell screens within the same laboratory. This situation is analogous to what we have also heard anecdotally for tuberculosis (TB) in

Table 5.1 HTS repurposing molecules for trypanosomal diseases.

Screening information	Library vendor	Compounds found	Reference
T. cruzi growth inhibition cell-based HTS	909 clinical compounds from Iconix, mostly FDA approved	55 hits, 17 with >5-fold selectivity; compounds not previously identified with trypanocidal activity included terconazole, azelastine, vinorelbine, mycophenolate, and dihydroergocristine	[5]
T. brucei luciferase assay	2160 Microsource Spectrum and Killer collection	35 hits with activity at $1\,\mu M$ or less includes drugs like orlistat	[4]
T. cruzi luciferase assay	303 286 MLPCN (Molecular Libraries Probe Production Centers) library screened first at the Broad Institute then a subset of compounds tested in house	23 compounds with $IC_{50} < 1.2\,\mu M$ and 100-fold activity versus cytotoxicity included verapamil, itraconazole, hexylresorcinol, and propiconazole; retesting showed 11 compounds failed and only two non-FDA-approved drugs had *in vivo* activity in mouse	[10]

several laboratories. In contrast, HTS of 197 861 compounds against cruzain, a thiol protease target for Chagas disease, led to 146 well-behaved, competitive ligands [11]. An emerging approach is to perform the whole-cell screens first on compounds that are putative hits or were designed for specific classes of targets, and then to fish out the targets once the researcher is at least confident that there will be whole-cell activity on the compound (or with greater confidence if within the compound class actual structure–activity relationship (SAR) trends are reproducibly observed).

Several groups have also used computational approaches to either assist in understanding SARs for compounds active against specific trypanosomal targets or to suggest compounds for testing (Table 5.2). These methods range from quantitative structure–activity relationships (QSARs) to docking and have been used widely elsewhere. We have recently described how such methods have been used for TB drug discovery [12]. From our literature review (Table 5.2), the number of studies using computational approaches is relatively smaller compared with those for TB, and could be reflective of the interest and funding differences in both diseases. As we observed for TB, the cheminformatics methods used have generally been used on a single target or compound series in *T. brucei* and *T. cruzi*, and rarely in combination with other computational tools [12]. Also, computational ADME/Tox (absorption, distribution, metabolism, elimination, and toxicity) methods appear not to have been used to either help select compounds or optimize them. There appear to be opportunities to combine HTS and cheminformatics to assist with finding active compounds for trypanosomal diseases.

CDD Database

We believe there is a need for a new approach to foster inter-group collaboration to speed up drug discovery. Neglected disease researchers represent a relatively small number, compared to scientists in cancer and cardiovascular research. However, in all cases they are plagued with the same challenges for effective collaboration, and thus need robust, intuitive tools for secure data mining and sharing. Recent research suggests that more collaborative drug discovery will be the future paradigm of biomedical research [13–16]. To facilitate this there are growing numbers of Internet based open-access chemistry databases and Internet-based collaborative tools [17,18] that are likely to enhance scientific research. The challenges associated with bringing chemists and biologists together for virtual drug discovery projects for neglected diseases [19] provides an arena for testing a new approach. Traditionally, biological data available for sharing is stored in an unstructured format (e.g., in single document or Excel^{TM} files). Compilation of data is sporadic with little, if any, standardization of the data formats (e.g., ontology creation) or critical information such as experimental procedures and statistical analysis to quantify data quality to quantitate reproducibility for comparisons between groups. Before collaborations begin, data security and integrity often is considered while intellectual property (IP) arrangements (Materials

Table 5.2 Computational approaches used for drug discovery against trypanosomal diseases.

Approach	Target	Notes	Reference
Docking	hypoxanthine phosphoribosyltransferase	using DOCK the Available Chemicals Directory (34 million compounds) was screened with flexible docking, 22 inhibitors acquired, 16 had K_i values of 0.5–17 μM	[33]
CoMFA-SIMCA	trypanothione reductase	18 nitrofurazones used and model suggests amide like group 7–9 Å from an easily reducible group.	[34]
FlexX docking	DHFR	936 compounds docked in human and *T. cruzi* enzymes, several 4-nM inhibitors developed.	[35]
Linear discriminant analysis	trypanothione reductase	58 compounds used to build a model with two- and three-dimensional descriptors, and BMDP and Statistica software used to screen 422 367 compounds to suggest compounds for testing	[36]
Catalyst and CoMSIA	hexokinase	17 compounds used for pharmacophore (two hydrophobes, neutral ring aromatic and two negative ionizable features), 24 for CoMSIA (electrostatic, hydrophobic, and steric interactions)	[37]
Two-dimensional and HQSAR	cruzain	45 thiosemicarbazones and semicarbazones used to build QSAR with DRAGON descriptors and Pirouette software, using MLR, GA, PLS; 10 compounds as a test set. HQSAR $r^2 = 0.95$, QSAR $r^2 = 0.91$	[38]
GOLD docking	*trans* sialidase	305 000 compounds docked, visually inspected 1819, 23 compounds selected, five inhibited subnanomolar	[39]
AM1 method, GOLD docking and HERMES	cruzain	N-acylhydrazones docked to visualize and evaluate binding	[40]
MOE docking	triosephosphate isomerase	methylbrevifolin docked to show interactions	[41]
SAR, DFT calculations, LUMO, ClogP	squalene epoxidase	5-nitrofuranes and 5-nitrothiophenes – electronic properties could have a role in accumulation of squalene; lipophilicity related to squalene accumulation	[42]
			[43]

	Target	Description	Reference
MLR QSAR Dragon descriptors		23 3-arylquinoxaline-2-carbonitrile di-N-oxides used to build MLR QSAR with 1497 Dragon descriptors; models used to predict 49 potential candidate compounds; three were described with predicted activities (low micomolar)	
PCA, Consensus PCA, PLS, VolSurf+, GRID	NADH oxidase	QSAR with 40 flavones and 128 descriptors, training set $N = 30$, test set $N = 10$, consensus $PCA = 71.23\%$, $PCA = 76.55\%$, $PLS = 100\%$, Test set $r^2 = 0.70$; hydrophobic tendency for most actives	[44]
iGemDock Molecular docking	DHFR	six compounds docked, ranks compounds well	[45]
Fujitsu Scigress Explorer Docking	FPPS	MBHA mechanism of action docking suggests it is weaker than residronate	[46]
QSAR		eight 1',4-dihydropyridines compounds with GETAWAY descriptors + GA; designed two new compounds	[47]
Docking with DOCK	cruzain	197 861 MLSMR compounds docked and parallel HTS screen; initial enrichment factor 3-fold; for competitive inhibitors the enrichment factor increases to 34-fold	[11]

CoMFA, comparative molecular field analysis; CoMSIA, comparative molecular similarity analysis; DHFR, dihydrofolate reductase; FPPS, farnesyl diphosphate synthase; GA, genetic algorithm; HQSAR, hologram QSAR; LUMO, lowest unoccupied molecular orbital; MLR, multiple linear regression; MLSMR, molecular libraries small molecules repository; PCA, principal component analysis; PLS, partial least squares.

Transfer and IP Rights Agreements) are often (at least in academia) seen as necessary, but generally as a hindrance to progress. In practice, groups initiate collaborations at all stages of the IP discussions – traditional (IP sensitive), collaborative (pre-IP), and open (post-IP).

Existing software tools, both commercial and public, do not address these issues. Available traditional chemistry and biology data management software offers no community-oriented data-sharing features; it can also be expensive to license, and difficult to deploy and support. To promote data exchange, it is essential to respect IP constraints. Existing databases can also be technically complex and challenging to use, so many academic researchers simply do not bother to adhere to the advanced data management practices that pharmaceutical discovery efforts mandate internally. Exploiting 8 years of experience of using cloud computing and Web 2.0 [17], Collaborative Drug Discovery, Inc. (CDD) has developed a unique web-based software currently helping scientists optimally identify and advance novel drug candidates. The software allows scientists to not only manage and analyze their data more effectively, but also to optionally share their data effortlessly and securely to the degree they want, with whomever they wish, at the time of their choosing [20]. It allows them to easily toggle between and simultaneously mine across private, shared, and public datasets. The CDD software and existing user network is uniquely positioned to improve collaborations in the neglected disease space, thereby increasing the efficiency of drug discovery and development [19].

The development of the CDD database has been described previously with applications for collaborative malaria research [20]. The CDD database brings the power of cloud computing to drug discovery, enabling collaborators to share research data securely within and across organizations without the need to install and maintain complex software. CDD has been funded by the Bill and Melinda Gates Foundation to build the Collaborative Drug Discovery Tuberculosis Database (http://www.collaborativedrug.com/register). The CDD database is also now part of the More Medicines for TB project (www.mm4tb.org) in which over 20 groups are collaborating to develop drugs for *Mycobacterium tuberculosis*. CDD hosts many *M. tuberculosis*-specific datasets representing well over 300 000 compounds derived from patents, literature, and HTS data. Access to such data enables cheminformatics analysis [21–25]. In addition, these large datasets can be used to create computational machine learning models that can identify active molecules against infectious diseases [23–25] such as TB, and databases like CDD may have a role for both target-based and phenotypic screening [25]. CDD is an integral part of many global TB researcher pilot laboratories (including many multigroup collaborations) and also facilitates collaborations with large global pharmaceutical companies. To date several research groups have deposited their screening data from *T. brucei* and *T. cruzi* in CDD (Table 5.3).

The CDD database can archive and mine a broad range of diverse objects that can later be selectively and securely shared with other researchers (or permanently kept private, which is the default behavior). The CDD database is a hosted collaborative system with an important advantage over traditional PC-based database systems

Table 5.3 Examples of relevant trypanosomal disease screening datasets available in CDD publicly.

Database name/source	Description	Molecules
Trypanosomal PDE Inhibitors – Northeastern University and Marine Biological Laboratory	this shared dataset contains the published biochemical and *T. brucei* screening data for the trypanosomal phosphodiesterase (*Tbr*PDEB1 and B2) inhibitor drug discovery project underway at Northeastern University (Michael Pollastri, PI) and the Marine Biological Laboratory (Robert Campbell, PI)	31
Sandler-UCSF Celera Cysteine Protease Inhibitor Library	*in vitro T. cruzi* and *T. brucei* parasite and specific enzyme screens (Jim McKerrow, PI)	1860
Malaria/Trypanosome: St Jude Public Data	open-access results from St Jude Children's Research Hospital including HTS of bioactives against malaria and *T. brucei* (Kip Guy, PI)	2426

since it can enable secure login into the database from any computer, using any common browser (e.g., Firefox, Internet Explorer, Chrome, or Safari). This unique capability for a database system provides flexibility for the users. The CDD Web-based database architecture handles a broad array of data types and is arranged as three integrated modules: the CDD Vault® securely stores and enables mining of data in a private data are hosted and managed by CDD; CDD Collaborate® enables the confidential exchange of data between vaults as selected by users; and CDD Public® hosts public datasets that can be mined. These modules are naturally integrated behind the scenes in the backend of the single CDD platform, so researchers conveniently look at whatever data or combinations of data are of interest, via a single front-end GUI (graphic user interface). One can zoom in and out of datasets, analogous to adjusting setting on a microscope or telescope (e.g., with one tool). The CDD platform incorporates Marvin, calculated plug-ins for physical chemical calculations, and the JChem Cartridge for structure searching from ChemAxon (Budapest, Hungary) within the application as the chemistry engine. This allows one to do sophisticated SAR analysis, including chemical pattern recognition (e.g., similarity and substructure searching), physical/chemical property calculations, Boolean search and save capabilities for potency, selectivity, toxicity, and other experimentally derived properties. The database can handle heterogeneous data files as well as standardized .csv and .sdf file convertible formats that represent the chemical and biological data. In particular, CDD is tailored for common data formats used by biologists such as Microsoft Excel™ (.xls) and text (.txt) files. The technology can mine against a variety of values including concentration, time, percent, real, integer, textline, cpm, rlu, Z/Z' plate statistics, and IC_{50}

(logIC$_{50}$, R^2 values, Hillslope, etc.). The outputs of such mining can be either saved, exported, shared inside CDD, or plotted with an integrated plug-in.

The researcher can control which data to keep 100% private, share with groups of individual researchers, or share more generally with the public. A further unique capability of CDD is the ability to compare all or subsets of public-access data with private data simultaneously together in a single container as well as analyze multiple vaults that the user has access to. The power of this collaborative approach to drug discovery can be seen in different types of community-based research projects. These range from traditional completely private collaborations, to temporally private collaborations which may become more open following a privacy escrow period, to completely open collaborations where researchers can blog about the experiments as they occur [20].

Ironically, we have observed that the more privacy controls and more refined options for controlling data privacy that are available to researchers, the more they are comfortable sharing or selectively sharing data. In hindsight, this is not surprising, as researchers traditionally share drug discovery information via publications and patents, albeit not in a directly useful, database format. Another catalyst has been to separate, and lower, the barrier to simply archiving data for private analysis. Once data is in a database format, tools can make the process for selective or public sharing of data much easier.

When users login to CDD they have the option to select the vault that they want to look at; once selected they will then see a dashboard that summarizes recent protocols and molecules that they have accessed, as well as a listing of recent activity and messages. Data import into CDD is currently a simple process from a . csv or .sdf file with reusable templates for efficiently mapping datasets to a user-defined protocol, molecule, and/or plate-well fields. A "best guess" algorithm even guesses the right field for data mapping in the vast majority of cases (the algorithm works as a function of the similarly of the data field name in the file and the database). Data can be readily mined in CDD (Figure 5.1a), and in addition the user can specify which private vaults and public datasets to use. One can quickly find if data is available in public datasets. For example, some of the trypanosomal phosphodiesterase inhibitors (Table 5.3) are also present in the PDSP dataset (Figure 5.1b). A full Boolean search is possible by specifying the protocol, run, readout, chemical properties, and/or keywords of interest. If molecules are selected, CDD also provides a link to find more information in external databases like ChemSpider. Data in CDD can also be plotted graphically using an interactive visualization which also provides a snapshot of the molecule and data upon mousing over a X,Y coordinate. These capabilities facilitate simple SAR analysis.

CDD has "Projects" – functionality that enhances the capability to share research data securely using CDD. This enables users of CDD to organize their data within a vault into projects and invite individual vault members to be able to access specific projects, allowing for more flexible data sharing and management both within a group as well as across groups. Put simply, molecules, batches, plates, and protocols (and intentionally invited people, with two levels of security to avoid accidental data sharing) all belong to specific projects.

(a)

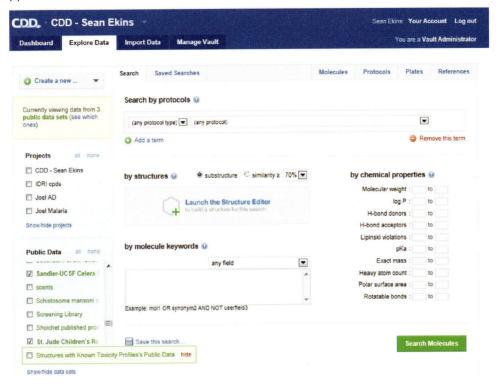

Figure 5.1 (a) CDD database screenshot showing data mining facilities. (b) *T. brucei* phosphodiesterase inhibitor compound with data in PDSP.

Using HTS Data for Machine Learning Models

Our analysis of the trypanosomal cheminformatics literature (Table 5.2) indicates how rarely groups to date use HTS and computational data from individual targets or the whole organism (Table 5.3). We have previously published studies that used large TB datasets to produce computational machine learning models that in turn have been used with other datasets to validate the models and to identify new hit compounds. For example, one study involved two large publicly available *M. tuberculosis* datasets with over 200 000 molecules and a second with over 100 000 molecules. We used Bayesian classifier models and predicted datasets from additional laboratories, and identified 4- and 10-fold enrichment factors [23–25]. These models were then used as part of an in-house drug discovery program with collaborators at Stanford Research International (SRI), which identified two new hits for TB [26].

Using the *T. brucei* data from two laboratories available in CDD it is possible to create Bayesian models in the same way as for TB. Laplacian-corrected Bayesian classifier models were generated using Discovery Studio using the St Jude's

(b)

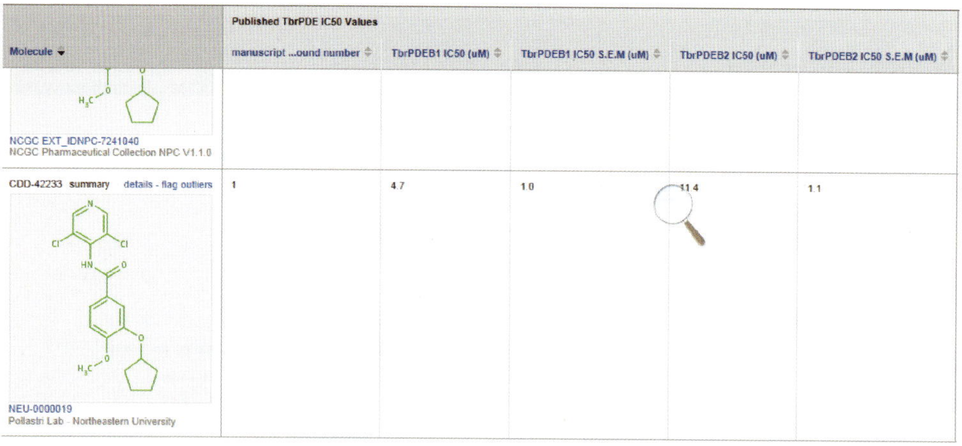

	Published TbrPDE IC50 Values				
Molecule ▾	manuscript ...ound number ⇕	TbrPDEB1 IC50 (uM) ⇕	TbrPDEB1 IC50 S.E.M (uM) ⇕	TbrPDEB2 IC50 (uM) ⇕	TbrPDEB2 IC50 S.E.M (uM) ⇕
NCGC EXT_IDNPC-7241040 NCGC Pharmaceutical Collection NPC V1.1.0					
CDD-42233 summary details - flag outliers	1	4.7	1.0	11.4	1.1
NEU-0000019 Pollastri Lab - Northeastern University					

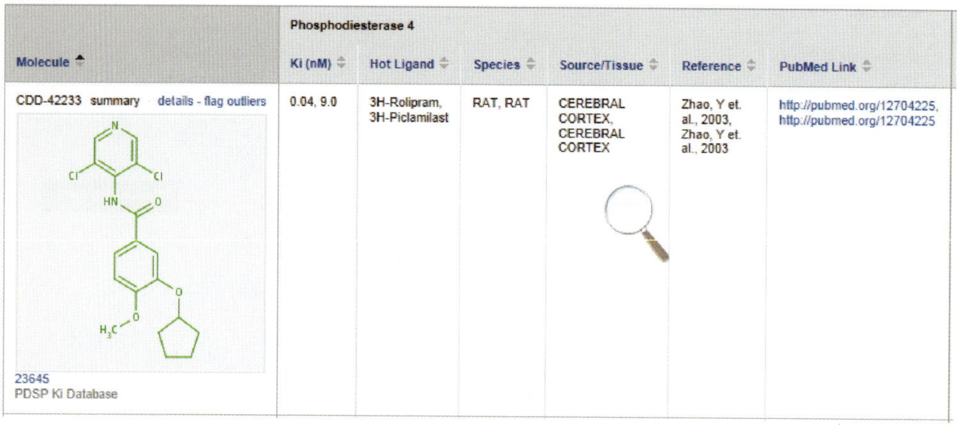

	Phosphodiesterase 4					
Molecule ▲	Ki (nM) ⇕	Hot Ligand ⇕	Species ⇕	Source/Tissue ⇕	Reference ⇕	PubMed Link ⇕
CDD-42233 summary details - flag outliers	0.04, 9.0	3H-Rolipram, 3H-Piclamilast	RAT, RAT	CEREBRAL CORTEX, CEREBRAL CORTEX	Zhao, Y et. al., 2003, Zhao, Y et. al., 2003	http://pubmed.org/12704225, http://pubmed.org/12704225
23645 PDSP Ki Database						

Figure 5.1 *(Continued)*

($N = 1994$) and UCSF datasets ($N = 1850$, Table 5.3). Molecular function class fingerprints of maximum diameter 6 (FCFP_6), Alog$P$, molecular weight, number of rotatable bonds, number of rings, number of aromatic rings, number of hydrogen bond acceptors, number of hydrogen bond donors, and molecular fractional polar surface area were calculated from input.sdf files using the "calculate molecular properties" protocol. The "create Bayesian model" protocol was used for model generation. The St Jude's model had a leave out 1 cross-validation receiver operating characteristic (ROC) value $= 0.79$ while the UCSF model had ROC $= 0.88$. Use of the molecular "function class fingerprints of maximum diameter 6" (FCFP_6) descriptors allowed the identification of molecular features that favored activity, as well as features that did not, for each model (Figures 5.2 and 5.3). These models can be used to quickly score compounds, and rank them for selection and future testing.

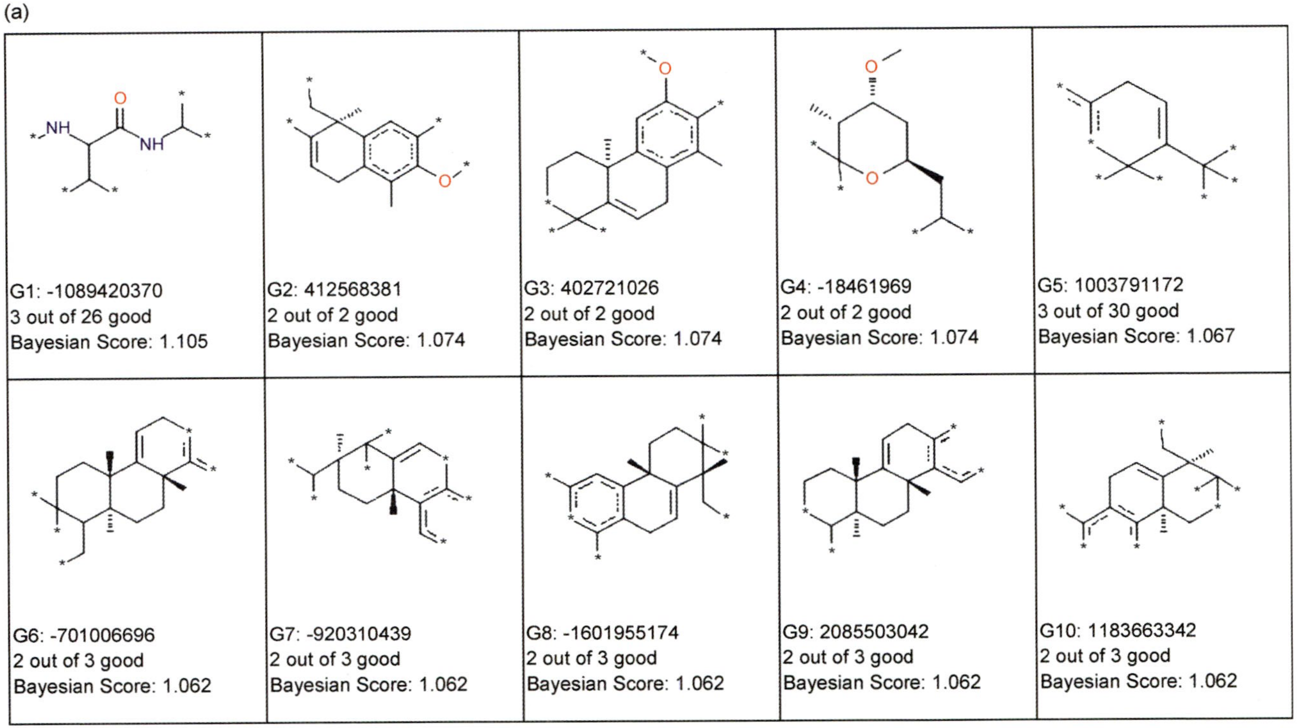

Figure 5.2 *T. brucei* St Jude's dataset: (a) good features for activity and (b) bad features for activity.

(a)

G1: -1089420370
3 out of 26 good
Bayesian Score: 1.105

G2: 412568381
2 out of 2 good
Bayesian Score: 1.074

G3: 402721026
2 out of 2 good
Bayesian Score: 1.074

G4: -18461969
2 out of 2 good
Bayesian Score: 1.074

G5: 1003791172
3 out of 30 good
Bayesian Score: 1.067

G6: -701006696
2 out of 3 good
Bayesian Score: 1.062

G7: -920310439
2 out of 3 good
Bayesian Score: 1.062

G8: -1601955174
2 out of 3 good
Bayesian Score: 1.062

G9: 2085503042
2 out of 3 good
Bayesian Score: 1.062

G10: 1183663342
2 out of 3 good
Bayesian Score: 1.062

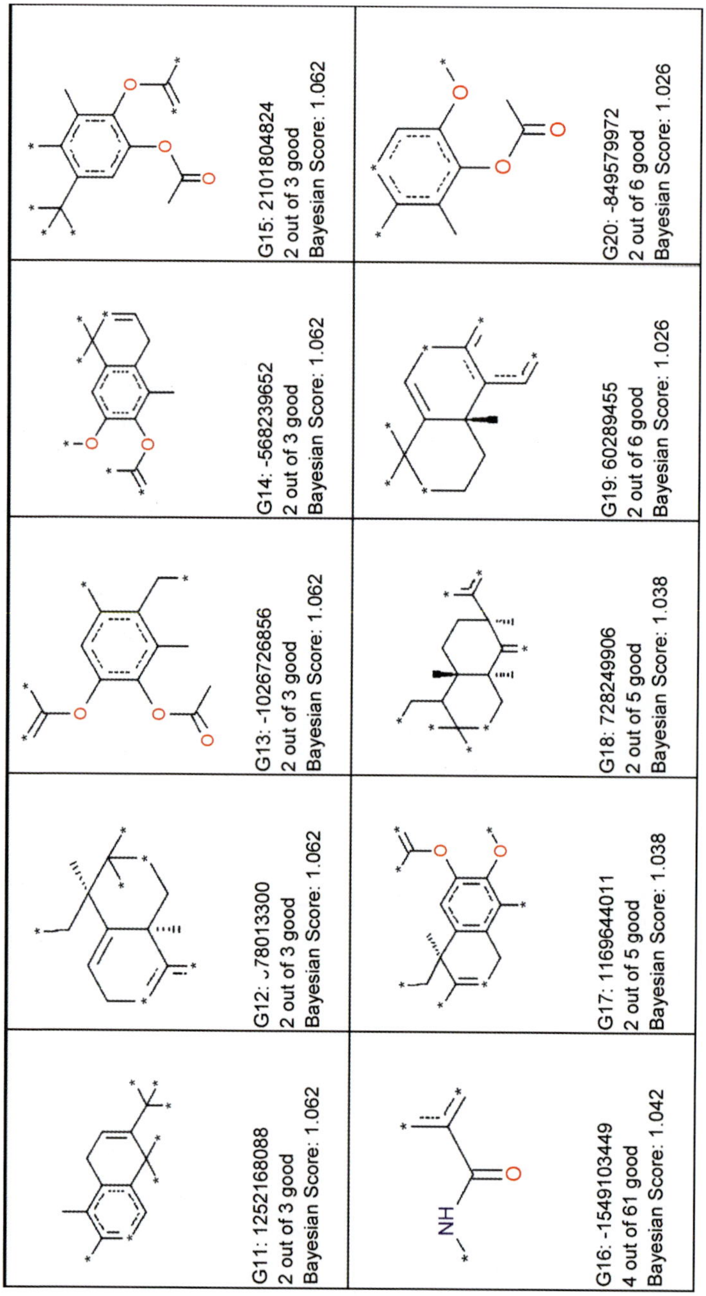

G11: 1252168088
2 out of 3 good
Bayesian Score: 1.062

G12: -78013300
2 out of 3 good
Bayesian Score: 1.062

G13: -1026726856
2 out of 3 good
Bayesian Score: 1.062

G14: -568239652
2 out of 3 good
Bayesian Score: 1.062

G15: 2101804824
2 out of 3 good
Bayesian Score: 1.062

G16: -1549103449
4 out of 61 good
Bayesian Score: 1.042

G17: 1169644011
2 out of 5 good
Bayesian Score: 1.038

G18: 728249906
2 out of 5 good
Bayesian Score: 1.038

G19: 60289455
2 out of 6 good
Bayesian Score: 1.026

G20: -849579972
2 out of 6 good
Bayesian Score: 1.026

Figure 5.2 *(Continued)*

(b)

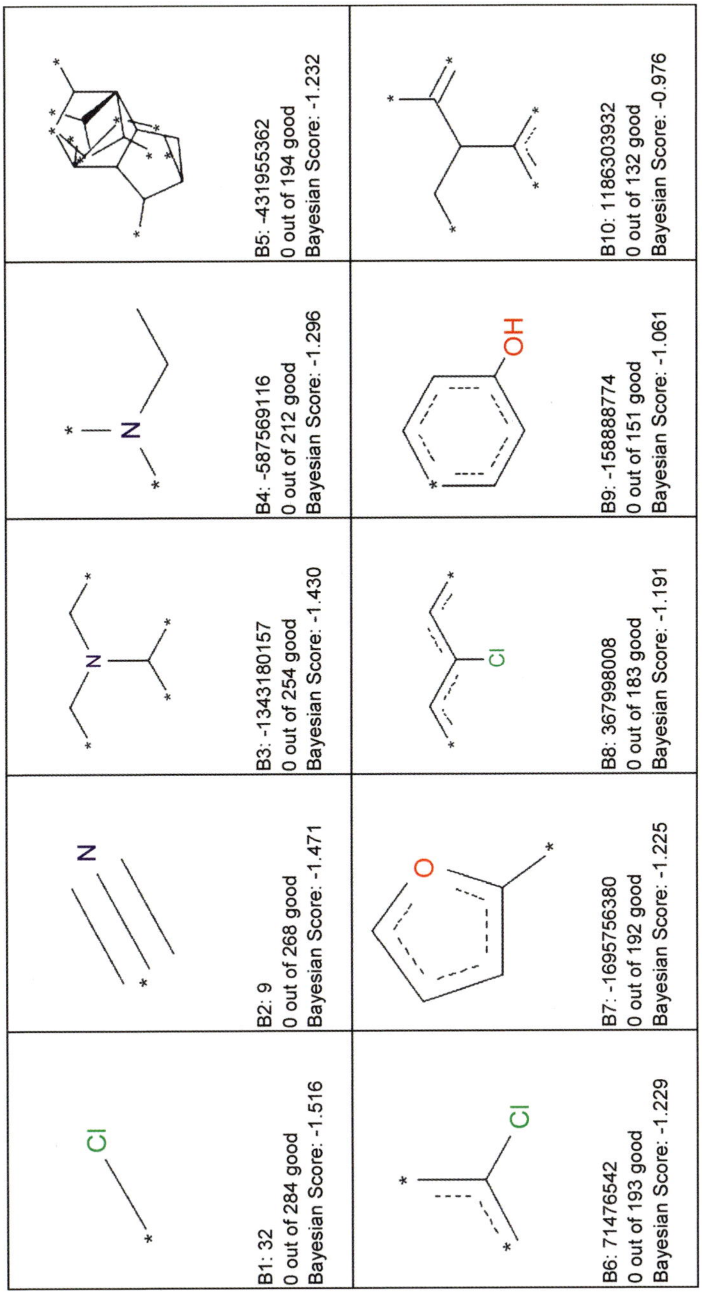

B1: 32
0 out of 284 good
Bayesian Score: -1.516

B2: 9
0 out of 268 good
Bayesian Score: -1.471

B3: -1343180157
0 out of 254 good
Bayesian Score: -1.430

B4: -587569116
0 out of 212 good
Bayesian Score: -1.296

B5: -431955362
0 out of 194 good
Bayesian Score: -1.232

B6: 71476542
0 out of 193 good
Bayesian Score: -1.229

B7: -1695756380
0 out of 192 good
Bayesian Score: -1.225

B8: 367998008
0 out of 183 good
Bayesian Score: -1.191

B9: -158888774
0 out of 151 good
Bayesian Score: -1.061

B10: 1186303932
0 out of 132 good
Bayesian Score: -0.976

Figure 5.2 (*Continued*)

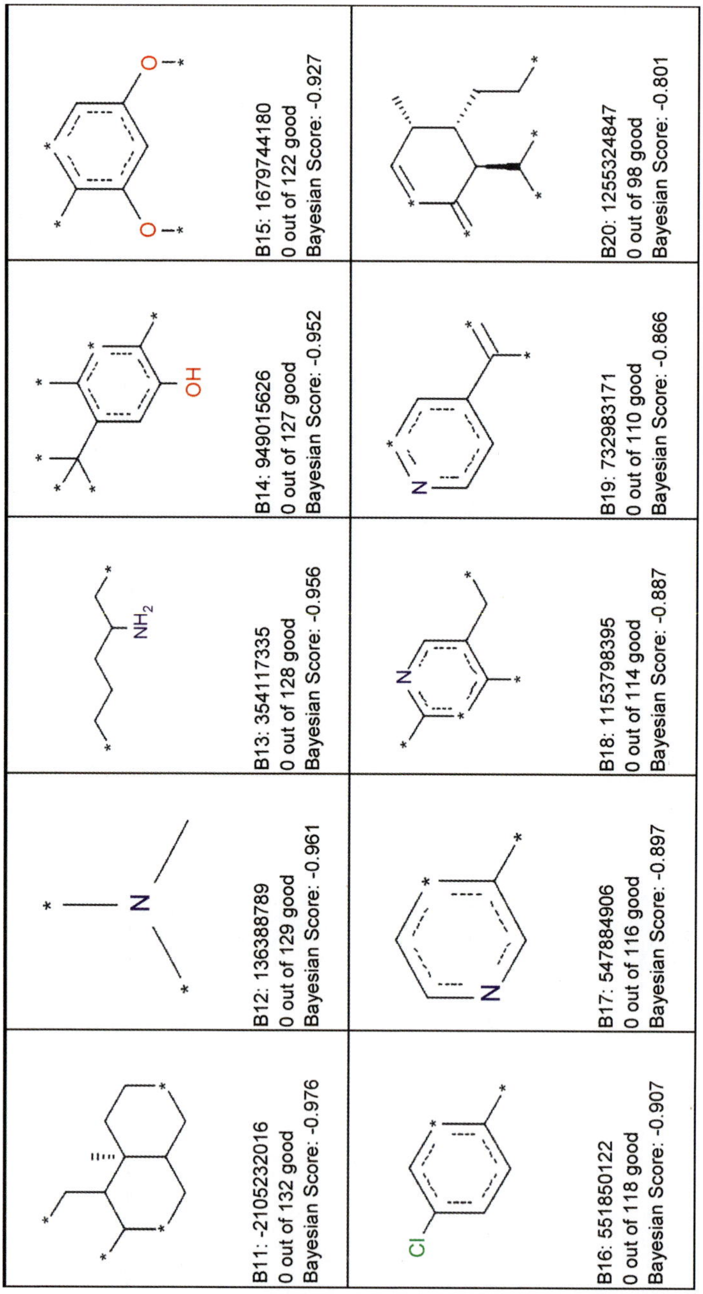

B11: -2105232016
0 out of 132 good
Bayesian Score: -0.976

B12: 136388789
0 out of 129 good
Bayesian Score: -0.961

B13: 3541117335
0 out of 128 good
Bayesian Score: -0.956

B14: 949015626
0 out of 127 good
Bayesian Score: -0.952

B15: 1679744180
0 out of 122 good
Bayesian Score: -0.927

B16: 551850122
0 out of 118 good
Bayesian Score: -0.907

B17: 547884906
0 out of 116 good
Bayesian Score: -0.897

B18: 1153798395
0 out of 114 good
Bayesian Score: -0.887

B19: 732983171
0 out of 110 good
Bayesian Score: -0.866

B20: 1255324847
0 out of 98 good
Bayesian Score: -0.801

Figure 5.2 (*Continued*)

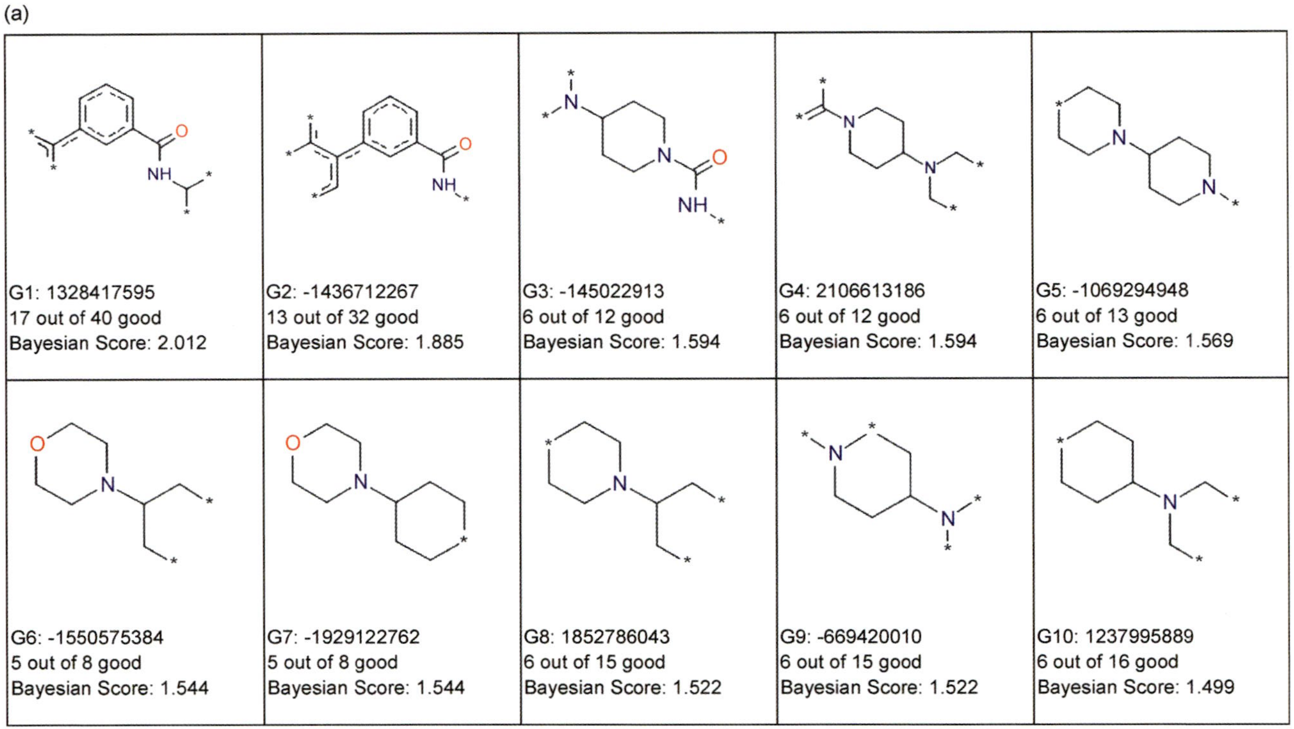

(a)

G1: 1328417595	G2: -1436712267	G3: -145022913	G4: 2106613186	G5: -1069294948
17 out of 40 good	13 out of 32 good	6 out of 12 good	6 out of 12 good	6 out of 13 good
Bayesian Score: 2.012	Bayesian Score: 1.885	Bayesian Score: 1.594	Bayesian Score: 1.594	Bayesian Score: 1.569
G6: -1550575384	G7: -1929122762	G8: 1852786043	G9: -669420010	G10: 1237995889
5 out of 8 good	5 out of 8 good	6 out of 15 good	6 out of 15 good	6 out of 16 good
Bayesian Score: 1.544	Bayesian Score: 1.544	Bayesian Score: 1.522	Bayesian Score: 1.522	Bayesian Score: 1.499

Figure 5.3 *T. brucei* UCSF dataset: (a) good features for activity and (b) bad features for activity.

G11: 1766792939
6 out of 17 good
Bayesian Score: 1.477

G12: -1459071555
8 out of 31 good
Bayesian Score: 1.460

G13: -496622026
6 out of 19 good
Bayesian Score: 1.434

G14: 277616995
7 out of 27 good
Bayesian Score: 1.412

G15: -469219613
7 out of 27 good
Bayesian Score: 1.412

G16: 1884057863
7 out of 27 good
Bayesian Score: 1.412

G17: -1448737182
5 out of 17 good
Bayesian Score: 1.323

G18: 1426409825
10 out of 56 good
Bayesian Score: 1.309

G19: -343334360
4 out of 10 good
Bayesian Score: 1.308

G20: -1171019670
5 out of 18 good
Bayesian Score: 1.301

Figure 5.3 *(Continued)*

(b)

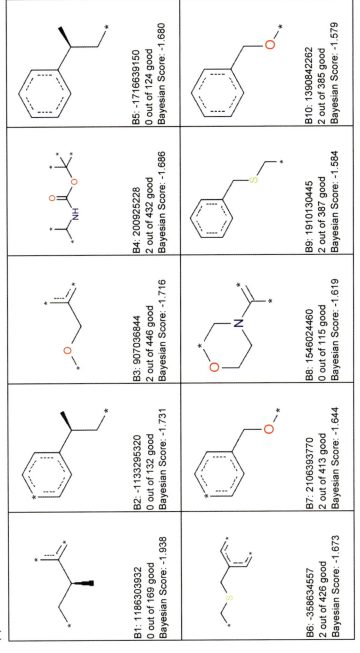

B1: 1186303932
0 out of 169 good
Bayesian Score: -1.938

B2: -1133295320
0 out of 132 good
Bayesian Score: -1.731

B3: 907036844
2 out of 446 good
Bayesian Score: -1.716

B4: 200925228
2 out of 432 good
Bayesian Score: -1.686

B5: -1716639150
0 out of 124 good
Bayesian Score: -1.680

B6: -358634557
2 out of 426 good
Bayesian Score: -1.673

B7: 2106393770
2 out of 413 good
Bayesian Score: -1.644

B8: 1546024460
0 out of 115 good
Bayesian Score: -1.619

B9: 1910130445
2 out of 387 good
Bayesian Score: -1.584

B10: 1390842262
2 out of 385 good
Bayesian Score: -1.579

Figure 5.3 (*Continued*)

B11: -1581865633
0 out of 106 good
Bayesian Score: -1.554

B12: -1525101452
1 out of 236 good
Bayesian Score: -1.537

B13: 1545215786
0 out of 102 good
Bayesian Score: -1.524

B14: 1572957466
2 out of 352 good
Bayesian Score: -1.496

B15: -363392379
0 out of 98 good
Bayesian Score: -1.493

B16: -252328621
2 out of 350 good
Bayesian Score: -1.490

B17: -1696815507
0 out of 94 good
Bayesian Score: -1.460

B18: -2104106152
0 out of 94 good
Bayesian Score: -1.460

B19: -344785855
2 out of 335 good
Bayesian Score: -1.450

B20: -1000107659
2 out of 333 good
Bayesian Score: -1.444

Figure 5.3 *(Continued)*

Discussion

We are clearly at the start of a new era for drug discovery involving more collaborative databases such as HEOS® (for all private data; http://accelrys.com/products/informatics/cheminformatics/heos.html) [27], and CDD (for private, collaborative, and open data) [20,23,24]. These technologies have become widely adopted, supporting thousands of researchers around the world who routinely trust these hosted systems. We have described the development of the CDD database in detail and suggest that, as with TB, it could be used to connect researchers working on finding inhibitors for trypanosomal disease and, more widely, protozoan diseases. In the space of 8 years this database has become a viable technology that has attracted many research foundations, academics, biotechs, and large pharma customers. In the process we have used it to provide new insights into the vast amounts of screening data being produced [24] as well as facilitate global collaborations [20] and provide a means for collaboration [28–31]. We have also described how the large datasets that are stored in CDD public can be used as a resource for machine learning models that may then be used to filter libraries of compounds for testing. We have highlighted molecular features that may be important for activity (Figures 5.2a and 5.3a) and those to avoid (Figures 5.2b and 5.3b). Based on analysis of the trypanosomal disease literature this represents the first example we are aware of in which this approach has been taken, in contrast to the docking and limited QSAR studies listed in Table 5.2. In the future, compounds described in the datasets in Table 5.2 could be collated and used to create additional trypanosomal disease related datasets in CDD.

Cloud-based technologies like CDD represent the future for drug discovery and this technology is being pioneered in the neglected disease community. We believe that the efficiencies possible using collaborative technologies for neglected disease drug discovery will be generally applicable to all commercial drug discovery too, because the data security and selective sharing needs of neglected disease researchers really do parallel those of commercial researchers. The mobility of researchers and technologies may also argue that such collaborative tools and datasets should be as functional as on the desktop when accessed by tablets and smart phones [32].

Acknowledgments

The authors gratefully acknowledge Drs Michael Pollastri, Robert Campbell, Jim McKerrow, and Kip Guy, our colleagues, and the many researchers in the CDD community who have collaborated with us and each other. S.E. gratefully acknowledges Accelrys for providing access to Discovery Studio. The CDD TB database is funded by the Bill and Melinda Gates Foundation (grant 49852 "Collaborative drug discovery for TB through a novel database of SAR data optimized to promote data archiving and sharing").

References

1 Jacobs, R.T., Nare, B., and Phillips, M.A. (2011) State of the art in African trypanosome drug discovery. *Curr. Top. Med. Chem.*, **11**, 1255–1274.

2 McKerrow, J.H., Doyle, P.S., Engel, J.C., Podust, L.M., Robertson, S.A., Ferreira, R., Saxton, T., Arkin, M., Kerr, I.D., Brinen, L.S., and Craik, C.S. (2009) Two approaches to discovering and developing new drugs for Chagas disease. *Mem. Inst. Oswaldo Cruz*, **104** (Suppl. 1), 263–269.

3 Muskavitch, M.A., Barteneva, N., and Gubbels, M.J. (2008) Chemogenomics and parasitology: small molecules and cell-based assays to study infectious processes. *Comb. Chem. High Throughput Screen*, **11**, 624–646.

4 Mackey, Z.B., Baca, A.M., Mallari, J.P., Apsel, B., Shelat, A., Hansell, E.J., Chiang, P.K., Wolff, B., Guy, K.R., Williams, J., and McKerrow, J.H. (2006) Discovery of trypanocidal compounds by whole-cell HTS of *Trypanosoma brucei. Chem. Biol. Drug Des.*, **67**, 355–363.

5 Engel, J.C., Ang, K.K., Chen, S., Arkin, M. R., McKerrow, J.H., and Doyle, P.S. (2010) Image-based high-throughput drug screening targeting the intracellular stage of *Trypanosoma cruzi*, the agent of Chagas' disease. *Antimicrob. Agents Chemother.*, **54**, 3326–3334.

6 Cho, Y., Vermeire, J.J., Merkel, J.S., Leng, L., Du, X., Bucala, R., Cappello, M., and Lolis, E. (2011) Drug repositioning and pharmacophore identification in the discovery of hookworm MIF inhibitors. *Chem. Biol.*, **18**, 1089–1101.

7 Abdulla, M.H., Ruelas, D.S., Wolff, B., Snedecor, J., Lim, K.C., Xu, F., Renslo, A. R., Williams, J., McKerrow, J.H., and Caffrey, C.R. (2009) Drug discovery for schistosomiasis: hit and lead compounds identified in a library of known drugs by medium-throughput phenotypic screening. *PLoS Negl. Trop. Dis.*, **3**, e478.

8 Ekins, S., Williams, A.J., Krasowski, M.D., and Freundlich, J.S. (2011) *In silico* repositioning of approved drugs for rare and neglected diseases. *Drug Discov. Today*, **16**, 298–310.

9 Ekins, S. and Williams, A.J. (2011) Finding promiscuous old drugs for new uses. *Pharm. Res.*, **28**, 1786–1791.

10 Andriani, G., Chessler, A.D., Courtemanche, G., Burleigh, B.A., and Rodriguez, A. (2011) Activity *in vivo* of anti-*Trypanosoma cruzi* compounds selected from a high throughput screening. *PLoS Negl. Trop. Dis.*, **5**, e1298.

11 Ferreira, R.S., Simeonov, A., Jadhav, A., Eidam, O., Mott, B.T., Keiser, M.J., McKerrow, J.H., Maloney, D.J., Irwin, J.J., and Shoichet, B.K. (2010) Complementarity between a docking and a high-throughput screen in discovering new cruzain inhibitors. *J. Med. Chem.*, **53**, 4891–4905.

12 Ekins, S., Freundlich, J.S., Choi, I., Sarker, M., and Talcott, C. (2011) Computational databases, pathway and cheminformatics tools for tuberculosis drug discovery. *Trends Microbiol.*, **19**, 65–74.

13 Carpy, A.J. and Marchand-Geneste, N. (2006) Structural e-bioinformatics and drug design. *SAR QSAR Environ. Res.*, **17**, 1–10.

14 Ertl, P. and Jelfs, S. (2007) Designing drugs on the internet? Free web tools and services supporting medicinal chemistry. *Curr. Top. Med. Chem.*, **7**, 1491–1501.

15 Munos, B. (2006) Can open-source R&D reinvigorate drug research? *Nat. Rev. Drug Discov.*, **5**, 723–729.

16 Tralau-Stewart, C.J., Wyatt, C.A., Kleyn, D. E., and Ayad, A. (2009) Drug discovery: new models for industry–academic partnerships. *Drug Discov. Today*, **14**, 95–101.

17 Williams, A.J. (2008) Internet-based tools for communication and collaboration in chemistry. *Drug Discov. Today*, **13**, 502–506.

18 Williams, A.J. (2008) A perspective of publicly accessible/open-access chemistry databases. *Drug Discov. Today*, **13**, 495–501.

19 Nwaka, S. and Ridley, R.G. (2003) Virtual drug discovery and development for neglected diseases through public–private partnerships. *Nat. Rev. Drug Discov.*, **2**, 919–928.

20 Hohman, M., Gregory, K., Chibale, K., Smith, P.J., Ekins, S., and Bunin, B. (2009)

Novel web-based tools combining chemistry informatics, biology and social networks for drug discovery. *Drug Discov. Today*, **14**, 261–270.

21 Metz, J.T., Huth, J.R., and Hajduk, P.J. (2007) Enhancement of chemical rules for predicting compound reactivity towards protein thiol groups. *J. Comput. Aided Mol Des.*, **21**, 139–144.

22 Huth, J.R., Mendoza, R., Olejniczak, E.T., Johnson, R.W., Cothron, D.A., Liu, Y., Lerner, C.G., Chen, J., and Hajduk, P.J. (2005) ALARM NMR: a rapid and robust experimental method to detect reactive false positives in biochemical screens. *J. Am. Chem. Soc.*, **127**, 217–224.

23 Ekins, S., Kaneko, T., Lipinksi, C.A., Bradford, J., Dole, K., Spektor, A., Gregory, K., Blondeau, D., Ernst, S., Yang, J., Goncharoff, N., Hohman, M., and Bunin, B. (2010) Analysis and hit filtering of a very large library of compounds screened against *Mycobacterium tuberculosis. Mol. BioSyst.*, **6**, 2316–2324.

24 Ekins, S., Bradford, J., Dole, K., Spektor, A., Gregory, K., Blondeau, D., Hohman, M., and Bunin, B. (2010) A collaborative database and computational models for tuberculosis drug discovery. *Mol. BioSystems*, **6**, 840–851.

25 Ekins, S. and Freundlich, J.S. (2011) Validating new tuberculosis computational models with public whole-cell screening aerobic activity datasets. *Pharm. Res.*, **28**, 1859–1869.

26 Sarker, M., Talcott, C., Madrid, P., Chopra, S., Bunin, B.A., Lamichhane, G., Freundlich, J.S., and Ekins, S. (2012) Combining Cheminformatics methods and pathway analysis to identify molecules with whole cell activity against Mycobacterium tuberculosis. *Pharm. Res.*, **29**, 2115–2127.

27 Bost, F., Jacobs, R.T., and Kowalczyk, P. (2010) Informatics for neglected diseases collaborations. *Curr. Opin. Drug Discov. Dev.*, **13**, 286–296.

28 Ekins, S. and Williams, A.J. (2010) Reaching out to collaborators: crowdsourcing for pharmaceutical research. *Pharm. Res.*, **27**, 393–395.

29 Williams, A.J., Tkachenko, V., Lipinski, C., Tropsha, A., and Ekins, S. (2009) Free online resources enabling crowdsourced drug discovery. *Drug Discov. World*, **10** (Winter), 33–38.

30 Louise-May, S., Bunin, B., and Ekins, S. (2009) Towards integrated web-based tools in drug discovery. *Touch Brief. Drug Discov.*, **6**, 17–21.

31 Bingham, A. and Ekins, S. (2009) Competitive collaboration in the pharmaceutical and biotechnology industry. *Drug Discov. Today*, **14**, 1079–1081.

32 Williams, A.J., Ekins, S., Clark, A.M., Jack, J.J., and Apodaca, R.L. (2011) Mobilizing chemistry in the world of drug discovery. *Drug Discov. Today*, **16**, 928–939.

33 Freymann, D.M., Wenck, M.A., Engel, J.C., Feng, J., Focia, P.J., Eakin, A.E., and Craig, S.P. (2000) Efficient identification of inhibitors targeting the closed active site conformation of the HPRT from *Trypanosoma cruzi. Chem. Biol.*, **7**, 957–968.

34 Martinez-Merino, V. and Cerecetto, H. (2001) CoMFA-SIMCA model for antichagasic nitrofurazone derivatives. *Bioorg. Med. Chem.*, **9**, 1025–1030.

35 Khabnadideh, S., Pez, D., Musso, A., Brun, R., Perez, L.M., Gonzalez-Pacanowska, D., and Gilbert, I.H. (2005) Design, synthesis and evaluation of 2,4-diaminoquinazolines as inhibitors of trypanosomal and leishmanial dihydrofolate reductase. *Bioorg. Med. Chem.*, **13**, 2637–2649.

36 Prieto, J.J., Talevi, A., and Bruno-Blanch, L. E. (2006) Application of linear discriminant analysis in the virtual screening of antichagasic drugs through trypanothione reductase inhibition. *Mol. Divers.*, **10**, 361–375.

37 Hudock, M.P., Sanz-Rodriguez, C.E., Song, Y., Chan, J.M., Zhang, Y., Odeh, S., Kosztowski, T., Leon-Rossell, A., Concepcion, J.L., Yardley, V., Croft, S.L., Urbina, J.A., and Oldfield, E. (2006) Inhibition of *Trypanosoma cruzi* hexokinase by bisphosphonates. *J. Med. Chem.*, **49**, 215–223.

38 Guido, R.V., Trossini, G.H., Castilho, M.S., Oliva, G., Ferreira, E.I., and Andricopulo, A.D. (2008) Structure–activity relationships for a class of selective inhibitors of the major cysteine protease from *Trypanosoma cruzi. J. Enzyme. Inhib. Med. Chem.*, **23**, 964–973.

39 Neres, J., Brewer, M.L., Ratier, L., Botti, H., Buschiazzo, A., Edwards, P.N., Mortenson, P.N., Charlton, M.H., Alzari, P.M., Frasch, A.C., Bryce, R.A., and Douglas, K.T. (2009) Discovery of novel inhibitors of *Trypanosoma cruzi* trans-sialidase from *in silico* screening. *Bioorg. Med. Chem. Lett.*, **19**, 589–596.

40 dos Santos Filho, J.M., Leite, A.C., de Oliveira, B.G., Moreira, D.R., Lima, M.S., Soares, M.B., and Leite, L.F. (2009) Design, synthesis and cruzain docking of 3-(4-substituted-aryl)-1,2,4-oxadiazole-*N*-acylhydrazones as anti-*Trypanosoma cruzi* agents. *Bioorg. Med. Chem.*, **17**, 6682–6691.

41 Gayosso-De-Lucio, J., Torres-Valencia, M., Rojo-Dominguez, A., Najera-Pena, H., Aguirre-Lopez, B., Salas-Pacheco, J., Avitia-Dominguez, C., and Tellez-Valencia, A. (2009) Selective inactivation of triosephosphate isomerase from *Trypanosoma cruzi* by brevifolin carboxylate derivatives isolated from *Geranium bellum* Rose. *Bioorg. Med. Chem. Lett.*, **19**, 5936–5939.

42 Gerpe, A., Alvarez, G., Benitez, D., Boiani, L., Quiroga, M., Hernandez, P., Sortino, M., Zacchino, S., Gonzalez, M., and Cerecetto, H. (2009) 5-Nitrofuranes and 5-nitrothiophenes with anti-*Trypanosoma cruzi* activity and ability to accumulate squalene. *Bioorg. Med. Chem.*, **17**, 7500–7509.

43 Vicente, E., Duchowicz, P.R., Benitez, D., Castro, E.A., Cerecetto, H., Gonzalez, M., and Monge, A. (2010) Anti-*T. cruzi* activities and QSAR studies of 3-arylquinoxaline-2-carbonitrile di-*N*-oxides. *Bioorg. Med. Chem. Lett.*, **20**, 4831–4835.

44 Scotti, L., Ferreira, E.I., Silva, M.S., and Scotti, M.T. (2010) Chemometric studies on natural products as potential inhibitors of the NADH oxidase from *Trypanosoma cruzi* using the VolSurf approach. *Molecules*, **15**, 7363–7377.

45 Schormann, N., Velu, S.E., Murugesan, S., Senkovich, O., Walker, K., Chenna, B.C., Shinkre, B., Desai, A., and Chattopadhyay, D. (2010) Synthesis and characterization of potent inhibitors of *Trypanosoma cruzi* dihydrofolate reductase. *Bioorg. Med. Chem.*, **18**, 4056–4066.

46 Sandes, J.M., Borges, A.R., Junior, C.G., Silva, F.P., Carvalho, G.A., Rocha, G.B., Vasconcellos, M.L., and Figueiredo, R.C. (2010) 3-Hydroxy-2-methylene-3-(4-nitrophenylpropanenitrile): a new highly active compound against epimastigote and trypomastigote form of *Trypanosoma cruzi*. *Bioorg. Chem.*, **38**, 190–195.

47 Reimao, J.Q., Scotti, M.T., and Tempone, A.G. (2010) Anti-leishmanial and anti-trypanosomal activities of 1,4-dihydropyridines: *in vitro* evaluation and structure-activity relationship study. *Bioorg. Med. Chem.*, **18**, 8044–8053.

Part Two
Metabolic Peculiarities in the Trypanosomatid Family Guiding Drug Discovery

Trypanosomatid Diseases: Molecular Routes to Drug Discovery, First edition. Edited by T. Jäger, O. Koch, and L. Flohé.
© 2013 Wiley-VCH Verlag GmbH & Co. KGaA. Published 2013 by Wiley-VCH Verlag GmbH & Co. KGaA.

6

Interaction of *Leishmania* Parasites with Host Cells and its Functional Consequences

*Uta Schurigt, Anita Masic, and Heidrun Moll**

Abstract

Research into the discovery of drugs and vaccines for leishmaniasis has been strongly hampered for many reasons, including the vast complexity of the interactions of *Leishmania* parasites with neutrophils, macrophages, and dendritic cells. These phagocytes represent some of the most important players in innate and adaptive immunity, and are largely responsible for elimination of intracellular pathogens. However, *Leishmania* developed successful strategies to escape the microbicidal effector mechanisms of these host cells and finally to manipulate the cellular immune response for their own benefit. Although leishmaniasis belongs to the so-called neglected diseases, there has been much progress in understanding the cell biology and immunology of *Leishmania*–host cell relationships during the last two decades. In this chapter, we address various aspects of *Leishmania*–host interactions and their effects on the outcome of infection. Furthermore, we discuss the mechanisms of parasite evasion of host cell functions, in particular with regard to the formation of parasitophorous vacuoles, manipulation of transcription factor activity, signal transduction pathways, and cytokine expression. The manipulation of host cell functions by secretion of parasitic molecules into the phagosomal compartment is also discussed. Other points of interest are the functional consequences of dendritic cell–*Leishmania* interaction with regard to T helper type 1 and type 2 responses. The majority of studies on *Leishmania*–host cell interactions are based on *in vitro* experiments with murine cells or *in vivo* experiments with *Leishmania*-infected mice. Altogether, the knowledge about *Leishmania*–host interactions collected in the murine model will facilitate the development of novel strategies to combat *Leishmania* infections in humans.

Life Cycle of *Leishmania*

The biphasic life cycle of *Leishmania* is relatively simple compared to other eukaryotic parasitic protozoa. There are two morphologically distinct main differentiation stages known as promastigotes and amastigotes, which replicate asexually [1].

* Corresponding Author

Trypanosomatid Diseases: Molecular Routes to Drug Discovery, First edition. Edited by T. Jäger, O. Koch, and L. Flohé.
© 2013 Wiley-VCH Verlag GmbH & Co. KGaA. Published 2013 by Wiley-VCH Verlag GmbH & Co. KGaA.

Promastigotes live in the midgut of female sandflies and are characterized by a long lancet-like cell body with a flagellum, which is responsible for motility [1]. Amastigotes – the clinically relevant form – are roundish and unflagellated, and replicate intracellularly in host cells. Leishmaniasis is an insect vector-transmitted infectious disease of humans and animals. Female sandflies – 2- to 3-mm-long blood-sucking insects (*Phlebotomus* species in the Old World: Europe, Africa, and Asia; *Lutzomyia* species in the New World: South and Central America) – acquire *Leishmania* parasites when they feed on an infected mammalian host. Amastigotes are released after host cell rupture into the insect midgut and differentiate into promastigotes. The weakly motile procyclic promastigotes colonize the insect midgut by fast replication and finally differentiate during metacyclogenesis into highly motile metacyclic promastigotes [1–3]. Metacyclic promastigotes, being infective for mammals, have an altered protein expression and their ability to modulate the host immune response is more pronounced than that of the procyclic form [4–7]. They are transmitted to a new mammalian host when an infected female sandfly takes a subsequent blood meal, and are ingested by recruited macrophages and other host cells including dendritic cells (DCs) and neutrophils. The differentiation into the amastigote stage takes place in endocytic vacuoles termed parasitophorous vacuoles (PVs). After replication by binary fission, amastigotes are released from macrophages and other host cells to infect new phagocytes.

Host Cells of *Leishmania*

Amastigotes live as intracellular parasites in a variety of mammalian cells, predominantly professional phagocytes such as neutrophils, macrophages, and DCs. However, recent studies demonstrated that *Leishmania* also infect skin and lymph node fibroblasts [8–10]. In addition, cells not harboring *Leishmania* contribute to disease outcome. Platelets in the blood pool at the inoculation site are among the first effector cells of the innate immune system interacting with *Leishmania* [11]. Keratinocytes in the epidermis also play a critical role in the initiation of a protective immune response to *Leishmania* by secretion of immunomodulating molecules [12]. This chapter will focus on interactions between *Leishmania* and its phagocytic host cells.

Neutrophils

Neutrophils are the major class of white blood cells in the peripheral blood and constitute the first line of host defense. Neutrophil granules contain preformed proteinases and antimicrobial proteins that are able to degrade pathogens [13]. Oxygen metabolites and lytic enzymes released from the granules kill invading microorganisms after phagocytosis [13]. *Leishmania* are able to manipulate neutrophil functions. However, it is a current subject of debate whether neutrophils play a protective or a non-protective role in leishmaniasis. Experimental findings with neutrophils seem to be dependent on the investigated *Leishmania* species and mouse strains, the antibodies selected for neutrophil depletion, and the infection state of neutrophils. Several potentially disease-promoting functions of neutrophils have been reported. An attractive hypothesis is the "Trojan horse" model describing the strategy of *L. major* promastigotes to infect macrophages without the induction of an immune response by hiding in neutrophils presenting non-danger surface signals of apoptotic cells [14]. Promastigotes release *Leishmania* chemotactic factor (LCF) to actively recruit neutrophils without subsequent activation of their lethal effector functions [15]. Other leukocytes, such as monocytes or natural killer (NK) cells, are not attracted [15]. A study investigating the interaction of naturally transmitted fluorescent *L. major* parasites with neutrophils and macrophages in living mice using two-photon microscopy confirmed that neutrophils are indeed the first cells that phagocytose *L. major* promastigotes [16]. *Leishmania* inhibits the spontaneous apoptosis of normally short-living neutrophils [17,18]. However, neutrophil apoptosis is induced after the influx of macrophages to the infection site to ensure a silent uptake of these *Leishmania*-infected host cells [19]. The induction of transforming growth factor (TGF)-β after phagocytosis of apoptotic infected neutrophils promotes additionally the replication of intracellular parasites in macrophages [20,21]. *Leishmania* downregulate the production of interferon (IFN)-γ–inducible protein (IP)-10 by neutrophils to avoid the recruitment of inflammatory anti-leishmanial NK cells and T helper (T_h) type 1 (T_h1) cells, and therefore a protective immune response [15]. *Leishmania*-infected neutrophils secrete macrophage inflammatory protein (MIP)-1β to recruit macrophages, the most important host cells for replication and survival of the parasite [22]. However, several experimental studies stand in strong contrast to these disease-promoting functions of neutrophils. Uninfected neutrophils significantly reduce the parasite load in macrophages infected with *L. braziliensis* in coculture experiments *in vitro* [23,24]. Depletion of neutrophils in *L. braziliensis*- or *L. donovani*-infected mice significantly increases the parasite load of macrophages *in vivo* [24,25]. Furthermore, neutrophils contribute to the elimination of *Leishmania* through the release of neutrophil extracellular traps [26,27]. However, even this mechanism normally involved in the elimination of microorganisms could facilitate the uptake of *Leishmania* by macrophages recruited to the site of inflammation and, therefore, increase the parasite load of macrophages.

Macrophages

Manipulation of Macrophage Functions

Macrophages are large mononuclear phagocytic cells that are important in innate immunity in the early non-adaptive phase of host defense. They act as scavengers that can engulf dead cells, foreign substances, other debris, and pathogens. Furthermore, macrophages also act as antigen-presenting cells and as effector cells in humoral and cell-mediated adaptive immunity. It is generally accepted that macrophages are the major host cells for *Leishmania* replication and long-term survival. A prerequisite is the ability of *Leishmania* to inhibit the microbicidal activities of macrophages in order to survive the harsh antimicrobial environment, to escape the lysosomal digestion in host cell phagolysosomes, and to subvert the innate and adaptive immune defense system.

Some of the most important macrophage effector mechanisms (e.g., the expression of inducible nitric oxide synthase (iNOS) and of major histocompatibility complex (MHC) class II) are induced by IFN-γ followed by protein phosphorylation in the Janus kinase/signal transducer and activator of transcription (JAK/STAT) and the mitogen-activated protein kinase (MAPK) pathways [28]. A key mechanism of *Leishmania* to manipulate these signal transduction cascades is the activation of host cell phosphatases and their expression [29,30]. *L. donovani* infection markedly up-regulates the expression of MAPK phosphatases (MKP)1, MKP3, and PP2A that dephosphorylate ERK1/2 and p38 [30]. In addition, the protein tyrosine phosphatase (PTP) SHP-1 is proteolytically activated by GP63 immediately after infection [29]. GP63 is a parasitic zinc metalloprotease that is the most abundant surface protein of *Leishmania* promastigotes [31,32]. A soluble form of GP63 with an acidic pH optimum is expressed by *Leishmania* amastigotes, suggesting a delivery into the acidic environment of amastigotes in the PV [31]. Activated SHP-1 dephosphorylates JAK1 and JAK2 in *Leishmania*-infected macrophages in response to IFN-γ [33,34]. In addition, the activity of iNOS that catalyzes the production of the microbicidal gas NO from the amino acid L-arginine is impaired after SHP-1 activation [34]. In agreement with this, NO synthesis cannot be completely inhibited in IFN-γ-activated *Leishmania*-infected macrophages generated from SHP-1-deficient mice [33,34].

Synthesis of NO by iNOS is one of the most important microbicidal mechanisms of innate immunity. Experiments with iNOS-deficient mice of a genetically resistant background becoming susceptible for *Leishmania* infections demonstrated the central role of NO for disease control [35]. L-Arginine cannot only be oxidized by host iNOS to produce NO, it can also be hydrolyzed by macrophage arginase 1 to ornithine and urea, which support parasite proliferation. Interestingly, *Leishmania* encode a parasitic arginase, which cooperates with host arginase activity to improve parasite survival [36]. The balance between activities of iNOS and arginases, enzymes that compete for the substrate L-arginine, is of crucial importance for the outcome of *L. major* infections and is influenced by the T_h cell cytokines IFN-γ and IL-4.

The phosphatidylinositol-3 kinase (PI3K) pathway is a signal transduction cascade that is central to a variety of basic physiological functions, including protein synthesis, apoptosis, and autophagy. Two important downstream effector molecules of PI3K are Akt and the mammalian target of rapamycin (mTOR). Interestingly, PI3K, Akt, and mTOR are involved in the regulation of anti-inflammatory (e.g., IL-10) and pro-inflammatory cytokines (e.g., IL-12 and tumor necrosis factor (TNF)-α) in infected and uninfected cells, and therefore control innate immune functions [37,38]. Infection of macrophages with *L. major*, *L. pifanoi*, and *L. amazonensis* activates the PI3K/Akt signaling pathway [39,40]. *L. amazonensis* stimulation of PI3K/Akt signaling results in a strong downregulation of IL-12 p70 at the level of its p40 subunit in macrophages [40]. Phosphorylated Akt is detectable in macrophages within a few minutes after infection with *L. amazonen*sis and is maintained throughout the first 24 h of infection [40]. Inhibition of Akt phosphorylation by the PI3K-specific inhibitor wortmannin in infected macrophages relieves IL-12 p40 production at the level of transcription [40]. Rapamycin-mediated mTOR inactivation increased IL-12 p40 production by *L. amazonensis-* and *L. donovani*-infected macrophages [38,40]. Furthermore, the resistance of *Leishmania*-infected macrophages to stauroporine-induced apoptosis can be reversed by application of PI3K- or Akt-specific inhibitors [39]. Treatment of macrophages with small interfering RNA against Akt also resulted in the inability of infected macrophages to resist apoptosis [39]. The pro-apoptotic molecule BAD – a well-characterized substrate of Akt – is phosphorylated during *L. major* and *L. amazonensis* infections, and, therefore, unable to promote the release of cytochrome *c* from mitochondria – a key event in apoptosis induction [39,41]. mTOR is a critical regulator of autophagy induction. Autophagic processes are frequently involved in the degradation of intracellular pathogens and the modulation of immune responses [42]. However, some microbes have developed multiple strategies to avoid autophagolysosomal degradation and, in some cases, intracellular microorganisms take advantage of this cellular process to support the infection [42]. mTOR activates protein synthesis at the translational level through the direct phosphorylation of the translation initiation factor 4E-binding protein 1 (4E-BP1) [43]. Proteolytical cleavage of mTOR by GP63 of *L. major* and, therefore, inhibition of 4E-BP1 phosphorylation leads to a decrease of translational activity in infected macrophages [44]. Furthermore, pharmacological inhibition of 4E-BP phosphorylation by the autophagy inducer rapamycin promotes *L. major* replication and survival [44,45]. Starvation – a further condition that stimulates autophagy – actually increases the intracellular load of *L. amazonensis* in BALB/c mice [45]. *L. mexicana* utilize the autophagic pathway to support intracellular survival by delivery of cytosolic macromolecules from host cells to the PV of *L. mexicana* via the autophagic pathway for catabolic degradation [46]. Currently, small inhibitors targeting the key players in the PI3K/Akt/mTOR pathway are in development to treat chronic and infectious diseases. Screening of these libraries with *Leishmania*-infected macrophages may allow the identification of new potential drug candidates to combat leishmaniasis. Blocking Akt and mTOR may be an attractive strategy to bypass the cytokine deviation by the parasite and boost the host immune response during leishmaniasis. The development of new leishmanicidal drugs interfering with the autophagic pathway may also be of great interest. However, the manipulation of the PI3K/Akt/mTOR pathway by *Leishmania* is very complex, has not been fully understood yet, and seems to be *Leishmania* species- and host cell-specific.

Proteolytical modification of transcription factors and cytokines by parasitic proteases is a further strategy of *Leishmania* to influence signal transduction cascades and the cytokine milieu during infection [47–49]. c-Jun, the central component of activated protein-1 (AP-1), an important transcription factor regulating the expression of pro-inflammatory cytokines and chemokines, is directly cleaved by GP63 [47]. The transcription factor nuclear factor "kappa light chain enhancer" of activated B cells (NF-κB) is a further substrate of GP63 and is also cleaved by cysteine protease B, resulting in the expression of disease-promoting chemokines and the inhibition of IL-12 expression [48,49]. TGF-β, a pro-leishmanial cytokine, is proteolytically activated by the cathepsin B-like cysteine cathepsin CPC [50,51]. In addition, the cytokine milieu during infection is influenced by the secretion of parasitic orthologs of host cell cytokines. Two macrophage migration inhibitory factor (MIF)-like proteins are expressed by *Leishmania* and modulate host macrophage responses [52]. The exact role of host MIF and parasitic MIF-like proteins, which also have tautomerase activity, is not fully understood yet. However, macrophage MIF plays an important role in infection outcome [53,54]. Pharmacological targeting of MIF-like proteins (e.g., with small tautomerase inhibitors) may offer therapeutic benefit. New technologies are applied to identify additional parasite molecules – potential drug targets – that are preferentially expressed in infected cells and secreted into the PV [55].

Parasitophorous Vacuoles in Macrophages
In macrophages, *Leishmania* survive and multiply within PVs. Two main types of PVs exist that differ significantly in morphology and depend on the infecting *Leishmania* species. The Old World *Leishmania* species (e.g., *L. tropica*, *L. donovani*, and *L. major*) occupy small individual vacuoles (i.e., type I vacuoles) in which host membranes are tightly wrapped around a single parasite [56,57]. The character of these single vacuoles is maintained during amastigote replication; no communal PVs after parasite replication are being generated [57]. In contrast, the New World *Leishmania* species (e.g., *L. mexicana*, *L. amazonensis*, and *L. pifanoi*) occupy large vacuoles (i.e., type II vacuoles) that contain up to 30 amastigotes [58–60]. In spite of their very different morphology, PVs of Old and New World *Leishmania* species in macrophages share some properties and features. PVs are acidic compartments as demonstrated using weak bases as dyes, for instance Neutral red and Acridine orange [61,62]. The parasites actively participate in the acidification of PVs [62–64]. This acidic pH in PVs is very important for the survival of *Leishmania*. The activity of some leishmanicidal compounds depends on their ability to increase the pH in PVs as it is, for instance, shown for tamoxifen, which is effective against several *Leishmania* species *in vitro* and *in vivo* [65–68]. PVs are hydrolytic compartments containing a range of potential carbon sources, proteins, and other essential nutrients, which are rapidly degraded by mammalian and parasitic enzymes to low-molecular-weight components. Glucose, amino acids, nucleosides, polyamines, and other degradation products are taken up by membrane transporters of amastigotes that are optimally active at acidic pH [69–71]. Cathepsins B, H, and D, proteases with pH optimum in the acidic range, that contribute to protein degradation are concentrated in macrophage PVs [72,73]. Collectively, these findings suggest that *Leishmania* PVs are nutritionally complex compartments with high enzymatic activities. Amastigotes are optimally adapted to these harsh conditions and escape the phagolysosomal digestion [7,63,64,74].

The first step of PV formation is the phagocytosis of *Leishmania* promastigotes. During this process, *Leishmania* promastigotes engage a variety of receptors of macrophages (e.g., complement receptors 1 and 3 (CR1 and 3), and Fcγ receptor (FcγR)) [75–79]. Phagocytosis of *Leishmania* promastigotes by macrophages is a relatively fast process occurring within a couple of minutes [73]. Finally, internalized promastigotes are located in very long narrow compartments limited by a membrane that adopted the exact shape of promastigotes [73]. These phagosomes fuse with late endosomes and lysosomes, which results in the formation of an acidified PV containing the markers of a mature phagolysosome. Finally, PVs in host macrophages are surrounded by a membrane enriched with late endosomal/lysosomal proteins, such as rab7p, LAMP-1, H^+-ATPase, and macrosialin [61,62,73,80]. Lysosomal enzymes such as cathepsins B and D are present [73,80]. PV maturation is transiently delayed by the promastigote stages of *L. major* and *L. donovani* to avoid intracellular digestion by lytic enzymes before the differentiation into the amastigote stage is completed. In particular, the presence of lipophosphoglycan (LPG) on the promastigote surface seems to be responsible for this delay [81,82]. *L. major* promastigotes lacking LPG survive poorly within the PV [82]. Amastigotes can also be internalized by macrophages in a CR3- and FcR-dependent fashion [83,84]. PV maturation after infection of macrophages with amastigotes, characterized by fusion with endosomes and lysosomes, is faster compared to promastigotes as expected by better adaption of this life cycle stage to acidic conditions [73]. Finally, also mature PVs containing *L. donovani* amastigotes are highly fusogenic with organelles of the endocytic pathway [81,85]. Knowledge of the functional state of the PVs such as the intravacuolar pH and the enzymatic composition in the vacuole are important for target-oriented development of new leishmanicidal drugs. The development of drug delivery systems carrying compounds exclusively by phagocytosis to the PV may open the possibility to reduce side-effects by decreasing the applied drug doses.

DCs

DCs are professional antigen-presenting cells specialized in antigen uptake and presentation to T cells within lymphoid organs, thus initiating cellular immunity to infection [86]. Mouse DCs are classified either as plasmacytoid DCs (pDCs) or myeloid DCs (mDCs), like dermal DCs and Langerhans cells (LCs), which act as migratory sentinels [87] being rapidly recruited by the neutrophil-derived chemokine CCL3 to the site of infection [88]. DC activation is characterized by the upregulation and increased expression of MHC class I and II molecules, costimulatory molecules, like CD40, CD80, and CD86, as well as enhanced IL-12 expression [89,90]. Activated DCs have the ability to present antigens via MHC class I to $CD8^+$ T lymphocytes as a result of Fcγ receptor-mediated phagocytosis and via MHC class II to $CD4^+$ T lymphocytes as a result of CR3-mediated phagocytosis of parasites [91]. $CD4^+$ T cells are the most important cell population mediating either susceptibility or resistance to *Leishmania* infections, depending on the predominating T_h subset [92]. Resistance against leishmaniasis is associated with a cytokine milieu dominated by TNF-α and T_h1-derived IFN-γ [93], whereas a T_h2 immune response characterized by IL-4, IL-5, IL-10, and IL-13 correlates with susceptibility [94]. The leishmanicidal activity of alternatively activated macrophages is suppressed upon IL-4-induced arginase 1 expression, consequently promoting early disease progression, while IL-4-induced arginase 1-expressing DCs promote progressive leishmaniasis during the onset of infection [95,96]. Interestingly, *Leishmania* parasites express arginase 1 themselves [97], highlighting one of many immune evasion strategies to ensure parasite survival. The complexity of *Leishmania* parasites leads to strain-specific differences. CD8[+] T cells are another source of IFN-γ, thus mediating immunity to *L. major* [98], but CD8[+] T cells have also been reported to aggravate acute infection with *L. braziliensis* [99] and to enhance the manifestation of chronic *L. donovani* infection [100]. *Leishmania* uptake by mDCs is a highly dynamic process occurring in a FcγR I- and III- or CR3-mediated manner within the first few hours of infection [91,101,102], enabling the parasites to modulate DC functions as well as the DC-induced immune response. *Leishmania* amastigotes are able to suppress DC activation and maturation by various mechanisms, termed "silent entry" [103]. *L. amazonensis*, *L. donovani*, *L. infantum*, *L. pifanoi*, and *L. mexicana* circumvent DC activation by targeting the C-type lectin receptor, ICAM-3-grabbing non-integrin (DC-SIGN) on the surface of DCs [104]. Another potent immune evasion mechanism used by *Leishmania* parasites is the manipulation of the migratory functions of DC. *L. major*-secreted products inhibit the motility of splenic DCs [105] and the skin emigration of LCs is diminished by purified *L. major* LPG [106], indicating the ability of *Leishmania* parasites to alter the transport of antigens to lymphoid tissues [107]. However, the DC maturation status influences the intracellular fate of *Leishmania* parasites. It has been shown that *L. major* promastigotes reduce lysosomal degradation in immature DCs as a consequence of decreased fusion activity of parasite-containing phagosomes with lysosomes, resulting in enhanced parasite survival within the host cell [108]. The fusion retardation in immature DCs allows the differentiation of promastigotes into amastigotes, which are more adapted to the harsh conditions within lysosomal compartments. In contrast, parasite degradation in mature DCs occurs after parasite-containing phagosomes acquire small GTPase Ras-related protein (Rab) 7 and fuse with lysosomes [108]. *Leishmania* amastigotes are potent suppressors of DC functions. Rapid phosphorylation of MAPK and ERK1/2 is mediated by *L. amazonensis* amastigote-derived proteases or proteasomes, whereas phosphorylation of MAPK/ERK occurs with a 4-h delay in DC infected with promastigotes, most likely associated with their differentiation into amastigotes [109]. In contrast to the activation of the MAPK/ERK pathway in *L. amazonensis*-infected DC resulting in the inhibition of IL-12 [110], *L. major* infection mediates the activation of NF-κB and the up-regulation and nuclear translocation of IRF-1 and IRF-8, thus promoting an IL-12- and type I IFN-induced protective T$_h$1 response [111]. PI3K negatively regulates excessive IL-12 secretion by DCs, thus preventing potential immunopathologic and pro-parasitic effects mediated by uncontrolled sensitization and disproportionate physiological responses [112]. These observations document that *Leishmania* parasites developed complex and wide-ranging immune evasion strategies to assure parasite survival within a hostile environment.

Conclusion

Leishmania is a genus of pathogenic trypanosomatid protozoa with a simple life cycle. Studies with various *Leishmania* spp. uncovered a vast complexity of pathogen–host cell interactions. The parasites manipulate effector mechanisms of neutrophils, macrophages, and DCs – some of the most important players of the innate and adaptive immune system, which communicate during infection by direct cell contact and cytokine/chemokine secretion. Manipulation strategies are often *Leishmania* species- and host cell-specific. Therefore, the mechanisms of manipulation of different host cells have to be investigated in more detail in cocultures of *Leishmania* with more than one host cell *in vitro* and particularly in *Leishmania* infection models *in vivo*. Results of these studies may accelerate the development of leishmanicidal drugs and drug delivery systems, which are not only efficient *in vitro* in drug screening assays but also *in vivo* without unexpected side-effects.

References

1 Bates, P.A. (2007) Transmission of *Leishmania* metacyclic promastigotes by phlebotomine sand flies. *Int. J. Parasitol.*, **37**, 1097–1106.

2 Saraiva, E.M., Pinto-da-Silva, L.H., Wanderley, J.L., Bonomo, A.C., Barcinski, M.A. *et al.* (2005) Flow cytometric assessment of *Leishmania* spp metacyclic differentiation: validation by morphological features and specific markers. *Exp. Parasitol.*, **110**, 39–47.

3 Sacks, D.L. (1989) Metacyclogenesis in *Leishmania* promastigotes. *Exp. Parasitol.*, **69**, 100–103.

4 Santos, M.G., Silva, M.F., Zampieri, R. A., Lafraia, R.M., and Floeter-Winter, L. M. (2011) Correlation of meta 1 expression with culture stage, cell morphology and infectivity in *Leishmania* (*Leishmania*) *amazonensis* promastigotes. *Mem. Inst. Oswaldo Cruz*, **106**, 190–193.

5 Matos, D.C., Faccioli, L.A., Cysne-Finkelstein, L., Luca, P.M., Corte-Real, S. *et al.* (2010) Kinetoplastid membrane protein-11 is present in promastigotes and amastigotes of *Leishmania amazonensis* and its surface expression increases during metacyclogenesis. *Mem. Inst. Oswaldo Cruz*, **105**, 341–347.

6 Sartori, A., Oliveira, M.A., Scott, P., and Trinchieri, G. (1997) Metacyclogenesis

modulates the ability of *Leishmania* promastigotes to induce IL-12 production in human mononuclear cells. *J. Immunol.*, **159**, 2849–2857.

7 Campbell, S.M. and Rainey, P.M. (1993) *Leishmania pifanoi*: kinetics of messenger RNA expression during amastigote to promastigote transformation *in vitro*. *Exp. Parasitol.*, **77**, 1–12.

8 Hespanhol, R.C., de Nazare, C.S.M., Meuser, M.B., de Nazareth, S.L.M.M., and Corte-Real, S. (2005) The expression of mannose receptors in skin fibroblast and their involvement in *Leishmania (L.) amazonensis* invasion. *J. Histochem. Cytochem.*, **53**, 35–44.

9 Bogdan, C., Donhauser, N., Doring, R., Röllinghoff, M., Diefenbach, A. *et al.* (2000) Fibroblasts as host cells in latent leishmaniosis. *J. Exp. Med.*, **191**, 2121–2130.

10 de Oliveira Cardoso, F., de Souza Cda, S., Mendes, V.G., Abreu-Silva, A.L., Goncalves da Costa, S.C. *et al.* (2010) Immunopathological studies of *Leishmania amazonensis* infection in resistant and in susceptible mice. *J. Infect. Dis.*, **201**, 1933–1940.

11 Goncalves, R., Zhang, X., Cohen, H., Debrabant, A., and Mosser, D.M. (2011) Platelet activation attracts a subpopulation of effector monocytes to sites of

Leishmania major infection. *J. Exp. Med.*, **208**, 1253–1265.

12 Ehrchen, J.M., Roebrock, K., Foell, D., Nippe, N., von Stebut, E. *et al.* (2010) Keratinocytes determine T_h1 immunity during early experimental leishmaniasis. *PLoS Pathog.*, **6**, e1000871.

13 Mantovani, A., Cassatella, M.A., Costantini, C., and Jaillon, S. (2011) Neutrophils in the activation and regulation of innate and adaptive immunity. *Nat. Rev. Immunol.*, **11**, 519–531.

14 Laskay, T., van Zandbergen, G., and Solbach, W. (2003) Neutrophil granulocytes – Trojan horses for *Leishmania major* and other intracellular microbes? *Trends Microbiol.*, **11**, 210–214.

15 van Zandbergen, G., Hermann, N., Laufs, H., Solbach, W., and Laskay, T. (2002) *Leishmania* promastigotes release a granulocyte chemotactic factor and induce interleukin-8 release but inhibit gamma interferon-inducible protein 10 production by neutrophil granulocytes. *Infect. Immun.*, **70**, 4177–4184.

16 Peters, N.C., Egen, J.G., Secundino, N., Debrabant, A., and Kimblin, N. (2008) *et al.In vivo* imaging reveals an essential role for neutrophils in leishmaniasis transmitted by sand flies. *Science*, **321**, 970–974.

17 Aga, E., Katschinski, D.M., van Zandbergen, G., Laufs, H., Hansen, B. *et al.* (2002) Inhibition of the spontaneous apoptosis of neutrophil granulocytes by the intracellular parasite *Leishmania major*. *J. Immunol.*, **169**, 898–905.

18 Gueirard, P., Laplante, A., Rondeau, C., Milon, G., and Desjardins, M. (2008) Trafficking of *Leishmania donovani* promastigotes in non-lytic compartments in neutrophils enables the subsequent transfer of parasites to macrophages. *Cell. Microbiol.*, **10**, 100–111.

19 Allenbach, C., Zufferey, C., Perez, C., Launois, P., Mueller, C. *et al.* (2006) Macrophages induce neutrophil apoptosis through membrane TNF, a process amplified by *Leishmania major*. *J. Immunol.*, **176**, 6656–6664.

20 Afonso, L., Borges, V.M., Cruz, H., Ribeiro-Gomes, F.L., DosReis, G.A. *et al.* (2008) Interactions with apoptotic but not with necrotic neutrophils increase parasite burden in human macrophages infected with *Leishmania amazonensis*. *J. Leukoc. Biol.*, **84**, 389–396.

21 Ribeiro-Gomes, F.L., Otero, A.C., Gomes, N.A., Moniz-De-Souza, M.C., Cysne-Finkelstein, L. *et al.* (2004) Macrophage interactions with neutrophils regulate *Leishmania major* infection. *J. Immunol.*, **172**, 4454–4462.

22 van Zandbergen, G., Klinger, M., Mueller, A., Dannenberg, S., Gebert, A. *et al.* (2004) Cutting edge: neutrophil granulocyte serves as a vector for *Leishmania* entry into macrophages. *J. Immunol.*, **173**, 6521–6525.

23 de Souza Carmo, E.V., Katz, S., and Barbieri, C.L. (2010) Neutrophils reduce the parasite burden in *Leishmania (Leishmania) amazonensis*-infected macrophages. *PLoS ONE*, **5**, e13815.

24 Novais, F.O., Santiago, R.C., Bafica, A., Khouri, R., Afonso, L. *et al.* (2009) Neutrophils and macrophages cooperate in host resistance against *Leishmania braziliensis* infection. *J. Immunol.*, **183**, 8088–8098.

25 McFarlane, E., Perez, C., Charmoy, M., Allenbach, C., Carter, K.C. *et al.* (2008) Neutrophils contribute to development of a protective immune response during onset of infection with *Leishmania donovani*. *Infect. Immun.*, **76**, 532–541.

26 Gabriel, C., McMaster, W.R., Girard, D., and Descoteaux, A. (2010) *Leishmania donovani* promastigotes evade the antimicrobial activity of neutrophil extracellular traps. *J. Immunol.*, **185**, 4319–4327.

27 Guimaraes-Costa, A.B., Nascimento, M.T., Froment, G.S., Soares, R.P., Morgado, F.N. *et al.* (2009) *Leishmania amazonensis* promastigotes induce and are killed by neutrophil extracellular traps. *Proc. Natl. Acad. Sci. USA*, **106**, 6748–6753.

28 Feng, G.J., Goodridge, H.S., Harnett, M.M., Wei, X.Q., Nikolaev, A.V. *et al.* (1999) Extracellular signal-related kinase (ERK) and p38 mitogen-activated protein (MAP) kinases differentially regulate the lipopolysaccharide-mediated induction of inducible nitric oxide synthase and IL-12

in macrophages: *Leishmania* phosphoglycans subvert macrophage IL-12 production by targeting ERK MAP kinase. *J. Immunol.*, **163**, 6403–6412.

29 Gomez, M.A., Contreras, I., Halle, M., Tremblay, M.L., McMaster, R.W. *et al.* (2009) *Leishmania* GP63 alters host signaling through cleavage-activated protein tyrosine phosphatases. *Sci. Signal,* **2**, ra58.

30 Kar, S., Ukil, A., Sharma, G., and Das, P. K. (2010) MAPK-directed phosphatases preferentially regulate pro- and anti-inflammatory cytokines in experimental visceral leishmaniasis: involvement of distinct protein kinase C isoforms. *J. Leukoc. Biol.*, **88**, 9–20.

31 Hsiao, C.H., Yao, C., Storlie, P., Donelson, J.E., and Wilson, M.E. (2008) The major surface protease (MSP or GP63) in the intracellular amastigote stage of *Leishmania chagasi*. *Mol. Biochem. Parasitol.*, **157**, 148–159.

32 Schneider, P., Rosat, J.P., Bouvier, J., Louis, J., and Bordier, C. (1992) *Leishmania major*: differential regulation of the surface metalloprotease in amastigote and promastigote stages. *Exp. Parasitol.*, **75**, 196–206.

33 Blanchette, J., Abu-Dayyeh, I., Hassani, K., Whitcombe, L., and Olivier, M. (2009) Regulation of macrophage nitric oxide production by the protein tyrosine phosphatase Src homology 2 domain phosphotyrosine phosphatase 1 (SHP-1). *Immunology*, **127**, 123–133.

34 Forget, G., Gregory, D.J., Whitcombe, L. A., and Olivier, M. (2006) Role of host protein tyrosine phosphatase SHP-1 in *Leishmania donovani*-induced inhibition of nitric oxide production. *Infect. Immun.*, **74**, 6272–6279.

35 Wei, X.Q., Charles, I.G., Smith, A., Ure, J., Feng, G.J. *et al.* (1995) Altered immune responses in mice lacking inducible nitric oxide synthase. *Nature*, **375**, 408–411.

36 Muleme, H.M., Reguera, R.M., Berard, A., Azinwi, R., Jia, P. *et al.* (2009) Infection with arginase-deficient *Leishmania major* reveals a parasite number-dependent and cytokine-independent regulation of host cellular arginase activity and disease

pathogenesis. *J. Immunol.*, **183**, 8068–8076.

37 Schmitz, F., Heit, A., Dreher, S., Eisenacher, K., Mages, J. *et al.* (2008) Mammalian target of rapamycin (mTOR) orchestrates the defense program of innate immune cells. *Eur. J. Immunol.*, **38**, 2981–2992.

38 Cheekatla, S.S., Aggarwal, A., and Naik, S. (2012) mTOR signaling pathway regulates the IL-12/IL-10 axis in *Leishmania donovani* infection. *Med. Microbiol. Immunol.*, **201**, 37–46.

39 Ruhland, A., Leal, N., and Kima, P.E. (2007) *Leishmania* promastigotes activate PI3K/Akt signalling to confer host cell resistance to apoptosis. *Cell. Microbiol.*, **9**, 84–96.

40 Ruhland, A. and Kima, P.E. (2009) Activation of PI3K/Akt signaling has a dominant negative effect on IL-12 production by macrophages infected with *Leishmania amazonensis* promastigotes. *Exp. Parasitol.*, **122**, 28–36.

41 Datta, S.R., Dudek, H., Tao, X., Masters, S., Fu, H. *et al.* (1997) Akt phosphorylation of BAD couples survival signals to the cell-intrinsic death machinery. *Cell*, **91**, 231–241.

42 Deretic, V. and Levine, B. (2009) Autophagy, immunity, and microbial adaptations. *Cell Host Microbe*, **5**, 527–549.

43 Zhou, H. and Huang, S. (2010) The complexes of mammalian target of rapamycin. *Curr. Protein Pept. Sci.*, **11**, 409–424.

44 Jaramillo, M., Gomez, M.A., Larsson, O., Shio, M.T., Topisirovic, I. *et al.* (2011) *Leishmania* repression of host translation through mTOR cleavage is required for parasite survival and infection. *Cell Host Microbe*, **9**, 331–341.

45 Pinheiro, R.O., Nunes, M.P., Pinheiro, C. S., D'Avila, H., Bozza, P.T. *et al.* (2009) Induction of autophagy correlates with increased parasite load of *Leishmania amazonensis* in BALB/c but not C57BL/6 macrophages. *Microbes Infect.*, **11**, 181–190.

46 Schaible, U.E., Schlesinger, P.H., Steinberg, T.H., Mangel, W.F., Kobayashi, T. *et al.* (1999) Parasitophorous vacuoles of *Leishmania mexicana* acquire

macromolecules from the host cell cytosol via two independent routes. *J. Cell Sci.*, **112**, 681–693.

47 Contreras, I., Gomez, M.A., Nguyen, O., Shio, M.T., McMaster, R.W. *et al.* (2010) *Leishmania*-induced inactivation of the macrophage transcription factor AP-1 is mediated by the parasite metalloprotease GP63. *PLoS Pathog.*, **6**, e1001148.

48 Gregory, D.J., Godbout, M., Contreras, I., Forget, G., and Olivier, M. (2008) A novel form of NF-kappaB is induced by *Leishmania* infection: involvement in macrophage gene expression. *Eur. J. Immunol.*, **38**, 1071–1081.

49 Cameron, P., McGachy, A., Anderson, M., Paul, A., Coombs, G.H. *et al.* (2004) Inhibition of lipopolysaccharide-induced macrophage IL-12 production by *Leishmania mexicana* amastigotes: the role of cysteine peptidases and the NF-kappaB signaling pathway. *J. Immunol.*, **173**, 3297–3304.

50 Gantt, K.R., Schultz-Cherry, S., Rodriguez, N., Jeronimo, S.M., Nascimento, E.T. *et al.* (2003) Activation of TGF-beta by *Leishmania chagasi*: importance for parasite survival in macrophages. *J. Immunol.*, **170**, 2613–2620.

51 Somanna, A., Mundodi, V., and Gedamu, L. (2002) Functional analysis of cathepsin B-like cysteine proteases from *Leishmania donovani* complex. Evidence for the activation of latent transforming growth factor beta. *J. Biol. Chem.*, **277**, 25305–25312.

52 Kamir, D., Zierow, S., Leng, L., Cho, Y., Diaz, Y. *et al.* (2008) A *Leishmania* ortholog of macrophage migration inhibitory factor modulates host macrophage responses. *J. Immunol.*, **180**, 8250–8261.

53 Satoskar, A.R., Bozza, M., Rodriguez Sosa, M., Lin, G., and David, J.R. (2001) Migration-inhibitory factor gene-deficient mice are susceptible to cutaneous *Leishmania major* infection. *Infect. Immun.*, **69**, 906–911.

54 Juttner, S., Bernhagen, J., Metz, C.N., Röllinghoff, M., Bucala, R. *et al.* (1998) Migration inhibitory factor induces killing of *Leishmania major* by macrophages:

dependence on reactive nitrogen intermediates and endogenous TNF-alpha. *J. Immunol.*, **161**, 2383–2390.

55 Kima, P.E., Bonilla, J.A., Cho, E., Ndjamen, B., Canton, J. *et al.* (2010) Identification of *Leishmania* proteins preferentially released in infected cells using change mediated antigen technology (CMAT). *PLoS Negl. Trop. Dis.*, **4**, e842.

56 Lang, T., Hellio, R., Kaye, P.M., and Antoine, J.C. (1994) *Leishmania donovani*-infected macrophages: characterization of the parasitophorous vacuole and potential role of this organelle in antigen presentation. *J. Cell. Sci.*, **107**, 2137–2150.

57 Castro, R., Scott, K., Jordan, T., Evans, B., Craig, J. *et al.* (2006) The ultrastructure of the parasitophorous vacuole formed by *Leishmania major*. *J. Parasitol.*, **92**, 1162–1170.

58 De Souza Leao, S., Lang, T., Prina, E., Hellio, R., and Antoine, J.C. (1995) Intracellular *Leishmania amazonensis* amastigotes internalize and degrade MHC class II molecules of their host cells. *J. Cell Sci.*, **108**, 3219–3231.

59 Antoine, J.C., Lang, T., Prina, E., Courret, N., and Hellio, R. (1999) H-2M molecules, like MHC class II molecules, are targeted to parasitophorous vacuoles of *Leishmania*-infected macrophages and internalized by amastigotes of *L. amazonensis* and *L. mexicana*. *J. Cell Sci.*, **112**, 2559–2570.

60 Russell, D.G., Xu, S., and Chakraborty, P. (1992) Intracellular trafficking and the parasitophorous vacuole of *Leishmania mexicana*-infected macrophages. *J. Cell Sci.*, **103**, 1193–1210.

61 Rabinovitch, M., Zilberfarb, V., and Ramazeilles, C. (1986) Destruction of *Leishmania mexicana amazonensis* amastigotes within macrophages by lysosomotropic amino acid esters. *J. Exp. Med.*, **163**, 520–535.

62 Antoine, J.C., Prina, E., Jouanne, C., and Bongrand, P. (1990) Parasitophorous vacuoles of *Leishmania amazonensis*-infected macrophages maintain an acidic pH. *Infect. Immun.*, **58**, 779–787.

63 Marchesini, N. and Docampo, R. (2002) A plasma membrane P-type H^+-ATPase regulates intracellular pH in *Leishmania mexicana amazonensis. Mol. Biochem. Parasitol.*, **119**, 225–236.

64 Glaser, T.A., Baatz, J.E., Kreishman, G.P., and Mukkada, A.J. (1988) pH homeostasis in *Leishmania donovani* amastigotes and promastigotes. *Proc. Natl. Acad. Sci. USA*, **85**, 7602–7606.

65 Eissa, M.M., Amer, E.I., and El Sawy, S.M. (2011) *Leishmania major*: activity of tamoxifen against experimental cutaneous leishmaniasis. *Exp. Parasitol.*, **128**, 382–390.

66 Miguel, D.C., Yokoyama-Yasunaka, J.K., Andreoli, W.K., Mortara, R.A., and Uliana, S.R. (2007) Tamoxifen is effective against *Leishmania* and induces a rapid alkalinization of parasitophorous vacuoles harbouring *Leishmania (Leishmania) amazonensis* amastigotes. *J. Antimicrob. Chemother.*, **60**, 526–534.

67 Miguel, D.C., Yokoyama-Yasunaka, J.K., and Uliana, S.R. (2008) Tamoxifen is effective in the treatment of *Leishmania amazonensis* infections in mice. *PLoS Negl. Trop. Dis.*, **2**, e249.

68 Miguel, D.C., Zauli-Nascimento, R.C., Yokoyama-Yasunaka, J.K., Katz, S., Barbieri, C.L. *et al.* (2009) Tamoxifen as a potential antileishmanial agent: efficacy in the treatment of *Leishmania braziliensis* and *Leishmania chagasi* infections. *J. Antimicrob. Chemother.*, **63**, 365–368.

69 Zilberstein, D. and Gepstein, A. (1993) Regulation of L-proline transport in *Leishmania donovani* by extracellular pH. *Mol. Biochem. Parasitol.*, **61**, 197–205.

70 Burchmore, R.J. and Hart, D.T. (1995) Glucose transport in amastigotes and promastigotes of *Leishmania mexicana mexicana. Mol. Biochem. Parasitol.*, **74**, 77–86.

71 Ortiz, D., Sanchez, M.A., Koch, H.P., Larsson, H.P., and Landfear, S.M. (2009) An acid-activated nucleobase transporter from *Leishmania major. J. Biol. Chem.*, **284**, 16164–16169.

72 Prina, E., Antoine, J.C., Wiederanders, B., and Kirschke, H. (1990) Localization and activity of various lysosomal proteases in *Leishmania amazonensis*-infected macrophages. *Infect. Immun.*, **58**, 1730–1737.

73 Courret, N., Frehel, C., Gouhier, N., Pouchelet, M., Prina, E. *et al.* (2002) Biogenesis of *Leishmania*-harbouring parasitophorous vacuoles following phagocytosis of the metacyclic promastigote or amastigote stages of the parasites. *J. Cell Sci.*, **115**, 2303–2316.

74 Lefurgey, A., Gannon, M., Blum, J., and Ingram, P. (2005) *Leishmania donovani* amastigotes mobilize organic and inorganic osmolytes during regulatory volume decrease. *J. Eukaryot. Microbiol.*, **52**, 277–289.

75 Mosser, D.M. and Edelson, P.J. (1985) The mouse macrophage receptor for C3bi (CR3) is a major mechanism in the phagocytosis of *Leishmania* promastigotes. *J. Immunol.*, **135**, 2785–2789.

76 Wozencraft, A.O. and Blackwell, J.M. (1987) Increased infectivity of stationary-phase promastigotes of *Leishmania donovani*: correlation with enhanced C3 binding capacity and CR3-mediated attachment to host macrophages. *Immunology*, **60**, 559–563.

77 Wozencraft, A.O., Sayers, G., and Blackwell, J.M. (1986) Macrophage type 3 complement receptors mediate serum-independent binding of *Leishmania donovani*. Detection of macrophage-derived complement on the parasite surface by immunoelectron microscopy. *J. Exp. Med.*, **164**, 1332–1337.

78 Talamas-Rohana, P., Wright, S.D., Lennartz, M.R., and Russell, D.G. (1990) Lipophosphoglycan from *Leishmania mexicana* promastigotes binds to members of the CR3, p150, 95 and LFA-1 family of leukocyte integrins. *J. Immunol.*, **144**, 4817–4824.

79 Da Silva, R.P., Hall, B.F., Joiner, K.A., and Sacks, D.L. (1989) CR1, the C3b receptor, mediates binding of infective *Leishmania major* metacyclic promastigotes to human macrophages. *J. Immunol.*, **143**, 617–622.

80 Rodriguez, N.E., Gaur Dixit, U., Allen, L. A., and Wilson, M.E. (2011) Stage-specific pathways of *Leishmania infantum chagasi* entry and phagosome maturation in macrophages. *PLoS ONE*, **6**, e19000.

81 Dermine, J.F., Scianimanico, S., Prive, C., Descoteaux, A., and Desjardins, M. (2000)

Leishmania promastigotes require lipophosphoglycan to actively modulate the fusion properties of phagosomes at an early step of phagocytosis. *Cell. Microbiol.*, **2**, 115–126.

82 Späth, G.F., Epstein, L., Leader, B., Singer, S.M., Avila, H.A. *et al.* (2000) Lipophosphoglycan is a virulence factor distinct from related glycoconjugates in the protozoan parasite *Leishmania major*. *Proc. Natl. Acad. Sci. USA*, **97**, 9258–9263.

83 Guy, R.A. and Belosevic, M. (1993) Comparison of receptors required for entry of *Leishmania major* amastigotes into macrophages. *Infect. Immun.*, **61**, 1553–1558.

84 Peters, C., Aebischer, T., Stierhof, Y.D., Fuchs, M., and Overath, P. (1995) The role of macrophage receptors in adhesion and uptake of *Leishmania mexicana* amastigotes. *J. Cell Sci.*, **108**, 3715–3724.

85 Desjardins, M. and Descoteaux, A. (1997) Inhibition of phagolysosomal biogenesis by the *Leishmania* lipophosphoglycan. *J. Exp. Med.*, **185**, 2061–2068.

86 Banchereau, J. and Steinman, R.M. (1998) Dendritic cells and the control of immunity. *Nature*, **392**, 245–252.

87 Wu, L. and Dakic, A. (2004) Development of dendritic cell system. *Cell. Mol. Immunol.*, **1**, 112–118.

88 Charmoy, M., Auderset, F., Allenbach, C., and Tacchini-Cottier, F. (2010) The prominent role of neutrophils during the initial phase of infection by *Leishmania* parasites. *J. Biomed. Biotechnol.*, **2010**, 719361.

89 Inaba, K., Turley, S., Iyoda, T., Yamaide, F., Shimoyama, S. *et al.* (2000) The formation of immunogenic major histocompatibility complex class II-peptide ligands in lysosomal compartments of dendritic cells is regulated by inflammatory stimuli. *J. Exp. Med.*, **191**, 927–936.

90 Moser, M. and Murphy, K.M. (2000) Dendritic cell regulation of T_H1–T_H2 development. *Nat. Immunol.*, **1**, 199–205.

91 Woelbing, F., Kostka, S.L., Moelle, K., Belkaid, Y., Sunderkoetter, C. *et al.* (2006) Uptake of *Leishmania major* by dendritic cells is mediated by Fcgamma receptors and facilitates acquisition of protective immunity. *J. Exp. Med.*, **203**, 177–188.

92 Sacks, D. and Noben-Trauth, N. (2002) The immunology of susceptibility and resistance to *Leishmania major* in mice. *Nat. Rev. Immunol.*, **2**, 845–858.

93 Murray, H.W., Hariprashad, J., and Coffman, R.L. (1997) Behavior of visceral *Leishmania donovani* in an experimentally induced T helper cell 2 (T_h2)-associated response model. *J. Exp. Med.*, **185**, 867–874.

94 Kane, M.M. and Mosser, D.M. (2001) The role of IL-10 in promoting disease progression in leishmaniasis. *J. Immunol.*, **166**, 1141–1147.

95 Holscher, C., Arendse, B., Schwegmann, A., Myburgh, E., and Brombacher, F. (2006) Impairment of alternative macrophage activation delays cutaneous leishmaniasis in nonhealing BALB/c mice. *J. Immunol.*, **176**, 1115–1121.

96 Munder, M., Eichmann, K., Moran, J.M., Centeno, F., Soler, G. *et al.* (1999) T_h1/T_h2-regulated expression of arginase isoforms in murine macrophages and dendritic cells. *J. Immunol.*, **163**, 3771–3777.

97 Roberts, S.C., Tancer, M.J., Polinsky, M.R., Gibson, K.M., Heby, O. *et al.* (2004) Arginase plays a pivotal role in polyamine precursor metabolism in *Leishmania*. Characterization of gene deletion mutants. *J. Biol. Chem.*, **279**, 23668–23678.

98 Belkaid, Y., Von Stebut, E., Mendez, S., Lira, R., Caler, E. *et al.* (2002) $CD8^+$ T cells are required for primary immunity in C57BL/6 mice following low-dose, intradermal challenge with *Leishmania major*. *J. Immunol.*, **168**, 3992–4000.

99 Faria, D.R., Souza, P.E., Duraes, F.V., Carvalho, E.M., Gollob, K.J. *et al.* (2009) Recruitment of $CD8^+$ T cells expressing granzyme A is associated with lesion progression in human cutaneous leishmaniasis. *Parasite Immunol.*, **31**, 432–439.

100 Joshi, T., Rodriguez, S., Perovic, V., Cockburn, I.A., and Stager, S. (2009) B7-H1 blockade increases survival of dysfunctional $CD8^+$ T cells and confers

protection against *Leishmania donovani* infections. *PLoS Pathog.*, **5**, e1000431.

101 Ng, L.G., Hsu, A., Mandell, M.A., Roediger, B., Hoeller, C. *et al.* (2008) Migratory dermal dendritic cells act as rapid sensors of protozoan parasites. *PLoS Pathog.*, **4**, e1000222.

102 Blank, C., Fuchs, H., Rappersberger, K., Röllinghoff, M., and Moll, H. (1993) Parasitism of epidermal Langerhans cells in experimental cutaneous leishmaniasis with *Leishmania major*. *J. Infect. Dis.*, **167**, 418–425.

103 Bennett, C.L., Misslitz, A., Colledge, L., Aebischer, T., and Blackburn, C.C. (2001) Silent infection of bone marrow-derived dendritic cells by *Leishmania mexicana* amastigotes. *Eur. J. Immunol.*, **31**, 876–883.

104 Colmenares, M., Corbi, A.L., Turco, S.J., and Rivas, L. (2004) The dendritic cell receptor DC-SIGN discriminates among species and life cycle forms of *Leishmania*. *J. Immunol.*, **172**, 1186–1190.

105 Jebbari, H., Stagg, A.J., Davidson, R.N., and Knight, S.C. (2002) *Leishmania major* promastigotes inhibit dendritic cell motility *in vitro*. *Infect. Immun.*, **70**, 1023–1026.

106 Ponte-Sucre, A., Heise, D., and Moll, H. (2001) *Leishmania major* lipophosphoglycan modulates the phenotype and inhibits migration of murine Langerhans cells. *Immunology*, **104**, 462–467.

107 Moll, H., Flohé, S., and Röllinghoff, M. (1995) Dendritic cells in *Leishmania major*-immune mice harbor persistent parasites and mediate an antigen-specific T cell immune response. *Eur. J. Immunol.*, **25**, 693–699.

108 Körner, U., Fuss, V., Steigerwald, J., and Moll, H. (2006) Biogenesis of *Leishmania major*-harboring vacuoles in murine dendritic cells. *Infect. Immun.*, **74**, 1305–1312.

109 Boggiatto, P.M., Jie, F., Ghosh, M., Gibson-Corley, K.N., Ramer-Tait, A.E. *et al.* (2009) Altered dendritic cell phenotype in response to *Leishmania amazonensis* amastigote infection is mediated by MAP kinase. *ERK. Am. J. Pathol.*, **174**, 1818–1826.

110 Xin, L., Li, K., and Soong, L. (2008) Down-regulation of dendritic cell signaling pathways by *Leishmania amazonensis* amastigotes. *Mol. Immunol.*, **45**, 3371–3382.

111 Jayakumar, A., Donovan, M.J., Tripathi, V., Ramalho-Ortigao, M., and McDowell, M. A. (2008) *Leishmania major* infection activates NF-kappaB and interferon regulatory factors 1 and 8 in human dendritic cells. *Infect. Immun.*, **76**, 2138–2148.

112 Fukao, T., Tanabe, M., Terauchi, Y., Ota, T., Matsuda, S. *et al.* (2002) PI3K-mediated negative feedback regulation of IL-12 production in DCs. *Nat. Immunol.*, **3**, 875–881.

7
Function of Glycosomes in the Metabolism of Trypanosomatid Parasites and the Promise of Glycosomal Proteins as Drug Targets

Melisa Gualdrón-López, Paul A.M. Michels, Wilfredo Quiñones, Ana J. Cáceres, Luisana Avilán, and Juan-Luis Concepción*

Abstract

Trypanosomatids have the unique feature of compartmentalizing the major part of the glycolytic pathway inside peroxisome-related organelles called glycosomes. However, these organelles also contain enzymes of several other important pathways involved in both catabolic and anabolic processes. The enzyme content and the metabolic role of glycosomes differ between trypanosomatid species and between their life cycle stages. Several of the glycosomal pathways have been shown to be important for the viability, pathogenicity, and/or virulence of different trypanosomatid parasites. Additionally, the correct compartmentalization of glycosomal enzymes inside the organelles appeared to be vital for these pathogens. Therefore, many of these enzymes, as well as the proteins involved in the translocation of metabolites across the glycosomal membrane and peroxins (PEXs), proteins responsible for the biogenesis of glycosomes, are candidate drug targets. Glycosomal enzymes and PEX proteins of *Trypanosoma brucei*, *T. cruzi*, and *Leishmania* spp. are being studied, and compounds that interfere with their functioning are being developed for use as lead drugs against the diseases caused by these parasites. Potent, selective inhibitors of several enzymes have been obtained that exert trypanocidal activity on parasites cultured *in vitro* and have no or only little effect on growth of human cells. In addition, some compounds showed anti-parasite activity in experimentally infected animals.

Introduction

Pathogenic trypanosomatids share with all other representatives of the clade Kinetoplastea studied, as well as with representatives of the evolutionary related Diplonemida, the presence of organelles called glycosomes. Glycosomes are authentic peroxisomes, as revealed by their route of biogenesis. The biogenesis occurs in a similar way for all members of this quite diverse organelle family and involves homologous proteins. However, glycosomes distinguish themselves from

---

* Corresponding Author

Trypanosomatid Diseases: Molecular Routes to Drug Discovery. First edition. Edited by T. Jäger, O. Koch, and L. Flohé.
© 2013 Wiley-VCH Verlag GmbH & Co. KGaA. Published 2013 by Wiley-VCH Verlag GmbH & Co. KGaA.

other peroxisomes by the unique presence of the majority of the enzymes of the glycolytic pathway. This was first detected in *Trypanosoma brucei* [1], and later also in other kinetoplastids and a diplonemid species [2]. Insight into the full metabolic repertoire sequestered inside glycosomes has been obtained for the human pathogenic trypanosomatids by detailed biochemical studies as well as by the sequencing of the genomes of different species of African trypanosomes responsible for human sleeping sickness and the related disease "nagana" in domestic animals, different strains of *T. cruzi*, responsible for Chagas disease in Latin America, and various species of *Leishmania* responsible for different manifestations of leishmaniasis [2]. The first six or seven (dependent on species and/or life cycle stage) enzymes of glycolysis, responsible for the conversion of glucose – or other hexoses – into 1,3-bisphosphoglycerate (1,3-PGA) or 3-phosphoglycerate (3-PGA), are found within the organelle, as well as other enzymes involved in carbohydrate metabolism, such as two enzymes of glycerol metabolism, and enzymes of the gluconeogenic, succinic fermentation, and pentose-phosphate pathways (PPP) (Figure 7.1). Most of these enzymes must have been acquired by peroxisomes in an ancestral kinetoplastid, leading to the formation of glycosomes. In subsequent evolution, the organelles also acquired enzymes of squalene and pyrimidine biosynthesis, purine salvage, and ascorbate metabolism, while typical peroxisomal enzymes such as H_2O_2-producing oxidases and catalase were lost [2]. Other typical peroxisomal enzymes such as those involved in fatty acid β-oxidation and ether-lipid biosynthesis were retained.

Glycosomes of *T. brucei*

The human pathogenic stage of African trypanosomes, which lives in the host's bloodstream, is completely dependent on the fermentation of glucose taken up from the blood. In contrast to the other life cycle stages, the repertoire of other metabolic enzymes is highly repressed in this bloodstream form; the mitochondrion does not have tricarboxylic acid (TCA) cycle enzymes, a functional respiratory chain, and the capacity for oxidative phosphorylation. Furthermore, African trypanosomes do not have any carbohydrate or other material serving as energy storage. Under aerobic conditions, they synthesize all their ATP from the free energy obtained by the conversion of the sugar into pyruvate: two molecules of pyruvate and ATP from one molecule of glucose. Within the glycosomes, glucose is broken down into two 3-PGA, while the investment of ATP in the hexokinase (HXK) and phosphofructokinase (PFK) reactions is balanced by the two ATP produced when the two 1,3-PGAs are converted into 3-PGAs by phosphoglycerate kinase (PGK) (Figure 7.1). The two 3-PGAs exit the glycosomes to the cytosol where the last three reactions, catalyzed by phosphoglycerate mutase (PGAM), enolase (ENO), and pyruvate kinase (PYK) occur. PYK is responsible for the net production of two ATP. The NADH formed during glycolysis inside the glycosomes, in the reaction catalyzed by glyceraldehyde-3-phosphate dehydrogenase (GAPDH), is reoxidized to NAD^+ by a system that shuttles the electrons to the mitochondrion where it reduces O_2 to H_2O without the

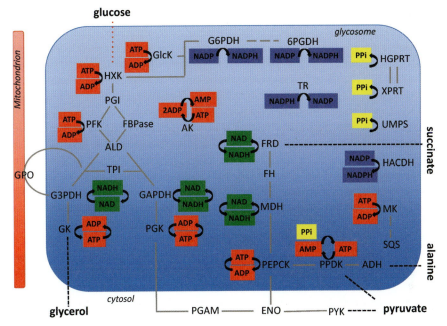

Figure 7.1 Diagram presenting enzymes of major metabolic pathways or parts of pathways found in glycosomes of different trypanosomatids and the cross-talk between these pathways by shared cofactors (NAD(H), NADP(H), ATP, ADP, and AMP) and PPi. The substrate glucose and the end-products of its catabolism are given in bold. For complete schemes of all reactions occurring or postulated to occur inside glycosomes, see [2,3]. Abbreviations of enzyme names: (glycolysis/gluconeogenic/succinate production pathways) HXK, hexokinase; GlcK, glucokinase; PGI, 6-phosphoglucose isomerase (or glucose-6-phosphate isomerase); PFK, phosphofructokinase; FBPase, fructose-1,6-bisphosphatase; ALD, aldolase; TPI, triosephosphate isomerase; G3PDH, glycerol-3-phosphate dehydrogenase; GK, glycerol kinase; GPO, glycerol-3-phosphate oxidase; GAPDH, glyceraldehyde-3-phosphate dehydrogenase; PGK, phosphoglycerate kinase; PGAM, phosphoglycerate mutase; ENO, enolase; PYK, pyruvate kinase; PEPCK, phosphoenolpyruvate carboxykinase; MDH, malate dehydrogenase; FH, fumarate hydratase (or fumarase); FRD, fumarate reductase; PPDK, pyruvate phosphate dikinase; ADH, alanine dehydrogenase; AK, adenylate kinase; (pentose phosphate pathway) G6PDH, glucose-6-phosphate dehydrogenase; 6PGDH, 6-phosphogluconate dehydrogenase; (purine salvage) HGPRT, hypoxanthine-guanine phosphoribosyltransferase; XPRT, xanthine phosphoribosyltransferase; (pyrimidine synthesis) UMPS, UMP synthase; (sterol synthesis) MK, mevalonate kinase; SQS, squalene synthase; (fatty acid β-oxidation) HACDH, 3-hydroxyacyl-CoA dehydrogenase; (pyrimidine synthesis); (antioxidant defense) TR, trypanothione reductase. Other abbreviation: PPi, inorganic pyrophosphate.

formation of a proton-motive force and ATP. The shuttle involves a glycosomal NADH-dependent glycerol-3-phosphate dehydrogenase (G3PDH), a putative glycerol 3-phosphate (G3P)/dihydroxyacetone phosphate (DHAP) exchange transporter in the glycosomal membrane and a glycerol-3-phosphate oxidase (GPO) system in the mitochondrial membrane. This GPO comprises a FAD-dependent G3PDH, ubiquinone-10, and an alternative oxidase (AO). Under anaerobic conditions, when the AO cannot function, NADH inside the glycosomes is still oxidized by the G3PDH, leading to G3P accumulation within the organelle. Glycosomes also contain a glycerol kinase (GK), whose normal function in cells is the ATP-dependent phosphorylation of glycerol to G3P. The equilibrium of the GK reaction favors strongly the phosphorylation; under physiological conditions the enzyme cannot convert G3P into glycerol with concomitant ATP formation. However, the important G3P accumulation within the glycosomes under anaerobic conditions allows the reversal by mass action. Consequently, glucose is then converted into one molecule of pyruvate and one molecule of glycerol. The intraglycosomal ATP/ADP balance is thus maintained, with, per molecule of glucose consumed, one ATP formed by the PGK reaction and another one by GK, but the net ATP production by PYK is then only one (Figure 7.1). This appears sufficient to keep the cells alive for some time, but not for growth. Consequently, the trypanosomes, which cannot sustain metabolic arrest, will die within hours under anaerobic conditions or when the GPO activity is inhibited by salicylhydroxamic acid (SHAM) [4].

Since bloodstream-form *T. brucei* is entirely dependent on sugar uptake and glycolysis for its free energy supply, both the uptake and glycolytic enzymes have already since several decades been considered as potential drug targets (reviewed in [5,6]). Indeed deprivation of these trypanosomes from glucose leads to death within minutes [7]. The essentiality, and thus the genetic validation as drug targets, has been obtained by RNA interference (RNAi) and conditional knockout experiments for the following glycosomal enzymes: HXK, PFK, aldolase (ALD), triosephosphate isomerase (TPI), and GAPDH, as well as the other enzymes PGAM, ENO, PYK, and AO, which are also involved in aerobic glycolysis in trypanosomes, but not present in the organelles [4,8,9]. The plasma membrane glucose transporter, as well as the pyruvate transporter that is responsible for the efflux of the trypanosome's glycolytic end-product into the blood, have been chemically validated as drug targets [7,10,11].

A control analysis study of the glycolytic flux in bloodstream-form *T. brucei* has been performed to determine the distribution of control exerted by the different enzymes and to identify which steps of the pathway need the least inhibition to block the flux and, from that perspective, are the most promising drug targets. This involved both an *in silico* analysis, using a validated computer model developed on the basis of the kinetic data determined for all enzymes involved [12], and an experimental approach in which the activities of enzymes and transporters were varied *in situ* by genetic methods and/or inhibitors. The results showed that, under physiological conditions, by far most control resides in the glucose transporter, whereas the remaining control is shared by various enzymes: ALD, GAPDH, G3PDH, PGK, PGAM and ENO. Surprisingly, HXK, PFK, and PYK are in excess, and consequently exert no control, and ATP demand appeared to have no control either unless PYK is inhibited [8–10,13,14]. Therefore, it was concluded that, from a network perspective, the glucose transporter is the most promising drug target, followed by ALD, GAPDH, G3PDH, PGK, PGAM, and ENO. These results were experimentally confirmed by titrating the activities of enzymes and the glucose transporter by RNAi and inhibitors, with the observation that the transporter has approximately 40% control at 5 mM glucose [8–10,13,14]. Partial inhibition of each of the enzymes appeared sufficient to inhibit the glycolytic flux and kill the cells, even in the case of the three kinases that are in excess. Importantly, a compilation of all data showed that a reduction of the glycolytic flux by 30–50% is already sufficient to arrest growth [15].

Interestingly, a control analysis performed for glycolysis in human erythrocytes, which reside in the same environment as the trypanosomes (i.e., the blood), showed that, in contrast to trypanosomes, the flux is controlled by the ATP demand, not by the ATP supply and that the glucose transporter has no control at all [16]. In consequence, a differential control analysis indicated that the transporter is an even more promising drug target [17].

Glycosomes of bloodstream-form *T. brucei* are nearly completely devoted to glycolysis; over 90% of their protein content is comprised of glycolytic enzymes, in contrast to the procyclic-form trypanosomes living in the tsetse fly's midgut where this number is estimated to be only 40–50% [18]. Little is known about the importance of the other glycosomal enzymes of the bloodstream form and the possibility to use them as drug targets. Only PPP enzymes such as glucose-6-phosphate dehydrogenase (G6PDH) and 6-phosphogluconate dehydrogenase (6PGDH) have been chemically and genetically validated as targets [19–21]. The enzymes of both the oxidative and non-oxidative branches of the PPP have a dual distribution in trypanosomatids, in glycosomes and cytosol, with the ratios varying dependent on enzyme, species, and life cycle stage. For *T. brucei* G6PDH, approximately 40% was located inside glycosomes. The characterization of G6PDH, its validation as a drug target, and its specific *in situ* inhibition by human steroids resulting in death of bloodstream-form cells have been reviewed elsewhere [22], and the PPP enzymes of trypanosomatids as drug targets are described in Chapter 16 of this volume.

Sugar nucleotides are needed for the majority of glycosylation reactions. For *T. brucei* they are mostly synthesized by *de novo* pathways (i.e., by the bioconversion of an existing sugar or sugar nucleotide). Whereas in most organisms these pathways are present in the cytosol, work by Ferguson et al. has shown that in trypanosomes several steps of the synthesis of GDP-fucose, UDP-glucose, UDP-galactose, and UDP-*N*-acetylglucosamine occur inside glycosomes (Figure 7.2) [23–28]. These enzymes, as well GDP-mannose pyrophosphorylase (of which the subcellular localization has not yet been reported and it has no recognizable PTS motif), which makes GDP-mannose [29], are essential for growth of bloodstream-form parasites and thus may be considered as validated drug-target candidates. No detailed studies of these pathways have been performed as yet for other trypanosomatids.

Glycosomes of *T. cruzi*

The life cycle of *T cruzi* involves four developmental stages: in the insect vector the epimastigotes and metacyclic trypomastigotes, and in the mammalian host the trypomastigotes living in the blood and amastigotes replicating intracellularly in different tissues and organs. The latter two are the clinically relevant forms for which

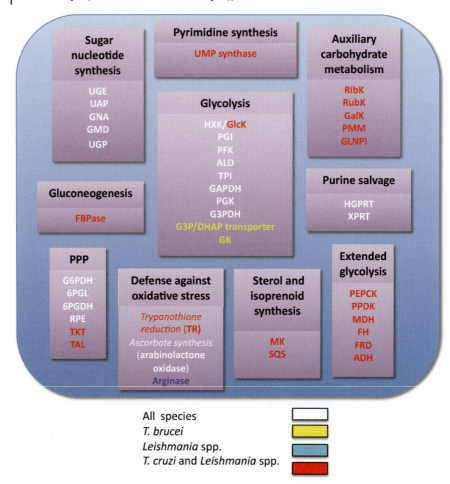

Figure 7.2 Inventory of the different metabolic processes and enzymes present inside glycosomes of the human pathogenic stages of the different trypanosomatids. The names of processes are given in black. The experimentally determined presence or inferred functionally importance of enzymes within glycosomes of the different trypanosomatid species (see main text and [2]) is indicated with different colors. Abbreviations: (glycolysis) HXK, hexokinase; GlcK, glucokinase; PGI, 6-phosphoglucose isomerase (or glucose-6-phosphate isomerase); PFK, phosphofructokinase; ALD, aldolase; TPI, triosephosphate isomerase; GAPDH, glyceraldehyde-3-phosphate dehydrogenase; PGK, phosphoglycerate kinase; G3PDH, glycerol-3-phosphate dehydrogenase; G3P, glycerol 3-phosphate; DHAP, dihydroxyacetone phosphate; GK, glycerol kinase; (gluconeogenesis) FBPase, fructose-1,6-bisphosphatase; (extended glycolysis) PEPCK, phosphoenolpyruvate carboxykinase; PPDK, pyruvate phosphate dikinase; MDH, malate dehydrogenase; FH, fumarate hydratase (or fumarase); FRD, fumarate reductase; ADH, alanine dehydrogenase; pentose phosphate pathway, PPP; G6PDH, glucose-6-phosphate dehydrogenase; 6PGL, 6-phosphogluconolactonase; 6PGDH, 6-phosphogluconate dehydrogenase; RPE, ribulose-5-phosphate-3-epimerase; TAL, transaldolase; TKT, transketolase; (auxiliary carbohydrate metabolism) RibK, ribosekinase; RubK, ribulosekinase; GalK, galactosekinase;

drugs are required. *T. cruzi* has to adapt its metabolism to the wide range of environments encountered during its life cycle. The nutritional conditions vary from amino acid-rich with transiently available glucose for epimastigotes living in the insect's gut, to glucose-rich for blood trypomastigotes, and to very low in sugars, but rich in a plethora of metabolites such as intermediates of carbohydrate metabolism, fatty acids, and amino acids as present in the mammalian cytosol for amastigotes. All developmental stages of *T. cruzi*, in contrast to *T. brucei*, possess a well-developed mitochondrion with a TCA cycle and a complete, functional electron transfer chain coupled to oxidative phosphorylation [30]. Nonetheless, when glucose is available, *T. cruzi* will oxidize it, but even under aerobic conditions only incompletely, to succinate, acetate, L-alanine, and CO_2 [31,32].

T. cruzi glycosomes contain, similarly to those of *T. brucei* (see the "Glycosomes of *T. brucei*" section) and other trypanosomatids, the glycolytic enzymes responsible for the conversion of glucose into 3-PGA [33]. The three final steps, converting 3-PGA into pyruvate, occur in the cytosol. The kinetic properties of the glycosomal enzymes of the different trypanosomatid species are also very similar, including the apparent lack of activity regulation of HXK and PFK. However, the glucose fermentation pathway in each of the *T. cruzi* life cycle stages and also in *Leishmania* spp. is extended to a succinate production pathway – also observed in procyclic *T. brucei* – in which the phosphoenolpyruvate (PEP), produced in the cytosol by ENO, enters the glycosomes, to be converted into succinate by the activities of a PEP carboxykinase (PEPCK), malate dehydrogenase (MDH), fumarate hydratase (FH), and a soluble, NAD-dependent fumarate reductase (FRD) [34,35] (Figures 7.1 and 7.2). Alternatively, PEP can be dephosphorylated inside the glycosomes to pyruvate by a pyruvate phosphate dikinase (PPDK) with the concomitant formation of ATP and inorganic phosphate (Pi) at the expense of AMP and inorganic pyrophosphate (PPi). This PPi is an energy-rich byproduct from glycosomal biosynthetic reactions; no pyrophosphatase is present to hydrolyze it. The pyruvate may be further reduced using NADH by a glycosomal alanine dehydrogenase (ADH). The presence of the additional NADH-dependent oxidoreductases (MDH, FRD, and ADH) and kinases (PEPCK and PPDK) contribute to the maintenance of the intraglycosomal NAD/NADH and ATP/ADP balances. Contrary to the situation in bloodstream-form *T. brucei*, G3PDH and GK, also present in glycosomes [3,36], seem not to play an important role in balancing these cofactors in *T. cruzi* and *Leishmania* spp., but may rather act to form G3P for lipid metabolism from either DHAP or glycerol.

◀──

PMM, phosphomannomutase; GLNPI, glucosamine-6-phosphate isomerase; (sugar nucleotide synthesis) UGE, UDP-glucose 4'-epimerase; UAP, UDP-N-acetylglucosamine pyrophosphorylase; GNA, glucosamine-6-phosphate N-acetyltransferase; GMD, GDP-mannose dehydratase; UGP, UDP-glucose pyrophosphorylase; (purine salvage) HGPRT, hypoxanthine-guanine phosphoribosyltransferase; XPRT, xanthine phosphoribosyltransferase; (pyrimidine synthesis) UMPS, UMP synthase; (sterol and isoprenoid synthesis) MK, mevalonate kinase; SQS, squalene synthase; (defense against oxidative stress) TR, trypanothione reductase.

Also different from bloodstream-form *T. brucei* is the fact that biosynthetic processes seem to play a quantitatively more important role in glycosomes of these other parasites (and in procyclic *T. brucei*) and are coupled to the catabolic processes by producing PPi, to be used by PPDK, and their requirement of NAD(P)H and ATP (see Figure 7.1 and below).

PEP is also a substrate of the cytosolic PEP mutase that catalyzes the conversion of PEP to phosphonopyruvate, the initial step in the formation of many naturally occurring phosphonate compounds in *T. cruzi* [37]. The amount of PEP that enters the glycosome would depend on the activity regulation of the allosteric enzyme PYK.

Glycolysis plays a less important role in *T. cruzi* than in bloodstream-form *T. brucei*. Epimastigotes live in an amino-rich environment, but nonetheless will preferentially use glucose as an energy substrate during the time when it is available after the insect's blood meal [38], similar to insect-stage procyclic *T. brucei*. In contrast, trypomastigotes, living in the blood, may rely considerably on glycolysis, although little data are available. Indeed, most enzymes of the extended glucose breakdown to succinate and pyruvate (via both PYK and PPDK) have been detected in cells of this life cycle stage (reviewed in [39]). Contradictory data have been reported about the energy metabolism of amastigotes. Early studies with an axenic culture model suggested an essentially glycolytic metabolism for this life cycle form, fermenting glucose to succinate and acetate for their ATP production [40]. Indeed, most enzymes are detectable in amastigotes (reviewed in [39]). However, recent studies showed no indications for the expression of the plasma membrane hexose transporter in amastigotes, contrary to epimastigotes and trypomastigotes where it was found to be active [41,42]. This would tally with the notion that free sugar levels are low in the cytosol of mammalian cells. It is feasible, however, that glycolytic intermediates such as phosphorylated hexoses or trioses are taken up from the cytosol of the host cell to be metabolized by the glycolytic pathway and, in addition to fatty acid and amino acid catabolism, contribute to the ATP supply. Indeed, the *T. cruzi* genome, but not those of *T. brucei* and *Leishmania* spp., codes for a hexose phosphate transporter similar to that present in the membranes of bacteria, plastids, and the mammalian endoplasmic reticulum (ER) [43]. Nonetheless, proteomic studies indicated that the transition of trypomastigotes to amastigotes is accompanied by a dramatic shift from carbohydrate- to lipid-dependent energy metabolism [41]. Therefore, the glycolytic enzymes detected in glycosomes of amastigotes are probably necessary for gluconeogenesis to synthesize glucoconjugates.

T. cruzi and *Leishmania* contain also other enzymes in carbohydrate metabolism, but not found *T. brucei*, that are probably all present inside glycosomes as inferred from the presence of a peroxisome-targeting signal (PTS): sugar kinases other than a hexokinase, such as a glucokinase (GlcK) to be discussed below, ribosekinase, ribulosekinase, and galactokinase, as well as phosphomannomutase and glucosamine-6-phosphate isomerase (Figure 7.2) [2,3]. These enzymes may be important for the use of alternative sugars as an energy source, but also for the formation of important or essential glucoconjugates.

Other pathways or parts of them are also present in *T. cruzi* glycosomes, such as the PPP, responsible for about 10% of the glucose consumption flux in *T. cruzi* epimastigotes, considerably higher than in bloodstream-form *T. brucei* [44]. All PPP enzymes were found in each of the four major life cycle stages and for each of the enzymes a predominantly cytosolic localization was reported, but also a presence in glycosomes. Also found inside glycosomes are purine salvage, pyrimidine biosynthesis, biosynthesis of ether lipids, β-oxidation of fatty acids, some isoprenoid biosynthesis enzymes [45], and enzymes involved in protection against oxidative stress (reviewed in [39]) (Figures 7.1 and 7.2).

All parasitic trypanosomatids are auxotrophic for purines. Purine bases are taken up from the host and interconverted into purine nucleotides by enzymes of the purine salvage pathway, of which several have been located inside glycosomes and/or identified as glycosomal enzymes by the presence of a PTS [3]. Hypoxanthine is the predominant salvageable purine in the host milieu, rendering the enzyme hypoxanthine-guanine phosphoribosyltransferase (HGPRT) a crucial enzyme in the metabolism of the parasites and thus a potential drug target. This enzyme is present in the glycosomes. The *T. cruzi* HGPRT [46], as well as its homolog from other trypanosomatids, have been studied in detail.

Isoprenoids are important for trypanosomatids, for the production of squalene and sterols. Isoprenoid synthesis in these parasites occurs via the mevalonate pathway. The ergosterol synthesis of *T. cruzi* has been studied in detail and several enzymes involved in it have been chemically validated in *in vitro* cultures (reviewed in [47,48]). About 45% of one of the enzymes, squalene synthase (SQS), has been located in the glycosomes of *T. cruzi* [45]. In addition, the likely synthesis of isoprenoids inside the glycosomes is supported by the presence of several intermediates such as squalene in the organelle's matrix and membrane [49], in agreement with similar observations made for mammalian peroxisomes [50]. More details about sterol synthesis in trypanosomatids will be presented in Chapter 26 of this volume.

The organization of the metabolic network in glycosomes of *T. cruzi* suggests that the role of these organelles in this organism is fundamentally different from that in bloodstream-form *T. brucei*. Whereas the organellar metabolism of the latter comprises almost only the catabolic process of glycolysis, that of *T. cruzi*, and also procyclic *T. brucei* and different *Leishmania* spp. life cycle stages, has the catabolism of glucose via glycolysis to succinate and alanine, and via the PPP connected to several biosynthetic pathways by the production and consumption of ATP and NAD(P)H and PPi (see Figure 7.1).

Interestingly, PPi seems not only to form a metabolic link by being a product and substrate in glycosomal anabolism and catabolism, respectively, but it may also regulate the distribution of fluxes through these pathways by modulating the activity of some *T. cruzi* enzymes, such as PEPCK and HXK [35,51]. An increase of intraglycosomal PPi by a high biosynthetic activity will inhibit PEPCK, and thus steer the PEP away from the succinate production towards PPDK and ADH, consequently using the PPi for ATP production and so increasing the free energy yield from glucose. Moreover, PPDK and ADH will in this situation become crucial for maintaining the energy and redox balance within the glycosomes and thus sustaining the glycolytic flux [35]. Simultaneous HXK inhibition by PPi may promote glucose phosphorylation by the PPi-insensitive GlcK, also present in glycosomes of *T. cruzi* and *Leishmania* spp., but not *T. brucei* [52]. This GlcK produces preferentially the β-anomer of glucose 6-phosphate (G6P) [53], the substrate of G6PDH. Since the substrate of the second enzyme of the glycolytic pathway, G6P isomerase, is α-G6P, the preferential product of HXK, the increase in PPi will thus lead to a rerouting of the glucose flux from glycolysis to the PPP, and consequently stimulate the NADPH production for biosynthetic processes.

Glycosomes of *Leishmania* spp.

During their life cycle, *Leishmania* parasites alternate between their motile promastigote stage and non-motile amastigote stage, respectively, in their invertebrate vector and mammalian host. In mammals, the parasites thrive inside the phagolysosomes of macrophages or other cells such as neutrophils and dendritic cells [54]. *Leishmania* are capable of performing multiple metabolic adaptations to cope with the distinct environments in both hosts. The adaptations involve several metabolic pathways in different cell compartments including the glycosomes. Although the medically relevant form is the amastigote, glycosomes and their enzymes have been more intensively studied in promastigotes because these are more easily cultured. These studies have allowed the identification of important features of the metabolism inside glycosomes. *In silico* studies with the genomes of different *Leishmania* spp. have also provided invaluable information about the metabolic capacity of the parasite's glycosomes [3]. These studies, together with transcriptomic and proteomic analyses of the amastigote form and the analysis of virulence phenotypes of *Leishmania* mutants [55], have been important to identify aspects of the glycosome that are essential for the physiology of the amastigote form and may thus be selected as candidate drug targets.

Leishmania amastigotes have a reduced metabolism and a slow growth rate in comparison with promastigotes [56]. However, amastigotes seem to have a comparable glycosome density as promastigotes [57] and, similar to the promastigote form, glycosomes are involved in several metabolic processes that appear to be crucial for the amastigote form. Among these processes are carbohydrate, polyamine, and lipid metabolism as well as purine salvage, pyrimidine synthesis, and protection against oxidant stress (Figure 7.2).

As with the glycosomes in other trypanosomatids, those of *Leishmania*, in both its promastigote and amastigote stage, contain all of the first seven enzymes of the glycolytic pathway [58–60], with the glycosomal glycolytic enzymes slightly upregulated, but the cytosolic enzymes of the final steps of glycolysis significantly downregulated in the amastigote stage [61]. Hexose uptake is essential for growth and viability of the amastigote form, despite the low level of hexoses in the phagolysosome [62]. A hexose transporter null mutant cannot survive as amastigote in macrophages [63,64], highlighting the importance of sugar as a carbon source. This importance of sugar metabolism and the involvement of glycosomes therein in amastigotes are also underscored by the fact that gluconeogenesis is increased in the amastigote form. The gluconeogenic enzymes PEPCK and fructose-1,6-bisphosphatase (FBPase), both localized in the glycosomes, are upregulated in this stage [61,65]. Indeed this latter enzyme, FBPase, is important for virulence in *L. major*. Parasites lacking this enzyme were unable to replicate in the macrophage's phagolysosome and failed to generate normal lesions [66], indicating that gluconeogenesis is essential for amastigotes. In addition, *Leishmania* amastigotes accumulate the reserve oligosaccharide mannogen (formerly known as mannan) in the cytosol [67]. This oligosaccharide, 4 to 40 mannose residues long, is required for a normal establishment of infection and survival in macrophages [68,69]. Mannose-α-1-phosphate, which is used for mannogen synthesis, is derived from hexose phosphates formed in the glycosomes. *Leishmania* amastigotes are also dependent on hexosamines [70] scavenged from the phagolysosome that may contain glucosamine and *N*-acetylglucosamine. These hexosamines can be products of matrix proteoglycans and glycosaminoglycans internalized and degraded by the macrophages or by chitinase secreted by the amastigotes [71]. These exogenous hexosamines are phosphorylated and can be converted into fructose 6-phosphate within the glycosomes. Catabolism of the amino sugars inside the glycosomes is important for growth in macrophages and establishment of infection [72]. However, the sugars and amino sugars are almost certainly not only essential for *N*-glycosylation and oligosaccharide biosynthesis, but also for sustaining the flux through the PPP. The NADPH produced by this process is needed for oxidative stress protection, which is very important in the hostile environment of the macrophage's phagolysosome, and for nucleotide synthesis.

Whereas sugar catabolism plays only a minor role in the energy supply of *Leishmania* amastigotes, β-oxidation of fatty acids appears to be the main source of energy in this intracellular stage, as is the case in *T. cruzi* amastigotes. *In silico* analysis of the *Leishmania* genome led to the prediction that several enzymes of this pathway are associated with glycosomes [3], in agreement with results from earlier cell fractionation studies [73]. Proteomic and enzymatic analyses have shown that levels of enzymes involved in this pathway are increased in amastigotes [61,65]. However, the upregulated enzymes of β-oxidation could not be clearly identified as glycosomal proteins [61,65,74]. Moreover, a correlated expression pattern was observed for β-oxidation of fatty acids with mitochondrial functions in differentiating *L. donovani* [61], suggesting that at least a major part of β-oxidation occurs in the mitochondrion. The fatty acids can be obtained from phospholipids through the upregulated phospholipase A_2 and monoglyceride lipase. These enzymes would also provide glycerol required for gluconeogenesis in the glycosome [61]. Glycosomes are also involved in the synthesis of isoprenoids for sterols and other products, for which the enzymes are distributed in different subcellular compartments [75,76]. The mevalonate kinase (MK) has been found associated with the glycosomal matrix in *L. major* and *T. brucei* [77].

Leishmania amastigotes are also able to use amino acids as a carbon source, but the glycosome is not directly involved in this metabolism. Nonetheless, glycosomes contain the enzyme arginase that catalyzes the conversion of arginine into ornithine and urea as the first step in the biosynthesis of polyamines [78], necessary for the synthesis of trypanothione. This latter molecule is essential for the defense against oxidative stress [79]. The function of arginase is also associated with decreasing arginine levels in the phagolysosome to interfere with the host's nitric oxide production. Mutant parasites of different species of *Leishmania* lacking this enzyme have a reduced virulence; the pathology emerges less rapidly than in infection with wild-type parasites [78,80–83]. *Trypanosoma* spp. lack the arginase [83].

The glycosome also contains arabinolactone oxidase [84,85], the last enzyme of the synthesis of ascorbate. In conjunction with ascorbate peroxidase, this could play a role in the antioxidant defense in *Leishmania* when residing within the phagolysosome. Indeed, *Leishmania* spp. contain an asorbate peroxidase, but its subcellular localization remains to be determined. In an *in vitro* infection model, a *L. donovani* strain overexpressing arabinonolactone oxidase showed a higher infection index than wild-type cells [85].

Like the other trypanosomatids, *Leishmania* is not able to synthesize purines *de novo* and scavenge them from the host. Four enzymes are required and two of them, HGPRT and xanthine phosphoribosyltransferase (XPRT), which have been located inside the glycosome [86,87], are critical for the infection of macrophages and mice [88]. Moreover, studies performed with *L. donovani* promastigotes have shown that the parasite responds rapidly to purine starvation by increasing the expression of the purine transporter and purine salvage enzymes, including HGPRT and XPRT [89]. This adaptation to purine starvation might occur in amastigotes as a response to changes in the phagolysosome. In contrast to purines, trypanosomatid parasites are able to synthesize pyrimidine nucleotides *de novo*. The last two enzymes of this pathway (orotate phosphoribosyltransferase and orotidine-5′-monophosphate decarboxylase) are fused into a bifunctional enzyme (uridine-5-monophosphate (UMP) synthase) that is also present inside the glycosome [83,90]. Promastigotes of *L. donovani* lacking UMP synthase were unable to proliferate in the absence of pyrimidine supplement [90]. However, whether this bifunctional enzyme is essential for amastigote physiology remains to be elucidated.

Essentiality of Controlled Communication Across the Glycosomal Membrane

Like peroxisomes in mammalian and plant cells and in yeasts, glycosomes seem to be distinct entities with a well-defined metabolic repertoire for specific environmental conditions of the cells. Moreover, these organelles are also synthesized and degraded as separate entities (see the "Essentiality of Correct Integration of Glycosomal Metabolism in the Overall Metabolism – Relation to Life Cycle Differentiation" section). Nonetheless, the metabolic network in the organelles should be well integrated in the overall network of the cell in order to function properly. Moreover, when the cell needs to change its metabolic repertoire to adapt to altered environmental conditions, such as occur during the life cycle-related differentiation of trypanosomatid parasites, the organellar network should change as well. Therefore, the cytosolic and glycosomal networks should be linked by devices for exchange of substrates, intermediates, and products, and these links should allow different transmembrane solute fluxes when the networks in both compartments change. How is this solute translocation across the glycosomal membrane achieved and would the translocation devices involved be suitable drug targets? Studies on these questions have so far been mostly restricted to bloodstream-form *T. brucei*.

Like peroxisomal membranes, the glycosomal membrane is an apparent permeability barrier. This notion seems firmly established for bulky compounds such as ATP, NADH, and fatty acids. The ATP consumption and synthesis are balanced inside the glycosome and an ATP/ADP ratio different from that in the cytosol is maintained (see the "Glycosomes of *T. brucei*" section) [12]. For bloodstream-form *T. brucei*, reoxidation of intraglycosomal NADH involves a mechanism by which the electrons are transferred from the cofactor to the mitochondrion by a shuttle mechanism. Three ABC transporters are present in the glycosomal membrane [91], one of them has been shown to import long-chain fatty acids such as oleoyl-CoA into the organelles [92]. Smaller compounds such as glycolytic intermediates also seem capable of crossing the glycosomal membrane, but only relatively slowly, suggestive of a low permeability. Upon addition of a pulse of radioactively labeled glucose to bloodstream trypanosomes, the label appears very rapidly in a small (20–30%) pool of intermediates, interpreted as those present inside the glycosomes, and in pyruvate, but only 60 times slower in a large (70–80%) pool of intermediates, the cytosol [93]. Also, the possibility to reverse the GK reaction under anaerobic conditions, due to the increase in the glycosomal G3P concentration, is indicative of a low permeability of the membrane for this metabolite [1,94,95]. Furthermore, simulation of glycolysis using the kinetic model indicated the essentiality of a defined pool of phosphorylated glycolytic intermediates within the glycosome, separate from the cytosol, to enable a functional glycolytic flux [12,96]. Nonetheless, like for the membranes of peroxisomes from plant and mammalian cells and yeast, channel-forming activities have been found in preparations from purified glycosomal membranes [97]. The data available from this study, together with inference from data obtained for peroxisomes, suggest the presence of various, distinct channels in the glycosomal membrane that allow the permeation of most low-molecular-mass metabolites, including charged compounds such as the glycolytic phosphorylated intermediates. The nonetheless observed low equilibration of many such intermediates between glycosomes and cytosol may be attributed to the existence of a multienzyme complex and channeling of metabolites directly between the active sites of successive enzymes without their release from the complex, as has similarly been observed for plant peroxisomes (reviewed in [98]). Additionally or alternatively, control of the fluxes through the channels by regulatory proteins or association of the channels with the enzymes and/or the presence of the Donnan potential due to the high intraglycosomal density of many proteins with a high pI may also be responsible for the low transmembrane exchange of many metabolites [97,99].

Despite the presence of channels, it cannot be yet excluded that the glycosomal membrane contains some transporter molecules for specific low-molecular-weight substrates that have not been recognized because of a low similarity with known transporters and/or difficult identification by biochemical approaches.

Any protein involved in metabolite translocation across the glycosomal membrane is a potential drug target for several reasons: (i) the unique compartmentalization of glycolysis and some other processes inside glycosomes; (ii) the proved essentiality of this compartmentalization, at least for glycolysis in bloodstream-form trypanosomes (reviewed in [100,101]) and probably also for other processes in the other parasites as well; (ii) the very low similarity between the glycosomal solute transporters identified so far and their human counterparts [91]; and (iv) the apparent absence of homologs of the so far only known peroxisomal channel protein, Pxmp2 [102], in the genomes of the trypanosomatids.

Essentiality of Correct Integration of Glycosomal Metabolism in the Overall Metabolism – Relation to Life Cycle Differentiation

As described in the previous sections, the metabolic networks within glycosomes, like in peroxisomes, are well integrated within the overall cell metabolic network, although these organelles are synthesized and degraded as separate entities. The biosynthesis of the organelles should be well coordinated with the growth of the cells for the proper functioning of the metabolism. Biosynthesis of peroxisomes/glycosomes occurs by growth and division of existing organelles, in which proteins are post-translationally imported from the cytosol into the matrix or inserted into the membrane, and lipids are obtained from the ER by non-vesicular transport. Moreover, both lipids and specific membrane proteins can also be recruited via membrane vesicles from distinct regions of the ER. These processes involve a number of specific proteins called peroxins (PEXs) that perform their functions through cascades of interactions and conformational changes (reviewed in [100,101]). Degradation of the organelles is achieved by a specific form of autophagy called pexophagy. Under normal growth conditions, the levels of autophagy and pexophagy in a cell, including trypanosomatid parasites, are relatively low. However, under conditions of stress or when there is a need for remodeling the structure or metabolic repertoire of a cell, these processes are upregulated. Indeed, autophagy is importantly increased during differentiation of trypanosomatids [103,104] and, in the case of *T. brucei*, also an increased turnover of glycosomes by pexophagy is observed [105]. Autophagy involves a considerable number of specific autophagy-related proteins (ATGs) as well as several proteins shared with other processes.

About 10 PEX proteins of *T. brucei* have been identified, most of them involved in import of matrix proteins, some others in insertion of proteins into the glycosomal membrane or in glycosome proliferation. Knockdown of the expression of each of these PEX proteins leads to arrest of glycosome biogenesis as shown by the presence of all or part of the newly synthesized matrix proteins in the cytosol, and growth retardation followed by death. The effect is particularly dramatic in bloodstream-form trypanosomes. An explanation why this is so detrimental for the cell was offered by the finding that the glycosomal enzymes involved in glucose metabolism, and probably also other enzymes, cannot function properly outside the organelles because of a lack of activity regulation mechanisms [95,96]. This, together with the low similarity of the trypanosome PEX amino acid sequences compared to that of their human counterparts (varying from about 35% until less than 15% or barely detectable [100]), renders these proteins promising drug targets. Some ATGs and other proteins involved in autophagy have also been shown to be essential for trypanosomatid parasites, particularly during their differentiation [103,104]. This has not yet been demonstrated for proteins specifically involved in glycosome degradation, but it is likely the case. Therefore, these ATGs, of which the sequences are not very well conserved [106], may also be interesting drug targets.

What Has Been Achieved So Far in Target Characterization?

The most prominent aspects of glycosomes are glycolysis and its reverse process of gluconeogenesis. As discussed in the previous sections, glycolysis is essential and thus a drug target in the pathogenic form of *T. brucei*. This is probably also the case for trypomastigotes of *T. cruzi*. Furthermore, the production of G6P for glucoconjugates and mannogen from sugars and fatty acids by HXK and gluconeogenic enzymes is vital for *Leishmania* amastigotes. The same is probably the case for *T. cruzi* amastigotes. Each of the enzymes shared by the glycolytic and gluconeogenic pathways is thus a validated potential drug target in the three parasites, and PFK and PYK also in *T. brucei*, while FBPase, PEPCK, and possibly also PPDK are targets in the intracellular trypanosomatids. Progress has been made in the characterization of many of these enzymes such as development of protein expression systems, detailed kinetic characterization, protein crystallization, and structure determination. Results are summarized in Table 7.1. Many proteins, particularly the glycolytic enzymes, are quite well conserved between the different trypanosomatids, while they are much more different from the corresponding proteins from other groups such as mammals. In some cases similar reactions are even catalyzed in the parasites and human by non-homologous enzymes, such as PGAM and – only in *T. brucei* – the enzyme eventually responsible for the reoxidation of glycolytically produced NADH, AO. This often offers the possibility to use information about unique structural and/or functional features from an enzyme of only one of the trypanosomatids to develop potent inhibitors that are effective on the corresponding enzyme of each of the parasites with no or little effect on the human counterpart. Nonetheless, for optimization of such inhibitors for a specific enzyme of each parasite by structure–activity relationship (SAR) analysis, structural information for each enzyme in some cases appeared advantageous to exploit its subtle, unique features.

HGPRT from both *T. cruzi* and *L. tarentolae* has been characterized in detail, and crystal structures are available for drug design [107,108].

The PPP is very important for each of the trypanosomatids, notably for the production of NADPH to deal with the host's oxidative defense by which the parasites are attacked. In *T. brucei*, G6PDH and 6PGDH, the NADPH-producing enzymes of the oxidative branch, have been validated as drug targets by RNAi, but not those of the non-oxidative branch; transketolase and transaldolase were even undetectable in bloodstream forms. G6PDH and 6PGDH have been characterized

Table 7.1 Potential drug targets in glycosomes of trypanosomatid parasites and the stage of drug development.

Enzyme	Target				Crystal structure available	Selective inhibitor available	Inhibitor with *in vitro* anti-parasite activity available	Inhibitors with *in vivo* anti-parasite activity available
	Tb		*Tc*	*L*				
	BF	T	A	A				
Glycolysis/gluconeogenesis/succinate production								
HXK	V	L	N	V	*Tc*	*Tb/Tc*	*Tb/Tc*	*Tc*
GlcK	–	N	N	L	*L*			
PGI	V	L	L	L				
PFK	V	P	U	U	*Tb*	*Tb*	*Tb*	
ALD	V	L	L	L	*Tb/L*	*Tb*		
TPI	V	L	L	L	*Tb/Tc/L*			
GAPDH	V	L	L	L	*Tb/Tc/L*	*Tb/Tc/L*	*Tb/Tc*	
PGK	V	L	L	L	*Tb*			
G3PDH	V	P	P	P	*L*			
GK	U	U	U	U				
(PGAM)	V	L	L	L	*Tb/L*			
(ENO)	V	L	L	L	*Tb*			
(PYK)	V	L	U	U	*Tb/L*	*Tb*	*Tb*	
PEPCK	–	P	U	P	*Tc*			
MDH	–	P	U	P				
FH	–	L	U	P				
FRD	–	P	U	P				
PPDK	–	P	U	p	*Tb*			

ADH	–	P	U	P			
FBPase	–	U	L	V			
(Glucose transporter)	V	L	U	V			
PPP							
G6PDH	V	L	L	L	Tc	Tb/Tc	Tb/Tc
6PGDH	V	L	L	L	L	Tb	Tb
Sterol synthesis							
SQS	U	V	V	V		Tc	Tc
Purine salvage							Tc
HGPRT	?	V	V	V	Tc	Tc/L	Tc/L
Sugar nucleotide synthesis							
UGE	V	L	L	L	Tb		
UAP	V	L	L	L			
GNA	V	L	L	L	Tb		
GMD	V	L	L	L			
UGP	L	L	L	L	Tb		

Abbreviations: *Tb, T. brucei; Tc, T. cruzi; L, Leishmania* spp.; BF, bloodstream form; T, trypomastigote; A, amastigote; V = validated; L = likely; P = possibly; U = unlikely (but likely or possibly in combination with another enzyme); N = not known; – = not present. For abbreviations of proteins, see main text and/or legends to Figures 7.1 and 7.2. Enzymes given in parentheses are glycolytic enzymes present exclusively in the cytosol but important for the glycolytic flux through the glycosome; similarly for the plasma membrane glucose transporter. The likelihood of enzymes as drug targets for *T. cruzi* trypomastigotes is in part inferred from knockdown and knockout studies on glucose-grown procyclic *T. brucei* that is considered a good model system for this *T. cruzi* life cycle stage (published data and personal communication by F. Bringaud, Université Bordeaux Segalen, France).

in detail (reviewed in [21,22]) and crystal structures are available for the *T. cruzi* and *T. brucei* enzymes, respectively. For further discussion of the PPP as a target, see Chapter 16 of this volume.

Four glycosomal enzymes involved in the biosynthesis of sugar nucleotides that are necessary for glycosylation reactions have been genetically validated as drug targets in *T. brucei* (UDP-glucose-4'-epimerase (UGE), UDP-*N*-acetylglucosamine pyrophosphorylase (UAP), glucosamine-6-phosphate *N*-acetyltransferase (GNA), and GDP-mannose dehydratase (GMD), see the "Glycosomes of *T. brucei*" section). These enzymes have been biochemically characterized and the crystal structures of UGE and GNA, as well as UDP-glucose pyrophosphorylase (UGP), have been determined at high resolution [27,28,109]. Of these, UGP catalyzes the condensation of glucose 1-phosphate with UTP, UGE interconverts UDP-glucose and UDP-galactose, and GNA acetylates glucosamine 6-phosphate using acetyl-CoA [27,28]. These structures will provide a framework for the design of inhibitors against the parasite enzymes.

What Has Been Achieved So Far in the Development of Inhibitors of Glycosomal Enzymes or Processes

Some drugs used against trypanosomatid-borne diseases appear to exert inhibitory actions on glycosomal enzymes *in vitro*. The most prominent example is the sleeping sickness drug suramin. It inhibits all seven glycolytic enzymes isolated from *T. brucei* glycosomes as well as the cytosolic PYK with IC_{50} values between 3 and $100\,\mu M$ [110,111]. That does not imply that this drug kills the parasite by inhibition of glycolysis; it is doubtful that such a large molecule (molecular mass 1297 Da) easily crosses the glycosomal membrane. Moreover, suramin has an effect on many more enzymes, also mammalian glycolytic and other enzymes, and it inhibits growth of cultured trypanosomes with an ED_{50} value as low as 50 nM.

New inhibitors for glycolytic enzymes from trypanosomatid glycosomes and cytosol are now being obtained by different approaches that involve synthesis after structure-based design and catalytic-mechanism based design, structure-based database mining, medium- or high-throughput screening (HTS) of compound libraries and combinations of these approaches. As mentioned in "What Has Been Achieved So Far in Target Characterization?" section, crystal structures are available for several of these enzymes from *T. brucei*, *T. cruzi*, and/or *L. mexicana* (Table 7.1). Based on these structures, fructose 6-phosphate analogs – furanose sugar amino amides – have been developed as inhibitors of *T. brucei* PFK that have IC_{50} values of about $25\,\mu M$ and trypanocidal activity on cultured parasites in the low micromolar range with much less effect on cultured human fibroblasts. These fructose 6-phosphate analogs were also tested on trypanosomatid PYKs, that have a binding site for the allosteric activator fructose 2,6-bisphosphate with a quite different architecture than the fructose 1,6-bisphosphate binding site of the human PYK isoenzymes. Indeed, some of these compounds also inhibited this enzyme and killed the parasites at similar IC_{50} and ED_{50} values, respectively [112], although the binding of the compounds in the effector-binding site has not been ascertained.

Crystal structures have been determined for both *T. brucei* and *L. mexicana* ALD. Although their active sites are quite similar to that of mammalian ALDs, the minimal differences that exists and knowledge of the catalytic mechanism has allowed the development of a quasi-irreversibly binding inhibitor, 5-formyl-6-hydroxy-2-naphthyl di-sodium phosphate, that inactivated the trypanosomatid enzymes at low micromolar concentrations without effect, or only very weakly on mammalian ALDs, even at 1 mM [113]. Pro-drug forms of this and similar charged compounds were able to kill cultured trypanosomes with ED_{50} values in the low micromolar range with no effect on mammalian cells [114].

High-resolution crystal structures have been determined for the glycosomal GAPDH of each of the three trypanosomatids. These GAPDHs are characterized by a unique binding site for the adenosine moiety of the cofactor NAD^+. Most striking among the various differences is a hydrophobic cleft adjacent to the 2'-OH group of the adenosine ribose. The combined differences have been exploited for the synthesis of adenosine analogs with ribosyl C2' and adenosyl N^6 substitutions that act as selective inhibitors of the parasite enzyme with IC_{50} values as low as 0.06 μM [115–117]. These inhibitors block pyruvate production of *T. brucei*, kill cultured bloodstream-form trypanosomes but not human fibroblasts and are also active on *Leishmania* axenic amastigotes and intracellular *T. cruzi*. N^6,N^2-substituted adenosine analogs also inhibited *T. brucei* PGK, with IC_{50} values of approximately 30 μM, and inhibited growth of *T. brucei* and intracellular *T. cruzi* at ED_{50}s of 20 μM. However, the selectivity compared to murine fibroblasts was only 2-fold [118].

For several trypanosomatid enzymes, assays have been developed for HTS of large libraries of small compounds. For *T. brucei* HXK this has resulted in the identification of 10 compounds with IC_{50} values between 0.05 and 41 μM, 20- to 17 000-fold and 2- to 1720-fold, respectively, more potent than the previously identified *T. brucei* HXK inhibitors londiamine and quercetin [119]. Seven of the compounds inhibited growth of bloodstream-form *T. brucei* with $0.03 \leq ED_{50} \leq 3$ μM, while the corresponding values for human cell lines were greater than 12.5 μM, suggesting at least a 400-fold greater toxicity toward parasites for the most potent inhibitor. For PFK and PYK, submicromolar inhibitors have been obtained with trypanocidal activity in the low micromolar range (unpublished results). The potency of these inhibitors is currently being optimized by SAR analysis.

Trypanosomatid HXKs are inhibited by PPi, although at quite different concentrations and by different mechanisms: for *T. cruzi* ($K_i = 0.5$ mM, mixed type), and *Leishmania* spp. ($K_i = 0.035$ mM, competitive with ATP) [51,60]. *T. brucei* possesses two almost identical HXK isoforms, HK1 and HK2. Oligomers of HK1 are active, whereas oligomers of HK2 are not. However, hetero-oligomers have even an increased activity, up to 3-fold. HK1 is not inhibited by PPi, but HK2 endows the oligomers sensitivity towards PPi [120]. These specific properties of trypanosomatid HXKs were used to develop bisphosphonates as inhibitors. Bisphosphonates are metabolically inert inorganic PPi analogs in which the oxygen bridge between the two phosphorus atoms has been replaced by a carbon substituted with various side-chains [121]. Aromatic amino-methylene bisphosphonate derivatives have been identified as potent and selective inhibitors of *T. cruzi* hexokinase. These compounds blocked glycolysis and growth of both extracellular epimastigotes and intracellular amastigotes, with a selectivity ratio of more than three orders of magnitude [122,123], and therefore constitute a promising new class of anti-*T. cruzi* agents. Bisphosphonates have been shown already to be active both *in vitro* and *in vivo* against *T. cruzi* without apparent toxicity to the host cells [48]. Since millions of people have already been treated with bisphosphonates and since they have proved anti-chagasic activity, such compounds as inhibitors of PPi-susceptible glycosomal enzymes appear attractive for further development as chemotherapeutic agents using structure-based drug design. A crystal structure of a trypanosomatid HXK that would allow, by SAR analysis, further optimization of any of the available inhibitors is not yet available. In contrast, a crystal structure has been determined for the *T. cruzi* GlcK [53], but this enzyme is not susceptible to PPi [52] and thus unlikely inhibited by the bisphosphonate compounds developed for the HXK. No GlcK inhibitors have been developed to date.

SQS, also involved in sterol synthesis and with a dual glycosomal and mitochondrial/microsomal localization in both *T. cruzi* and *L. mexicana* [45], has been chemically validated as a chemotherapeutic target in both parasites [47]. *T. cruzi* SQS has been produced as a soluble, fully active, recombinant enzyme and used to identify quinuclidine derivatives acting as parasite enzyme-specific inhibitors [124,125]. Two of such compounds, E5700 and ER-119884, display very potent anti-*T. cruzi* activity *in vitro*, and one of them (E5700) was able to provide full protection against death and completely arrested development of parasitemia in a murine model of acute disease when given orally [126]. This was the first report of an orally active SQS inhibitor as an anti-infection agent [48]. A new class of anti-*T. cruzi* agents, aryloxyethylthiocyanates, comprises 4-phenoxyphenoxyethylthiocyanate (WC-9); it acts also by selectively inhibiting the parasite's SQS [48,127]. Sterol synthesis of *T. cruzi* as a drug target is discussed in much greater detail in Chapter 26 of this volume.

Several enzymes involved in the trypanosomatids' unique peroxide detoxification cascade involving trypanothione have PTS motifs, indicating a potentially glycosomal localization, although most or almost all activity seems to be present in the cytosol (reviewed in [3]). For *T. cruzi*, but not *T. brucei*, the activity was partially associated with glycosomes, whereas the situation for *Leishmania* spp. is unknown [128,129]. The design and tests of specific trypanothione reductase (TR) inhibitors has received much attention from several research groups in the last 15 years, and many families of compounds have been identified as TR inhibitors and trypanocidal agents *in vitro* (reviewed in [48]). Thioridazine, a known inhibitor of TR *in vitro* [130], is able to reduce the parasitemia, increase survival, and prevent cardiac damage in murine models of acute Chagas disease [131,132]. For a more detailed discussion of the trypanothione system as a drug target in trypanosomatids, the reader is referred to Chapters 9, 21, and 22 in this volume.

Inhibitors with trypanocidal activity at micro- and submicromolar concentrations, respectively, are also available for the partially in glycosomes located PPP enzymes G6PDH and 6PGDH [22,133], and are discussed in more detail in Chapter 16 of this volume.

The glycosomal enzyme HGPRT, involved in purine salvage, has been proposed as a target for anti-parasitic chemotherapy. The enzyme has already been used in the development of trypanocidals, by exploiting the fact that it can phosphoribosylate the hypoxanthine analog allopurinol (4-hydroxypyrazolo(3,4-*d*)pyrimidine); the ribonucleotide analog produced is incorporated into RNA during transcription, resulting in its degradation and consequently a decreased protein synthesis in the trypanosomatids [134]. Although the allopurinol is also metabolized by the human enzyme, its selectivity against trypanosomatids is attributed to the higher specific activity of the enzyme in the parasites as well as the fact that humans can synthesize purines *de novo* [135]. In leishmaniasis, the efficacy of this molecule alone is not sufficient for routine clinical use, but combined with meglumine antimoniate it is applied as a parasitostatic in infected dogs [136,137]. Allopurinol was shown to be active in murine models of acute Chagas disease [138], and has also been used to treat patients with the chronic form of the disease [139].

The available *T. cruzi* and *L. tarentolae* HGPRT crystal structures [107,108] may allow us to exploit differences between the active site of the parasite and human enzymes for the design of parasite enzyme-selective inhibitors or improved subversive substrates as better trypanocidals. Purine and pyrimidine analogs have been tested with IC_{50} values in the micromolar range, including allopurinol [108]. Allopurinol appeared to be more efficient for inhibition of the *Leishmania* than the *T. cruzi* enzyme [107,108]. A docking program was used to screen the Available Chemicals Directory for ligands of the active site of the *T. cruzi* enzyme [140]. This yielded inhibitors with K_is between 0.5 and 17 µM, some of them being effective in inhibiting growth of parasites in infected mammalian cells at low micromolar concentration. Further optimization of HGPRT ligands as trypanocidals seems warranted.

Discussion and Conclusions

In each of the trypanosomatid parasites, glycosomes are very important. In the pathogenic stages of all of them, several glycosomal processes or functions have been shown to be essential for viability or pathogenic virulence. The organelles offer potential drug targets at several levels: (i) in the enzymes they harbor, (ii) in metabolic communication between their matrix and the cytosol via solute transporters and channels, and (iii) in their biogenesis and degradation.

Although glycolysis remains the most remarkable process inside glycosomes, research during the last 30 years has demonstrated that additionally a considerable number of other metabolic processes, involving many enzymes, are present inside these organelles (reviewed in [2]). An increasing number of these processes and enzymes also appeared to be essential for the viability or virulence of the pathogenic stages of one or all of the trypanosomatid parasites. In this chapter, we described the processes and enzymes that have been shown to be essential or at least important, the progress made in the characterization of a considerable number of these candidate drug targets, and the state of the art in the development of compounds that, in a selective manner, inhibit such target enzymes of the parasites, growth of parasites, and decrease or cure infections in animal models.

An aspect of glycosomes that has not yet been a topic of drug discovery-related research concerns the connection between the metabolism processes in the glyco-somal matrix and the cytosol. Until very recently nothing was known about how metabolic substrates, intermediates, and products cross the glycosomal membrane. Nonetheless, such solute translocation is essential for the proper functioning of the parasites' metabolism and thus their viability. Recently obtained data discussed in this chapter show that almost certainly, bulky solutes are translocated by specific transporters, while the majority of the metabolites that have to cross the membrane and have a molecular mass smaller than 400 Da do so via some channels with low substrate selectivity [91,92,97,99]. Furthermore, the solute transporters have a very low sequence similarity with their human counterparts and no homologs can be found of the known human peroxisomal solute channel in the trypanosomatid genome databases. Therefore, the glycosomal solute transporters and channels also offer interesting perspectives for future drug discovery. A corollary of the existence of channels in the glycosomal membrane is that drugs targeted to glycosomal matrix proteins should preferably have a mass that permits their translocation through the aqueous pore formed by the channel-forming proteins, thus not larger than approximately 400 Da.

For *T. brucei*, the proper compartmentalization of glycolysis has been shown to be essential. Due to the peculiar properties of some glycolytic enzymes, the process can only function inside glycosomes; even partial mislocalization is detrimental to the cell. This will certainly also be the case under glycolytic growth conditions of the other parasites, such as is probably the case for *T. cruzi* trypomastigotes, but glycolysis seems not very important for the intracellular *T. cruzi* and *Leishmania* spp. amastigotes. However, it is conceivable that also other glycosomal processes that are essential for the parasites need complete compartmentalization for proper functioning, but this remains to be established. The essentiality of proper sequestering of enzymes inside glycosomes implies that the organelle's biogenesis and thus the PEX proteins mediating this process are good drug targets. This approach of drug discovery is currently actively being pursued, because PEX proteins are not well conserved between human and trypanosomatid. Indeed, preliminary results are promising. Similarly, the degradation of glycosomes by autophagy, and thus autophagy-related proteins involved in it, are probably promising drug targets in those pathogenic stages where reprogramming of glycosomal metabolism during life cycle differentiation plays a role for viability or virulence. This notion has been extensively discussed in [104], but needs further research to substantiate it.

Glycosomes were first described 35 years ago, as microbodies containing gly-colytic enzymes in *T. brucei* [1]. Since then much research has been devoted to the demonstration of the organelles in other Kinetoplastea, the identification of other metabolic processes inside the organelles, and the characterization of the glycolytic and some other glycosomal enzymes of the human parasitic trypanosomatid species. In the last 10–15 years our knowledge of the organelle has increased enormously thanks to the systems biology and reverse genetics approaches being used in the understanding of its functioning, the studies of its biogenesis, and all of the information that became available through the sequence of the trypanosomatid genomes and functional genomics projects. Together with the advances made in the drug discovery process by improvement of structure-based drug design and mining methods, and the introduction of HTS of large compound libraries, this has led to a situation that research on drug discovery for glycosomal enzymes has accelerated significantly in recent years. It is hoped that this research will soon lead to compounds for clinical trials and eventually to therapies for people suffering from trypanosomatid infections.

Acknowledgments

We thank Professor Michael Ferguson (University of Dundee, UK) for providing detailed information about sugar-nucleotide biosynthesis in *T. brucei* glycosomes. M.G.L. gratefully acknowledges a PhD scholarship from the "Fonds pour la formation à la Recherche dans l'Industrie et dans l'Agriculture" (FRIA) and the "Patrimoine de Faculté Médicine, Université catholique de Louvain." L.A., W.Q., and J.L.C. thank the "Fondo Nacional de Ciencia, Tecnología e Innovación" for financial support for projects MC-2007000960 (L.A.) and MC-2007001425 (J.L.C. and W.Q.), and P.A.M.M. acknowledges the support from the "Fonds de la Recherche Scientifique" (FRS-FNRS) and the Belgian Interuniversity Attraction Poles–Federal Office for Scientific, Technical, and Cultural Affairs.

References

1 Opperdoes, F.R. and Borst, P. (1977) Localization of nine glycolytic enzymes in a microbody-like organelle in *Trypanosoma brucei*: the glycosome. *FEBS Lett.*, **80**, 360–364.

2 Gualdrón-López, M., Brennand, A., Hannaert, V., Quiñones, W., Cáceres, A.J., Bringaud, F., Concepción, J.L., and Michels, P.A.M. (2012) When, how and why glycolysis became compartmentalised in the Kinetoplastea. A new look at an ancient organelle. *Int. J. Parasitol.*, **42**, 1–20.

3 Opperdoes, F.R. and Szikora, J.P. (2006) *In silico* prediction of the glycosomal enzymes of *Leishmania major* and trypanosomes. *Mol. Biochem. Parasitol.*, **147**, 193–206.

4 Helfert, S., Estévez, A.M., Bakker, B., Michels, P., and Clayton, C. (2001) Roles of triosephosphate isomerase and aerobic

metabolism in *Trypanosoma brucei*. *Biochem. J.*, **357**, 117–125.

5 Verlinde, C.L.M.J., Hannaert, V., Blonski, C., Willson, M., Périé, J.J., Fothergill-Gilmore, L.A., Opperdoes, F.R. *et al.* (2001) Glycolysis as a target for the design of new anti-trypanosome drugs. *Drug Resist. Updat.*, **4**, 50–65.

6 Opperdoes, F.R. and Michels, P.A.M. (2001) Enzymes of carbohydrate metabolism as potential drug targets. *Int. J. Parasitol.*, **31**, 482–490.

7 Seyfang, A. and Duszenko, M. (1991) Specificity of glucose transport in *Trypanosoma brucei*. Effective inhibition by phloretin and cytochalasin B. *Eur. J. Biochem.*, **202**, 191–196.

8 Albert, M.A., Haanstra, J.R., Hannaert, V., Van Roy, J., Opperdoes, F.R., Bakker, B. M., and Michels, P.A.M. (2005) Experimental and *in silico* analyses of

glycolytic flux control in bloodstream form *Trypanosoma brucei*. *J. Biol. Chem.*, **280**, 28306–28315.

9 Cáceres, A.J., Michels, P.A.M., and Hannaert, V. (2010) Genetic validation of aldolase and glyceraldehyde-3-phosphate dehydrogenase as drug targets in *Trypanosoma brucei*. *Mol. Biochem. Parasitol.*, **169**, 50–54.

10 Bakker, B.M., Walsh, M.C., Ter Kuile, B.H., Mensonides, F.I., Michels, P.A.M., Opperdoes, F.R., and Westerhoff, H.V. (1999) Contribution of glucose transport to the control of the glycolytic flux in *Trypanosoma brucei*. *Proc. Natl. Acad. Sci. USA*, **96**, 10098–10103.

11 Wiemer, E.A.C., Michels, P.A.M., and Opperdoes, F.R. (1995) The inhibition of pyruvate transport across the plasma membrane of the bloodstream form of *Trypanosoma brucei* and its metabolic implications. *Biochem. J.*, **312**, 479–484.

12 Bakker, B.M., Michels, P.A.M., Opperdoes, F.R., and Westerhoff, H.V. (1997) Glycolysis in bloodstream form *Trypanosoma brucei* can be understood in terms of the kinetics of the glycolytic enzymes. *J. Biol. Chem.*, **272**, 3207–3215.

13 Bakker, B.M., Michels, P.A.M., Opperdoes, F.R., and Westerhoff, H.V. (1999) What controls glycolysis in bloodstream form *Trypanosoma brucei*? *J. Biol.Chem.*, **274**, 14551–14559.

14 Bakker, B.M., Westerhoff, H.V., Opperdoes, F.R., and Michels, P.A.M. (2000) Metabolic control analysis of glycolysis in trypanosomes as an approach to improve selectivity and effectiveness of drugs. *Mol. Biochem. Parasitol.*, **106**, 1–10.

15 Haanstra, J.R., Kerkhoven, E.J., Van Tuijl, A., Blits, M., Wurst, M., Van Nuland, R., Albert, M.A. *et al.* (2011) A domino effect in drug action: from metabolic assault towards parasite differentiation. *Mol. Microbiol.*, **79**, 94–108.

16 Schuster, R. and Holzhütter, H.G. (1995) Use of mathematical models for predicting the metabolic effect of large-scale enzyme activity alterations. Application to enzyme deficiencies of red blood cells. *Eur. J. Biochem.*, **229**, 403–418.

17 Hornberg, J.J., Bruggeman, F.J., Bakker, B.M., and Westerhoff, H.V. (2007) Metabolic control analysis to identify optimal drug targets. *Prog. Drug. Res.*, **64**, 172–189.

18 Misset, O., Bos, O.J.M., and Opperdoes, F.R. (1986) Glycolytic enzymes of *Trypanosoma brucei*. Simultaneous purification intraglycosomal concentrations and physical properties. *Eur. J. Biochem.*, **157**, 441–453.

19 Cordeiro, A.T., Thiemann, O.H., and Michels, P.A.M. (2009) Inhibition of *Trypanosoma brucei* glucose-6-phosphate dehydrogenase by human steroids and their effects on the viability of cultured parasites. *Bioorg. Med. Chem.*, **17**, 2483–2489.

20 Gupta, S., Cordeiro, A.T., and Michels, P.A.M. (2011) Glucose-6-phosphate dehydrogenase is the target for the trypanocidal action of human steroids. *Mol. Biochem. Parasitol.*, **176**, 112–115.

21 Hanau, S., Rinaldi, E., Dallocchio, F., Gilbert, I.H., Dardonville, C., Adams, M.J., Gover, S., and Barrett, M.P. (2004) 6-Phosphogluconate dehydrogenase: a target for drugs in African trypanosomes. *Curr. Med. Chem.*, **11**, 2639–2650.

22 Gupta, S., Igoillo-Esteve, M., Michels, P.A.M., and Cordeiro, A.T. (2011) Glucose-6-phosphate dehydrogenase of trypanosomatids: characterization target validation and drug discovery. *Mol. Biol. Int.*, **2011**, 135701.

23 Roper, J.R., Güther, M.L.S., Milne, K.G., and Ferguson, M.A.J. (2002) Galactose metabolism is essential for the African sleeping sickness parasite *Trypanosoma brucei*. *Proc. Natl. Acad. Sci. USA*, **99**, 5884–5889.

24 Roper, J.R., Güther, M.L.S., MacRae, J.I., Prescott, A.R., Hallyburton, I., Acosta-Serrano, A., and Ferguson, M.A.J. (2005) The suppression of galactose metabolism in procylic form *Trypanosoma brucei* causes cessation of cell growth and alters procyclin glycoprotein structure and copy number. *J. Biol. Chem.*, **280**, 19728–19736.

25 Turnock, D.C., Izquierdo, L., and Ferguson, M.A. (2007) The *de novo* synthesis of GDP-fucose is essential for flagellar adhesion and cell growth in *Trypanosoma brucei*. *J. Biol. Chem.*, **282**, 28853–28863.

26 Stokes, M.J., Güther, M.L.S., Turnock, D.C., Prescott, A.R., Martin, K.L., Alphey, M.S., and Ferguson, M.A.J. (2008) The synthesis of UDP-N-acetylglucosamine is essential for bloodstream form *Trypanosoma brucei in vitro* and *in vivo* and UDP-N-acetylglucosamine starvation reveals a hierarchy in parasite protein glycosylation. *J. Biol. Chem.*, **283**, 16147–16161.

27 Mariño, K., Güther, M.L., Wernimont, A.K., Amani, M., Hui, R., and Ferguson, M.A. (2010) Identification subcellular localization biochemical properties and high-resolution crystal structure of *Trypanosoma brucei* UDP-glucose pyrophosphorylase. *Glycobiology*, **20**, 1619–1630.

28 Mariño, K., Güther, M.L., Wernimont, A.K., Qiu, W., Hui, R., and Ferguson, M.A. (2011) Characterization localization essentiality and high-resolution crystal structure of glucosamine-6-phosphate N-acetyltransferase from *Trypanosoma brucei*. *Eukaryot. Cell*, **10**, 985–997.

29 Denton, H., Fyffe, S., and Smith, T.K. (2010) GDP-mannose pyrophosphorylase is essential in the bloodstream form of *Trypanosoma brucei*. *Biochem. J.*, **425**, 603–614.

30 Stoppani, A.O., Docampo, R., de Boiso, J. F., and Frasch, A.C. (1980) Effect of inhibitors of electron transport and oxidative phosphorylation on *Trypanosoma cruzi* respiration and growth. *Mol. Biochem. Parasitol.*, **2**, 3–21.

31 Cannata, J.J. and Cazzulo, J.J. (1984) The aerobic fermentation of glucose by *Trypanosoma cruzi*. *Comp. Biochem. Physiol. B*, **79**, 297–308.

32 Sanchez-Moreno, M., Fernandez-Becerra, M.C., Castilla-Calvente, J.J., and Osuna, A. (1995) Metabolic studies by ¹H NMR of different forms of *Trypanosoma cruzi* as obtained by 'in vitro' culture. *FEMS Microbiol. Lett.*, **133**, 119–125.

33 Taylor, M.B. and Gutteridge, W.E. (1987) *Trypanosoma cruzi*: subcellular distribution of glycolytic and some related enzymes of epimastigotes. *Exp. Parasitol.*, **63**, 84–97.

34 Besteiro, S., Biran, M., Biteau, N., Coustou, V., Baltz, T., Canioni, P., and Bringaud, F. (2002) Succinate secreted by *Trypanosoma brucei* is produced by a novel and unique glycosomal enzyme NADH-dependent fumarate reductase. *J. Biol. Chem.*, **277**, 38001–38012.

35 Acosta, H., Dubourdieu, M., Quiñones, W., Cáceres, A., Bringaud, F., and Concepción, J.L. (2004) Pyruvate phosphate dikinase and pyrophosphate metabolism in the glycosome of *Trypanosoma cruzi* epimastigotes. *Comp. Biochem. Physiol. B Biochem. Mol. Biol.*, **138**, 347–356.

36 Concepción, J.L., Acosta, H., Quiñones, W., and Dubourdieu, M. (2001) An α-glycerophosphate dehydrogenase is present in *Trypanosoma cruzi* glycosomes. *Mem. Inst. Oswaldo Cruz*, **96**, 697–701.

37 Sarkar, M., Hamilton, C.J., and Fairlamb, A.H. (2003) Properties of phosphoenolpyruvate mutase the first enzyme in the aminoethylphosphonate biosynthetic pathway in *Trypanosoma cruzi*. *J. Biol. Chem.*, **278**, 22703–22708.

38 Kollien, A.H. and Schaub, G.A. (2000) The development of *Trypanosoma cruzi* in Triatominae. *Parasitol. Today*, **16**, 381–387.

39 Maugeri, D.A., Cannata, J.J., and Cazzulo, J.J. (2011) Glucose metabolism in *Trypanosoma cruzi*. *Essays Biochem.*, **51**, 15–30.

40 Engel, J.C., Franke de Cazzulo, B.M., Stoppani, A.O.M., Cannata, J.J.B., and Cazzulo, J.J. (1987) Aerobic glucose fermentation by *Trypanosoma cruzi* axenic culture amastigote-like forms during growth and differentiation to epimastigotes. *Mol. Biochem. Parasitol.*, **26**, 1–10.

41 Atwood, J.A.3rd, Weatherly, D.B., Minning, T.A., Bundy, B., Cavola, C., Opperdoes, F.R., Orlando, R., and Tarleton, R.L. (2005) The *Trypanosoma cruzi* proteome. *Science*, **309**, 473–476.

42 Silber, A.M., Tonelli, R.R., Lopes, C.G., Cunha-e-Silva, N., Torrecilhas, A.C., Schumacher, R.I., Colli, W., and Alves, M.J. (2009) Glucose uptake in the mammalian stages of *Trypanosoma cruzi*. *Mol. Biochem. Parasitol.*, **168**, 102–108.

43 Berriman, M., Ghedin, E., Hertz-Fowler, C., Blandin, G., Renauld, H., Bartholomeu, D.C., Lennard, N.J. *et al.*

(2005) The genome of the African trypanosome *Trypanosoma brucei*. *Science*, **309**, 416–422.

44 Maugeri, D.A. and Cazzulo, J.J. (2004) The pentose phosphate pathway in *Trypanosoma cruzi*. *FEMS Microbiol. Lett.*, **234**, 117–123.

45 Urbina, J.A., Concepción, J.L., Rangel, S., Visbal, G., and Lira, R. (2002) Squalene synthase as a chemotherapeutic target in *Trypanosoma cruzi* and *Leishmania mexicana*. *Mol. Biochem. Parasitol.*, **125**, 35–45.

46 Allen, T.E. and Ullman, B. (1994) Molecular characterization and overexpression of the hypoxanthine-guanine phosphoribosyltransferase gene from *Trypanosoma cruzi*. *Mol. Biochem. Parasitol.*, **65**, 233–245.

47 Urbina, J.A. and Docampo, R. (2003) Specific chemotherapy of Chagas disease: controversies and advances. *Trends Parasitol.*, **19**, 495–501.

48 Urbina, J.A. (2010) Specific chemotherapy of Chagas disease: relevance current limitations and new approaches. *Acta Trop.*, **115**, 55–68.

49 Quiñones, W., Urbina, J.A., Dubourdieu, M., and Concepción, J.L. (2004) The glycosome membrane of *Trypanosoma cruzi* epimastigotes: protein and lipid composition. *Exp. Parasitol.*, **106**, 135–149.

50 Aboushadi, N., Engfelt, W.H., Paton, V.G., and Krisans, S.K. (1999) Role of peroxisomes in isoprenoid biosynthesis. *J. Histochem. Cytochem.*, **47**, 1127–1132.

51 Cáceres, A.J., Portillo, R., Acosta, H., Rosales, D., Quiñones, W., Avilan, L., Salazar, L. *et al.* (2003) Molecular and biochemical characterization of hexokinase from *Trypanosoma cruzi*. *Mol. Biochem. Parasitol.*, **126**, 251–262.

52 Cáceres, A.J., Quiñones, W., Gualdrón, M., Cordeiro, A., Avilán, L., Michels, P.A. M., and Concepción, J.L. (2007) Molecular and biochemical characterization of novel glucokinases from *Trypanosoma cruzi* and *Leishmania* spp. *Mol. Biochem. Parasitol.*, **156**, 235–245.

53 Cordeiro, A.T., Cáceres, A.J., Vertommen, D., Concepción, J.L., Michels, P.A.M., and Versées, W. (2007) The crystal structure of *Trypanosoma cruzi* glucokinase reveals features determining oligomerization and anomer specificity of hexose-phosphorylating enzymes. *J. Mol. Biol.*, **372**, 1215–1226.

54 Murray, H.W., Berman, J.D., Davies, C.R., and Saravia, N.G. (2005) Advances in leishmaniasis. *Lancet*, **366**, 1561–1577.

55 Naderer, T. and McConville, M.J. (2011) Intracellular growth and pathogenesis of *Leishmania* parasites. *Essays Biochem.*, **51**, 81–95.

56 McConville, M.J. and Naderer, T. (2011) Metabolic pathways required for the intracellular survival of *Leishmania*. *Annu. Rev. Microbiol.*, **65**, 543–561.

57 Coombs, G.H., Tetley, L., Moss, V.A., and Vickerman, K. (1986) Three dimensional structure of the *Leishmania* amastigote as revealed by computer-aided reconstruction from serial sections. *Parasitology*, **92**, 13–23.

58 Coombs, G.H., Craft, J.A., and Hart, D.T. (1982) A comparative study of *Leishmania mexicana* amastigotes and promastigotes. Enzyme activities and subcellular locations. *Mol. Biochem. Parasitol.*, **5**, 199–211.

59 Mottram, J.C. and Coombs, G.H. (1985) *Leishmania mexicana*: subcellular distribution of enzymes in amastigotes and promastigotes. *Exp. Parasitol.*, **59**, 265–274.

60 Pabón, M.A., Cáceres, A.J., Gualdrón, M., Quiñones, W., Avilán, L., and Concepción, J.L. (2007) Purification and characterization of hexokinase from *Leishmania mexicana*. *Parasitol. Res.*, **100**, 803–810.

61 Rosenzweig, D., Smith, D., Opperdoes, F., Stern, S., Olafson, R.W., and Zilberstein, D. (2008) Retooling *Leishmania* metabolism: from sand fly gut to human macrophage. *FASEB J.*, **22**, 590–602.

62 Naderer, T. and McConville, M.J. (2008) The *Leishmania*-macrophage interaction: a metabolic perspective. *Cell Microbiol.*, **10**, 301–308.

63 Burchmore, R.J., Rodriguez-Contreras, D., McBride, K., Merkel, P., Barrett, M.P., Modi, G., Sacks, D., and Landfear, S.M. (2003) Genetic characterization of glucose

transporter function in *Leishmania mexicana*. *Proc. Natl. Acad. Sci. USA*, **100**, 3901–3906.

64 Feng, X., Rodriguez-Contreras, D., Buffalo, C., Bouwer, H.G., Kruvand, E., Beverley, S.M., and Landfear, S.M. (2009) Amplification of an alternate transporter gene suppresses the avirulent phenotype of glucose transporter null mutants in *Leishmania mexicana*. *Mol. Microbiol.*, **71**, 369–381.

65 Brotherton, M.C., Racine, G., Foucher, A. L., Drummelsmith, J., Papadopoulou, B., and Ouellette, M. (2010) Analysis of stage-specific expression of basic proteins in *Leishmania infantum*. *J. Proteome Res.*, **9**, 3842–3853.

66 Naderer, T., Ellis, M.A., Sernee, M.F., De Souza, D.P., Curtis, J., Handman, E., and McConville, M.J. (2006) Virulence of *Leishmania major* in macrophages and mice requires the gluconeogenic enzyme fructose-1,6-bisphosphatase. *Proc. Natl. Acad. Sci. USA*, **103**, 5502–5507.

67 Keegan, F.P. and Blum, J.J. (1992) Utilization of a carbohydrate reserve comprised primarily of mannose by *Leishmania donovani*. *Mol. Biochem. Parasitol.*, **53**, 193–200.

68 Ralton, J.E., Naderer, T., Piraino, H.L., Bashtannyk, T.A., Callaghan, J.M., and McConville, M.J. (2003) Evidence that intracellular β1–2 mannan is a virulence factor in *Leishmania* parasites. *J. Biol. Chem.*, **278**, 40757–40763.

69 Garami, A. and Ilg, T. (2001) Disruption of mannose activation in *Leishmania mexicana*: GDP-mannose pyrophosphorylase is required for virulence but not for viability. *EMBO J.*, **20**, 3657–3666.

70 Naderer, T., Wee, E., and McConville, M.J. (2008) Role of hexosamine biosynthesis in *Leishmania* growth and virulence. *Mol. Microbiol.*, **69**, 858–869.

71 Joshi, M.B., Rogers, M.E., Shakarian, A. M., Yamage, M., Al-Harthi, S.A., Bates, P. A., and Dwyer, D.M. (2005) Molecular characterization, expression, and *in vivo* analysis of *LmexCht1*. The chitinase of the human pathogen, *Leishmania mexicana*. *J. Biol. Chem.*, **280**, 3847–3861.

72 Naderer, T., Heng, J., and McConville, M. J. (2010) Evidence that intracellular stages of *Leishmania major* utilize amino sugars as a major carbon source. *PLoS Pathog.*, **6**, e1001245.

73 Hart, D.T. and Opperdoes, F.R. (1984) The occurrence of glycosomes (microbodies) in the promastigote stage of four major *Leishmania* species. *Mol. Biochem. Parasitol.*, **13**, 159–172.

74 Paape, D., Lippuner, C., Schmid, M., Ackermann, R., Barrios-Llerena, M.E., Zimny-Arndt, U., Brinkmann, V. *et al.* (2008) Transgenic fluorescent *Leishmania mexicana* allow direct analysis of the proteome of intracellular amastigotes. *Mol. Cell Proteomics*, **7**, 1688–1701.

75 Peña-Diaz, J., Montalvetti, A., Flores, C.L., Constan, A., Hurtado-Guerrero, R., De Souza, W., Gancedo, C. *et al.* (2004) Mitochondrial localization of the mevalonate pathway enzyme 3-hydroxy-3-methyl-glutaryl-CoA reductase in the Trypanosomatidae. *Mol. Biol. Cell*, **15**, 1356–1363.

76 Ginger, M.L., McFadden, G.I., and Michels, P.A.M. (2010) Rewiring and regulation of cross-compartmentalized metabolism in protists. *Philos. Trans. R. Soc. Lond. B Biol. Sci.*, **365**, 831–845.

77 Carrero-Lérida, J., Pérez-Moreno, G., Castillo-Acosta, V.M., Ruiz-Pérez, L.M., and González-Pacanowska, D. (2009) Intracellular location of the early steps of the isoprenoid biosynthetic pathway in the trypanosomatids *Leishmania major* and *Trypanosoma brucei*. *Int. J. Parasitol.*, **39**, 307–314.

78 Colotti, G. and Ilari, A. (2011) Polyamine metabolism in *Leishmania*: from arginine to trypanothione. *Amino Acids*, **40**, 269–285.

79 Krauth-Siegel, L.R., Comini, M.A., and Schlecker, T. (2007) The trypanothione system. *Subcell. Biochem.*, **44**, 231–251.

80 Gaur, U., Roberts, S.C., Dalvi, R.P., Corraliza, I., Ullman, B., and Wilson, M. E. (2007) An effect of parasite-encoded arginase on the outcome of murine cutaneous leishmaniasis. *J. Immunol.*, **179**, 8446–8453.

81 Balaña-Fouce, R., Calvo-Alvarez, E., Alvarez-Velilla, R., Prada, C.F.,

Pérez-Pertejo, Y., and Reguera, R.M. (2012) Role of trypanosomatid's arginase in polyamine biosynthesis and pathogenesis. *Mol. Biochem. Parasitol.*, **181**, 85–93.

82 Das, P., Lahiri, A., Lahiri, A., and Chakravortty, D. (2010) Modulation of the arginase pathway in the context of microbial pathogenesis: a metabolic enzyme moonlighting as an immune modulator. *PLoS Pathog.*, **6**, e1000899.

83 Opperdoes, F.R. and Michels, P.A.M. (2008) The metabolic repertoire of *Leishmania* and implications for drug discovery, in *Leishmania: After the Genome* (eds P.J. Myler and N. Fasel), Caister Academic Press, Norwich, pp. 123–158.

84 Wilkinson, S.R., Prathalingam, S.R., Taylor, M.C., Horn, D., and Kelly, J.M. (2005) Vitamin C biosynthesis in trypanosomes: a role for the glycosome. *Proc. Natl. Acad. Sci. USA*, **102**, 11645–11650.

85 Biyani, N. and Madhubala, R. (2011) *Leishmania donovani* encodes a functional enzyme involved in vitamin C biosynthesis: arabino-1,4-lactone oxidase. *Mol. Biochem. Parasitol.*, **180**, 76–85.

86 Hassan, H.F., Mottram, J.C., and Coombs, G.H. (1985) Subcellular localisation of purine-metabolising enzymes in *Leishmania mexicana mexicana*. *Comp. Biochem. Physiol. B*, **81**, 1037–1040.

87 Zarella-Boitz, J.M., Rager, N., Jardim, A., and Ullman, B. (2004) Subcellular localization of adenine and xanthine phosphoribosyltransferases in *Leishmania donovani*. *Mol. Biochem. Parasitol.*, **134**, 43–51.

88 Boitz, J.M. and Ullman, B. (2006) A conditional mutant deficient in hypoxanthine-guanine phosphoribosyltransferase and xanthine phosphoribosyltransferase validates the purine salvage pathway of *Leishmania donovani*. *J. Biol. Chem.*, **281**, 16084–16089.

89 Carter, N.S., Yates, P.A., Gessford, S.K., Galagan, S.R., Landfear, S.M., and Ullman, B. (2010) Adaptive responses to purine starvation in *Leishmania donovani*. *Mol. Microbiol.*, **78**, 92–107.

90 French, J.B., Yates, P.A., Soysa, D.R., Boitz, J.M., Carter, N.S., Chang, B., Ullman, B., and Ealick, S.E. (2011) The *Leishmania donovani* UMP synthase is essential for promastigote viability and has an unusual tetrameric structure that exhibits substrate-controlled oligomerization. *J. Biol. Chem.*, **286**, 20930–20941.

91 Yernaux, C., Fransen, M., Brees, C., Lorenzen, S., and Michels, P.A.M. (2006) *Trypanosoma brucei* glycosomal ABC transporters: identification and membrane targeting. *Mol. Membr. Biol.*, **23**, 157–172.

92 Igoillo-Esteve, M., Mazet, M., Deumer, G., Wallemacq, P., and Michels, P.A.M. (2011) Glycosomal ABC transporters of *Trypanosoma brucei*: characterisation of their expression topology and substrate specificity. *Int. J. Parasitol.*, **41**, 429–438.

93 Visser, N., Opperdoes, F.R., and Borst, P. (1981) Subcellular compartmentation of glycolytic intermediates in *Trypanosoma brucei*. *Eur. J. Biochem.*, **118**, 521–526.

94 Hammond, D.J., Aman, R.A., and Wang, C.C. (1985) The role of compartmentation and glycerol kinase in the synthesis of ATP within the glycosome of *Trypanosoma brucei*. *J. Biol. Chem.*, **260**, 15646–15654.

95 Haanstra, J.R., Van Tuijl, A., Kessler, P., Reijnders, W., Michels, P.A.M., Westerhoff, H.V., Parsons, M., and Bakker, B.M. (2008) Compartmentation prevents a lethal turbo-explosion of glycolysis in trypanosomes. *Proc. Natl. Acad. Sci. USA*, **105**, 17718–17723.

96 Bakker, B.M., Mensonides, F.I., Teusink, B., Van Hoek, P., Michels, P.A.M., and Westerhoff, H.V. (2000) Compartmentation protects trypanosomes from the dangerous design of glycolysis. *Proc. Natl. Acad. Sci. USA*, **97**, 2087–2092.

97 Gualdrón-López, M., Vapola, M.H., Miinalainen, I.J., Hiltunen, J.K., Michels, P.A., and Antonenkov, V.D. (2012) Channel-forming activities in the glycosomal fraction from the bloodstream form of *Trypanosoma brucei*. *PLoS ONE*, **7**, e34530.

98 Reumann, S. (2000) The structural properties of plant peroxisomes and their

metabolic significance. *Biol. Chem.*, **381**, 639–648.

99 Antonenkov, V.D. and Hiltunen, J.K. (2012) Transfer of metabolites across the peroxisomal membrane. *Biochim. Biophys. Acta*, **1822**, 1374–1386.

100 Moyersoen, J., Choe, J., Fan, E., Hol, W.G.J., and Michels, P.A.M. (2004) Biogenesis of peroxisomes and glycosomes: trypanosomatid glycosome assembly is a promising new drug target. *FEMS Microbiol. Rev.*, **28**, 603–643.

101 Galland, N. and Michels, P.A.M. (2010) Comparison of the peroxisomal matrix protein import system of different organisms. Exploration of possibilities for developing inhibitors of the import system of trypanosomatids for anti-parasite chemotherapy. *Eur. J. Cell Biol.*, **89**, 621–637.

102 Rokka, A., Antonenkov, V.D., Soininen, R., Immonen, H.L., Pirilä, P.L., Bergmann, U., Sormunen, R.T. *et al.* (2009) Pxmp2 is a channel-forming protein in mammalian peroxisomal membrane. *PLoS ONE*, **4**, e5090.

103 Duszenko, M., Ginger, M.L., Brennand, A., Gualdrón-López, M., Colombo, M.I., Coombs, G.H., Coppens, I. *et al.* (2011) Autophagy in protists. *Autophagy*, **7**, 127–158.

104 Brennand, A., Gualdrón-López, M., Coppens, I., Rigden, D.J., Ginger, M.L., and Michels, P.A.M. (2011) Autophagy in parasitic protists: unique features and drug targets. *Mol. Biochem. Parasitol.*, **177**, 83–99.

105 Herman, M., Pérez-Morga, D., Schtickzelle, N., and Michels, P.A.M. (2008) Turnover of glycosomes during differentiation of *Trypanosoma brucei*. *Autophagy*, **4**, 294–308.

106 Herman, M., Gillies, S., Michels, P.A.M., and Rigden, D.J. (2006) Autophagy and related processes in trypanosomatids: insight from genomic and bioinformatics analyses. *Autophagy*, **2**, 107–118.

107 Eakin, A.E., Guerra, A., Focia, P.J., Torres-Martinez, J., and Craig, S.P. (1997) Hypoxanthine phosphoribosyltransferase from *Trypanosoma cruzi* as a target for structure-based inhibitor design: crystallization and inhibition studies with purine analogs. *Antimicrob. Agents Chemother.*, **41**, 1686–1692.

108 Monzani, P.S., Trapani, S., Thiemann, O. H., and Oliva, G. (2007) Crystal structure of *Leishmania tarentolae* hypoxanthine-guanine phosphoribosyltransferase. *BMC Struct. Biol.*, **7**, 59.

109 Shaw, M.P., Bond, C.S., Roper, J.R., Gourley, D.G., Ferguson, M.A.J., and Hunter, W.N. (2003) High-resolution crystal structure of *Trypanosoma brucei* UDP-galactose 4′-epimerase: a potential target for structure-based development of novel trypanocides. *Mol. Biochem. Parasitol.*, **126**, 173–180.

110 Willson, M., Callens, M., Kuntz, D.A., Périé, J., and Opperdoes, F.R. (1993) Synthesis and activity of inhibitors highly specific for the glycolytic enzymes from *Trypanosoma brucei*. *Mol. Biochem. Parasitol.*, **59**, 201–210.

111 Morgan, H.P., McNae, I.W., Nowicki, M. W., Zhong, W., Michels, P.A.M., Auld, D. S., Fothergill-Gilmore, L.A., and Walkinshaw, M.D. (2011) The trypanocidal drug suramin and other trypan blue mimetics are inhibitors of pyruvate kinases and bind to the adenosine site. *J. Biol. Chem.*, **286**, 31232–31240.

112 Nowicki, M.W., Tulloch, L.B., Worrall, L., McNae, I.W., Hannaert, V., Michels, P.A. M., Fothergill-Gilmore, L.A. *et al.* (2008) Design synthesis and trypanocidal activity of lead compounds based on inhibitors of parasite glycolysis. *Bioorg. Med. Chem.*, **16**, 5050–5061.

113 Dax, C., Duffieux, F., Chabot, N., Coincon, M., Sygush, J., Michels, P.A.M., and Blonski, C. (2006) Selective irreversible inhibition of fructose-1,6-bisphosphate aldolase from *Trypanosoma brucei*. *J. Med. Chem.*, **49**, 1499–1502.

114 Azéma, L., Lherbet, C., Baudoin, C., and Blonski, C. (2006) Cell permeation of a *Trypanosoma brucei* aldolase inhibitor: evaluation of different enzyme-labile phosphate protecting groups. *Bioorg. Med. Chem. Lett.*, **16**, 3440–3444.

115 Aronov, A.M., Suresh, S., Buckner, F.S., Van Voorhis, W.C., Verlinde, C.L., Opperdoes, F.R., Hol, W.G.J., and Gelb, M.H. (1999) Structure-based design of submicromolar biologically active inhibitors of trypanosomatid glyceraldehyde-3-phosphate dehydrogenase. *Proc. Natl. Acad. Sci. USA*, **96**, 4273–4278.

116 Bressi, J.C., Verlinde, C.L., Aronov, A.M., Shaw, M.L., Shin, S.S., Nguyen, L.N., Suresh, S. *et al.* (2001) Adenosine analogues as selective inhibitors of glyceraldehyde-3-phosphate dehydrogenase of Trypanosomatidae via structure-based drug design. *J. Med. Chem.*, **44**, 2080–2093.

117 Kennedy, K.J., Bressi, J.C., and Gelb, M.H. (2001) A disubstituted NAD analogue is a nanomolar inhibitor of trypanosomal glyceraldehyde-3-phosphate dehydrogenase. *Bioorg. Med. Chem. Lett.*, **11**, 95–98.

118 Bressi, J.C., Choe, J., Hough, M.T., Buckner, F.S., Van Voorhis, W.C., Verlinde, C.L., Hol, W.G.J., and Gelb, M. H. (2000) Adenosine analogues as inhibitors of *Trypanosoma brucei* phosphoglycerate kinase: elucidation of a novel binding mode for a 2-amino-N^6-substituted adenosine. *J. Med. Chem.*, **43**, 4135–4150.

119 Sharlow, E.R., Lyda, T.A., Dodson, H.C., Mustata, G., Morris, M.T., Leimgruber, S.S., Lee, K.H. *et al.* (2010) A target-based high throughput screen yields *Trypanosoma brucei* hexokinase small molecule inhibitors with antiparasitic activity. *PLoS Negl. Trop. Dis.*, **4**, e659.

120 Chambers, J.W., Kearns, M.T., Morris, M.T., and Morris, J.C. (2008) Assembly of heterohexameric trypanosome hexokinases reveals that hexokinase 2 is a regulable enzyme. *J. Biol. Chem.*, **283**, 14963–14970.

121 Montalvetti, A., Bailey, B.N., Martin, M.B., Severin, G.W., Oldfield, E., and Docampo, R. (2001) Bisphosphonates are potent inhibitors of *Trypanosoma cruzi* farnesyl pyrophosphate synthase. *J. Biol. Chem.*, **276**, 33930–33937.

122 Hudock, M.P., Sanz-Rodríguez, C.E., Song, Y., Chan, J.M., Zhang, Y., Odeh, S., Kosztowski, T. *et al.* (2006) Inhibition of *Trypanosoma cruzi* hexokinase by bisphosphonates. *J. Med. Chem.*, **49**, 215–223.

123 Sanz-Rodríguez, C.E., Concepción, J.L., Pekerar, S., Oldfield, E., and Urbina, J.A. (2007) Bisphosphonates as inhibitors of *Trypanosoma cruzi* hexokinase: kinetic and metabolic studies. *J. Biol. Chem.*, **282**, 12377–12387.

124 Orenes Lorente, S., Gómez, R., Jiménez, C., Cammerer, S., Yardley, V., de Luca-Fradley, K., Croft, S.L. *et al.* (2005) Biphenylquinuclidines as inhibitors of squalene synthase and growth of parasitic protozoa. *Bioorg. Med. Chem.*, **13**, 3519–3529.

125 Sealey-Cardona, M., Cammerer, S., Jones, S., Ruiz-Pérez, L.M., Brun, R., Gilbert, I. H., Urbina, J.A., and González-Pacanowska, D. (2007) Kinetic characterization of squalene synthase from *Trypanosoma cruzi*: selective inhibition by quinuclidine derivatives. *Antimicrob. Agents Chemother.*, **51**, 2123–2129.

126 Urbina, J.A., Concepción, J.L., Caldera, A., Payares, G., Sanoja, C., Otomo, T., and Hiyoshi, H. (2004) *In vitro* and *in vivo* activities of E5700 and ER-119884, two novel orally active squalene synthase inhibitors against *Trypanosoma cruzi*. *Antimicrob. Agents Chemother.*, **48**, 2379–2387.

127 Urbina, J.A., Concepción, J.L., Montalvetti, A., Rodriguez, J.B., and Docampo, R. (2003) Mechanism of action of 4-phenoxyphenoxyethyl thiocyanate (WC-9) against *Trypanosoma cruzi* the causative agent of Chagas' disease. *Antimicrob. Agents Chemother.*, **7**, 2047–2050.

128 Wilkinson, S.R., Meyer, D.J., Taylor, M.C., Bromley, E.V., Miles, M.A., and Kelly, J.M. (2002) The *Trypanosoma cruzi* enzyme TcGPXI is a glycosomal peroxidase and can be linked to trypanothione reduction by glutathione or tryparedoxin. *J. Biol. Chem.*, **277**, 17062–17071.

129 Wilkinson, S.R. and Kelly, J.M. (2003) The role of glutathione peroxidases in trypanosomatids. *Biol. Chem.*, **384**, 517–525.

130 Gutierrez-Correa, J., Fairlamb, A.H., and Stoppani, A.O. (2001) *Trypanosoma cruzi* trypanothione reductase is inactivated by peroxidase-generated phenothiazine cationic radicals. *Free Radic. Res.*, **34**, 363–378.

131 Rivarola, H.W., Fernández, A.R., Enders, J.E., Fretes, R., Gea, S., Suligoy, M., Palma, J.A., and Paglini-Oliva, P. (1999) Thioridazine treatment modifies the evolution of *Trypanosoma cruzi* infection in mice. *Ann. Trop. Med. Parasitol.*, **93**, 695–702.

132 Lo Presti, M.S., Rivarola, H.W., Bustamante, J.M., Fernández, A.R., Enders, J.E., Fretes, R., Gea, S., and Paglini-Oliva, P.A. (2004) Thioridazine treatment prevents cardiopathy in *Trypanosoma cruzi* infected mice. *Int. J. Antimicrob. Agents*, **23**, 634–636.

133 Ruda, G.F., Wong, P.E., Alibu, V.P., Norval, S., Read, K.D., Barrett, M.P., and Gilbert, I.H. (2010) Aryl phosphoramidates of 5-phospho erythronohydroxamic acid a new class of potent trypanocidal compounds. *J. Med. Chem.*, **53**, 6071–6078.

134 Marr, J.J. and Berens, R.L. (1983) Pyrazolopyrimidine metabolism in the pathogenic Trypanosomatidae. *Mol. Biochem. Parasitol.*, **7**, 339–356.

135 Ullman, B. and Carter, D. (1997) Molecular and biochemical studies on the hypoxanthine-guanine phosphoribosyltransferases of the pathogenic haemoflagellates. *Int. J. Parasitol.*, **27**, 203–213.

136 Koutinas, A.F., Saridomichelakis, M.N., Mylonakis, M.E., Leontides, L., Polizopoulou, Z., Billinis, C., Argyriadis, D. *et al.* (2001) A randomised blinded placebo-controlled clinical trial with allopurinol in canine leishmaniosis. *Vet. Parasitol.*, **98**, 247–261.

137 Torres, M., Bardagí, M., Roura, X., Zanna, G., Ravera, I., and Ferrer, L. (2011) Long term follow-up of dogs diagnosed with leishmaniosis (clinical stage II) and treated with meglumine antimoniate and allopurinol. *Vet. J.*, **188**, 346–351.

138 Gobbi, P., Lo Presti, M.S., Fernández, A. R., Enders, J.E., Fretes, R., Gea, S., Paglini-Oliva, P.A., and Rivarola, H.W. (2007) Allopurinol is effective to modify the evolution of *Trypanosoma cruzi* infection in mice. *Parasitol. Res.*, **101**, 1459–1462.

139 Apt, W., Aguilera, X., Arribada, A., Pérez, C., Miranda, C., Sánchez, G., Zulantay, I. *et al.* (1998) Treatment of chronic Chagas' disease with itraconazole and allopurinol. *Am. J. Trop. Med. Hyg.*, **59**, 133–138.

140 Freymann, D.M., Wenck, M.A., Engel, J.C., Feng, J., Focia, P.J., Eakin, A.E., and Craig, S.P. (2000) Efficient identification of inhibitors targeting the closed active site conformation of the HPRT from *Trypanosoma cruzi*. *Chem. Biol.*, **7**, 957–968.

8
Glyoxalase Enzymes in Trypanosomatids

Marta Sousa Silva, António E.N. Ferreira, Ricardo Gomes, Ana M. Tomás,
Ana Ponces Freire, and Carlos Cordeiro[*]

Abstract

The glyoxalase pathway catalyzes the formation of D-lactate from methylglyoxal – a non-enzymatic glycolytic byproduct with toxic effects. This pathway comprises two enzymes, glyoxalase I and glyoxalase II, and usually uses glutathione as catalytic cofactor. In trypanosomatids, this system makes no exception in respect of the functional replacement of glutathione by trypanothione. Structural analysis of both glyoxalase enzymes revealed key amino acids for glutathione binding, explaining why glyoxalase I is a more promiscuous enzyme. Glyoxalase II shows absolute specificity towards trypanothione. Changing two residues at the active site enables the enzyme to also use the glutathione as substrate. Although it was tempting to propose that the inhibition of this pathway might impair the parasite's viability, due to methylglyoxal accumulation and potential toxic effects, several studies indicate that the glyoxalases are unlike targets for this purpose. Indeed, there are alternative catabolic routes for methylglyoxal in both *Leishmania* and *Trypanosoma*, and the system is not complete in *T. brucei*, where only glyoxalase II was found. Sensitivity analysis using a complete model of the methylglyoxal metabolism in *L. infantum* revealed that inhibition of both the glyoxalase pathway and aldose reductase by 90% only causes a negligible increase of the steady-state concentration of methylglyoxal. The activities of these enzymes change during the life cycle of *L. infantum* and *T. brucei*, but the robustness and regulation of the metabolism of these parasites keeps the intracellular concentration of methylglyoxal way below toxic values.

Glyoxalase Pathway

Methylglyoxal and the glyoxalase pathway remain one of the most elusive challenges of modern biochemistry. Once considered to be an integral part of glycolysis [1] and proposed to be essential for the regulation of cell division [2], this 2-oxoaldehyde is presently believed to be a toxic compound and the glyoxalase

[*] Corresponding Author

Trypanosomatid Diseases: Molecular Routes to Drug Discovery, First edition. Edited by T. Jäger, O. Koch, and L. Flohé.
© 2013 Wiley-VCH Verlag GmbH & Co. KGaA. Published 2013 by Wiley-VCH Verlag GmbH & Co. KGaA.

pathway would thus have a detoxification role [3]. This latter view is supported by the high reactivity of methylglyoxal towards amino groups in proteins and nucleic acids, and its involvement in human pathologies, most notably in diabetes mellitus [4–6] and in amyloidotic-type neurodegenerative diseases, like Alzheimer, Parkinson, and Andrade's syndrome [7–10].

In eukaryotic cells, methylglyoxal is mainly formed from the β-elimination of the phosphate group from dihydroxyacetone phosphate (DHAP) and D-glyceraldehyde-3-phosphate (GAP) during glycolysis [11]. It is catabolized through the sequential action of the enzymes glyoxalase I (lactoylglutathione methylglyoxal-lyase, EC 4.4.1.5; GLO1) and glyoxalase II (hydroxyacylglutathione hydrolase, EC 3.1.2.6; GLO2) with glutathione as cofactor [3].

The first study of the glyoxalase system in trypanosomatids pointed to a similar enzyme activity, namely conversion of methylglyoxal to D-lactate in the presence of reduced glutathione [12]. However, 16 years later, the characterization of glyoxalase I

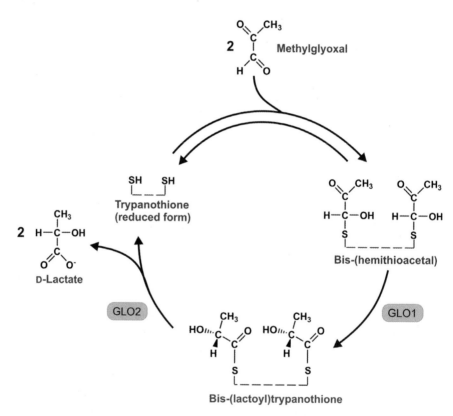

Figure 8.1 Trypanothione-dependent glyoxalase pathway. Methylglyoxal reacts non-enzymatically with trypanothione, forming a hemithioacetal that is isomerized to the thioester S-D-lactoyltrypanothione by glyoxalase I (GLO1). S-D-Lactoyltrypanothione is then hydrolyzed to D-lactate and trypanothione by glyoxalase II (GLO2). Only the thiol groups (—SH) of trypanothione are represented.

in *Leishmania major* [13] and glyoxalase II in *Trypanosoma brucei* [14] revealed that trypanothione was a better substrate for these enzymes. Glyoxalase I uses reduced trypanothione to convert methylglyoxal into *S*-D-lactoyltrypanothione. This thioester is then hydrolyzed to D-lactate by glyoxalase II, which regenerates the thiol [14–17] (Figure 8.1). The functional replacement of glutathione by trypanothione, a unique bis(glutathione)spermidine conjugate [18–20], and consequently the dependence of homologous enzymes on this thiol [18], is a unique specialized feature developed by trypanosomatids along evolution. The glyoxalase pathway follows this pattern in trypanosomatids.

Glyoxalase I

Glyoxalase I is the first enzyme of the thiol-dependent glyoxalase pathway, essential for the detoxification of methylglyoxal. This compound reacts with trypanothione, forming a hemithioacetal that is converted into the thioester *S*-D-lactoyltrypanothione.

The GLO1-encoding gene was already identified and cloned in different trypanosomatid species [13,21–23]. In *Leishmania* there is a single copy of the glyoxalase I gene in the parasite genomes, sharing a high homology between species (over 95%) and about 30% identity to the human homolog. In *Trypanosoma* species, there is only one *GLO1* gene in *T. cruzi* [22], but no gene is found in *T. brucei* genome, while GLO2 is present. However, the absence of the first enzyme of the pathway in *T. brucei* casts serious doubts about the system's functionality in this trypanosomatid [24].

The deduced protein sequence of trypanosomatid GLO1 enzymes contains the glyoxalase I signature 1 [25] located at the N-terminal region, a signature that has been found in all known glyoxalase I sequences. The corresponding proteins are active in these parasites and produce *S*-D-lactoyltrypanothione from methylglyoxal and reduced trypanothione in an irreversible reaction [13,17,22,23]. Although the GLO1 enzyme in trypanosomatids can also use glutathione as substrate, albeit with less affinity, the main physiological thiol substrate is trypanothione [17,22,26]. The analysis of the first solved structure of a trypanosomatid glyoxalase I (from *L. major*, Figure 8.2a) revealed that, most likely, this enzyme binds trypanothione through its glutathione moiety [15], explaining the reaction with both substrates. This is in striking contrast with the highly selective glyoxalase II from *L. infantum*, which does not use the glutathione-derived thioester and the substrate binding occurs through the spermidine moiety of the trypanothione molecule [16]. In the recently solved structure of *L. infantum* glyoxalase I [21] both substrates can be accommodated. However, the active site allows a better fitting of trypanothione than of glutathione, showing that structural differences determine the enzyme's substrate preference (our work, unpublished data).

Glyoxalase I enzymes are typically homodimers, containing about 140 residues and 16–18 kDa per monomer, with the active site located at the interface of the two subunits [15,21,27–29]. The most notable exceptions are the glyoxalase I enzymes

(a)   PDB 2C21   (b)   PDB 2P18

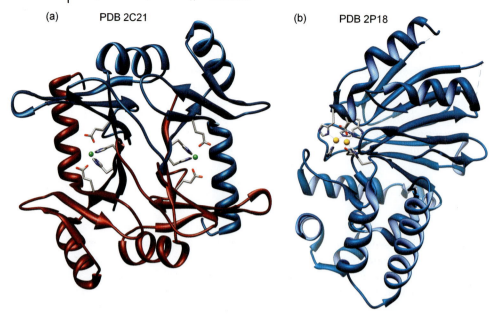

Figure 8.2 X-ray crystallographic structures of trypanosomatid glyoxalases. Metal binding sites and secondary structure elements are shown. (a) Structure of *L. major* glyoxalase I (Protein Data Bank (PDB) ID: 2C21). The protein is dimeric, and the subunits are colored red and blue. Nickel atoms are colored green. (b) Structure of *L. infantum* glyoxalase II (PDB ID: 2P18). Zinc atoms are colored in yellow.

from *Saccharomyces cerevisiae* [30] and *Plasmodium falciparum* [31], both being monomeric with two active sites. We may speculate that these trypanosomatid enzymes might have evolved through gene duplication. The overall structures of the two known trypanosomatid GLO1 proteins, from *L. major* [15] and *L. infantum* [21], are very similar, with three dimers in the asymmetric unit of the orthorhombic crystal form (unpublished data for *Li*GLO1). GLO1s are metalloenzymes that contain a metal center, with either zinc or nickel, which are essential for activity. In general, the Zn^{2+}-dependent enzymes comprise the eukaryotic ones, including human [27] and yeast [32], while the Ni^{2+}-dependent proteins comprise the prokaryotic GLO1s from *Escherichia coli*, *Pseudomonas aeruginosa*, *Yersinia pestis*, and *Neisseria meningitides* [28]. Nevertheless, exceptions have been found, such as Zn^{2+} in the prokaryotic *Pseudomonas putida* GLO1 [33], and Ni^{2+} in the eukaryotic GLO1s of *T. cruzi* [22] and *L. major* [13,15]. These findings in the trypanosomatid enzymes, and the fact that bacterial and *Leishmania* GLO1s sequences share about 50% identity, had suggested that the glyoxalase I from *L. major* has a prokaryotic origin [13]. However, the recent structure of *L. infantum* glyoxalase I challenges this view. As mentioned, both *L. major* and *L. infantum* GLO1 structures are very similar, and even the predicted metal-biding residues are conserved in the two enzymes. *L. infantum* glyoxalase I, like the eukaryotic GLO1 enzymes, contains zinc at the metal binding site (our work, unpublished results). In the genus *Pseudomonas*, a different metal content was reported for two species: nickel in *P. aeruginosa* [28] and zinc in *P. putida* [33]. The sequences of the two *Pseudomonas* proteins significantly differ, with additional regions in the *P. putida* enzyme [28]. In *Leishmania* this is not observed and *Li*GLO1 shares a high degree of sequence identity with *Lm*GLO1 (97% identity). The biological effects of this change in metal specificity of GLO1s are still unknown, but it is tempting to relate it to the distinct forms of leishmaniasis caused by these parasites, cutaneous for *L. major* and visceral for *L. infantum*. However, significant differences between these two species were observed in gene expression profiles, which may also differentiate *L. major* and *L. infantum* as pathogens [34].

Glyoxalase II

Glyoxalase II, the second enzyme of the glyoxalase pathway, hydrolyses the thioester *S*-D-lactoyltrypanothione into D-lactate and regenerates the thiol.

The GLO2-encoding gene was the first of the glyoxalase system to be isolated and characterized in a trypanosomatid, the African trypanosome *T. brucei* [14]. In the genome of *T. brucei* there are two putative *GLO2* genes (the characterized AJ492819 and the putative second *GLO2* AC091702, 25% identity), which share about 30–36% identity with the human glyoxalase II [14]. However, only one (AJ492819) seems to encode a functional enzyme, since GLO2-deficient parasites do not have a detectable glyoxalase II activity [24]. It is though intriguing that two genes coding for glyoxalase II are present in *T. brucei* and glyoxalase I is absent. Recently, another function was attributed to *T. brucei* GLO2: a thioesterase activity that is unrelated to methylglyoxal detoxification, since the enzyme is able to hydrolyze a wide variety of other trypanothione-derived thioesters [24]. Hence, methylglyoxal detoxification in *T. brucei* was proposed to mainly occur through the methylglyoxal reductase pathway, forming L-lactate [35]. In *T. cruzi* there is only one copy of *GLO2*, sharing about 60% identity with the *T. brucei* genes. In *Leishmania* species, also a single copy of *GLO2* was found, which share between 99 and 96% identity within *Leishmania*, and close to 50% with the human homolog.

Glyoxalase II enzymes are monomeric proteins, of approximately 29–33 kDa. An analysis of the deduced protein sequence of trypanosomatid GLO2 enzymes clearly identifies them as a (hydroxyacyl)glutathione hydrolases belonging to the metallo-β-lactamase superfamily. A characteristic feature of the zinc-containing members of this family [36], and of all glyoxalase II enzymes, is the highly conserved metal-binding motif THxHxDH, which is equally present in all trypanosomatid GLO2s [14,16,37]. Like all known GLO2s, trypanosomatid glyoxalase II enzymes contain a binuclear metal center essential for substrate binding and catalysis, zinc being the main metal present, although the enzymes are able to bind either zinc or iron [14,16].

Unlike the GLO1s, trypanosomatid GLO2s show absolute specificity towards the trypanothione-derived substrate. The first solved structure of a trypanosomatid glyoxalase II, from *L. infantum* (Figure 8.2b), revealed the substrate-binding mechanisms through the spermidine moiety of the trypanothione-thioester [16]. In fact, the replacement of two essential residues for substrate binding, Tyr291 and Cys294, by the corresponding ones on the human enzyme (positively charged Arg and Lys), produced a mutant *Li*GLO2 that is able to hydrolyze the glutathione-derived thioester [38]. This mutein still reacts with the *S*-D-lactoyltrypanothione through the spermidine-interacting residues Tyr212 and Phe219 (Figure 8.3) [16], which are conserved across all known structures of glyoxalase I and glyoxalase II from *Leishmania* and absent from the human homologues ([15,16]; data not published for *L. infantum* glyoxalase I).

Glyoxalase Pathway Regulation

Trypanosomatids have a very robust metabolism, regulated by the differential expression of its enzymes. One of the most marked examples is glycolysis. In *Leishmania* and *Trypanosoma* species, the first steps of the glycolytic pathway occur inside the glycosome, an organelle unique to these parasites [39,40]. Since the main methylglyoxal formation system is from DHAP and GAP of glycolysis, the glyoxalase pathway enzymes were also assumed to be located inside this special organelle [39]. A fact supporting this hypothesis is the presence of a D-lactate dehydrogenase-like protein in *Leishmania* that contains a signal sequence to the glycosome [41]. This enzyme, which converts D-lactate into pyruvate, is, however, absent from *Trypanosoma* species. The glyoxalases do not contain the glycosome-targeting sequence and their presence in the glycosome was not proven yet. Moreover, the triose phosphate DHAP can be transported across the glycosomal membrane to the cytosol, via the glycerol-3-phosphate/DHAP shuttle [26,42]. It is therefore possible that methylglyoxal detoxification through the glyoxalase pathway occurs in the cytosol and, indeed, a recent study with *L. donovani* parasites expressing a GLO1–Green Fluorescent Protein construct suggests a cytosolic location [43].

Trypanosomatids have complex life cycles, alternating between an insect vector and a vertebrate host. The activity of glyoxalase enzymes along a parasite's life cycle was analyzed in *T. brucei* [35] and, more recently, in *L. infantum* (our work, unpublished results). In the study with African trypanosomes, although they lack GLO1, the production of D-lactate upon methylglyoxal stimulation was measured in both procyclic and bloodstream forms, and was higher (about 4-fold) in the latter [35]. Also, these parasites produce much more L-lactate, suggesting that they might catabolize methylglyoxal through a NADPH-dependent methylglyoxal reductase and a lactaldehyde dehydrogenase system [35]. Again, the produced L-lactate, either with or without the addition of methylglyoxal, is higher in bloodstream forms. In a transgenic cell line expressing glyoxalase I from *T. cruzi*, the GLO1 activity increased by 1.6-fold in the bloodstream forms of the parasite. In this stage, *T. brucei* exclusively depends on glycolysis for ATP production [42,44]. With an increased

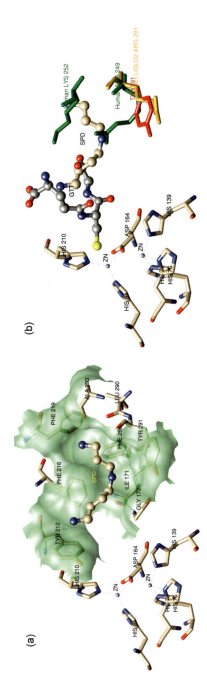

Figure 8.3 Trypanothione specificity in *L. infantum* glyoxalase II. (a) Zinc-binding site and spermidine (SPD) molecular surface "pocket" in *L. infantum* glyoxalase II (PDB ID: 2P18). (b) Superposition of spermidine and glutathione (GTT) binding residues, from human (PDB ID: 1QH3) and *L. infantum* (PDB ID: 2P18) glyoxalases II, and the homology model of mutated *L. infantum* glyoxalase II. The two residues of the human enzyme (Lys and Arg, colored in green) block the binding of the spermidine moiety and, consequently, trypanothione. In the *L. infantum* glyoxalase II, after replacement of Tyr291 (red) for an Arg (yellow) the enzyme is able to bind the glutathione-derived thioester.

glycolytic flux, the methylglyoxal formation rate also increases [45]. The intracellular concentration of this 2-oxoaldehyde is even higher in bloodstream stationary parasites [24], in line with the higher activity of methylglyoxal catabolizing enzymes in these forms of African trypanosomes.

In *L. infantum*, changes in the activity of glyoxalase I and II were also observed during the different life cycle stages (our work, unpublished results). Activities were measured in promastigotes, at exponential and stationary phases of growth, and in amastigotes. The activity of both glyoxalase enzymes increases during the stationary growth phase, when compared to the exponential phase, when promastigotes are enriched in infective forms, and further in amastigotes. This activity pattern is similar to *L. infantum* detoxification enzymes, namely tryparedoxin 1 [46] involved in parasite resistance to host-derived hydrogen peroxide and trypanothione reductase [47], a NADPH-dependent oxidoreductase crucial for thiol metabolism in all trypanosomatids, that plays a fundamental role on detoxification of reactive oxygen and nitrogen species by keeping the thiol pool reduced. In all cases, enzyme expression is upregulated in stationary-phase promastigotes and in axenic amastigotes. An alternative catabolic system for methylglyoxal is also present in *L. infantum*, the NADPH-dependent aldose reductase (EC 1.1.1.21 [48]) that reduces methylglyoxal to 1,2-propanediol in a NADPH-dependent two-step reaction [49]. *L. infantum* aldo-keto reductase is active and catabolizes methylglyoxal with an activity 10- to 20-fold lower than glyoxalase I, depending on the life cycle stage. This does not imply, however, that the glyoxalase pathway is more relevant in these parasites. Only a sensitivity analysis based on a detailed kinetic model of methylglyoxal catabolism can enlighten the relative importance of these two pathways. Interestingly, during the *L. infantum* life cycle, the two catabolic routes for methylglyoxal have different behaviors. Aldose reductase activity is higher in exponentially growing promastigotes, decreasing during the stationary phase and at the amastigote stage. It is tempting to speculate that, in stationary-phase promastigotes and in amastigotes, the parasite decreases the activity of aldose reductase to reduce NADPH consumption, in dare need for thiol reduction and anti-oxidative defenses. The increase of glyoxalase I and II activities in amastigotes would compensate for the decrease of the aldose reductase activity, to efficiently eliminate methylglyoxal.

Glyoxalase Pathway as a Therapeutic Target

The ultimate goal of recent studies on methylglyoxal metabolism in trypanosomatids is to find new pharmacological opportunities based on the plain rationale that inhibition of the glyoxalase pathway might lead to an increase of methylglyoxal intracellular concentration with harmful effects to the parasite. However, considering the robustness of metabolic pathways, it is highly unlikely that targeting a single enzyme or protein will produce the desired results.

A previous sensitivity analysis performed in *L. infantum* promastigotes, assuming the elimination of methylglyoxal exclusively by the glyoxalase pathway, revealed that the inhibition of the glyoxalase enzymes has no significant effects on the steady-state concentration of methylglyoxal and, therefore, would not be a good therapeutic target [17]. In fact, the existence of alternative methylglyoxal catabolizing systems in both *Leishmania* and *Trypanosoma* and the absence of a GLO1 enzyme in *T. brucei*, indicates that the glyoxalase pathways is not essential for parasite survival. Even the double knockout of *GLO2* in *T. brucei* had no effect in parasite growth or phenotype [24]. A recent study in *L. donovani* using GLO1 gene deletion mutants contradicts this view, showing that mutant parasites have more difficulty to grow [43]. The authors report that the growth of these parasites is inhibited by 50% with methylglyoxal concentrations around 0.4 mM, while the same effect was obtained in wild-type parasites with 1 mM methylglyoxal. However, these concentrations are not physiological and the methylglyoxal used is of low purity, containing considerable amounts of formaldehyde. In trypanosomatids, intracellular methylglyoxal concentration does not exceed the micromolar range, even in the African trypanosome lacking GLO1 [17,24].

Methylglyoxal metabolism in *L. infantum* was revisited, now including both glyoxalase pathway enzymes and aldose reductase. Since these methylglyoxal catabolic systems have different activity patterns during the *L. infantum* life cycle, this study enlightens the relative importance of each system along the parasite life cycle. Upon GLO1 removal, methylglyoxal concentration would, at most, increase by 1.5-fold (Figure 8.4a). Aldose reductase activity has a greater effect on methylglyoxal concentration (Figure 8.4b), but, in the absence of this enzyme, only a 2-fold increase in stationary promastigotes and a 4-fold increase in exponential promastigotes and amastigotes is predicted. Using this model, even a total depletion of trypanothione does not result in a marked effect on methylglyoxal steady-state concentration (Figure 8.4c), in contrast to the previously reported results based on a simpler model without aldose reductase [17]. In the context of methylglyoxal detoxification, the two pathways fulfill a role of mutual backup. In exponential-phase promastigotes, as well as in amastigotes, about 80% of methylglyoxal is eliminated by aldose reductase, and only 20% is catabolized by the glyoxalase pathway. However, the model predicts that in stationary promastigotes around 40% of methylglyoxal is eliminated via the glyoxalase pathway with 60% going through the aldose reductase. A simultaneous inhibition of glyoxalase I and aldose reductase would only have a significant effect at the exponential phase of growth, but even in this case a 90% inhibition of both enzymes would be required to achieve a 5-fold increase in methylglyoxal steady-state concentration (Figure 8.4d). To reach the same variation in amastigotes, both enzymes would have to be inhibited by 99%. In this life cycle stage, parasites are resilient and the inhibition of these specific enzymes is a difficult task. Even though, if successful, we would just achieve a meager increase of the steady-state concentration of methylglyoxal and it is difficult to predict whether this increase would have a toxic effect on *L. infantum*.

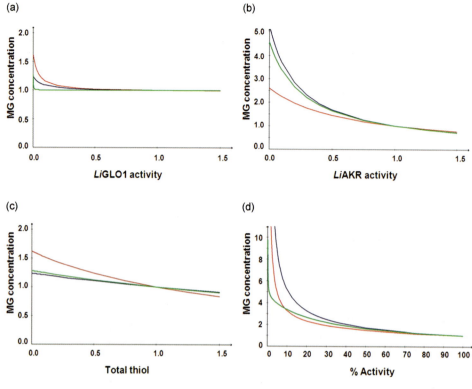

Figure 8.4 Sensitivity analysis of methylglyoxal (MG) metabolism in promastigotes, exponential (blue line) and stationary (red line) growth phases, and amastigotes (green line) of *L. infantum*. All values are normalized to the reference state. Parameters scanned are: (a) glyoxalase I (*Li*GLO1) activity, (b) aldose reductase (*Li*AKR) activity, and (c) total trypanothione concentration. The effect of simultaneous inhibition of glyoxalase I and aldose reductase on the steady-state concentration of methylglyoxal is also shown (d).

Conclusion

Trypanosomatids undergo complex life cycles, associated with major morphological and biochemical changes. They activate some pathways and inhibit other processes to invade and survive inside their host, some of them in hostile environments such as the lysosome-like vesicles in macrophages replete with hydrolytic enzymes and a characteristically low pH. During this process, key metabolic changes are expected, being therefore important to have an integrative view of the parasite metabolism along its life cycle.

The glyoxalase pathway is an important piece of the methylglyoxal catabolic puzzle. The discovery of other methylglyoxal detoxifying systems adds new elements

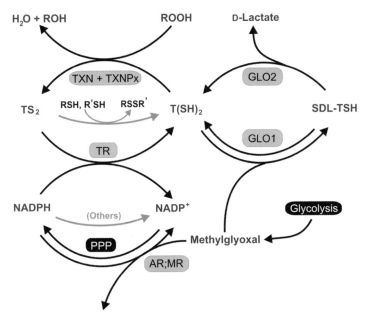

Figure 8.5 Connection between carbonyl and redox stresses in trypanosomatids. This model links the trypanothione redox cycle, NADPH oxidation-reduction and methylglyoxal catabolism. The NADPH, cofactor of aldose reductase (AR) and methylglyoxal reductase (MR) enzymes, is needed for the reduction of oxidized trypanothione (TS_2). Carbonylic stress may imbalance redox metabolism, showing potential for a synergistic effect of both stresses. GLO1, glyoxalase I; GLO2, glyoxalase II T(SH)$_2$, trypanothione; TS_2, trypanothione disulfide; SDL-TSH, S-D-lactoyltrypanothione TR, trypanothione reductase; TXN, tryparedoxin; TXNPx, tryparedoxin peroxidases; RSH and R′SH, reduced cellular thiols (glutathione, ovothiol A); RSSR′, oxidized cellular thiols; ROOH, hydroperoxide; PPP, pentose phosphate pathway.

in the quest for novel potential therapeutic targets related to the metabolism of this 2-oxoaldehyde.

The presence of a NADPH-dependent methylglyoxal reductase in *T. brucei* [35] and a novel NADPH-dependent aldose reductase in *L. infantum* [48] suggests a direct connection between carbonylic and oxidative stresses (Figure 8.5). This vision is supported by the tight regulation of methylglyoxal catabolism during the life cycle of *L. infantum*, most likely to meet the demands of adaptation to different life cycle stages. Disrupting this cycle might lead to a synergistic impairment of the parasite viability, offering the opportunity to develop new and effective enzyme inhibitors with potential therapeutic value. Thiol metabolism, particularly trypanothione, remains the most promising research landscape for novel drug target candidates, with potential differential effects at different stages of the parasite's life cycle. Trypanothione-dependent enzymes can also be exploited for drug design, but certainly the glyoxalases are unlikely to be adequate targets.

References

1 Neuberg, C. and Kobel, M. (1928) On the question of evidence of methyl-glyoxal as an intermediate product of glycolysis. *Biochem. Z.*, **193**, 464–467.

2 Szent-Gyorgyi, A. (1977) The living state and cancer. *Proc. Natl. Acad. Sci. USA*, **74**, 2844–2847.

3 Thornalley, P.J. (1990) The glyoxalase system: new developments towards functional characterization of a metabolic pathway fundamental to biological life. *Biochem. J.*, **269**, 1–11.

4 Couturier, M., Amman, H., Des Rosiers, C., and Comtois, R. (1997) Variable glycation of serum proteins in patients with diabetes mellitus. *Clin. Invest. Med.*, **20**, 103–109.

5 Sensi, M., Pricci, F., Pugliese, C., De Rossi, M.G., Celi, F.S., Cristina, A., Mokano, S., Andreani, D., and Di Mario, U. (1992) Enhanced nonenzymatic glycation of eye lens proteins in experimental diabetes mellitus: an approach for the study of protein alterations as mediators of normal aging phenomena. *Arch. Gerontol. Geriatr.*, **15** (Suppl. 1), 333–337.

6 van Boekel, M.A. (1991) The role of glycation in aging and diabetes mellitus. *Mol. Biol. Rep.*, **15**, 57–64.

7 Vitek, M.P., Bhattacharya, K., Glendening, J.M., Stopa, E., Vlassara, H., Bucala, R., Manogue, K., and Cerami, A. (1994) Advanced glycation end products contribute to amyloidosis in Alzheimer disease. *Proc. Natl. Acad. Sci. USA*, **91**, 4766–4770.

8 Yan, S.D., Chen, X., Schmidt, A.M., Brett, J., Godman, G., Zou, Y.S., Scott, C.W., Caputo, C., Frappier, T., Smith, M.A. *et al.* (1994) Glycated tau protein in Alzheimer disease: a mechanism for induction of oxidant stress. *Proc. Natl. Acad. Sci. USA*, **91**, 7787–7791.

9 Castellani, R., Smith, M.A., Richey, P.L., and Perry, G. (1996) Glycoxidation and oxidative stress in Parkinson disease and diffuse Lewy body disease. *Brain Res.*, **737**, 195–200.

10 Gomes, R., Sousa Silva, M., Quintas, A., Cordeiro, C., Freire, A., Pereira, P., Martins, A., Monteiro, E., Barroso, E., and Ponces Freire, A. (2005) Argpyrimidine, a methylglyoxal-derived advanced glycation end-product in familial amyloidotic polyneuropathy. *Biochem. J.*, **385**, 339–345.

11 Lohman, K. and Meyerhof, O. (1934) Über die enzymatische Umwandlung von Phosphoglyzerinsäure in Brenztraubensäure und Phosphorsäure [Enzymatic transformation of phosphoglyceric acid into pyruvic and phosphoric acid]. *Biochem. Z.*, **273**, 60–72.

12 Darling, T.N. and Blum, J.J. (1988) D-Lactate production by *Leishmania braziliensis* through the glyoxalase pathway. *Mol. Biochem. Parasitol.*, **28**, 121–127.

13 Vickers, T.J., Greig, N., and Fairlamb, A.H. (2004) A trypanothione-dependent glyoxalase I with a prokaryotic ancestry in *Leishmania major*. *Proc. Natl. Acad. Sci. USA*, **101**, 13186–13191.

14 Irsch, T. and Krauth-Siegel, R.L. (2004) Glyoxalase II of African trypanosomes is trypanothione-dependent. *J. Biol. Chem.*, **279**, 22209–22217.

15 Ariza, A., Vickers, T.J., Greig, N., Armour, K.A., Dixon, M.J., Eggleston, I.M., Fairlamb, A.H., and Bond, C.S. (2006) Specificity of the trypanothione-dependent *Leishmania major* glyoxalase I: structure and biochemical comparison with the human enzyme. *Mol. Microbiol.*, **59**, 1239–1248.

16 Silva, M.S., Barata, L., Ferreira, A.E., Romao, S., Tomas, A.M., Freire, A.P., and Cordeiro, C. (2008) Catalysis and structural properties of *Leishmania infantum* glyoxalase II: trypanothione specificity and phylogeny. *Biochemistry*, **47**, 195–204.

17 Sousa Silva, M., Ferreira, A.E., Tomas, A.M., Cordeiro, C., and Ponces Freire, A. (2005) Quantitative assessment of the glyoxalase pathway in *Leishmania infantum* as a therapeutic target by modelling and computer simulation. *FEBS J.*, **272**, 2388–2398.

18 Muller, S., Liebau, E., Walter, R.D., and Krauth-Siegel, R.L. (2003) Thiol-based redox metabolism of protozoan parasites. *Trends Parasitol.*, **19**, 320–328.

19 Ariyanayagam, M.R. and Fairlamb, A.H. (2001) Ovothiol and trypanothione as antioxidants in trypanosomatids. *Mol. Biochem. Parasitol.*, **115**, 189–198.

20 Fairlamb, A.H., Blackburn, P., Ulrich, P., Chait, B.T., and Cerami, A. (1985) Trypanothione: a novel bis(glutathionyl) spermidine cofactor for glutathione reductase in trypanosomatids. *Science*, **227**, 1485–1487.

21 Barata, L., Sousa Silva, M., Schuldt, L., da Costa, G., Tomas, A.M., Ferreira, A.E., Weiss, M.S., Ponces Freire, A., and Cordeiro, C. (2010) Cloning, expression, purification, crystallization and preliminary X-ray diffraction analysis of glyoxalase I from *Leishmania infantum*. *Acta. Crystallogr. F*, **66**, 571–574.

22 Greig, N., Wyllie, S., Vickers, T.J., and Fairlamb, A.H. (2006) Trypanothione-dependent glyoxalase I in *Trypanosoma cruzi*. *Biochem. J.*, **400**, 217–223.

23 Padmanabhan, P.K., Mukherjee, A., Singh, S., Chattopadhyaya, S., Gowri, V.S., Myler, P.J., Srinivasan, N., and Madhubala, R. (2005) Glyoxalase I from *Leishmania donovani*: a potential target for anti-parasite drug. *Biochem. Biophys. Res. Commun.*, **337**, 1237–1248.

24 Wendler, A., Irsch, T., Rabbani, N., Thornalley, P.J., and Krauth-Siegel, R.L. (2009) Glyoxalase II does not support methylglyoxal detoxification but serves as a general trypanothione thioesterase in African trypanosomes. *Mol. Biochem. Parasitol.*, **163**, 19–27.

25 de Castro, E., Sigrist, C.J., Gattiker, A., Bulliard, V., Langendijk-Genevaux, P.S., Gasteiger, E., Bairoch, A., and Hulo, N. (2006) ScanProsite: detection of PROSITE signature matches and ProRule-associated functional and structural residues in proteins. *Nucleic Acids Res.*, **34**, W362–W365.

26 Wyllie, S. and Fairlamb, A.H. (2011) Methylglyoxal metabolism in trypanosomes and *Leishmania*. *Semin. Cell Dev. Biol.*, **22**, 271–277.

27 Cameron, A.D., Olin, B., Ridderstrom, M., Mannervik, B., and Jones, T.A. (1997) Crystal structure of human glyoxalase I – evidence for gene duplication and 3D domain swapping. *EMBO J.*, **16**, 3386–3395.

28 Sukdeo, N., Clugston, S.L., Daub, E., and Honek, J.F. (2004) Distinct classes of glyoxalase I: metal specificity of the *Yersinia pestis*, *Pseudomonas aeruginosa* and *Neisseria meningitidis* enzymes. *Biochem. J.*, **384**, 111–117.

29 He, M.M., Clugston, S.L., Honek, J.F., and Matthews, B.W. (2000) Determination of the structure of *Escherichia coli* glyoxalase I suggests a structural basis for differential metal activation. *Biochemistry*, **39**, 8719–8727.

30 Marmstal, E., Aronsson, A.C., and Mannervik, B. (1979) Comparison of glyoxalase I purified from yeast (*Saccharomyces cerevisiae*) with the enzyme from mammalian sources. *Biochem. J.*, **183**, 23–30.

31 Iozef, R., Rahlfs, S., Chang, T., Schirmer, H., and Becker, K. (2003) Glyoxalase I of the malarial parasite *Plasmodium falciparum*: evidence for subunit fusion. *FEBS Lett.*, **554**, 284–288.

32 Aronsson, A.C., Marmstal, E., and Mannervik, B. (1978) Glyoxalase I, a zinc metalloenzyme of mammals and yeast. *Biochem. Biophys. Res. Commun.*, **81**, 1235–1240.

33 Saint-Jean, A.P., Phillips, K.R., Creighton, D.J., and Stone, M.J. (1998) Active monomeric and dimeric forms of *Pseudomonas putida* glyoxalase I: evidence for 3D domain swapping. *Biochemistry*, **37**, 10345–10353.

34 Rochette, A., Raymond, F., Ubeda, J.M., Smith, M., Messier, N., Boisvert, S., Rigault, P., Corbeil, J., Ouellette, M., and Papadopoulou, B. (2008) Genome-wide gene expression profiling analysis of *Leishmania major* and *Leishmania infantum* developmental stages reveals substantial differences between the two species. *BMC Genomics*, **9**, 255.

35 Greig, N., Wyllie, S., Patterson, S., and Fairlamb, A.H. (2009) A comparative study of methylglyoxal metabolism in trypanosomatids. *FEBS J.*, **276**, 376–386.

36 Concha, N.O., Rasmussen, B.A., Bush, K., and Herzberg, O. (1996) Crystal structure of the wide-spectrum binuclear zinc

beta-lactamase from *Bacteroides fragilis.
Structure*, **4**, 823–836.

37 Padmanabhan, P.K., Mukherjee, A., and
Madhubala, R. (2006) Characterization of
the gene encoding glyoxalase II from
Leishmania donovani: a potential target for
anti-parasite drugs. *Biochem. J.*, **393**,
227–234.

38 Barata, L., Sousa Silva, M., Schuldt, L.,
Ferreira, A.E., Gomes, R.A., Tomas, A.M.,
Weiss, M.S., Ponces Freire, A., and
Cordeiro, C. (2011) Enlightening the
molecular basis of trypanothione specificity
in trypanosomatids: mutagenesis of
Leishmania infantum glyoxalase II.
Exp. Parasitol., **129**, 402–408.

39 Opperdoes, F.R. and Coombs, G.H. (2007)
Metabolism of *Leishmania*: proven and
predicted. *Trends Parasitol.*, **23**, 149–158.

40 Opperdoes, F.R. and Borst, P. (1977)
Localization of nine glycolytic enzymes in a
microbody-like organelle in *Trypanosoma
brucei*: the glycosome. *FEBS Lett.*, **80**,
360–364.

41 Myler, P.J. and Fasel, N. (2008) *Leishmania:
After the Genome*, Caister Academic Press,
Norwich.

42 Bakker, B.M., Michels, P.A., Opperdoes,
F.R., and Westerhoff, H.V. (1997)
Glycolysis in bloodstream form
Trypanosoma brucei can be understood in
terms of the kinetics of the glycolytic
enzymes. *J. Biol. Chem.*, **272**, 3207–3215.

43 Chauhan, S.C. and Madhubala, R. (2009)
Glyoxalase I gene deletion mutants of
Leishmania donovani exhibit reduced
methylglyoxal detoxification. *PLoS One*, **4**,
e6805.

44 Bakker, B.M., Westerhoff, H.V.,
Opperdoes, F.R., and Michels, P.A. (2000)
Metabolic control analysis of glycolysis
in trypanosomes as an approach to
improve selectivity and effectiveness
of drugs. *Mol. Biochem. Parasitol.*,
106, 1–10.

45 Gomes, R.A., Sousa Silva, M., Vicente
Miranda, H., Ferreira, A.E., Cordeiro, C.A.,
and Freire, A.P. (2005) Protein glycation
in *Saccharomyces cerevisiae*. Argpyrimidine
formation and methylglyoxal catabolism.
FEBS J., **272**, 4521–4531.

46 Castro, H., Sousa, C., Novais, M., Santos,
M., Budde, H., Cordeiro-da-Silva, A.,
Flohé, L., and Tomas, A. (2004) Two linked
genes of *Leishmania infantum* encode
tryparedoxins localised to cytosol and
mitochondrion. *Mol. Biochem. Parasitol.*,
136, 137–147.

47 Castro-Pinto, D.B., Echevarria, A.,
Genestra, M.S., Cysne-Finkelstein, L.,
and Leon, L.L. (2004) Trypanothione
reductase activity is prominent in
metacyclic promastigotes and axenic
amastigotes of *Leishmania amazonesis*.
Evaluation of its potential as a
therapeutic target. *J. Enzyme. Inhib. Med.
Chem.*, **19**, 57–63.

48 Barata, L., Silva, M.S., da Costa, G.,
Schuldt, L., Ferreira, A.E., Tomas, A.M.,
Weiss, M.S., Freire, A.P., and Cordeiro, C.
(2009) *Leishmania Infantum* aldose
reductase: expression with molecular
chaperones, purification and kinetic
studies. *Am. J. Trop. Med. Hyg.*, **81**,
139–139.

49 Vander Jagt, D.L., Han, L.P., and Lehman,
C.H. (1972) Kinetic evaluation of substrate
specificity in the glyoxalase-I-catalyzed
disproportionation of a-ketoaldehydes.
Biochemistry, **11**, 3735–3740.

9
Trypanothione-Based Redox Metabolism of Trypanosomatids

Marcelo A. Comini* and Leopold Flohé

Abstract

The intracellular redox balance largely depends on thiol-dependent reactions, and is pivotal to survival and proliferation of all living organisms. Most eukaryotes and prokaryotes use glutathione and thioredoxin complemented with pertinent reductases to maintain their reducing capacity. Strikingly, trypanosomatids lack glutathione reductase and thioredoxin reductase, and have developed a unique thiol-based redox metabolism that differs substantially in some of its molecular entities. The system that controls the thiol redox homeostasis in these parasites comprises N^1,N^8-bis(glutathionyl)spermidine called trypanothione, the NADPH-dependent trypanothione reductase, multipurpose oxidoreductases called tryparedoxins, other redoxins, and tryparedoxin-dependent peroxidases of different classes. Moreover, trypanothione itself, or assisted by enzymes such as tryparedoxins, glutaredoxins, glyoxalases, and methionine sulfoxide reductase, acts as reductant, cofactor or ligand in a plethora of key biological reactions encompassing DNA replication, antioxidant defense, assembly of iron–sulfur clusters, and detoxification of ketoaldehydes, xenobiotics, and heavy metals. In consequence, several components of the trypanothione system proved to be critical for the viability and virulence of *Trypanosoma* and *Leishmania* species. The absence of trypanothione-independent backup systems in the parasites and lacking conservation of trypanothione and related reactions in the mammalian hosts render several system components promising drug targets. This chapter updates functional aspects of the trypanothione metabolism and ranks drug target candidates for the development of novel therapies against trypanosomiasis and leishmaniasis.

Thiol Redox Metabolism of Trypanosomatids: A Brief Historical Overview

Trypanosomatids are exposed to reactive oxygen and nitrogen species, which are metabolic byproducts or stem from the host's defense mechanisms. An uncontrolled production or insufficient detoxification of these compounds alters the cellular redox balance, which may cause a wide range of damage to macromolecules, ultimately leading to cell death. Redox-active thiol groups present in proteins or low-molecular-mass

* Corresponding Author

Trypanosomatid Diseases: Molecular Routes to Drug Discovery, First edition. Edited by T. Jäger, O. Koch, and L. Flohé.
© 2013 Wiley-VCH Verlag GmbH & Co. KGaA. Published 2013 by Wiley-VCH Verlag GmbH & Co. KGaA.

compounds play a key role in reducing these oxidants or acting as redox sensors to regulate diverse cellular functions [1]. Long before the components of the thiol redox system of trypanosomatids were identified, the relevance of this metabolism for pathogenic trypanosomatids was recognized by chemotherapeutic approaches employing compounds known to directly (e.g., buthionine sulfoximine, nifurtimox, melarsoprol, and benznidazole) [2–8] or indirectly (e.g., antimonials) [9,10] interfere with cellular redox balance. Historically, the elucidation of the thiol-dependent redox system of trypanosomatids resembles a puzzle game. Some of the components had been identified long ago, but their interconnection remained obscure for decades. Indeed, soon after the presence of an unusual thiol-polyamine conjugate (i.e., mono(glutathionyl)spermidine (Gsp)) had been reported in *Escherichia coli* [11], Fairlamb and Cerami [12] laid the foundation stone in trypanosomatid redox metabolism by the discovery of trypanothione (T(SH)$_2$), the bis(glutathionyl)-conjugate of spermidine (Spd). T(SH)$_2$ is almost exclusively found in the order *Kinetoplastida* and there represents the main low-molecular-mass thiol [13,14]. One year after the discovery of T(SH)$_2$, its biosynthesis from Spd and GSH [15] and regeneration from its oxidized cyclic disulfide form [16] was clarified in principle, and in the following year the enzyme responsible for T(SH)$_2$ regeneration, trypanothione reductase (TR), was in-depth characterized and crystallized [17]. In contrast, it took more than a decade to identify the enzymatic entities responsible for the removal of hydroperoxides, the oxidoreductase tryparedoxin (TXN) [18,19] and two types of peroxidases (see next sections) and, more importantly, to recognize their dependence on T(SH)$_2$ [18,20]. Furthermore, earlier experimental evidence supporting the lack in trypanosomatids of the major reductases that control the thiol redox homeostasis in most eukaryotes and prokaryotes (i.e., glutathione reductase and thioredoxin reductase) was confirmed by sequencing the parasites' genomes [21–23]. The final elucidation of T(SH)$_2$ biosynthesis was only achieved in the last decade [24–27]. Not surprisingly, the trypanothione system did not remain as simple as seemingly clarified towards the end of the last century, but became enriched with multiple isoenzymes of mostly unknown specialization [28–31] and with unexpected ramifications, such as ribonucleotide reduction [32], iron–sulfur cluster (ISC) metabolism [33–35], and methionine sulfoxide reduction [36] (Figure 9.1). Finally, the development of fast and reliable genetic tools enabling the functional characterization of different components of this system and, thus, validating their putative essentiality for parasites survival and/or virulence was lagging behind and still remains a challenge [37–39].

These and other deficiencies in basic knowledge and experimental tools represented major obstacles in the exploitation of the trypanothione system for the development of novel drugs. Progress in recent years, however, has substantially enriched related knowledge: (i) by RNA interference (RNAi) and other techniques of inverse genetics, most of the system components could be demonstrated to be of vital importance, mostly for *T. brucei*; (ii) subcellular location and metabolic context has been clarified to a large extent; (iii) structures were elucidated for at least one representative of each system component; and (iv) reliable molecular models could be generated for the orthologs of other species. Collectively, available data (Table 9.1 and references therein) now promises a safe

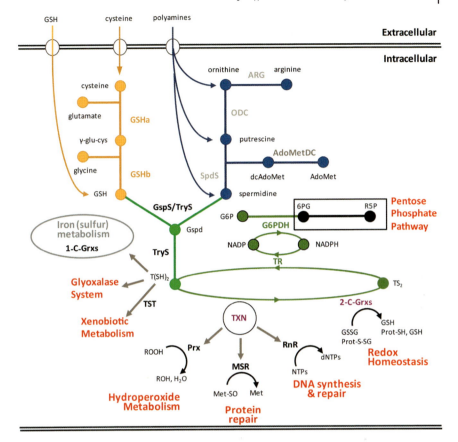

Figure 9.1 Trypanothione metabolism. Scheme summarizing metabolic pathways involved in synthesis, reduction, and utilization of trypanothione. Metabolites and enzymes involved in: (i) glutathione (GSH) uptake and biosynthesis are depicted in yellow with GSHa, γ-glutamylcysteine synthetase; GSHb, glutathione synthetase; (ii) polyamine uptake and biosynthesis are shown in blue with ARG, arginase; ODC, ornithine decarboxylase; AdoMetDC, S-adenosinylmethionine decarboxylase; SpdS, spermidine synthase; (iii) trypanothione synthesis is shown in light green with GspS, mono(glutathionyl)spermidine synthetase; TryS, trypanothione synthetase; (iv) trypanothione reduction is highlighted in green olive with TR, trypanothione reductase; TS₂, trypanothione disulfide; G6PDH, glucose-6-phosphate dehydrogenase; G6P, glucose-6-phosphate; and other metabolites (6PG, 6-phosphogluconate; R5P, ribose-5-phosphate) of the pentose phosphate pathway (box); (v) trypanothione-dependent pathways with trypanothione as cofactor (e.g., removal of methylglyoxal by glyoxalase system and thiol ligand of iron-sulfur clusters by glutaredoxins; 1-C-Grxs, monothiol glutaredoxins) or nucleophile (e.g., addition to xenobiotics such as electrophile drugs in reactions catalyzed or not by trypanothione S-transferase, TST). The trypanothione-dependent redoxin-mediated (shown in magenta) pathways involve those catalyzed by the main oxidoreductase of trypanosomatids, tryparedoxin (TXN) (e.g., reduction of distinct types of peroxidases (Prx) that decompose different hydroperoxides (ROOH) to the corresponding alcohol (ROH) and water, reduction of methionine sulfoxide reductase (MSR) that regenerates methionine (Met) from its sulfoxide form (Met-SO), and reduction of ribonucleotide reductase (RnR), which produces desoxinucleotides (dNTPs) from nucleotides (NTPs), and dithiol glutaredoxins (2-C-Grxs) (e.g., reduction of glutathione disulfide (GSSG) and protein/GSH-mixed disulfides (Prot-S-SG)).

Table 9.1 Components of trypanothione-related pathways as drug target candidates.

Metabolic pathway	Protein[a]	Species	Validation method	Phenotype	Structure (Protein Data Bank ID)	Druggable	References
T(SH)₂ synthesis	GshA	T. brucei	genetic, chemical in vitro, and mouse model	indispensable	2WYO		[6,40,41]
		T. cruzi	chemical in vitro, and mouse model	increased susceptibility to nifurtimox and benznidazole		ND[b]	[42,43]
		L. infantum L. donovani	genetic and chemical in vitro	indispensable decreased infectivity	ND		[44,45]
	ODC	T. brucei brucei	genetic and chemical in vitro, mouse model and clinically	indispensable	2TOD, 1QU4, 1F3T		[46–53]
		T. brucei gambiense			1NJJ	Yes	
		L. donovani	genetic	indispensable	ND		[54]
	AdoMetC	T. brucei, L. donovani	genetic and chemical	indispensable	ND	Yes	[55–64]
	SpdS	T. brucei	genetic	indispensable	no		[52,65–69] and Bosch unpublished
		Leishmania	genetic and chemical			ND	
		T. cruzi	ND	ND	3BWB, 3BWC		
	TryS	T. brucei	genetic and chemical in vitro and mouse model	indispensable	ND	Yes	[70–74]
		L. major	ND	ND	2VOB, 2VPM, 2VPS		

		Species	Method	Phenotype	PDB		References
T(SH)$_2$ recycling	TR	*T. brucei*	genetic	indispensable	2WOI, 2WOV, 2WOW, 2WP5, 2WP6, 2WPC, 2WPE, 2WPF, 2WBA	Yes	[17,75–83]
		L. donovani. L. major, L. infantum	genetic	decreased infectivity	2X5O, 2YAU, 2WOH, 2JK6		
		T. cruzi	ND	ND	1AOG, 1BZL, 1NDA		
	G6PDH	*T. brucei*	genetic	indispensable	ND	Yes	[84] and Chapter 16
		T. cruzi	chemical *in vitro* and mouse model		4EM5/4E9I		
T(SH)$_2$ utilization	cTXN	*T. brucei*	genetic and chemical	indispensable	1O73	Yes	[85–87] and Fiorillo
		L. infantum			ND		unpublished
		L. major	ND	ND	3S9F		
	mTXN	*L. infantum*	genetic	dispensable	ND	No	[88]
	Trx	*T. brucei*	genetic	dispensable	1R26	ND	[89,90]
	2-C-Grxs	*T. brucei*	genetic	dispensable	ND	ND	[33]
	cTXNPx	*T. brucei*	genetic	indispensable	ND	No	[85]
		L. amazonensis	genetic	protection against oxidants	ND		[91]
		T. cruzi			1UUL		[92,93]
		T. brucei		dispensable	ND		[85]
	mTXNPx	*L. amazonensis*	genetic	protection against oxidants	ND	No	[91]
		L. infantum		dispensable *in vitro*, but loss of virulence *in vivo*	ND		[88]

Metabolic pathway	Protein[a]	Species	Validation method	Phenotype	Structure (Protein Data Bank ID)	Druggable[b]	References
	GPx-type TXNPx	T. brucei	genetic	indispensable (cytosolic isoform)	3DWV, 2RM5, 2RM6, 2VUP	No	[94–97]
		T. cruzi	ND	ND	3EOU		
	GLXI	L. donovani	genetic	reduced methylglyoxal detoxification	ND	No	[98–101]
		L. major		ND	2C21		
	GLXII	L. infantum	ND	ND	2P18, 2P1E		
		T. brucei	genetic	None	ND		
	1-C-Grx1	T. brucei	genetic in vitro and mouse model	indispensable	2LTK	ND	[34,102]
	MSR	T. cruzi	genetic	protection against H2O2	ND	ND	[36]

a) GshA, γ-glutamylcysteine synthetase; ODC, ornithine decarboxylase; TryS, trypanothione synthetase; TR, trypanothione reductase; cTXN and mTXN, cytosolic and mitochondrial tryparedoxin, respectively; Trx, thioredoxin; cPrx and mPrx, cytosolic and mitochondrial 2-Cys-peroxiredoxin-type tryparedoxin peroxidase, respectively; GPx, glutathione peroxidase-type tryparedoxin peroxidases; GLX I/II, glyoxalase I and II; 1-C-Grx1, mitochondrial monothiol glutaredoxin 1; MSR, methionine sulfoxide reductase.
b) ND, not determined.

prediction how to most effectively hit the system without affecting vital targets in the host, thus paving the way to create more efficacious and safer trypanocidal drugs.

Trypanothione Biosynthesis

The biosynthesis of T(SH)$_2$ demands the supply of GSH and Spd, metabolites that, depending on the trypanosomatid species, are synthesized *de novo* as in mammals or taken up from the extracellular medium. The final step involves the addition of two GSH molecules to Spd – a reaction catalyzed by one or, in certain trypanosomatids perhaps, by two related enzymes (Figure 9.1). This link between the polyamine and GSH metabolism is unique to trypanosomatids and, *a priori* therefore, offers exceptional chances for drug development.

Glutathione Synthesis

The first and rate-limiting step in GSH biosynthesis is catalyzed by γ-glutamylcysteine synthetase (GshA), which ligates L-glutamate and L-cysteine to produce γ-glutamylcysteine. Glutathione synthetase (GshB) then catalyzes the reaction between γ-glutamylcysteine and L-glycine to yield GSH. Both reactions are ATP-dependent. Chemical inhibition of GshA with the irreversible inhibitor L-buthionine-*S,R*-sulfoximine (BSO) provided the first evidence for the indispensability of the thiol metabolism in African trypanosomes [6]. Subsequent studies conducted in different trypanosomatid species and using BSO as model drug confirmed the chemotherapeutic potential of GSH synthesis and its contribution to drug sensitivity (see sections below) [42–44,103]. The importance of this pathway was further validated by genetic approaches. RNAi-mediated downregulation of GshA in procyclic *T. brucei* depleted the cellular pools of GSH and T(SH)$_2$ with subsequent parasite death [40]. *L. infantum* mutants with impaired levels of GshA were more susceptible to oxidative and xenobiotic stress, and showed decreased survival inside activated macrophages [45]. Kinetic characterization of recombinant *T. brucei* GshA suggested the existence of important molecular differences with respect to the mammalian enzyme [104,105]. However, analysis of the *Tb*GshA crystal structure disclosed a high similarity with its human counterpart, shedding doubt on *Tb*GshA being a useful target for specific inhibitors [41]. Moreover, the ability of *T. brucei* to incorporate GSH from the extracellular medium implies that an effective therapy should also target the uptake mechanism (transporter), as, for instance, BSO does [40]. Although the TriTryp genomes contain sequences coding for putative GshB [21–23], the gene products await characterization, before their potential as targets for selective inhibition can be forecasted.

Polyamine Synthesis, Salvage, and Uptake

The acquisition of Spd varies among different trypanosomatids (Figure 9.1). African trypanosomes depend entirely on *de novo* synthesis of Spd [68], due to their negligible polyamine uptake capability, which probably remained undeveloped due to the scarce polyamine availability in the host's bloodstream. In contrast, *T. cruzi* is auxotrophic for polyamines, and relies on high-affinity transporters to scavenge putrescine and cadaverine from the host [106–108]. *Leishmania* parasites are more versatile being capable of both synthesis and transport-mediated uptake of polyamines from the extracellular environment [109–111].

The biosynthetic pathway for polyamine production starts from arginine and involves its decarboxylation. The genomes of TriTryps harbor sequences encoding putative arginases, but none of them has yet been functionally characterized. Nevertheless, a role in polyamine synthesis can be envisaged for arginase from *Leishmania* species and *T. brucei* in the light of their metabolic output (urea excretion) or needs (extreme dependence on *de novo* polyamine synthesis), respectively. The occurrence of an arginase gene in *T. cruzi* is probably irrelevant for polyamine metabolism, since this parasite lacks ornithine decarboxylase (ODC) [22,112,113]. In contrast, ODC is present and indispensable for *Leishmania* and *T. brucei* grown in polyamine-deficient media [48,52,54]; reviewed in [114,115]. Recent phylogenetic studies propose that parasites from the *T. brucei* clade replaced, probably by horizontal gene transfer, their protozoan ODC gene by one of vertebrate origin [116]. Despite the high similarity of sequence (around 60% identity) and structure between mammalian and *Tb*ODC [27,49,51], the therapeutic approach based on an irreversible inhibitor (difluoromethylornithine (DFMO)) successfully survived laboratory and clinical validations [46,47] and, for two decades already, has become a therapeutic routine to treat both early- and late-stage sleeping sickness caused by *T. b. gambiense*. The effectiveness of DFMO towards *T. b. gambiense* infections is, in part, explained by the longer half-life of the trypanosomal ODC as compared to the human ortholog (18 h *versus* 8–30 min, respectively), and the resulting shortage in polyamines in the parasite that causes (i) cell growth arrest, (ii) decreased synthesis of macromolecules (e.g., components of the glycoprotein coat that allows the parasite to escape from host immune recognition), (iii) aberrant methylation due to accumulation of decarboxylated *S*-adenosylmethionine (dcAdoMet), and (iv) limited antioxidant capacity due to trypanothione depletion. The failure of DFMO to act on the more aggressive *T. b. rhodesiense* has been ascribed to the higher activity (3-fold) and shorter half-life (around 4 h) of its ODC as compared to its counterpart in *T. b. gambiense* [117], and, probably, to a reduced drug uptake [118]. Recent studies have identified the amino acid transporter *Tb*AAT6 as the solely responsible for laboratory-induced DFMO resistance in trypanosomes [119]. This finding together with the increasing failures reported for DFMO treatment of human African trypanosomiasis [119] raises concerns about the mid-term success of a currently implemented melarsoprol–DFMO combined therapy. Nevertheless, this situation might be reverted if some of the recently discovered potent and selective *T. brucei* ODC inhibitors overcome successfully clinical trials [53].

Also the ODC of *L. donovani* exhibits a long-half life (greater than 20 h) [120,121]. However, *Leishmania* species are mostly tolerant to DFMO, which in part has been ascribed to increased ODC activity in DFMO-resistant strains [122], but also to the intracellular life style of *Leishmania*, which favors polyamine uptake from the host cell [110,123]. On this background, the development of polyamine-targeting inhibitors to treat leishmaniasis remains a challenge, since a successful strategy would likely have to target both transport-mediated uptake and endogenous synthesis.

AdoMetDC is expressed in all three trypanosomatids, shares a low sequence identity with the mammalian enzymes (around 30%), and has been shown to be essential for *L. donovani* promastigotes and *T. brucei* species by means of genetic or chemical approaches [55–59,61,62]. The mechanism of cell death in parasites treated with AdoMetDC inhibitors appears rather to be associated with aberrant methylation due to AdoMet accumulation than with polyamine depletion [57,58]. Early promising therapeutic data on AdoMetDC inhibitors in experimental *T. b. rhodesiense* infection [56,60] has recently been corroborated by novel more potent drug candidates [63,64]. Resolution of the three-dimensional structure of Kinetoplastida AdoMetDC and a thorough comparison with the human ortholog [124] might reanimate related drug design efforts.

Spermidine synthase (SpdS) has been biochemically characterized, and shown to be indispensable for the growth of *T. brucei*, *L. donovani*, and *T. cruzi* in the presence and the absence of exogenous Spd, respectively [52,65–69]. Inhibition of SpdS may be a suitable monotherapeutic option for *T. brucei*, because of its dependency on *de novo* polyamine synthesis, while in trypanosomatids that rely on polyamine uptake the transporters have to be targeted simultaneously. Unfortunately, potent and specific inhibitors have not yet been identified for this enzyme [65], and the sequence similarities with mammalian SpdS (40–50% identities) are not particularly encouraging.

Many eukaryotes also use an alternative pathway to synthesize putrescine that depends on the concerted action of arginine decarboxylase (ADC), which produces agmatine from arginine, followed by agmatine hydrolysis by agmatinase to finally yield putrescine and urea. Agmatinase-like sequences are present in the genome of the trypanosomatids [21–23]. However, the corresponding agmatinase activities have not yet been detected [125], and the submicromolar concentration of agmatine in mammalian tissues and fluids [126] would require highly efficient transporters to fulfill the parasites' needs for polyamine synthesis in the absence of ADC.

Trypanothione Synthesis

The first step in the biosynthesis of $T(SH)_2$ consists in the ATP-dependent addition of GSH to one of the amino groups of Spd, preferentially to the N^1, to form Gsp. Depending on the genetic background of the trypanosomatid this reaction can be catalyzed by either glutationylspermidine synthetase (GspS) or trypanothione synthetase (TryS). The addition of a second GSH molecule to Gsp is a reaction exclusively catalyzed by TryS. These proteins have no counterpart in mammals, their closest and ancestral relative being a GspS from γ-proteobacteria [127]. Although the genomes of *T. cruzi* and *L. brasiliensis* contain putative genes for GspS (www. tritrypdb.org), GspS activity has not yet been reported for any of these species. The role of a GspS in pathogenic trypanosomatids remains uncertain, since TryS from several species have been shown to produce $T(SH)_2$ from GSH and Spd. In fact, *T. brucei* [70,128], *L. major* [27], and probably *L. infantum* (Castro and Tomas, unpublished observations) rely entirely on TryS for $T(SH)_2$ biosynthesis irrespective of the presence of a GspS. The gene encoding GspS, thus, may be on the way to be lost, if it does not meet specific requirement other than $T(SH)_2$ synthesis (see below).

GspS and TryS are composed of two functional domains harboring opposite catalytic activities. The N-terminal domain presents a typical Cys-protease motif that confers hydrolytic activity to convert Gsp and $T(SH)_2$ back to the building blocks, GSH and Spd. The C-terminal synthetase domain belongs to the ATP-grasp enzyme family (i.e., GSHb, Ala–Ala synthetase, and other ATP-dependent C–N ligases) [129]. The biological role of the amidase activity of these enzymes remains obscure. In infective *T. brucei*, the amidase activity of TryS does not appear to confer any advantage in respect to *in vivo* survival [72]. However, the strict conservation of catalytic residues in the amidase domain of GspS and TryS from different trypanosomatids is suggestive of a peculiar biological role. Otherwise, this activity would simply maintain a costly futile cycle of $T(SH)_2$ synthesis and degradation. The amidase activity may, for instance, contribute to Spd salvage in *Leishmania* parasites, since ODC-null mutants have decreased levels of putrescine and $T(SH)_2$, but not of Spd [54], suggesting that either Spd transport or back conversion from Gsp or $T(SH)_2$ may suffice to maintain Spd homeostasis. In contrast, the synthetase activity of TryS is considered to be essential. TryS downregulation by RNAi or conditional knockout in *T. brucei* resulted in depletion of Gsp and $T(SH)_2$ and accumulation of GSH and, at the biological level, in growth arrest, impaired antioxidant capacity, and infectivity, and ultimately in death. Although the essentiality of TryS has so far been demonstrated for African trypanosomes only [70,72,128], the enzyme may be considered to be equally indispensable for species that lack a GspS. However, the phenotype of TryS depletion or inhibition may substantially differ in trypanosomatids expressing a GspS, since at least *in vitro* Gsp has been shown to be a reasonable substrate and reducing agent for TR and TXN, respectively [130,131]. In *L. major*, *T. cruzi*, and *T. brucei* TryS presents a non-uniform cytosolic distribution ([(27)] Medeiros and Comini, unpublished observations). In this respect, the $T(SH)_2$ requirement of specific organelles such as the mitochondrion still poses intriguing questions [132,133].

The crystal structure of *L. major* TryS has been solved at 2.8 Å [71]. Modeling of substrates and analogs to the presumed active site revealed well-structured binding sites for ATP and GSH, while the one for Spd appears less characteristic. In agreement with functional data [26], the substrate orientations comply with a mechanism by which GSH is first activated by phosphorylation at its glycine carboxylate for conjugation to N^1 of Spd. Interestingly, the Spd binding site extends into a second binding site for GSH, which suggests that the N^1-glutathionylated Spd formed in the initial step of $T(SH)_2$ synthesis flips around and is then re-bound in a way that its still free N^8 can also be glutathionylated (Koch and Flohé, unpublished). The detailed information on mechanism and substrate binding sites predict an excellent druggability of TryS and certainly will prove to be of outstanding importance for rational drug design. Before these structural and mechanistic insights, the design of TryS inhibitors was only possible on the basis of substrate similarity [134–136]. Inhibitors thus obtained showed indeed convincing trypanocidal activities with cultured parasites, but their peptidic character remained an obstacle for further development. More recently, novel drug-like TryS inhibitors have been identified by means of high-throughput drug screening [73,74], which confirms the druggability of TryS.

Collectively, therefore, TryS proved to be a most attractive drug target by several criteria: (i) uniqueness of sequence, (ii) low abundance, (iii) genetic proof of essentiality, and (iv) demonstrated druggability by chemical validation [26,31,70,73,74]. The only disadvantage of this target that emerges from ongoing drug design efforts is its species–specific susceptibility for inhibition. In fact, differences in IC_{50} of more than three orders of magnitude have been observed for the very same inhibitor for TryS of different trypanosomatid species [137,138].

Trypanothione Recycling

The maintenance of steady-state levels of dihydrotrypanothione (reduced form) is warranted in trypanosomatids by the presence of an NADPH-dependent flavoenzyme named TR. Although sharing homology with mammalian glutathione reductase (around 40% protein identity), TR has a remarkable specificity for the disulfide form of trypanothione and Gsp [130]. The protein has been shown to be essential for infective *T. brucei* [80], and to be important for the proliferation of *L. donovani* and *L. major* inside activated macrophages [77,78]. The crystal structure has been solved for TR from *T. cruzi* [17,75,76,79,139], *L. infantum* [83], and *T. brucei* [81,82], also in complex with ligands and inhibitors (for review, see [140] and references therein). A recent thorough comparative study reveals that the *T. brucei* and *T. cruzi* homologs are almost indistinguishable in terms of kinetics and active site structure, which facilitates the design of a promiscuous compound targeting the enzymes of both species [141]. Since its identification in the early 1990s, TR has been investigated as the preferred drug target candidate of trypanothione-dependent metabolism and, despite structural similarity with several mammalian flavoproteins, numerous specific TR inhibitors with good *in vitro* activities have been synthesized (reviewed in [140,141]). Nevertheless, none of these inhibitors was potent enough *in vivo* to warrant drug development. A likely explanation of this disappointing situation is offered by the conditional knockout of TR in *T. brucei* [80]. Although this genetic approach convincingly demonstrated the essentiality of TR, it simultaneously revealed that a more than 95% inhibition of the enzyme is required to critically affect the parasite's redox homeostasis. Evidently, such degree of enzyme inhibition is not easily sustained long enough by any kind of reversible inhibitor to achieve an efficient trypanocidal action *in vivo*.

The alternate option to interfere with $T(SH)_2$ regeneration, inhibition of the oxidative part of the pentose phosphate pathway, has not yet been intensively explored. The NADPH required for regeneration of $T(SH)_2$ is considered to be largely derived from glucose-6-phosphate dehydrogenase and 6-phosphoglunoco-lactone dehydrogenase of the pentose phosphate shunt. The role of carbohydrate metabolism in trypanosomatids and the potential use of related enzymes as drug targets are discussed in Chapters 7 and 16 of this volume.

Trypanothione Utilization

Redoxin-Independent Functions of Trypanothione

Trypanothione has been shown to be largely more efficient than GSH in: (i) reducing small molecules such as dehydroascorbate, hydrogen peroxide, and peroxynitrite [142–144], (ii) reducing protein disulfides such as those of Trx, TXN, RnR, and glutaredoxins [18,19,32,33,35,145,146], (iii) scavenging radiation-induced radicals [147,148], (iv) acting as cofactor of the trypanosomatid glyoxylase system [149,150], and ligand of ISCs bound to *T. brucei* 1-C-Grx1 and 2-C-Grx1 [33–35] and of nitrosyl-iron complexes [151], and (v) reacting with electrophilic xenobiotics [9]. Some of these functions will be shortly discussed here.

Trypanothione-Dependent Ligation of Iron–NO Complexes and ISCs

Nitric oxide ($^\bullet NO$) is a highly reactive gas that can be produced by endothelial and immune cells. If not neutralized rapidly, $^\bullet NO$ can modify proteins (nitrosylation) [152] or, in the presence of O_2^-, can originate peroxynitrite – a highly reactive and cytotoxic oxidant that mediates intracellular killing of *T. cruzi* [153,154]. $T(SH)_2$ has been shown to form a stable dinitrosyl-iron complex (DNIC) with a 600-fold higher efficiency than GSH. Interestingly, the complex formed with $T(SH)_2$, even at millimolar concentrations, did not inactivate TR in comparison to the potent inhibitory effect exerted by micromolar concentrations of dinitrosyl-diglutathionyl-iron complex on human glutathione reductase [155]. Formation of the DNIC–$T(SH)_2$ complex was demonstrated in *T. brucei* and *L. infantum* exposed to $^\bullet NO$, which led to the proposal for a protective role of $T(SH)_2$ in defense against macrophage-derived reactive nitrogen species [151].

As for other cells, ISCs are important structural elements and redox-active cofactors of iron–sulfur proteins of trypanosomatids [156,157]. A role in iron homeostasis has recently been recognized for certain dithiol and most monothiol glutaredoxins from distantly related organisms [158], which was, at least in part, linked to their capacity to assemble an ISC at the expense of their active-site cysteine and GSH as additional low-molecular-mass thiol ligand. Analogous protein–ISC holocomplexes have been reported for *T. brucei* 2-C-Grx1 and 1-C-Grx1 with the novelty that in these proteins T(SH)$_2$ efficiently replaced GSH as thiol ligand [33–35,102]. The ISC assembled by 2-C-Grx1 is supposed to play a regulatory role in enzyme activity with the holo-form of the protein being redox inactive [33]. 1-C-Grx1 fulfills an indispensable role in the mitochondrion of *T. brucei* [34], probably participating in the final step of iron–sulfur protein biogenesis that involves the transfer of the bound ISC to apo-proteins [102]. Recent structural characterization of *T. brucei* 1-C-Grx1 has pinpointed important differences with its human counterpart [34]. Moreover, these studies revealed that even in the absence of scaffold proteins, T(SH)$_2$ alone can coordinate and transfer an ISC to 2-C-Grx1 [33,34] raising the possibility for a new physiological role for the low-molecular-mass dithiol as a putative ISC carrier or ligand in trypanosomes [35].

Trypanothione-Dependent Detoxification Reactions and Drug Resistance

Methylglyoxal is a highly reactive and mutagenic byproduct of glycolysis that demands dedicated enzymes for its efficient detoxification. Trypanosomatids metabolize this oxoaldehyde through different pathways. *T. cruzi*, *L. major*, and *L. donovani* have a fully active glyoxalase system that uses T(SH)$_2$ as a reaction cofactor [98,100,101,150,159–161], while *T. brucei* lacks a complete glyoxalase system; the glyoxalase I gene is missing and glyoxalase II appears to be dispensable [99,100]. An alternative pathway to metabolize methylglyoxal relies on the concerted action of a NADPH-dependent methylglyoxal reductase that produces lactaldehyde, which is further converted into L-lactate by a NAD(P)H-dependent lactaldehyde dehydrogenase. Both activities were detected in cell extracts of trypanosomatids [100,160,162], but the enzymatic entities have not yet been isolated. The problem of oxoaldehyde detoxification is the subject of Chapter 8 in this volume. Based on metabolic modeling, the authors conclude that the trypanosomatid oxoaldehyde metabolism is likely too robust to be critically inhibited by targeting a single enzyme [163].

The role of T(SH)$_2$ in the detoxification of the trivalent arsenic compound melarsoprol, the trivalent antimonial triostam, and the nitroheterocyclic compounds nifurtimox, megazol, and benznidazole, has been studied intensively, and the hints toward T(SH)$_2$-dependent drug resistance are numerous [8,103,128,164–169]. The mechanisms by which T(SH)$_2$ interferes with different drugs may comprise (i) direct binding of trivalent arsenicals and likely antimonials, (ii) spontaneous or (iii) enzyme-catalyzed conjugation with electrophiles, but (iv) also the TXN/TXN-dependent Prx (TXNPx)-mediated removal of hydroperoxides generated from redox-cycling drugs, as outlined in the next section. To what extent drug resistance is due to direct or enzyme-mediated actions of T(SH)$_2$ appears to be far from clear. Certainly, electrophilic drugs or metabolites may be conjugated by T(SH)$_2$ directly, but more likely this detoxification is accelerated by a trypanothione-*S*-transferase, an enzyme found in different trypanosomatids and showing similarity with the eukaryotic elongation factor 1B (eEF1B) [170,171]. Also genes encoding an eEF1B homolog and a putative glutathione-*S*-transferase-related glutaredoxin are present in the *T. brucei* genome [21], but none of these enzymes have been characterized sufficiently to justify an attempt to overcome drug resistance by a targeted inhibition.

Also the seemingly straightforward binding of arsenicals and antimonials by $T(SH)_2$ turns out to be more complex than anticipated. For sure, trivalent arsenicals and antimonials can covalently bind to the dithiol $T(SH)_2$, but it does not imply that such mode of action is the only or the therapeutically relevant one. They could equally attack any of the exposed thiols in TR, as discussed [164], or the thiols of the various thiol peroxidases or of redoxins, which are the prototype of proteins preferentially labeled with arsenicals [172,173]. In line with this reasoning, resistance to arsenicals, benznidazole, and antimonials was found to be associated with natural or experimental elevation of TXNPx in *Leishmania* species [91,174–177]. However, recent studies on *Leishmania spp.* have revealed a more complex scenario for the mechanism of drug resistance generated in laboratories *versus* those occurring in the field [178,179].

Redoxin-Dependent Functions of Trypanothione

Without the assistance of thiol/disulfide oxidoreductases, the flow of reducing equivalents from $T(SH)_2$ to its different protein targets would likely be too slow to cope with cellular demands. Accordingly, trypanosomatids encode three types of dithiol oxidoreductases that are characterized by a CxxC active-site motif, belong to the thioredoxin (Trx) superfamily and are now commonly called "redoxins:" (i) typical Trx(s) with an active site WCGPCK motif, (ii) glutaredoxin(s) with a CPYC (exceptionally CQFC) motif [33], and (iii) tryparedoxin(s) characterized by a WCPPCR motif. The latter have so far only been detected in trypanosomatids. A typical Trx was found in *T. brucei* and *T. cruzi*, but proved to be functionally dispensable in *T. brucei* by inverse genetics [89,90,180,181]. Moreover, the TriTryp genomes completely lack sequences encoding for a thioredoxin reductase homolog gene, suggesting that Trx is a phylogenetic relict in trypanosomatids. In fact, all functions known of Trx in other organisms appear to be exerted by the trypanosomatid-specific TXN.

Two dithiol glutaredoxins (2-C-Grxs) were identified in *T. cruzi* [182] and *T. brucei* [33]. Although displaying different efficiencies and specificities, cytosolic Grx1 and mitochondrial Grx2 from *T. brucei* were able to not only reduce GSSG, but also protein–GSH mixed disulfides (deglutathionylation) as well as inter- or intramolecular disulfides [33]. Not surprisingly for organisms that lack glutathione reductase and strictly depend on $T(SH)_2$ to maintain the intracellular thiol/disulfide milieu, the trypanosomatid 2-C-Grxs evolved as catalysts for the reduction of GSSG by $T(SH)_2$ [33]. Although 2-C-Grxs cannot compete with TXN in the reduction of protein disulfides, except the former would have specific protein targets, they largely surpass TXN in their capacity to deglutathionylate proteins [33]. Protein glutathionylation is discussed as a reversible modification of thiols that protects proteins against loss of function associated with overoxidation of cysteines [152,183]. Cysteine-specific glutathionylation of recombinant forms of different trypanosomatid proteins has recently been reported [184]. However, and regardless of the physiological role of 2-C-Grxs in trypanosomes (e.g., kinetic control of GSSG reduction or protein deglutathionylation), none of the Grx activities appear critical for the viability of infective forms of *T. brucei* cultured *in vitro* [33].

In the parasite cytosol, TXN is the most abundant redoxin [18,26]. Despite belonging to the Trx superfamily, several functional and structural studies corroborate the preference of the enzyme for T(SH)$_2$ and Gsp, and the negligible capacity of GSH to act as reducing substrate [19,20,131,185–187]. In contrast to Trxs and 2-C-Grxs, downregulation of cytosolic TXN was detrimental for the proliferation of bloodstream *T. brucei* grown under optimal conditions [85,86]. TXN was equally indispensable for *L. infantum* where knockout of both chromosomal TXN1 alleles was only possible upon complementation with an episomal copy of the gene [87]. TXN has been shown to mediate important cellular processes such as the synthesis of deoxyribonucleotides [32], the decomposition of hydroperoxides [18,85,86,94,131,188,189], and the repair of (methionine) oxidized proteins [36]. By these and other suggested roles, TXN supports parasite virulence [13,87,190]. Altogether, this highlights the dominant role of the parasite-specific redoxin TXN in mastering the trypanothione-dependent intracellular redox homeostasis.

Hydroperoxide Metabolism

In trypanosomatids, TXNs as well as peroxiredoxin-type peroxidases (Prx) and cysteine-homologs of the classical selenocysteine-containing glutathione peroxidase-type proteins (GPx), complemented in certain species with a heme-type ascorbate peroxidase [191,192], form a most complex antioxidant defense system (for extensive reviews see [28,29,193–195], and Chapters 10 and 11 of this volume). TXNs, Prxs, and GPxs occur in multiple isoforms that display discrete differences in substrate specificities and are localized in different subcellular compartments. The link between TXN and peroxidases was first disclosed in *Crithidia fasciculata* [18], and then found to be common to all trypanosomatids [131,196–198]. The novel redoxin, thereby, emerged as the "missing factor" responsible for the reduction of hydroperoxides by the vaguely defined trypanothione-dependent peroxidase activity of trypanosomatids [18], which were later recognized to belong to the Prx type. The increased sensitivity towards hydrogen peroxide or the organic *tert*-butyl hydroperoxide exhibited by bloodstream *T. brucei* with a low content of TryS and TXN further confirmed the exclusive dependence of the hydroperoxide metabolism of trypanosomatids on the T(SH)$_2$/TXN couple [70,86].

Noticeably, trypanosomatids are endowed with Prxs only from the typical 2-Cys class [199] that are characterized by the formation of an intermolecular disulfide upon oxidation by hydroperoxide and by assembling into large quaternary structures (decamers and stacks of decamers) [92,200]. Different isoforms of TXNPx have been shown to be important for parasite survival and virulence [85,93,201–203]. Their biochemical, kinetic, and biological features are treated elsewhere in this volume (Chapters 10 and 11).

TXN also substitutes for Trx in the reduction of GPxs. The unexpected redoxin specificity of GPx-type proteins was first detected for a "glutathione peroxidase" from *Plasmodium falciparum* [204], and soon after in various plants, yeasts, insects, bacteria, and finally by Wilkinson *et al.* [205] and Hillebrand *et al.* [198] in kinetoplasts. It is likely more common to this type of proteins than the name-giving GPx activity of the mammalian prototype GPx1 [206]. The redoxin-specific GPxs are characterized as monomeric non-selenium GPxs having a second cysteine located in a flexible loop that forms an intramolecular disulfide bridge with the active-site (or peroxidatic) cysteine upon oxidation by a hydroperoxide [95–97,207], thus presenting a typical substrate structure for a redoxin-type disulfide reductase [208]. Similarly to GPx from other organisms, the parasite proteins showed specificity for reducing lipid hydroperoxides [94,188,195]. RNAi-mediated gene silencing depleted transcripts from all three gene copies present in the genome of *T. brucei*, and revealed the indispensability of GPx-type peroxidases for parasite growth [188]. Recently, targeted gene replacement (knockout) of GPx-type peroxidases demonstrated that the cytosolic isoforms of these proteins were major determinants for cell viability [94]. Interestingly, the detrimental effect caused by the lack of cytosolic GPx activity could be reverted by cultivating the GPx-deficient parasites in the presence of Trolox, a water-soluble version of α-tocopherol and well-known hydrophobic antioxidant, thus confirming that the main function of these proteins is to provide protection against lipid peroxidation and membrane damage. Knockout of the third GPx-type isoform localized in the parasite mitochondrion revealed an increase in cardiolipin oxidation, but only a transitory growth arrest [94].

Redoxin and DNA Synthesis

Ribonucleotide reductase (RnR) is the enzyme that catalyzes the reduction of the 2′-hydroxyl group of ribonucleotides to the corresponding deoxyribonucleotides and thus is indispensible for DNA synthesis [209]. RnRs require Trx or Grx as reducing cosubstrate in practically all organisms [210,211]. Trypanosomatid RnR had for long been measured with non-physiological thiols or with T(SH)$_2$. Finally, cytosolic *Tb*TXN was shown to be a much more efficient reductant of RnR than any other thiol previously applied and, thus, is likely the physiological RnR reductant [32]. Later attempts to replace TXN as RnR substrate by *Tb*Trx [212] or 2-C-Grxs [33] did not challenge this conclusion, since they were less active. In line with the assumption that TXN is the relevant substrate of RnR, *T. brucei* depleted in TXN or trypanothione displayed a decreased proliferation rate under normal culture conditions [70,86], whereas knockout of Trx and RNAi of cytosolic Tb 2-C-Grx1 remained without any obvious phenotype [33,89]. It is, however, hard to decide to what extent growth retardation in TXN- or T(SH)$_2$-deficient *T. brucei* results from deoxynucleotide shortage or a disturbed redox metabolism, since the RnR is under redox control, being inhibited by oxidized trypanothione [32]. RnR remains as an attractive drug target candidate out of the redoxin-dependent enzymes. Orthologs of this enzyme in other species have attracted considerable interest, particularly in the context of anti-cancer drug research, but so far not for the design of trypanocidal drugs.

New Putative Functions for TXN and Peroxidases

Methionine sulfoxide reductase (MSR) is a ubiquitous enzyme that catalyzes the reduction of methionine sulfoxide to methionine. MSR is considered to be part of the antioxidant armamentarium of cells by participating in the second line of defense that includes the repair of oxidized proteins [213]. The reaction mechanism is mediated by redox active thiols: subtraction of a single oxygen atom from methionine sulfoxide by a nucleophilic cysteine of MSR leads to formation of a sulfenic acid on the thiol and reduced methionine; a second cysteine from the same MSR subunit attacks the sulfenic acid with concomitant formation of an intra-molecular disulfide, which is typically reduced by Trx(s). Recent work has reported on the characterization of genes encoding for putative MSR type A in *T. cruzi* (*Tc*MSR10 and *Tc*MSR180) and *T. brucei* (*Tb*MSR) [36]. The recombinant proteins from all three isoforms displayed specificity for L-Met(S) sulfoxide and cytosolic *T. cruzi* TXN I as substrate. Active expression of the proteins was detected only in the replicative forms of *T. cruzi* (e.g., epimastigotes and amastigotes) and in both life stages of *T. brucei*. A 15- to 20-fold overexpression of *Tc*MSR10 in non-infective epimastigotes conferred a 2-fold resistance against H_2O_2, supporting a role of the protein in antioxidant protection. Although the biological relevance of MSR for parasite survival remains to be elucidated this work adds a new target to the list of $T(SH)_2$/TXN-dependent functions in trypanosomatids.

Admittedly, the complexity of the trypanothione-dependent hydroperoxide metab-olism may be underestimated when only regarded as a defense system that protects the parasites against the hostile environment created by the host's innate immune response. The substrates of TXNPxs and GPxs such as H_2O_2, lipid hydroperoxides, or peroxynitrite (for reviews, see [214,215]) are no longer considered just as toxic compounds responsible for oxidative cell damage, but are increasingly recognized as signaling molecules [1,183,216,217]. Like the GPx-type ORP1 of *Saccharomyces cerevisiae* [218] and the Prx-type TPx1 of *Schizosaccharomyces pombe* [219], a TXNPx of *C. fasciculata* was also reported to act as sensor for H_2O_2 and, as oxidized peroxidase, to oxidize a transcription factor, here the "universal mini circle sequence binding protein" implicated in replication of mitochondrial DNA [220]. The role of TXN in this context would be to prevent signaling by reducing the oxidized peroxidase and to reverse the signaling event by regenerating the reduced transcription factor. So far, however, the *in vivo* relevance of this regulatory concept could not be demonstrated, since knockdown of the mitochondrial TXNPx in *T. brucei* [85], as well as knockout in *L. infantum* [88], did not affect the proliferation rate of the parasites.

The reaction mechanism common to redoxins – attack of a (protein) disulfide by means of their exposed active-site cysteine residue followed by further thiol disulfide exchange – can be used to identify TXN targets in the form of disulfide-linked heterodimers, if the redoxin's coreacting ("resolving") cysteine is mutated to serine [207,221]. By means of this technology, several putative reaction partners of *Tc*TXN1C43S could be trapped from *T. cruzi* [190] and *T. brucei* ([13] and Comini unpublished), *inter alia* proteins involved in cysteine biosynthesis (cystathionase), methionine/adenine salvage (methylthioadenosine phosphorylase), and protein synthesis/degradation (eIF4AI, a subunit of the eukaryotic translation initiation factor eIFaF and ubiquitin-activating enzyme e1). Although further validations of these interactions are required, these results open up novel perspectives for further cellular functions of TXN and ultimately of $T(SH)_2$.

Redoxins and Peroxidases as Drug Targets?

In general, redoxins are considered to be pleiotropic, which means they are designed by nature to interact with multiple partners without being entirely unspecific. The most prominent example of pleiotropism is represented by Trx, which, apart from being a cosubstrate of RnR and peroxidases, is implicated as a transducer or terminator in signaling cascades, as a universal disulfide reductant and, extracellularly, as a kind of cytokine [210,217,222,223]. Its trypanosomal counterpart, TXN, appears not to make an exception to this rule: as outlined above, it can interact covalently with RnR, structurally distinct peroxidases, new protein partners engaged in different metabolic processes a and with its peptidic substrate $T(SH)_2$. This functional diversification is hard to understand on the basis of a highly specific enzyme substrate interaction according to the "lock and key" model and, indeed, TXN structures do not reveal any characteristic substrate-binding pockets. Instead, substrate interaction studies suggest that substrate recognition is essentially based on electrostatic interactions [185,187,199,224]. Recently, however, high-throughput screening against the components of the hydroperoxide-detoxifying cascade of African trypanosomes (i.e., TR, TXN, GPx and $T(SH)_2$) with around 80 000 chemicals identified a few system inhibitors [225]. Surprisingly, the most active compounds were time-dependent inhibitors of TXN that reacted irreversibly with its exposed N-terminal active-site cysteine. Although the molecules (e.g., thienopyrimidine-4-ones and purine-2,6-diones) interacted also with recombinant human Trx they displayed an at least greater than 10-fold cytotoxic potency against infective *T. brucei* than towards mammalian HeLa cells. These results may again place TXN into the previously discussed rank of useful targets [26].

Also, GPx-type proteins do not have any characteristic binding pocket for their reducing substrates and, with the exception of mammalian GPx1, are not particularly specific enzymes. As far as investigated, their interaction with substrates is also dominated by weak electrostatic attraction [208]. *In vitro* studies with knockout cell lines of *T. brucei* rule out a "moonlighting" function for the trypanosomatid GPxs, as was observed with mammalian and yeast orthologs [216,218,226–228]. In contrast, their crucial role appears to be restricted to the detoxification of lipid hydroperoxides and, hence, in protecting parasites against membrane damage [94]. The druggability of trypanosomatid non-selenium GPx may, indeed, be questioned based on the negative results obtained in a recent high-throughput screening approach [225].

Pleiotropism is also a hallmark of Prxs. Long before the discovery of their peroxidase nature, they were identified in different biological contexts [229,230], and "moonlighting," here between peroxidase and chaperone function, appears to be a common feature [88]. Thus far, TXNPx inhibitors have not been reported and the design of specific ones appears to be a highly challenging task. Nevertheless, synthetic (conoidin A) and natural (adenanthin) compounds have recently been reported to inhibit PrxII of *Toxoplasma gondii* and/or mammalian PrxI and PrxII, respectively [231,232]. These compounds might therefore be considered as first structural scaffolds for developing specific Prxs inhibitors.

In respect of target selection, it can be stated that cTXN, cTXNPx, and the GPx-type TXNPx were shown to be essential by inverse genetics for survival of *Trypanosoma* and/or *Leishmania* species (Table 9.1 and references therein), and knockout of the mTXNPx in *L. infantum* at least impaired virulence in an animal infection model [88]. However, all these proteins share a more or less pronounced pleiotropism. In line with this functional versatility, they are devoid of any well-structured substrate-binding pocket, where a high-affinity inhibitor could be accommodated with a specificity that reliably excludes cross-reaction with mammalian homologs. In short, Prxs and GPx-type peroxidases are not easily druggable.

Conclusions

The trypanothione system is indeed a unique feature of trypanosomatids, and it is of outstanding importance for the parasite's viability and virulence. Accordingly, its exploitation for therapeutic intervention merits consideration. The uniqueness of the system, however, does not imply that all of its components are unique nor are its individual components equally essential. If target druggability is also taken into account as an additional criterion for target selection, the following conclusions appear justified:

- Trypanosomatid glyoxalases and *S*-transferases should be disregarded as drug target because of lacking evidence of essentiality.
- Redoxins and peroxidases may be disregarded as preferred drug targets because of lack of essentiality, uniqueness, and/or poor druggability.
- Enzymes of polyamine synthesis and RnR deserve more attention, but selectivity of inhibition will remain a challenge.
- TR as target for reversible inhibitors disappointed, but irreversible inhibition remains a realistic option, if adequate selectivity can be achieved.
- To consider GspS as a drug target appears premature with regard to its still obscure biological role.
- TryS is the target of choice because of the uniqueness of its sequence and structure, low abundance, genetic support of essentiality, and structural evidence as well as chemical proof of druggability. Moreover, TryS shares with TR the important target criterion of controlling the metabolic flux through the entire pathway [163,233].

Acknowledgments

M.A.C. acknowledges Agencia Nacional de Investigación e Innovación (grant Innova Uruguay, agreement DCI-ALA/2007/19.040 between Uruguay and the European Commission) for financial support.

References

1 Flohé, L. (2010) Changing paradigms in thiology from antioxidant defense toward redox regulation. *Methods Enzymol.*, **473**, 1–39.

2 Thomas, H.W. and Breinl, A. (1905) *Trypanosomes, Trypanosomiasis, and Sleeping Sickness. Memoir XVI*, Liverpool School of Tropical Medicine, Liverpool.

3 Jacobs, W.A. and Heidelberger, M. (1919) Chemotherapy of trypanosome and spirochete infections: chemical series. I. *N*-phenylglycineamide *p*-arsonic acid. *J. Exp. Med.*, **30**, 411–415.

4 Friedheim, E.A. (1949) Mel B in the treatment of human trypanosomiasis. *Am. J. Trop. Med. Hyg.*, **29**, 173–180.

5 Docampo, R. and Stoppani, A.O. (1979) Generation of superoxide anion and hydrogen peroxide induced by nifurtimox in *Trypanosoma cruzi*. *Arch. Biochem. Biophys.*, **197**, 317–321.

6 Arrick, B.A., Griffith, O.W., and Cerami, A. (1981) Inhibition of glutathione synthesis as a chemotherapeutic strategy for trypanosomiasis. *J. Exp. Med.*, **153**, 720–725.

7 Docampo, R. and Moreno, S.N. (1984) Free radical metabolites in the mode of action of chemotherapeutic agents and phagocytic cells on *Trypanosoma cruzi*. *Rev. Infect. Dis.*, **6**, 223–238.

8 Fairlamb, A.H., Henderson, G.B., and Cerami, A. (1989) Trypanothione is the primary target for arsenical drugs against African trypanosomes. *Proc. Natl. Acad. Sci. USA*, **86**, 2607–2611.

9 Fairlamb, A.H. and Cerami, A. (1992) Metabolism and functions of trypanothione in the Kinetoplastida. *Annu. Rev. Microbiol.*, **46**, 695–729.

10 Mukhopadhyay, R., Dey, S., Xu, N., Gage, D., Lightbody, J., Ouellette, M., and Rosen, B.P. (1996) Trypanothione overproduction and resistance to antimonials and arsenicals in *Leishmania. Proc. Natl. Acad. Sci. USA*, **93**, 10383–10387.

11 Tabor, H. and Tabor, C.W. (1975) Isolation, characterization, and turnover of glutathionylspermidine from *Escherichia coli. J. Biol. Chem.*, **250**, 2648–2654.

12 Fairlamb, A.H., Blackburn, P., Ulrich, P., Chait, B.T., and Cerami, A. (1985) Trypanothione: a novel bis(glutathionyl) spermidine cofactor for glutathione reductase in trypanosomatids. *Science*, **227**, 1485–1487.

13 Krauth-Siegel, R.L. and Comini, M.A. (2008) Redox control in trypanosomatids, parasitic protozoa with trypanothione-based thiol metabolism. *Biochim. Biophys. Acta*, **1780**, 1236–1248.

14 Krauth-Siegel, R.L. and Leroux, A.E. (2012) Low-molecular-mass antioxidants in parasites. *Antioxid. Redox Signal.*, **17**, 583–607.

15 Fairlamb, A.H., Henderson, G.B., and Cerami, A. (1986) The biosynthesis of trypanothione and N^1-glutathionylspermidine in *Crithidia fasciculata. Mol. Biochem. Parasitol.*, **21**, 247–257.

16 Shames, S.L., Fairlamb, A.H., Cerami, A., and Walsh, C.T. (1986) Purification and characterization of trypanothione reductase from *Crithidia fasciculata*, a newly discovered member of the family of disulfide-containing flavoprotein reductases. *Biochemistry*, **25**, 3519–3526.

17 Krauth-Siegel, R.L., Enders, B., Henderson, G.B., Fairlamb, A.H., and Schirmer, R.H. (1987) Trypanothione reductase from *Trypanosoma cruzi*. Purification and characterization of the crystalline enzyme. *Eur. J. Biochem.*, **164**, 123–128.

18 Nogoceke, E., Gommel, D.U., Kiess, M., Kalisz, H.M., and Flohé, L. (1997) A unique cascade of oxidoreductases catalyses trypanothione-mediated peroxide metabolism in *Crithidia fasciculata*. *Biol. Chem.*, **378**, 827–836.

19 Lüdemann, H., Dormeyer, M., Sticherling, C., Stallmann, D., Follmann, H., and Krauth-Siegel, R.L. (1998) *Trypanosoma brucei* tryparedoxin, a thioredoxin-like protein in African trypanosomes. *FEBS Lett.*, **431**, 381–385.

20 Gommel, D.U., Nogoceke, E., Morr, M., Kiess, M., Kalisz, H.M., and Flohé, L. (1997) Catalytic characteristics of tryparedoxin. *Eur. J. Biochem.*, **248**, 913–918.

21 Berriman, M. *et al.* (2005) The genome of the African trypanosome *Trypanosoma brucei*. *Science*, **309**, 416–422.

22 El-Sayed, N.M. (2005) *et al.*The genome sequence of *Trypanosoma cruzi*, etiologic agent of Chagas disease. *Science*, **309**, 409–415.

23 Ivens, A.C. *et al.* (2005) The genome of the kinetoplastid parasite, *Leishmania major*. *Science*, **309**, 436–442.

24 Oza, S.L., Tetaud, E., Ariyanayagam, M.R., Warnon, S.S., and Fairlamb, A.H. (2002) A single enzyme catalyses formation of trypanothione from glutathione and spermidine in *Trypanosoma cruzi*. *J. Biol. Chem.*, **277**, 35853–35861.

25 Comini, M., Menge, U., and Flohé, L. (2003) Biosynthesis of trypanothione in *Trypanosoma brucei brucei*. *Biol. Chem.*, **384**, 653–656.

26 Comini, M., Menge, U., Wissing, J., and Flohé, L. (2005) Trypanothione synthesis in crithidia revisited. *J. Biol. Chem.*, **280**, 6850–6860.

27 Oza, S.L., Shaw, M.P., Wyllie, S., and Fairlamb, A.H. (2005) Trypanothione biosynthesis in *Leishmania major*. *Mol. Biochem. Parasitol.*, **139**, 107–116.

28 Krauth-Siegel, L.R., Comini, M.A., and Schlecker, T. (2007) The trypanothione system. *Subcell. Biochem.*, **44**, 231–251.

29 Castro, H. and Tomas, A.M. (2008) Peroxidases of trypanosomatids. *Antioxid. Redox Signal.*, **10**, 1593–1606.

30 Flohé, L. (2012) The trypanothione system and its implications in the therapy of trypanosomatid diseases. *Int. J. Med. Microbiol.*, **302**, 216–220.

31 Flohé, L. (2012) The trypanothione system and the opportunities it offers to create drugs for the neglected kinetoplast diseases. *Biotechnol. Adv.*, **30**, 294–301.

32 Dormeyer, M., Reckenfelderbäumer, N., Lüdemann, H., and Krauth-Siegel, R.L. (2001) Trypanothione-dependent synthesis of deoxyribonucleotides by *Trypanosoma brucei* ribonucleotide reductase. *J. Biol. Chem.*, **276**, 10602–10606.

33 Ceylan, S., Seidel, V., Ziebart, N., Berndt, C., Dirdjaja, N., and Krauth-Siegel, R.L. (2010) The dithiol glutaredoxins of African trypanosomes have distinct roles and are closely linked to the unique trypanothione metabolism. *J. Biol. Chem.*, **285**, 35224–35237.

34 Manta, B., Pavan, C., Sturlese, M., Medeiros, A., Crispo, M., Berndt, C., Krauth-Siegel, R.L., Bellanda, M., and Comini, M.A. (2012) Iron-sulfur cluster (ISC) binding by mitochondrial monothiol glutaredoxin-1 of Trypanosoma brucei: molecular basis of ISC coordination and relevance for parasite infectivity, Antioxid. Redox Signal. doi:10.1089/ars.2012.4859.

35 Comini, M.A., Krauth-Siegel, R.L., and Bellanda, M. (2012) Mono- and dithiol glutaredoxins in the trypanothione-based redox metabolism of pathogenic trypanosomes. *Antioxid. Redox Signal*, doi: 10.1089/ars.2012.4932.

36 Arias, D.G., Cabeza, M.S., Erben, E.D., Carranza, P.G., Lujan, H.D., Téllez Iñón, M.T., Iglesias, A.A., and Guerrero, S.A. (2011) Functional characterization of methionine sulfoxide reductase A from *Trypanosoma* spp. *Free Radic. Biol. Med.*, **50**, 37–46.

37 Meissner, M., Agop-Nersesian, C., and Sullivan, W.J.Jr. (2007) Molecular tools for analysis of gene function in parasitic microorganisms. *Appl. Microbiol. Biotechnol.*, **75**, 963–975.

38 Bellofatto, V. and Palenchar, J.B. (2008) RNA interference as a genetic tool in trypanosomes. *Methods Mol. Biol.*, **442**, 83–94.

39 Taylor, M.C., Huang, H., and Kelly, J.M. (2011) Genetic techniques in *Trypanosoma cruzi*. *Adv. Parasitol.*, **75**, 231–250.

40 Huynh, T.T., Huynh, V.T., Harmon, M.A., and Phillips, M.A. (2003) Gene knockdown of gamma-glutamylcysteine synthetase by RNAi in the parasitic protozoa *Trypanosoma brucei* demonstrates that it is an essential enzyme. *J. Biol. Chem.*, **278**, 39794–39800.

41 Fyfe, P.K., Alphey, M.S., and Hunter, W. N. (2010) Structure of *Trypanosoma brucei* glutathione synthetase: domain and loop alterations in the catalytic cycle of a highly conserved enzyme. *Mol. Biochem. Parasitol.*, **170**, 93–99.

42 Faundez, M., Pino, L., Letelier, P., Ortiz, C., López, R., Seguel, C., Ferreira, J., Pavani, M., Morello, A., and Maya, J.D. (2005) Buthionine sulfoximine increases the toxicity of nifurtimox and benznidazole to *Trypanosoma cruzi*. *Antimicrob. Agents Chemother.*, **49**, 126–130.

43 Faúndez, M., López-Muñoz, R., Torres, G., Morello, A., Ferreira, J., Kemmerling, U., Orellana, M., and Maya, J.D. (2008) Buthionine sulfoximine has anti-*Trypanosoma cruzi* activity in a murine model of acute Chagas' disease and enhances the efficacy of nifurtimox. *Antimicrob. Agents Chemother.*, **52**, 1837–1839.

44 Kapoor, P., Sachdev, M., and Madhubala, R. (2000) Inhibition of glutathione synthesis as a chemotherapeutic strategy for leishmaniasis. *Trop. Med. Int. Health*, **5**, 438–442.

45 Mukherjee, A., Roy, G., Guimond, C., and Ouellette, M. (2009) The gamma-glutamylcysteine synthetase gene of *Leishmania* is essential and involved in response to oxidants. *Mol. Microbiol.*, **74**, 914–927.

46 Bacchi, C.J., Nathan, H.C., Hutner, S.H., McCann, P.P., and Sjoerdsma, A. (1980) Polyamine metabolism: a potential therapeutic target in trypanosomes. *Science*, **210**, 332–334.

47 Van Nieuwenhove, S., Schechter, P.J., Declercq, J., Boné, G., Burke, J., and Sjoerdsma, A. (1985) Treatment of gambiense sleeping sickness in the Sudan with oral DFMO (DL-alpha-difluoromethylornithine), an inhibitor of ornithine decarboxylase; first field trial. *Trans. R. Soc. Trop. Med. Hyg.*, **79**, 692–698.

48 Li, F., Hua, S.B., Wang, C.C., and Gottesdiener, K.M. (1998) *Trypanosoma brucei brucei*: characterization of an ODC null bloodstream form mutant and the action of alpha-difluoromethylornithine. *Exp. Parasitol.*, **88**, 255–257.

49 Grishin, N.V., Osterman, A.L., Brooks, H.B., Phillips, M.A., and Goldsmith, E.J. (1999) X-ray structure of ornithine decarboxylase from *Trypanosoma brucei*: the native structure and the structure in complex with alpha-difluoromethylornithine. *Biochemistry*, **38**, 15174–15184.

50 Jackson, L.K., Brooks, H.B., Osterman, A. L., Goldsmith, E.J., and Phillips, M.A. (2000) Altering the reaction specificity of eukaryotic ornithine decarboxylase. *Biochemistry*, **39**, 11247–11257.

51 Jackson, L.K., Goldsmith, E.J., and Phillips, M.A. (2003) X-ray structure determination of *Trypanosoma brucei* ornithine decarboxylase bound to D-ornithine and to G418: insights into substrate binding and ODC conformational flexibility. *J. Biol. Chem.*, **278**, 22037–22043.

52 Xiao, Y., McCloskey, D.E., and Phillips, M. A. (2009) RNA interference-mediated silencing of ornithine decarboxylase and spermidine synthase genes in *Trypanosoma brucei* provides insight into regulation of polyamine biosynthesis. *Eukaryot. Cell*, **8**, 747–755.

53 Smithson, D.C., Lee, J., Shelat, A.A., Phillips, M.A., and Guy, R.K. (2010) Discovery of potent and selective inhibitors of *Trypanosoma brucei* ornithine decarboxylase. *J. Biol. Chem.*, **285**, 16771–16781.

54 Jiang, Y., Roberts, S.C., Jardim, A., Carter, N.S., Shih, S., Ariyanayagam, M., Fairlamb, A.H., and Ullman, B. (1999) Ornithine decarboxylase gene deletion mutants of *Leishmania donovani*. *J. Biol. Chem.*, **274**, 3781–3788.

55 Bitonti, A.J., Dumont, J.A., and McCann, P.P. (1986) Characterization of

Trypanosoma brucei brucei S-adenosyl-L-methioninedecarboxylase and its inhibition by Berenil, pentamidine and methylglyoxal bis(guanylhydrazone). *Biochem. J.*, **237**, 685–689.

56 Bitonti, A.J., Byers, T.L., Bush, T.L., Casara, P.J., Bacchi, C.J., Clarkson, A.B. Jr., McCann, P.P., and Sjoerdsma, A. (1990) Cure of *Trypanosoma brucei brucei* and *Trypanosoma brucei rhodesiense* infections in mice with an irreversible inhibitor of S-adenosyl methionine decarboxylase. *Antimicrob. Agents Chemother.*, **34**, 1485–1490.

57 Byers, T.L., Bush, T.L., McCann, P.P., and Bitonti, A.J. (1991) Antitrypanosomal effects of polyamine biosynthesis inhibitors correlate with increases in *Trypanosoma brucei brucei* S-adenosyl-L-methionine. *Biochem. J.*, **274**, 527–533.

58 Yakubu, M.A., Majumder, S., and Kierszenbaum, F. (1993) Inhibition of S-adenosyl-L-methionine (AdoMet) decarboxylase by the decarboxylated AdoMet analog 5'-([(Z)-4-amino-2-butenyl] methylamino)-5'-deoxyadenosine (MDL 73811) decreases the capacities of *Trypanosoma cruzi* to infect and multiply within a mammalian host cell. *J. Parasitol.*, **79**, 525–532.

59 Brun, R., Bühler, Y., Sandmeier, U., Kaminsky, R., Bacchi, C.J., Rattendi, D., Lane, S., Croft, S.L., Snowdon, D., Yardley, V., Caravatti, G., Frei, J., Stanek, J., and Mett, H. (1996) *In vitro* trypanocidal activities of new S-adenosylmethionine decarboxylase inhibitors. *Antimicrob. Agents Chemother.*, **40**, 1442–1447.

60 Bacchi, C.J., Brun, R., Croft, S.L., Alicea, K., and Bühler, Y. (1996) *In vivo* trypanocidal activities of new S-adenosylmethionine decarboxylase inhibitors. *Antimicrob Agents Chemother.*, **40**, 1448–1453.

61 Persson, K., Aslund, L., Grahn, B., Hanke, J., and Heby, O. (1998) *Trypanosoma cruzi* has not lost its S-adenosylmethionine decarboxylase: characterization of the gene and the encoded enzyme. *Biochem. J.*, **333**, 527–537.

62 Roberts, S.C., Scott, J., Gasteier, J.E., Jiang, Y., Brooks, B., Jardim, A., Carter, N. S., Heby, O., and Ullman, B. (2002) S-adenosylmethionine decarboxylase from *Leishmania donovani*. Molecular, genetic, and biochemical characterization of null mutants and overproducers. *J. Biol. Chem.*, **277**, 5902–5909.

63 Bacchi, C.J., Barker, R.H.Jr., Rodriguez, A., Hirth, B., Rattendi, D., Yarlett, N., Hendrick, C.L., and Sybertz, E. (2009) Trypanocidal activity of 8-methyl-5'-{[(Z)-4-aminobut-2-enyl]-(methylamino)}adenosine (Genz-644131), an adenosylmethionine decarboxylase inhibitor. *Antimicrob. Agents Chemother.*, **53**, 3269–3272.

64 Barker, R.H.Jr., Liu, H., Hirth, B., Celatka, C.A., Fitzpatrick, R., Xiang, Y., Willert, E. K., Phillips, M.A., Kaiser, M., Bacchi, C.J., Rodriguez, A., Yarlett, N., Klinger, J.D., and Sybertz, E. (2009) Novel S-adenosylmethionine decarboxylase inhibitors for the treatment of human African trypanosomiasis. *Antimicrob. Agents Chemother.*, **53**, 2052–2058.

65 Bitonti, A.J., Kelly, S.E., and McCann, P.P. (1984) Characterization of spermidine synthase from *Trypanosoma brucei brucei*. *Mol. Biochem. Parasitol.*, **13**, 21–28.

66 González, N.S., Huber, A., and Algranati, I.D. (2001) Spermidine is essential for normal proliferation of trypanosomatid protozoa. *FEBS Lett.*, **508**, 323–326.

67 Roberts, S.C., Jiang, Y., Jardim, A., Carter, N.S., Heby, O., and Ullman, B. (2001) Genetic analysis of spermidine synthase from *Leishmania donovani*. *Mol. Biochem. Parasitol.*, **115**, 217–226.

68 Taylor, M.C., Kaur, H., Blessington, B., Kelly, J.M., and Wilkinson, S.R. (2008) Validation of spermidine synthase as a drug target in African trypanosomes. *Biochem. J.*, **409**, 563–569.

69 Gilroy, C., Olenyik, T., Roberts, S.C., and Ullman, B. (2011) Spermidine synthase is required for virulence of *Leishmania donovani*. *Infect. Immun.*, **79**, 2764–2769.

70 Comini, M.A., Guerrero, S.A., Haile, S., Menge, U., Lünsdorf, H., and Flohé, L. (2004) Validation of *Trypanosoma brucei* trypanothione synthetase as drug target. *Free Radic.Biol. Med.*, **36**, 1289–1302.

71 Fyfe, P.K., Oza, S.L., Fairlamb, A.H., and Hunter, W.N. (2008) *Leishmania* trypanothione synthetase-amidase structure reveals a basis for

regulation of conflicting synthetic and hydrolytic activities. *J. Biol. Chem.*, **283**, 17672–17680.

72 Wyllie, S., Oza, S.L., Patterson, S., Spinks, D., Thompson, S., and Fairlamb, A.H. (2009) Dissecting the essentiality of the bifunctional trypanothione synthetase-amidase in *Trypanosoma brucei* using chemical and genetic methods. *Mol. Microbiol.*, **74**, 529–540.

73 Torrie, L.S., Wyllie, S., Spinks, D., Oza, S. L., Thompson, S., Harrison, J.R., Gilbert, I.H., Wyatt, P.G., Fairlamb, A.H., and Frearson, J.A. (2009) Chemical validation of trypanothione synthetase: a potential drug target for human trypanosomiasis. *J. Biol. Chem.*, **284**, 36137–36145.

74 Spinks, D., Torrie, L.S., Thompson, S., Harrison, J.R., Frearson, J.A., Read, K.D., Fairlamb, A.H., Wyatt, P.G., and Gilbert, I.H. (2012) Design, synthesis and biological evaluation of *Trypanosoma brucei* trypanothione synthetase inhibitors. *Chem. Med. Chem.*, **7**, 95–106.

75 Lantwin, C.B., Schlichting, I., Kabsch, W., Pai, E.F., and Krauth-Siegel, R.L. (1994) The structure of *Trypanosoma cruzi* trypanothione reductase in the oxidized and NADPH reduced state. *Proteins*, **18**, 161–173.

76 Zhang, Y., Bond, C.S., Bailey, S., Cunningham, M.L., Fairlamb, A.H., and Hunter, W.N. (1996) The crystal structure of trypanothione reductase from the human pathogen *Trypanosoma cruzi* at 2.3 A resolution. *Protein Sci.*, **5**, 52–61.

77 Dumas, C., Ouellette, M., Tovar, J., Cunningham, M.L., Fairlamb, A.H., Tamar, S., Olivier, M., and Papadopoulou, B. (1997) Disruption of the trypanothione reductase gene of *Leishmania* decreases its ability to survive oxidative stress in macrophages. *EMBO J.*, **16**, 2590–2598.

78 Tovar, J., Wilkinson, S., Mottram, J.C., and Fairlamb, A.H. (1998) Evidence that trypanothione reductase is an essential enzyme in *Leishmania* by targeted replacement of the tryA gene locus. *Mol. Microbiol.*, **29**, 653–660.

79 Bond, C.S., Zhang, Y., Berriman, M., Cunningham, M.L., Fairlamb, A.H., and

Hunter, W.N. (1999) Crystal structure of *Trypanosoma cruzi* trypanothione reductase in complex with trypanothione, and the structure-based discovery of new natural product inhibitors. *Structure*, **7**, 81–89.

80 Krieger, S., Schwarz, W., Ariyanayagam, M.R., Fairlamb, A.H., Krauth-Siegel, R.L., and Clayton, C. (2000) Trypanosomes lacking trypanothione reductase are avirulent and show increased sensitivity to oxidative stress. *Mol. Microbiol.*, **35**, 542–552.

81 Jones, D.C., Ariza, A., Chow, W.H., Oza, S.L., and Fairlamb, A.H. (2010) Comparative structural, kinetic and inhibitor studies of *Trypanosoma brucei* trypanothione reductase with *T. cruzi*. *Mol. Biochem. Parasitol.*, **169**, 12–19.

82 Patterson, S., Alphey, M.S., Jones, D.C., Shanks, E.J., Street, I.P., Frearson, J.A., Wyatt, P.G., Gilbert, I.H., and Fairlamb, A.H. (2011) Dihydroquinazolines as a novel class of *Trypanosoma brucei* trypanothione reductase inhibitors: discovery, synthesis, and characterization of their binding mode by protein crystallography. *J. Med. Chem.*, **54**, 6514–6530.

83 Baiocco, P., Franceschini, S., Ilari, A., and Colotti, G. (2009) Trypanothione reductase from *Leishmania infantum*: cloning, expression, purification, crystallization and preliminary X-ray data analysis. *Protein Pept. Lett.*, **16**, 196–200.

84 Ortíz, C., Larrieux, N., Medeiros, A., Botti, H., Comini, M., and Buschiazzo, A. (2011) Expression, crystallization and preliminary X-ray crystallographic analysis of glucose-6-phosphate dehydrogenase from the human pathogen *Trypanosoma cruzi* in complex with substrate. *Acta Crystallogr. F*, **67**, 1457–1461.

85 Wilkinson, S.R., Horn, D., Prathalingam, S.R., and Kelly, J.M. (2003) RNA interference identifies two hydroperoxide metabolizing enzymes that are essential to the bloodstream form of the African trypanosome. *J. Biol. Chem.*, **278**, 31640–31646.

86 Comini, M.A., Krauth-Siegel, R.L., and Flohé, L. (2007) Depletion of the

thioredoxin homologue tryparedoxin impairs antioxidative defence in African trypanosomes. *Biochem. J.*, **402**, 43–49.

87 Romao, S., Castro, H., Sousa, C., Carvalho, S., and Tomás, A.M. (2009) The cytosolic tryparedoxin of *Leishmania infantum* is essential for parasite survival. *Int. J. Parasitol.*, **39**, 703–711.

88 Castro, H., Teixeira, F., Romao, S., Santos, M., Cruz, T., Florido, M., Appelberg, R., Oliveira, P., Ferreira-da-Silva, F., and Tomas, A.M. (2011) *Leishmania* mitochondrial peroxiredoxin plays a crucial peroxidase-unrelated role during infection: insight into its novel chaperone activity. *PLoS Pathog.*, **7**, e1002325.

89 Schmidt, A., Clayton, C.E., and Krauth-Siegel, R.L. (2002) Silencing of the thioredoxin gene in *Trypanosoma brucei brucei*. *Mol. Biochem. Parasitol.*, **125**, 207–210.

90 Friemann, R., Schmidt, H., Ramaswamy, S., Forstner, M., Krauth-Siegel, R.L., and Eklund, H. (2003) Structure of thioredoxin from *Trypanosoma brucei brucei*. *FEBS Lett.*, **554**, 301–305.

91 Lin, Y.C., Hsu, J.Y., Chiang, S.C., and Lee, S.T. (2005) Distinct overexpression of cytosolic and mitochondrial tryparedoxin peroxidases results in preferential detoxification of different oxidants in arsenite-resistant *Leishmania amazonensis* with and without DNA amplification. *Mol. Biochem. Parasitol.*, **142**, 66–75.

92 Piñeyro, M.D., Pizarro, J.C., Lema, F., Pritsch, O., Cayota, A., Bentley, G.A., and Robello, C. (2005) Crystal structure of the tryparedoxin peroxidase from the human parasite *Trypanosoma cruzi*. *J. Struct. Biol.*, **150**, 11–22.

93 Piacenza, L., Peluffo, G., Alvarez, M.N., Kelly, J.M., Wilkinson, S.R., and Radi, R. (2008) Peroxiredoxins play a major role in protecting *Trypanosoma cruzi* against macrophage- and endogenously-derived peroxynitrite. *Biochem. J.*, **410**, 359–368.

94 Diechtierow, M. and Krauth-Siegel, R.L. (2011) A tryparedoxin-dependent peroxidase protects African trypanosomes from membrane damage. *Free Radic. Biol. Med.*, **51**, 856–868.

95 Melchers, J., Diechtierow, M., Fehér, K., Sinning, I., Tews, I., Krauth-Siegel, R.L., and Muhle-Goll, C. (2008) Structural basis

for a distinct catalytic mechanism in *Trypanosoma brucei* tryparedoxin peroxidase. *J. Biol. Chem.*, **283**, 30401–30411.

96 Alphey, M.S., König, J., and Fairlamb, A.H. (2008) Structural and mechanistic insights into type II trypanosomatid tryparedoxin-dependent peroxidases. *Biochem. J.*, **414**, 375–381.

97 Patel, S., Hussain, S., Harris, R., Sardiwal, S., Kelly, J.M., Wilkinson, S.R., Driscoll, P.C., and Djordjevic, S. (2010) Structural insights into the catalytic mechanism of *Trypanosoma cruzi* GPXI (glutathione peroxidase-like enzyme I). *Biochem. J.*, **425**, 513–522.

98 Ariza, A., Vickers, T.J., Greig, N., Armour, K.A., Dixon, M.J., Eggleston, I.M., Fairlamb, A.H., and Bond, C.S. (2006) Specificity of the trypanothione-dependent *Leishmania major* glyoxalase I: structure and biochemical comparison with the human enzyme. *Mol. Microbiol.*, **59**, 1239–1248.

99 Wendler, A., Irsch, T., Rabbani, N., Thornalley, P.J., and Krauth-Siegel, R.L. (2009) Glyoxalase II does not support methylglyoxal detoxification but serves as a general trypanothione thioesterase in African trypanosomes. *Mol. Biochem. Parasitol.*, **163**, 19–27.

100 Greig, N., Wyllie, S., Patterson, S., and Fairlamb, A.H. (2009) A comparative study of methylglyoxal metabolism in trypanosomatids. *FEBS J.*, **276**, 376–386.

101 Chauhan, S.C. and Madhubala, R. (2009) Glyoxalase I gene deletion mutants of *Leishmania donovani* exhibit reduced methylglyoxal detoxification. *PLoS ONE*, **4**, e6805.

102 Comini, M.A., Rettig, J., Dirdjaja, N., Hanschmann, E.M., Berndt, C., and Krauth-Siegel, R.L. (2008) Monothiol glutaredoxin-1 is an essential iron–sulfur protein in the mitochondrion of African trypanosomes. *J. Biol. Chem.*, **283**, 27785–27798.

103 Carter, K.C., Sundar, S., Spickett, C., Pereira, O.C., and Mullen, A.B. (2003) The *in vivo* susceptibility of *Leishmania donovani* to sodium stibogluconate is drug specific and can be reversed by inhibiting glutathione biosynthesis. *Antimicrob. Agents Chemother.*, **47**, 1529–1535.

104 Lueder, D.V. and Phillips, M.A. (1996) Characterization of *Trypanosoma brucei* gamma-glutamylcysteine synthetase, an essential enzyme in the biosynthesis of trypanothione (diglutathionylspermidine). *J. Biol. Chem.*, **271**, 17485–17490.

105 Brekken, D.L. and Phillips, M.A. (1998) *Trypanosoma brucei* gamma-glutamylcysteine synthetase. Characterization of the kinetic mechanism and the role of Cys-319 in cystamine inactivation. *J. Biol. Chem.*, **273**, 26317–26322.

106 Ariyanayagam, M.R. and Fairlamb, A.H. (1997) Diamine auxotrophy may be a universal feature of *Trypanosoma cruzi* epimastigotes. *Mol. Biochem. Parasitol.*, **84**, 111–121.

107 Carrillo, C., Canepa, G.E., Algranati, I.D., and Pereira, C.A. (2006) Molecular and functional characterization of a spermidine transporter TcPAT12 from *Trypanosoma cruzi. Biochem. Biophys. Res. Commun.*, **344**, 936–940.

108 Hasne, M.P., Coppens, I., Soysa, R., and Ullman, B. (2010) A high-affinity putrescine-cadaverine transporter from *Trypanosoma cruzi. Mol. Microbiol.*, **76**, 78–91.

109 Hasne, M.P. and Ullman, B. (2005) Identification and characterization of a polyamine permease from the protozoan parasite *Leishmania major. J. Biol. Chem.*, **280**, 15188–15194.

110 Hasne, M.P. and Ullman, B. (2011) Genetic and biochemical analysis of protozoal polyamine transporters. *Methods Mol. Biol.*, **720**, 309–326.

111 Colotti, G. and Ilari, A. (2011) Polyamine metabolism in *Leishmania*: from arginine to trypanothione. *Amino Acids*, **40**, 269–285.

112 Carrillo, C., Cejas, S., González, N.S., and Algranati, I.D. (1999) *Trypanosoma cruzi* epimastigotes lack ornithine decarboxylase but can express a foreign gene encoding this enzyme. *FEBS Lett.*, **454**, 192–196.

113 Carrillo, C., Cejas, S., Huber, A., González, N.S., and Algranati, I.D. (2003) Lack of arginine decarboxylase in

Trypanosoma cruzi epimastigotes. *J. Eukaryot. Microbiol.*, **50**, 312–316.

114 Heby, O., Roberts, S.C., and Ullman, B. (2003) Polyamine biosynthetic enzymes as drug targets in parasitic protozoa. *Biochem. Soc. Trans.*, **31**, 415–419.

115 Müller, S., Coombs, G.H., and Walter, R.D. (2001) Targeting polyamines of parasitic protozoa in chemotherapy. *Trends Parasitol.*, **17**, 242–249.

116 Steglich, C. and Schaeffer, S.W. (2006) The ornithine decarboxylase gene of *Trypanosoma brucei*: evidence for horizontal gene transfer from a vertebrate source. *Infect. Genet. Evol.*, **6**, 205–219.

117 Iten, M., Mett, H., Evans, A., Enyaru, J.C., Brun, R., and Kaminsky, R. (1997) Alterations in ornithine decarboxylase characteristics account for tolerance of *Trypanosoma brucei rhodesiense* to D,L-alpha-difluoromethylornithine. *Antimicrob. Agents Chemother.*, **41**, 1922–1925.

118 Bacchi, C.J., Garofalo, J., Ciminelli, M., Rattendi, D., Goldberg, B., McCann, P.P., and Yarlett, N. (1993) Resistance to DL-alpha-difluoromethylornithine by clinical isolates of *Trypanosoma brucei rhodesiense* – role of *S*-adenosylmethionine. *Biochem. Pharmacol.*, **46**, 471–481.

119 Vincent, I.M., Creek, D., Watson, D.G., Kamleh, M.A., Woods, D.J., Wong, P.E., Burchmore, R.J., and Barrett, M.P. (2010) A molecular mechanism for eflornithine resistance in African trypanosomes. *PLoS Pathog.*, **6**, e1001204.

120 Hanson, S., Adelman, J., and Ullman, B. (1992) Amplification and molecular cloning of the ornithine decarboxylase gene of *Leishmania donovani. J. Biol. Chem.*, **267**, 2350–2359.

121 Persson, L., Jeppsson, A., and Nasizadeh, S. (2003) Turnover of trypanosomal ornithine decarboxylases. *Biochem. Soc. Trans.*, **31**, 411–414.

122 Coons, T., Hanson, S., Bitonti, A.J., McCann, P.P., and Ullman, B. (1990) Alpha-difluoromethylornithine resistance in *Leishmania donovani* is associated with increased ornithine decarboxylase activity. *Mol. Biochem. Parasitol.*, **39**, 77–89.

123 Opperdoes, F.R. and Coombs, G.H. (2007) Metabolism of *Leishmania*: proven and predicted. *Trends Parasitol.*, **23**, 149–158.

124 Bale, S. and Ealick, S.E. (2010) Structural biology of *S*-adenosylmethionine decarboxylase. *Amino Acids*, **38**, 451–460.

125 Algranati, I.D. (2010) Polyamine metabolism in *Trypanosoma cruzi*: studies on the expression and regulation of heterologous genes involved in polyamine biosynthesis. *Amino Acids*, **38**, 645–651.

126 Zhao, S., Wang, B., Yuan, H., and Xiao, D. (2006) Determination of agmatine in biological samples by capillary electro-phoresis with optical fiber light-emitting-diode-induced fluorescence detection. *J. Chromatogr. A*, **1123**, 138–141.

127 Bollinger, J.M.Jr., Kwon, D.S., Huisman, G.W., Kolter, R., and Walsh, C.T. (1995) Glutathionylspermidine metabolism in *Escherichia coli*. Purification, cloning, overproduction, and characterization of a bifunctional glutathionylspermidine synthetase/amidase. *J. Biol. Chem.*, **270**, 14031–14041.

128 Ariyanayagam, M.R., Oza, S.L., Guther, M.L., and Fairlamb, A.H. (2005) Phenotypic analysis of trypanothione synthetase knockdown in the African trypanosome. *Biochem. J.*, **391**, 425–432.

129 Fawaz, M.V., Topper, M.E., and Firestine, S.M. (2011) The ATP-grasp enzymes. *Bioorg. Chem.*, **39**, 185–191.

130 Jockers-Scherubl, M.C., Schirmer, R.H., and Krauth-Siegel, R.L. (1989) Trypanothione reductase from *Trypanosoma cruzi*. Catalytic properties of the enzyme and inhibition studies with trypanocidal compounds. *Eur. J. Biochem.*, **180**, 267–272.

131 Tetaud, E. and Fairlamb, A.H. (1998) Cloning, expression and reconstitution of the trypanothione-dependent peroxidase system of *Crithidia fasciculata*. *Mol. Biochem. Parasitol.*, **96**, 111–123.

132 Castro, H., Romao, S., Gadelha, F.R., and Tomás, A.M. (2008) *Leishmania infantum*: provision of reducing equivalents to the mitochondrial tryparedoxin/tryparedoxin peroxidase system. *Exp. Parasitol.*, **120**, 421–423.

133 Castro, H., Romao, S., Carvalho, S., Teixeira, F., Sousa, C., and Tomás, A.M.

(2010) Mitochondrial redox metabolism in trypanosomatids is independent of tryparedoxin activity. *PLoS ONE*, **5**, e12607.

134 Amssoms, K., Oza, S.L., Ravaschino, E., Yamani, A., Lambeir, A., Rajan, P., Bal, G., Rodriguez, J., Fairlamb, A.H., Augustyns, K., and Haemers, A. (2002) Glutathione-like tripeptides as inhibitors of glutathionylspermidine synthetase. Part 1: substitution of the glycine carboxylic acid group. *Bioorg. Med. Chem. Lett.*, **12**, 2553–2556.

135 Amssoms, K., Oza, S.L., Augustyns, K., Yamani, A., Lambeir, A.M., Bal, G., Van der Veken, P., Fairlamb, A.H., and Haemers, A. (2002) Glutathione-like tripeptides as inhibitors of glutathionylspermidine synthetase. Part 2: substitution of the glycine part. *Bioorg. Med. Chem. Lett.*, **12**, 2703–2705.

136 Ravaschino, E.L., Docampo, R., and Rodriguez, J.B. (2006) Design, synthesis, and biological evaluation of phosphinopeptides against *Trypanosoma cruzi* targeting trypanothione biosynthesis. *J. Med. Chem.*, **49**, 426–435.

137 Koch, O., Jaeger, T., Heller, K., Stuhlmann, F., Flohé, L., and Selzer, P. (2009) What makes the difference? A computational approach to explain varying paulone inhibition activity on trypanopthione synthetse from different species, presented at *10th Drug Design and Development Seminar and COST Action CM0801 Workshop "New Drugs for Neglected Diseases"*, Rauischholzhausen Castle, p. 44.

138 Benítez, D., Charquero, D., and Comini, M.A. (2012) The inhibitory activity of organic compounds against trypanothione synthetase from pathogenic trypanosomatids is specie-specific, presented at *Structural Biology & Medicinal Chemistry WG1/WG3 Meeting COST Action CM0801*, Certosa di Pontignano, Siena, p. 2.

139 Saravanamuthu, A., Vickers, T.J., Bond, C.S., Peterson, M.R., Hunter, W.N., and Fairlamb, A.H. (2004) Two interacting binding sites for quinacrine derivatives in the active site of trypanothione reductase: a template for drug design. *J. Biol. Chem.*, **279**, 29493–29500.

140 Krauth-Siegel, R.L., Bauer, H., and Schirmer, R.H. (2005) Dithiol proteins as guardians of the intracellular redox milieu in parasites: old and new drug targets in trypanosomes and malaria-causing plasmodia. *Angew. Chem. Int. Ed. Engl.*, **44**, 690–715.

141 Spinks, D., Shanks, E.J., Cleghorn, L.A., McElroy, S., Jones, D., James, D., Fairlamb, A.H., Frearson, J.A., Wyatt, P.G., and Gilbert, I.H. (2009) Investigation of trypanothione reductase as a drug target in *Trypanosoma brucei*. *Chem. Med. Chem.*, **4**, 2060–2069.

142 Thomson, L., Denicola, A., and Radi, R. (2003) The trypanothione-thiol system in *Trypanosoma cruzi* as a key antioxidant mechanism against peroxynitrite-mediated cytotoxicity. *Arch. Biochem. Biophys.*, **412**, 55–64.

143 Carnieri, E.G., Moreno, S.N., and Docampo, R. (1993) Trypanothione-dependent peroxide metabolism in *Trypanosoma cruzi* different stages. *Mol. Biochem. Parasitol.*, **61**, 79–86.

144 Krauth-Siegel, R.L. and Lüdemann, H. (1996) Reduction of dehydroascorbate by trypanothione. *Mol. Biochem. Parasitol.*, **80**, 203–208.

145 Schmidt, H. and Krauth-Siegel, R.L. (2003) Functional and physicochemical characterization of the thioredoxin system in *Trypanosoma brucei*. *J. Biol. Chem.*, **278**, 46329–46336.

146 Filser, M., Comini, M.A., Molina-Navarro, M.M., Dirdjaja, N., Herrero, E., and Krauth-Siegel, R.L. (2008) Cloning, functional analysis, and mitochondrial localization of *Trypanosoma brucei* monothiol glutaredoxin-1. *Biol. Chem.*, **389**, 21–32.

147 Awad, S., Henderson, G.B., Cerami, A., and Held, K.D. (1992) Effects of trypanothione on the biological activity of irradiated transforming DNA. *Int. J. Radiat. Biol.*, **62**, 401–407.

148 Fitzgerald, M.P., Madsen, J.M., Coleman, M.C., Teoh, M.L., Westphal, S.G., Spitz, D.R., Radi, R., and Domann, F.E. (2010) Transgenic biosynthesis of trypanothione protects *Escherichia coli* from radiation-induced toxicity. *Radiat. Res.*, **174**, 290–296.

149 Irsch, T. and Krauth-Siegel, R.L. (2004) Glyoxalase II of African trypanosomes is trypanothione-dependent. *J. Biol. Chem.*, **279**, 22209–22217.

150 Vickers, T.J., Greig, N., and Fairlamb, A.H. (2004) A trypanothione-dependent glyoxalase I with a prokaryotic ancestry in *Leishmania major*. *Proc. Natl. Acad. Sci. USA*, **101**, 13186–13191.

151 Bocedi, A., Dawood, K.F., Fabrini, R., Federici, G., Gradoni, L., Pedersen, J.Z., and Ricci, G. (2010) Trypanothione efficiently intercepts nitric oxide as a harmless iron complex in trypanosomatid parasites. *FASEB J.*, **24**, 1035–1042.

152 Martinez-Ruiz, A. and Lamas, S. (2007) Signalling by NO-induced protein *S*-nitrosylation and *S*-glutathionylation: convergences and divergences. *Cardiovasc. Res.*, **75**, 220–228.

153 Alvarez, M.N., Piacenza, L., Irigoín, F., Peluffo, G., and Radi, R. (2004) Macrophage-derived peroxynitrite diffusion and toxicity to *Trypanosoma cruzi*. *Arch. Biochem. Biophys.*, **432**, 222–232.

154 Alvarez, M.N., Peluffo, G., Piacenza, L., and Radi, R. (2011) Intraphagosomal peroxynitrite as a macrophage-derived cytotoxin against internalized *Trypanosoma cruzi*: consequences for oxidative killing and role of microbial peroxiredoxins in infectivity. *J. Biol. Chem.*, **286**, 6627–6640.

155 Keese, M.A., Bose, M., Mulsch, A., Schirmer, R.H., and Becker, K. (1997) Dinitrosyl-dithiol-iron complexes, nitric oxide (NO) carriers *in vivo*, as potent inhibitors of human glutathione reductase and glutathione-S-transferase. *Biochem. Pharmacol.*, **54**, 1307–1313.

156 Taylor, M.C. and Kelly, J.M. (2010) Iron metabolism in trypanosomatids, and its crucial role in infection. *Parasitology*, **137**, 899–917.

157 Manta, B., Fleitas, L., and Comini, M.A. (2012) Iron metabolism in pathogenic trypanosomes, in *Iron Metabolism* (ed. S. Arora), InTech Press, Rijeka, pp. 147–186.

158 Rouhier, N., Couturier, J., Johnson, M.K., and Jacquot, J.P. (2010) Glutaredoxins: roles in iron homeostasis. *Trends Biochem. Sci.*, **35**, 43–52.

159 Greig, N., Wyllie, S., Vickers, T.J., and Fairlamb, A.H. (2006) Trypanothione-dependent glyoxalase I in *Trypanosoma cruzi*. *Biochem. J.*, **400**, 217–223.

160 Padmanabhan, P.K., Mukherjee, A., and Madhubala, R. (2006) Characterization of the gene encoding glyoxalase II from *Leishmania donovani*: a potential target for anti-parasite drug. *Biochem. J.*, **393**, 227–234.

161 Silva, M.S., Barata, L., Ferreira, A.E., Romão, S., Tomás, A.M., Freire, A.P., and Cordeiro, C. (2008) Catalysis and structural properties of *Leishmania infantum* glyoxalase II: trypanothione specificity and phylogeny. *Biochemistry*, **47**, 195–204.

162 Ghoshal, K., Banerjee, A.B., and Ray, S. (1989) Methylglyoxal-catabolizing enzymes of *Leishmania donovani* promastigotes. *Mol. Biochem. Parasitol.*, **35**, 21–29.

163 Sousa Silva, M., Ferreira, A.E., Tomás, A.M., Cordeiro, C., and Ponces Freire, A. (2005) Quantitative assessment of the glyoxalase pathway in *Leishmania infantum* as a therapeutic target by modelling and computer simulation. *FEBS J.*, **272**, 2388–2398.

164 Fairlamb, A.H., Carter, N.S., Cunningham, M., and Smith, K. (1992) Characterisation of melarsen-resistant *Trypanosoma brucei brucei* with respect to cross-resistance to other drugs and trypanothione metabolism. *Mol. Biochem. Parasitol.*, **53**, 213–222.

165 Wyllie, S., Cunningham, M.L., and Fairlamb, A.H. (2004) Dual action of antimonial drugs on thiol redox metabolism in the human pathogen *Leishmania donovani*. *J. Biol. Chem.*, **279**, 39925–39932.

166 Maya, J.D., Bollo, S., Nuñez-Vergara, L.J., Squella, J.A., Repetto, Y., Morello, A., Périé, J., and Chauvière, G. (2003) *Trypanosoma cruzi*: effect and mode of action of nitroimidazole and nitrofuran derivatives. *Biochem. Pharmacol.*, **65**, 999–1006.

167 Maya, J.D., Cassels, B.K., Iturriaga-Vásquez, P., Ferreira, J., Faúndez, M., Galanti, N., Ferreira, A., and Morello, A. (2007) Mode of action of natural and synthetic drugs against *Trypanosoma cruzi* and their interaction with the mammalian host. *Comp. Biochem.Physiol. A Mol. Integr. Physiol.*, **146**, 601–620.

168 Shahi, S.K., Krauth-Siegel, R.L., and Clayton, C.E. (2002) Overexpression of the putative thiol conjugate transporter TbMRPA causes melarsoprol resistance in *Trypanosoma brucei. Mol. Microbiol.*, **43**, 1129–1138.

169 Mäser, P., Lüscher, A., and Kaminsky, R. (2003) Drug transport and drug resistance in African trypanosomes. *Drug Resist. Updat.*, **6**, 281–290.

170 Vickers, T.J. and Fairlamb, A.H. (2004) Trypanothione S-transferase activity in a trypanosomatid ribosomal elongation factor 1B. *J. Biol. Chem.*, **279**, 27246–27256.

171 Vickers, T.J., Wyllie, S., and Fairlamb, A.H. (2004) *Leishmania major* elongation factor 1B complex has trypanothione S-transferase and peroxidase activity. *J. Biol. Chem.*, **279**, 49003–49009.

172 Gitler, C., Mogyoros, M., and Kalef, E. (1994) Labeling of protein vicinal dithiols: role of protein-S_2 to protein-$(SH)_2$ conversion in metabolic regulation and oxidative stress. *Methods Enzymol.*, **233**, 403–415.

173 Kalef, E. and Gitler, C. (1994) Purification of vicinal dithiol-containing proteins by arsenical-based affinity chromatography. *Methods Enzymol.*, **233**, 395–403.

174 Andrade, H.M., Murta, S.M., Chapeaurouge, A., Perales, J., Nirdé, P., and Romanha, A.J. (2008) Proteomic analysis of *Trypanosoma cruzi* resistance to benznidazole. *J. Proteome Res.*, **7**, 2357–2367.

175 Wyllie, S., Vickers, T.J., and Fairlamb, A.H. (2008) Roles of trypanothione S-transferase and tryparedoxin peroxidase in resistance to antimonials. *Antimicrob. Agents Chemother.*, **52**, 1359–1365.

176 Hsu, J.Y., Lin, Y.C., Chiang, S.C., and Lee, S.T. (2008) Divergence of trypanothionedependent tryparedoxin cascade into cytosolic and mitochondrial pathways in arsenite-resistant variants of *Leishmania amazonensis. Mol. Biochem. Parasitol.*, **157**, 193–204.

177 Wyllie, S., Mandal, G., Singh, N., Sundar, S., Fairlamb, A.H., and Chatterjee, M. (2010) Elevated levels of tryparedoxin-peroxidase in antimony unresponsive *Leishmania donovani* field isolates. *Mol. Biochem. Parasitol.*, **173**, 162–164.

178 Cruz, K.K., Fonseca, S.G., Monteiro, M. C., Silva, O.S., Andrade, V.M., Cunha, F. Q., and Romão, P.R. (2008) The influence of glutathione modulators on the course of *Leishmania major* infection in susceptible and resistant mice. *Parasite Immunol.*, **30**, 171–174.

179 Goyeneche-Patino, D.A., Valderrama, L., Walker, J., and Saravia, N.G. (2008) Antimony resistance and trypanothione in experimentally selected and clinical strains of *Leishmania panamensis*. *Antimicrob. Agents Chemother.*, **52**, 4503–4506.

180 Reckenfelderbäumer, N., Lüdemann, H., Schmidt, H., Steverding, D., and Krauth-Siegel, R.L. (2000) Identification and functional characterization of thioredoxin from *Trypanosoma brucei brucei*. *J. Biol. Chem.*, **275**, 7547–7552.

181 Piattoni, C.V., Blancato, V.S., Miglietta, H., Iglesias, A.A., and Guerrero, S.A. (2006) On the occurrence of thioredoxin in *Trypanosoma cruzi*. *Acta Trop.*, **97**, 151–160.

182 Marquez, V.E., Arias, D.G., Piattoni, C.V., Robello, C., Iglesias, A.A., and Guerrero, S.A. (2010) Cloning, expression, and characterization of a dithiol glutaredoxin from *Trypanosoma cruzi*. *Antioxid. Redox Signal.*, **12**, 787–792.

183 Forman, H.J., Maiorino, M., and Ursini, F. (2010) Signaling functions of reactive oxygen species. *Biochemistry*, **49**, 835–842.

184 Melchers, J., Dirdjaja, N., Ruppert, T., and Krauth-Siegel, R.L. (2007) Glutathionylation of trypanosomal thiol redox proteins. *J. Biol. Chem.*, **282**, 8678–8694.

185 Hofmann, B., Budde, H., Bruns, K., Guerrero, S.A., Kalisz, H.M., Menge, U., Montemartini, M., Nogoceke, E., Steinert, P., Wissing, J.B., Flohé, L., and Hecht, H. J. (2001) Structures of tryparedoxins revealing interaction with trypanothione. *Biol. Chem.*, **382**, 459–471.

186 Alphey, M.S., Gabrielsen, M., Micossi, E., Leonard, G.A., McSweeney, S.M., Ravelli, R.B., Tetaud, E., Fairlamb, A.H., Bond, C. S., and Hunter, W.N. (2003) Tryparedoxins from *Crithidia fasciculata* and *Trypanosoma brucei*: photoreduction of the redox disulfide using synchrotron radiation and evidence for a conformational switch implicated in function. *J. Biol. Chem.*, **278**, 25919–25925.

187 Krumme, D., Budde, H., Hecht, H.J., Menge, U., Ohlenschläger, O., Ross, A., Wissing, J., Wray, V., and Flohé, L. (2003) NMR studies of the interaction of tryparedoxin with redox-inactive substrate homologues. *Biochemistry*, **42**, 14720–14728.

188 Schlecker, T., Schmidt, A., Dirdjaja, N., Voncken, F., Clayton, C., and Krauth-Siegel, R.L. (2005) Substrate specificity, localization, and essential role of the glutathione peroxidase-type tryparedoxin peroxidases in *Trypanosoma brucei*. *J. Biol. Chem.*, **280**, 14385–14394.

189 Barr, S.D. and Gedamu, L. (2001) Cloning and characterization of three differentially expressed peroxidoxin genes from *Leishmania chagasi*. Evidence for an enzymatic detoxification of hydroxyl radicals. *J. Biol. Chem.*, **276**, 34279–34287.

190 Piñeyro, M.D., Parodi-Talice, A., Portela, M., Arias, D.G., Guerrero, S.A., and Robello, C. (2011) Molecular characterization and interactome analysis of *Trypanosoma cruzi* tryparedoxin 1. *J. Proteomics*, **74**, 1683–1692.

191 Wilkinson, S.R., Obado, S.O., Mauricio, I. L., and Kelly, J.M. (2002) *Trypanosoma cruzi* expresses a plant-like ascorbate-dependent hemoperoxidase localized to the endoplasmic reticulum. *Proc. Natl. Acad. Sci. USA*, **99**, 13453–13458.

192 Adak, S. and Pal, S. (2012) Ascorbate peroxidase acts as a novel determiner of redox homeostasis in *Leishmania*. *Antioxid. Redox Signal.*, doi: 10.1089/ ars.2012.4745.

193 Irigoín, F., Cibils, L., Comini, M.A., Wilkinson, S.R., Flohé, L., and Radi, R. (2008) Insights into the redox biology of *Trypanosoma cruzi*: trypanothione metabolism and oxidant detoxification. *Free Radic. Biol. Med.*, **45**, 733–742.

194 Wilkinson, S.R. and Kelly, J.M. (2003) The role of glutathione peroxidases in trypanosomatids. *Biol. Chem.*, **384**, 517–525.

195 Wilkinson, S.R., Taylor, M.C., Touitha, S., Mauricio, I.L., Meyer, D.J., and Kelly, J.M. (2002) TcGPXII, a glutathione-dependent *Trypanosoma cruzi* peroxidase with substrate specificity restricted to fatty acid and phospholipid hydroperoxides, is localized to the endoplasmic reticulum. *Biochem. J.*, **364**, 787–794.

196 Lopez, J.A., Carvalho, T.U., de Souza, W., Flohé, L., Guerrero, S.A., Montemartini, M., Kalisz, H.M., Nogoceke, E., Singh, M., Alves, M.J., and Colli, W. (2000) Evidence for a trypanothione-dependent peroxidase system in *Trypanosoma cruzi*. *Free Radic. Biol. Med.*, **28**, 767–772.

197 Flohé, L., Budde, H., Bruns, K., Castro, H., Clos, J., Hofmann, B., Kansal-Kalavar, S., Krumme, D., Menge, U., Plank-Schumacher, K., Sztajer, H., Wissing, J., Wylegalla, C., and Hecht, H.J. (2002) Tryparedoxin peroxidase of *Leishmania donovani*: molecular cloning, heterologous expression, specificity, and catalytic mechanism. *Arch. Biochem. Biophys.*, **397**, 324–335.

198 Hillebrand, H., Schmidt, A., and Krauth-Siegel, R.L. (2003) A second class of peroxidases linked to the trypanothione metabolism. *J. Biol. Chem.*, **278**, 6809–6815.

199 Hofmann, B., Hecht, H.J., and Flohé, L. (2002) Peroxiredoxins. *Biol. Chem.*, **383**, 347–364.

200 Budde, H., Flohé, L., Hecht, H.J., Hofmann, B., Stehr, M., Wissing, J., and Lünsdorf, H. (2003) Kinetics and redox-sensitive oligomerisation reveal negative subunit cooperativity in tryparedoxin peroxidase of *Trypanosoma brucei brucei*. *Biol. Chem.*, **384**, 619–633.

201 Castro, H., Sousa, C., Santos, M., Cordeiro-da-Silva, A., Flohé, L., and Tomás, A.M. (2002) Complementary antioxidant defense by cytoplasmic and mitochondrial peroxiredoxins in *Leishmania infantum*. *Free Radic. Biol. Med.*, **33**, 1552–1562.

202 Barr, S.D. and Gedamu, L. (2003) Role of peroxidoxins in *Leishmania chagasi* survival. Evidence of an enzymatic defense against nitrosative stress. *J. Biol. Chem.*, **278**, 10816–10823.

203 Iyer, J.P., Kaprakkaden, A., Choudhary, M.L., and Shaha, C. (2008) Crucial role of cytosolic tryparedoxin peroxidase in *Leishmania donovani* survival, drug response and virulence. *Mol. Microbiol.*, **68**, 372–391.

204 Sztajer, H., Gamain, B., Aumann, K.D., Slomianny, C., Becker, K., Brigelius-Flohé, R., and Flohé, L. (2001) The putative glutathione peroxidase gene of Plasmodium falciparum codes for a thioredoxin peroxidase. *J. Biol. Chem.*, **276**, 7397–7403.

205 A) Wilkinson, S.R., Meyer, D.J., Taylor, M.C., Bromley, E.V., Miles, M.A., and Kelly, J.M. (2002) The *Trypanosoma cruzi* enzyme TcGPXI is a glycosomal peroxidase and can be linked to trypanothione reduction by glutathione or tryparedoxin. *J. Biol. Chem.*, **277**, 17062–17071.

206 Maiorino, M., Ursini, F., Bosello, V., Toppo, S., Tosatto, S.C., Mauri, P., Becker, K., Roveri, A., Bulato, C., Benazzi, L., De Palma, A., and Flohé, L. (2007) The thioredoxin specificity of *Drosophila* GPx: a paradigm for a peroxiredoxin-like mechanism of many glutathione peroxidases. *J. Mol. Biol.*, **365**, 1033–1046.

207 Schlecker, T., Comini, M.A., Melchers, J., Ruppert, T., and Krauth-Siegel, R.L. (2007) Catalytic mechanism of the glutathione peroxidase-type tryparedoxin peroxidase of *Trypanosoma brucei*. *Biochem. J.*, **405**, 445–454.

208 Flohé, L., Toppo, S., Cozza, G., and Ursini, F. (2011) A comparison of thiol peroxidase mechanisms. *Antioxid. Redox Signal.*, **15**, 763–780.

209 Reichard, P., Baldesten, A., and Rutberg, L. (1961) Formation of deoxycytidine phosphates from cytidine phosphates in extracts from *Escherichia coli*. *J. Biol. Chem.*, **236**, 1150–1157.

210 Holmgren, A. (1985) Thioredoxin. *Annu. Rev. Biochem.*, **54**, 237–271.

211 Nordlund, P. and Reichard, P. (2006) Ribonucleotide reductases. *Annu. Rev. Biochem.*, **75**, 681–706.

212 Krauth-Siegel, R.L. and Schmidt, H. (2002) Trypanothione and tryparedoxin in ribonucleotide reduction. *Methods Enzymol.*, **347**, 259–266.

213 Moskovitz, J. (2005) Methionine sulfoxide reductases: ubiquitous enzymes involved in antioxidant defense, protein regulation, and prevention of aging-associated diseases. *Biochim. Biophys. Acta*, **1703**, 213–219.

214 Trujillo, M., Ferrer-Sueta, G., Thomson, L., Flohé, L., and Radi, R. (2007) Kinetics of peroxiredoxins and their role in the decomposition of peroxynitrite. *Subcell. Biochem.*, **44**, 83–113.

215 Toppo, S., Flohé, L., Ursini, F., Vanin, S., and Maiorino, M. (2009) Catalytic mechanisms and specificities of glutathione peroxidases: variations of a basic scheme. *Biochim. Biophys. Acta*, **1790**, 1486–1500.

216 Brigelius-Flohé, R. and Flohé, L. (2011) Basic principles and emerging concepts in the redox control of transcription factors. *Antioxid. Redox Signal.*, **15**, 2335–2381.

217 Morgan, B.A. and Veal, E.A. (2007) Functions of typical 2-Cys peroxiredoxins in yeast. *Subcell. Biochem.*, **44**, 253–265.

218 Toledano, M.B., Delaunay, A., Monceau, L., and Tacnet, F. (2004) Microbial H_2O_2 sensors as archetypical redox signaling modules. *Trends Biochem. Sci.*, **29**, 351–357.

219 Delaunay, A., Pflieger, D., Barrault, M.B., Vinh, J., and Toledano, M.B. (2002) A thiol peroxidase is an H_2O_2 receptor and redox-transducer in gene activation. *Cell*, **111**, 471–481.

220 Shlomai, J. (2010) Redox control of protein-DNA interactions: from molecular mechanisms to significance in signal transduction, gene expression, and DNA replication. *Antioxid. Redox Signal.*, **13**, 1429–1476.

221 Budde, H., Flohé, L., Hofmann, B., and Nimtz, M. (2003) Verification of the interaction of a tryparedoxin peroxidase with tryparedoxin by ESI-MS/MS. *Biol. Chem.*, **384**, 1305–1309.

222 Wakasugi, N., Tagaya, Y., Wakasugi, H., Mitsui, A., Maeda, M., Yodoi, J., and Tursz, T. (1990) Adult T-cell leukemia-derived factor/thioredoxin, produced by both human T-lymphotropic virus type I- and Epstein–Barr virus-transformed lymphocytes, acts as an autocrine growth factor and synergizes with interleukin 1 and interleukin 2. *Proc. Natl. Acad. Sci. USA*, **87**, 8282–8286.

223 Follmann, H. and Häberlein, I. (1995) Thioredoxins: universal, yet specific thiol-disulfide redox cofactors. *Biofactors*, **5**, 147–156.

224 Alphey, M.S., Leonard, G.A., Gourley, D. G., Tetaud, E., Fairlamb, A.H., and Hunter, W.N. (1999) The high resolution crystal structure of recombinant *Crithidia fasciculata* tryparedoxin-I. *J. Biol. Chem.*, **274**, 25613–25622.

225 Fueller, F., Jehle, B., Putzker, K., Lewis, J.D., and Krauth-Siegel, R.L. (2012) High-throughput screening against the peroxidase cascade of African trypanosomes identifies antiparasitic compounds that inactivate tryparedoxin. *J. Biol. Chem.*, **287**, 8792–8802.

226 Ursini, F., Heim, S., Kiess, M., Maiorino, M., Roveri, A., Wissing, J., and Flohé, L. (1999) Dual function of the selenoprotein PHGPx during sperm maturation. *Science*, **285**, 1393–1396.

227 Pfeifer, H., Conrad, M., Roethlein, D., Kyriakopoulos, A., Brielmeier, M., Bornkamm, G.W., and Behne, D. (2001) Identification of a specific sperm nuclei selenoenzyme necessary for protamine thiol cross-linking during sperm maturation. *FASEB J.*, **15**, 1236–1238.

228 Nguyen, V.D., Saaranen, M.J., Karala, A. R., Lappi, A.K., Wang, L., Raykhel, I.B., Alanen, H.I., Salo, K.E., Wang, C.C., and Ruddock, L.W. (2011) Two endoplasmic reticulum PDI peroxidases increase the efficiency of the use of peroxide during disulfide bond formation. *J. Mol. Biol.*, **406**, 503–515.

229 Rhee, S.G., Chae, H.Z., and Kim, K. (2005) Peroxiredoxins: a historical overview and speculative preview of novel mechanisms and emerging concepts in cell signaling. *Free Radic. Biol. Med.*, **38**, 1543–1552.

230 Flohé, L. and Harris, J.R. (2007) Introduction. *Subcell. Biochem.*, **44**, 1–25.

231 Haraldsen, J.D., Liu, G., Botting, C.H., Walton, J.G., Storm, J., Phalen, T.J., Kwok, L.Y., Soldati-Favre, D., Heintz, N. H., Müller, S., Westwood, N.J., and Ward, G.E. (2009) Identification of conoidin A as a covalent inhibitor of peroxiredoxin II. *Org. Biomol. Chem.*, **7**, 3040–3048.

232 Liu, C.X., Yin, Q.Q., Zhou, H.C., Wu, Y.L., Pu, J.X., Xia, L., Liu, W., Huang, X., Jiang, T., Wu, M.X., He, L.C., Zhao, Y.X., Wang, X.L., Xiao, W.L., Chen, H.Z., Zhao, Q., Zhou, A.W., Wang, L.S., Sun, H.D., and Chen, G.Q. (2012) Adenanthin targets peroxiredoxin I and II to induce differentiation of leukemic cells. *Nat. Chem. Biol.*, **8**486–493.

233 Olin-Sandoval, V., Moreno-Sánchez, R., and Saavedra, E. (2010) Targeting trypanothione metabolism in trypanosomatid human parasites. *Curr. Drug Targets*, **11**, 1614–1630.

10
Thiol Peroxidases of Trypanosomatids

Helena Castro and Ana M. Tomás*

Abstract

Hydroperoxide-reducing enzymes of pathogenic parasites of the family Trypanosomatidae, including *Leishmania* spp., *Trypanosoma cruzi*, and *T. brucei*, are regarded as potential targets for therapeutic intervention owing to their unique and essential character. This chapter reviews the thiol peroxidases of trypanosomatids (i.e., peroxiredoxins and non-selenium glutathione peroxidases), exploring their mechanisms, specificities, and functions.

Thiol-Dependent Peroxidases in Trypanosomatids

Hydroperoxide elimination in trypanosomatids is mainly accomplished by thiol-dependent peroxidases. These are enzymes whose hydroperoxide-reducing activity does not require any cofactor or prosthetic group (such as heme or flavin) and, instead, depends on the reactivity of specific cysteine residues. This group of enzymes comprises members of the peroxiredoxin (PRX) and of the glutathione peroxidase (GPX) families of proteins. The latter also includes selenocysteine GPXs, which, for being absent from trypanosomatids, will not be considered in this chapter. The abbreviation nsGPX will be used here to designate the thiol-dependent, non-selenium GPXs.

Similar to thiol peroxidases of other organisms, trypanosomatid PRXs and nsGPXs reduce a broad spectrum of hydroperoxides (ROOH). PRXs react preferentially with hydrogen peroxide (H_2O_2), organic hydroperoxides [1–7], and peroxynitrite ($ONOO^-$) [6,8], also accepting thymine hydroperoxide as substrate [5]. They react poorly with lipid hydroperoxides and are even susceptible to inactivation by these compounds [1–3,5]. This is not the case of nsGPXs, which readily reduce lipophilic hydroperoxides [4,5,9–11]. Some nsGPXs are also oxidized by H_2O_2, small organic, and thymine hydroperoxides [4,5,9,12]. Rate constants between 10^5 and $10^7 \, M^{-1} s^{-1}$ [1–4,7–9,13] have been reported for the reaction of trypanosomatid PRXs and nsGPXs with their hydroperoxide substrates, which are within the range of values reported for thiol peroxidases of other

---

* Corresponding Author

Trypanosomatid Diseases: Molecular Routes to Drug Discovery, First edition. Edited by T. Jäger, O. Koch, and L. Flohé.
© 2013 Wiley-VCH Verlag GmbH & Co. KGaA. Published 2013 by Wiley-VCH Verlag GmbH & Co. KGaA.

organisms [14]. These reaction rates are considerably high when compared to that of free cysteine with H_2O_2 ($26\,M^{-1}\,s^{-1}$) [15] and result from the active-site architecture of thiol peroxidases [14,16].

Mechanism of Reaction of Thiol Peroxidases

Thiol peroxidases react following an "enzyme substitution mechanism," and trypanosomatid PRXs and nsGPXs are no exception to this rule, as evidenced by their ping-pong kinetics [1,2,4,9,12,13,17,18]. This means that the catalytic steps of the peroxidase reaction are sequential, with the substrates reacting consecutively with the enzyme (Figure 10.1). In the first of these steps, the peroxidatic cysteine in its thiolate form ($-S^-$) reacts with ROOH to yield ROH and sulfenic acid ($-SOH$). This is followed by the formation of a disulfide bond between the oxidized cysteine and a resolving thiol group, with concomitant release of a molecule of water. In nsGPX the peroxidatic and resolving cysteines are within the same enzyme subunit and, when oxidized, form an intramolecular S–S bridge [17,20–22]. This is not the case for trypanosomatid PRXs, wherein each of those cysteine residues sits in adjacent enzyme subunits and the disulfide is thus formed intermolecularly [23,24]. The crucial character of both Cys residues to the catalytic cycle of trypanosomatid PRXs and nsGPXs has been demonstrated by site-directed mutagenesis [1,3,20,25]. Noticeably, in both classes of enzymes, the peroxidatic and the resolving Cys residues are too far away from each other in the three-dimensional structure [3,17,20–24] and formation of the S–S bridge entails the occurrence of a conformational change around the active site of the enzymes [17,23,24]. Irrespective of the intra- or intermolecular nature of the disulfide, this is subsequently attacked by a cysteine thiol from a different protein (the "reducing substrate"), in order to restore the peroxidatic cysteine to its reduced form. A catalytic intermediate, in which the resolving cysteine is covalently bound via an S–S bridge to the cysteine of the reducing substrate, is generated in this step. The reaction cycle is finally completed by a thiol–disulfide exchange, in which the mixed disulfide is resolved by a second thiol group (usually a second Cys residue of the reducing substrate), thus releasing the fully reduced peroxidase and the

Figure 10.1 Schematic representation of the mechanism of action of 2-Cys PRXs and nsGPXs. (1) The peroxidatic cysteine (P) of the thiol peroxidase is oxidized by the hydroperoxide substrate (ROOH) with concomitant generation of the corresponding alcohol (ROH). (2) The oxidized Cys ($-SOH$) is attacked by the resolving thiol group (R) of either a different enzyme subunit (in PRXs) or of the same molecule (in nsGPXs). Formation of the S–S bridge requires a conformational change around the active site of the enzyme to shorten the distance between both Cys residues (P and R). (3) The peroxidase disulfide is attacked by the proximal Cys (Cys 40; *L. infantum* TXN1 numbering [19]) of TXN. (4) A mixed disulfide intermediate is formed, in which Cys40 of TXN is covalently bound to the resolving Cys of the peroxidase. (5) A thiol–disulfide exchange reaction involving the distal redox active Cys of TXN (Cys43) results in the release of the reduced peroxidase and of the oxidized TXN.

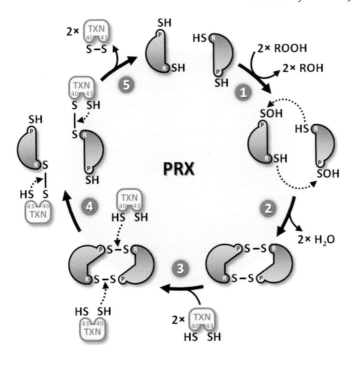

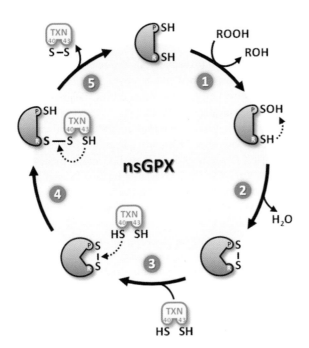

reducing agent in its oxidized (S–S) form. The reducing substrates of thiol peroxidases are typically CxxC-containing oxidoreductases of the thioredoxin family (including thioredoxins and glutaredoxins) or proteins containing thioredoxin-like active sites, such as the bacterial AhpF [14]. In trypanosomatids, however, PRXs and nsGPXs are preferentially reduced by tryparedoxin (TXN) [1–4,9,12,13,17,26], a specific oxidoreductase whose active-site signature reads WCPPCR instead of WC(G/A)PCK found in most thioredoxins. The proximal Cys of TXNs, which is solvent-exposed [27], attacks the disulfide of thiol peroxidases and forms an intermolecular S–S bridge with the latter enzymes [20,25]. Importantly, TXNs carry a network of acidic residues around their redox active site [27], which is absent from thioredoxins. These negatively charged amino acids were suggested to interact with positively charged residues in the vicinity of the PRX active site, thus explaining the preference of the trypanosomatid enzymes for reduction by TXN [24]. Likewise, the redox active site region of nsGPXs lies in a predominantly positively charged region of the proteins [17,21], the highly conserved basic Lys residues sitting 2 and 4 residues downstream from the resolving Cys having been suggested to interact with the TXN substrate [21]. Unlike thioredoxins, which are reduced enzymatically by thioredoxin reductase, TXNs are specifically reduced by the trypanosomatids' unique thiol, trypanothione (N^1,N^8-bis(glutathionyl)spermidine; T(SH)$_2$) [28], a conjugate of glutathione and spermidine that largely replaces glutathione functions in these parasites.

Trypanosomatid PRXs

PRXs were the first enzymes reported to display TXN-dependent peroxidase activity [7] and, for that reason, they were coined the acronym TXNPx. Among the six categories of PRXs found in nature [29], trypanosomatid PRXs fall in the Prx1/AhpC subfamily [30], also known as typical 2-Cys PRXs.

All trypanosomatids harbor one mitochondrial (mTXNPx) and at least one cytosolic (cTXNPx) PRX. Mitochondrial PRXs differ from their cytosolic counterparts in having the resolving Cys embedded in an IPC motif (instead of VCP described for most of the typical 2-Cys PRXs), resembling the LPC signature found in two cytosolic PRX isoenzymes of yeast [31,32]. Also, while mTXNPxs are encoded by single-copy genes, the cytosolic enzymes may include closely related genes clustered within the same chromosomal locus. In some species of *Leishmania*, one of the cytosolic isoforms carries a glycosomal targeting signal (SKL), suggesting that the enzyme localizes to this peroxisome-like organelle as well.

Irrespective of the different attributes of mitochondrial and cytosolic enzymes, they both preserve the structural signature that is common to all PRXs, namely the sulfur group of the peroxidatic cysteine coordinated to the guanidino group of an arginine and the OH of a threonine or, less frequently, of a serine [14]. The threonine is part of the highly conserved motif Pxxx(T/S)xxC of PRXs and the arginine residue is usually located 76 residues downstream the peroxidatic cysteine. The interaction of the peroxidatic cysteine with its surrounding residues within the active site acts in part to lower the pK_a of the thiol group for nucleophilic attack on the peroxyl bond of the hydroperoxide [33], as well as to maintain the proper orientation of the active site for reaction with the hydroperoxide [34]. Moreover, as proposed by Hall *et al.* [35], the organization of the active site helps in stabilizing the transition state of the reaction, in this way contributing to the high efficiency of PRXs as hydroperoxide-reducing enzymes. The relevance of the active-site triad for the activity of trypanosomatid PRXs has been demonstrated by site-directed mutagenesis [1,3,25] and by dissection of the crystal structures of cTXNPxs from *Trypanosoma cruzi* [23] and the related non-pathogenic parasite *Crithidia fasciculata* [24].

One factor that affects the reactivity of PRXs is their oligomeric structure. While in theory the minimal structure required for activity of typical 2-Cys PRXs is the dimer, these proteins can oligomerize into decamers in solution and in crystals [36]. The decameric proteins are built up of five inverted dimers arranged in a ring-like structure, which usually exhibit higher activities than the isolated dimers. Likewise, trypanosomatid PRXs are capable of associating into decamers [1,2,23,24], that, as shown for the *Leishmania infantum* mTXNPx [2], enhances peroxidase activity.

Typical 2-Cys PRXs are prone to overoxidation – a phenomenon that results from reaction of the cysteine sulfenic acid with a second hydroperoxide molecule to yield an inactive sulfinic acid ($-SO_2H$). Inactivation of PRXs by overoxidation has been proposed to act as a mechanism that allows transient accumulation of H_2O_2 and consequently enables this peroxide to mediate cell signaling [34]. Another function suggested for overoxidation was the conversion of PRXs from active peroxidases into highly efficient chaperones [37]. In the case of trypanosomatids, most PRXs conserve the GGLG and the YF motifs that render this family of peroxidases prone to overoxidation [34]. Using an antibody that specifically recognizes overoxidized PRXs, *T. cruzi* TXNPx enzymes were shown to be overoxidized upon treatment with ONOO$^-$ [38]. Moreover, based on the principle that overoxidized PRXs run as monomers in non-reducing sodium dodecylsulfate–polyacrylamide gel electrophoresis, *Leishmania* TXNPxs were also suggested to be prone to over-oxidation [39,40].

Trypanosomatid GPXs

Based on their primary structure, trypanosomatid nsGPXs can be classified as nsGPXAs and nsGPXBs [41]. The former are encoded by a cluster of open reading frames, whereas the latter are single-copy genes. Type B nsGPXs share only 30% identity with nsGPXAs and, unlike these, present amino acid modifications at canonical nsGPX motifs. The only report on trypanosomatid nsGPXBs refers to a *T. cruzi* enzyme [11], which was found to localize to the endoplasmic reticulum and to metabolize fatty acid and phospholipid hydroperoxides. Owing to the limited information on type B nsGPXs, only the well-characterized nsGPXA members will be dealt with below.

Trypanosomatids possess up to three genes arranged in tandem that encode almost identical nsGPXA proteins. In *T. cruzi* one of these isoforms is glycosomal, a small fraction possibly localizing to the cytosol as well [26]. Regarding the other two *T. cruzi* nsGPXA sequences, the absence of any obvious organelle endorsement signal suggests that they are cytosolic, as further confirmed by Wilkinson *et al.* [26]. In both, *T. brucei* and *Leishmania* spp., the nsGPXA molecules differ only in their N- and C-terminal regions, which may either possess or lack signal peptides to glycosomes and/or to the mitochondrion. Some of the predicted proteins carry both peptide endorsement sequences. This is the case of the *T. brucei* nsGPXA3 enzyme, which was verified to be mitochondrial [5,9]. The other two *T. brucei* isoforms (nsGPXA1 and 2) are cytosolic [9].

The amino acid sequences of parasitic nsGPXAs preserve the catalytic tetrad that is common to other GPXs, namely the redox active Cys located in a NVAxxCG environment, the last Gln residue of the FPCNQFGxQ motif (which in trypanosomatids is FPCN(Q/E)F(G/A)xQ), and the Trp and Asn residues of the C-terminal WNF sequence [14]. Noticeably, the nsGPXA1 enzyme of the 427 strain of *T. b. brucei* carries a NVACKAG stretch embedding the peroxidatic Cys [5]. This sequence alteration, which apparently hampers peroxidase activity [5], is also present in the cytosolic nsGPXA1 gene of *T. b. gambiense* (tritrypdb.org/tritrypdb).

In the three-dimensional structure of GPXs the residues of the catalytic tetrad sit close to each other, with Gln, Trp, and Asn acting together to lower the pK_a of the redox active chalcogene. While the Trp has the lowest impact on GPX activity [14,20], the carboxamide groups of Gln and particularly of the Asn appear most important to promote oxidation of the peroxidatic sulfhydryl group, in this way surpassing the need for a positively charged residue in the active site, which in PRXs is provided by the Arg residue of the catalytic of triad. In the case of trypanosomatid nsGPXs, as likely in most invertebrate GPXs, this architecture of the catalytic tetrad is not preserved over the entire catalytic circle. The typical tetrad rather represents the reduced enzyme form optimized for the reaction with a hydroperoxide. Formation of an intramolecular disulfide, which is characteristic of the trypanosomatid nsGPXs and a prerequisite for the reductive part of the catalysis (Figure 10.1), demands a substantial disintegration of the typical active-site architecture [14]. Even though the crystal structure of *Tb*GPXA2 does not disclose any critical alterations of the tetrad [17], nuclear magnetic resonance investigations of reduced *Tb*GPXA3 and *Tc*GPXA1 revealed the peroxidatic Cys to be remotely located from the tetrad residues proposed to participate in its activation [21,22]. These structures resembled those of oxidized nsGPXs in showing the resolving cysteine in the vicinity of the peroxidatic one, thus suggesting an inherent flexibility of these nsGPXs that allows shuttling between the conformations of the reduced and oxidized enzymes irrespective of their redox state [14,22].

Trypanosomatid nsGPXs share highest degree of similarity with plant nsGPXs, which belong to the phospholipid hydroperoxide GPX (PHGPX) clade. Like PHGPXs, trypanosomatid nsGPXs contain deletions [41] in regions that mediate protein oligomerization [42] and that limit substrate accessibility to the active site

[43]. Not surprisingly, trypanosomatid nsGPXs are monomeric [4,12,17,20] and, as mentioned earlier, have a broad specificity for hydroperoxide substrates. The monomeric nature of some GPXs may also be a prerequisite for interaction with thioredoxin and related CxxC-containing proteins [44]. This, added to the fact that the amino acid sequences of these enzymes harbor a thioredoxin recognition site (EPGxxxx(I/V)xx(F/M)(V/A)CT(R/K)FK) [45], likely explains why trypanosomatid nsGPXs are reduced by TXN [4,9,12,17,26] and, albeit less efficiently, by thioredoxin [12]. Such recognition motif is not conserved in type B nsGPXs, possibly accounting for their inability to be reduced by TXN [11]. Glutathione is a poor reductant of trypanosomatid nsGPXs [4,10,12], one possible reason being the absence of typical residues implicated in glutathione binding by mammalian GPXs [41].

Function of Thiol Peroxidases in Trypanosomatids

The existence of an efficient hydroperoxide-reducing apparatus in the cytosol of trypanosomatids is of particular relevance for *Leishmania* spp. and *T. cruzi*, which must invade phagocytic cells in order to establish a successful infection. The contribution of macrophage-derived superoxide anion ($O_2^{\bullet-}$, the precursor of H_2O_2) and of peroxynitrite (resulting from the reaction of $O_2^{\bullet-}$ with $^{\bullet}NO$) in parasite clearance is well documented [46,47] and, not surprisingly, virulence of *Leishmania* spp. and *T. cruzi* was found to be associated with the parasites ability to eliminate hydroperoxides [39,48–51] and $ONOO^-$ [51]. Interestingly, this phenotype was in some studies associated with differential expression of cTXNPxs [39,49–53]. Moreover, genetic studies have shown that overexpression of these enzymes enhances survival of *L. chagasi* and *L. donovani* within macrophages [54,55], and of *T. cruzi* within phagocytic and non-phagocytic cells [56], as well as in an animal model of infection [57]. Proof for cTXNPxs essentiality by reverse genetics was up to now obtained only for *T. brucei* [58]. By employing RNA interference (RNAi), the authors demonstrated that, apart from affecting survival, downregulation of cTXNPxs also impaired the resistance of bloodstream forms of *T. brucei* towards bolus H_2O_2. Despite being overlooked as virulence factors, cytosolic nsGPXs are also crucial for parasite survival, as demonstrated for the nsGPXA2 enzyme of *T. brucei* using a gene targeting approach [5]. This enzyme does not function as a general antioxidant, rather it is implicated in the detoxification of membrane-bound lipid hydroperoxides [5]. An overall indirect proof of the essentiality of both cytosolic TXNPx and nsGPXs was the observation that their reductant (i.e., the cytosolic TXN) is crucial for *T. brucei* and *L. infantum* survival [59,60]. Downregulation of cytosolic TXN decreased the antioxidant capacity of these parasites [59,60] and, in the case of *L. infantum*, reduced infectivity in macrophage monolayers [60]. In short, cytosolic TXNPx and nsGPX activity is essential to trypanosomatids, and both classes of thiol peroxidases play complementary roles in these organisms – the former being implicated in protection against endogenous and exogenously derived H_2O_2 and $ONOO^-$, and the latter in detoxification of lipid hydroperoxides.

Within the mitochondrion, mTXNPx has long been regarded as an important device to eliminate locally generated hydroperoxides [61,62] and ONOO$^-$ [38]. The observation that overexpression of mTXNPx confers protection towards exogenously added and macrophage-derived H$_2$O$_2$ and ONOO$^-$ [38,61–63] has suggested that these enzymes might also contribute to shield trypanosomatids from the oxidative challenge induced by their hosts. Apart from general antioxidant defense, mTXNPx has also been implicated in other oxidoreductase-related functions, namely prevention of H$_2$O$_2$-induced programmed cell death [64] and regulation of kinetoplast DNA replication [65]. Indirect evidence suggesting that mTXNPx is relevant for parasite survival in mammalian hosts came from the observations that the enzyme is downregulated in an attenuated *L. infantum* strain [49] and upregulated in virulent *T. cruzi* strains [51] or upon differentiation into metacyclic, infective forms [66]. Consistent with this assumption, mTXNPx overexpression conferred to *T. cruzi* enhanced capacity to survive in phagocytic and non-phagocytic cells [56]. Unequivocal proof that mTXNPx is essential was provided by a recent report showing that depletion of the enzyme rendered *L. infantum* parasites unable to persist in a murine model of infection [40]. Unexpectedly, however, the avirulent phenotype of these mTXNPx-depleted mutants could be rescued by a peroxidase-inactive version of the enzyme, thus revealing that the crucial role played by this enzyme during infection is unrelated to its oxidoreductase activity. Based on the observation that purified recombinant mTXNPx exhibits an oxidoreductase-independent chaperone-like activity, this was suggested to be the critical function of this enzyme in the mammalian stage of the parasite. In contrast to the data obtained for *L. infantum*, downregulation of the *T. brucei* enzyme by RNAi did not impact on survival of the mammalian stage of the parasite [58]. Also, the other mitochondrial thiol peroxidase, nsGPX, was found to be dispensable for *T. brucei* survival [5]. This observation is not entirely surprising if one takes into consideration that *T. cruzi* and *Leishmania braziliensis* lack an obvious candidate for a mitochondrial nsGPXA (tritrypdb.org/tritrypdb). The findings indicating that the peroxidase function of both mitochondrial enzymes is not essential in trypanosomatids could be explained by a mutual compensation of function. However, the activities of these two classes of thiol peroxidases do not always overlap, as illustrated by the use of lipid hydroperoxides as substrates. These, while being metabolized by the mitochondrial nsGPX both *in vitro* and in the parasite context [5], inhibit mTXNPx peroxidase activity [2]. In summary, none of the mitochondrial thiol peroxidases is crucial as an antioxidant device in these parasites. This is in line with the report of Castro *et al.* [67] showing that also the mitochondrial TXN is a non-essential enzyme in *Leishmania* spp.

PRXs are also involved in the generation of drug resistance. Illustrating this, benznidazole-resistant *T. cruzi* strains and *L. amazonensis* resistant to arsenite revealed an increased expression of cTXNPxs and mTXNPx [63,68–70]. Likewise, the cytosolic enzyme was found to be overexpressed in antimonial-resistant *L. tarentolae* [71] and *L. donovani* [72]. Finally, resistance to some of these drugs could be induced by artificially overexpressing cTXNPxs [55,71]. One possible explanation for implication of TXNPxs in drug resistance is their ability to enhance the cell antioxidant capacity, as corroborated by the observations that (i) these anti-parasitic compounds can directly or indirectly generate reactive oxygen species [68,73–75] and (ii) overexpression of an enzymatically inactive cTXNPx failed to confer antimony resistance [71].

Conclusions

Trypanosomatid hydroperoxide-reducing enzymes are mainly thiol peroxidases of two different classes, PRXs and nsGPXs. These enzymes have long been looked upon as prone to selective inhibition. As reviewed above, some of these enzymes are essential to the parasites, thus fulfilling one of the requisites for a drug target. From a structural and mechanistic point of view, however, trypanosomatid thiol peroxidases are akin of their mammalian homologs, suggesting that successful selective inhibition of these enzymes must exploit their exclusive specificity for TXNs.

References

1 Budde, H., Flohé, L., Hecht, J.H., Hofmann, B., Stehr, M., Wissing, J., and Lünsdorf, H. (2003) Kinetics and redox-sensitive oligomerisation reveal negative subunit cooperativity in tryparedoxin peroxidase of *Trypanosoma brucei brucei*. *Biol. Chem.*, **384**, 619–633.

2 Castro, H., Budde, H., Flohé, L., Hofmann, B., Lünsdorf, H., Wissing, J., and Tomás, A.M. (2002) Specificity and kinetics of a mitochondrial peroxiredoxin of *Leishmania infantum*. *Free Radic. Biol. Med.*, **33**, 1563–1574.

3 Flohé, L., Budde, H., Bruns, K., Castro, H., Clos, J., Hofmann, B., Kansal-Kalavar, S., Krumme, D., Menge, U., Plank-Schumacher, K. *et al.* (2002) Tryparedoxin peroxidase of *Leishmania donovani*: molecular cloning, heterologous expression, specificity, and catalytic mechanism. *Arch. Biochem. Biophys.*, **397**, 324–335.

4 König, J. and Fairlamb, A.H. (2007) A comparative study of type I and type II tryparedoxin peroxidases in *Leishmania major*. *FEBS J.*, **274**, 5643–5658.

5 Diechtierow, M. and Krauth-Siegel, R.L. (2011) A tryparedoxin-dependent peroxidase protects African trypanosomes from membrane damage. *Free Radic. Biol. Med.*, **51**, 856–868.

6 Piñeyro, M.D., Arcari, T., Robello, C., Radi, R., and Trujillo, M. (2011) Tryparedoxin peroxidases from *Trypanosoma cruzi*: high efficiency in the catalytic elimination of hydrogen peroxide and peroxynitrite. *Arch. Biochem. Biophys.*, **507**, 287–295.

7 Nogoceke, E., Gommel, D.U., Kiess, M., Kalisz, H.M., and Flohé, L. (1997) A unique cascade of oxidoreductases catalyses trypanothione-mediated peroxide metabolism in *Crithidia fasciculata*. *Biol. Chem.*, **378**, 827–836.

8 Trujillo, M., Budde, H., Piñeyro, M.D., Stehr, M., Robello, C., Flohé, L., and Radi, R. (2004) *Trypanosoma brucei* and *Trypanosoma cruzi* tryparedoxin peroxidases catalytically detoxify peroxynitrite via oxidation of fast reacting thiols. *J. Biol. Chem.*, **279**, 34175–34182.

9 Schlecker, T., Schmidt, A., Dirdjaja, N., Voncken, F., Clayton, C., and Krauth-Siegel, R.L. (2005) Substrate specificity, localization, and essential role of the glutathione peroxidase-type tryparedoxin peroxidases in *Trypanosoma brucei*. *J. Biol. Chem.*, **280**, 14385–14394.

10 Wilkinson, S.R., Meyer, D.J., and Kelly, J.M. (2000) Biochemical characterization of a trypanosome enzyme with glutathione-dependent peroxidase activity. *Biochem. J.*, **352**, 755–761.

11 Wilkinson, S.R., Taylor, M.C., Touitha, S., Mauricio, I.L., Meyer, D.J., and Kelly, J.M. (2002) TcGPXII, a glutathione-dependent *Trypanosoma cruzi* peroxidase with substrate specificity restricted to fatty acid and phospholipid hydroperoxides, is localized to the endoplasmic reticulum. *Biochem. J.*, **364**, 787–794.

12 Hillebrand, H., Schmidt, A., and Krauth-Siegel, R.L. (2003) A second class of peroxidases linked to the trypanothione metabolism. *J. Biol. Chem.*, **278**, 6809–6815.

13 Guerrero, S.A., Lopez, J.A., Steinert, P., Montemartini, M., Kalisz, H.M., Colli, W., Singh, M., Alves, M.J., and Flohé, L. (2000) His-tagged tryparedoxin peroxidase of *Trypanosoma cruzi* as a tool for drug screening. *Appl. Microbiol. Biotechnol.*, **53**, 410–414.

14 Flohé, L., Toppo, S., Cozza, G., and Ursini, F. (2011) A comparison of thiol peroxidase mechanisms. *Antioxid. Redox Signal.*, **15**, 763–780.

15 Winterbourn, C.C. and Metodiewa, D. (1999) Reactivity of biologically important thiol compounds with superoxide and hydrogen peroxide. *Free Radic. Biol. Med.*, 27, 322–328.

16 Ferrer-Sueta, G., Manta, B., Botti, H., Radi, R., Trujillo, M., and Denicola, A. (2011) Factors affecting protein thiol reactivity and specificity in peroxide reduction. *Chem. Res. Toxicol.*, **24**, 434–450.

17 Alphey, M.S., König, J., and Fairlamb, A.H. (2008) Structural and mechanistic insights into type II trypanosomatid tryparedoxin-dependent peroxidases. *Biochem. J.*, **414**, 375–381.

18 Montemartini, M., Nogoceke, E., Singh, M., Steinert, P., Flohé, L., and Kalisz, H.M. (1998) Sequence analysis of the tryparedoxin peroxidase gene from *Crithidia fasciculata* and its functional expression in *Escherichia coli. J. Biol. Chem.*, **273**, 4864–4871.

19 Castro, H., Sousa, C., Novais, M., Santos, M., Budde, H., Cordeiro-da-Silva, A., Flohé, L., and Tomás, A.M. (2004) Two linked genes of *Leishmania infantum* encode tryparedoxins localised to cytosol and mitochondrion. *Mol. Biochem. Parasitol.*, **136**, 137–147.

20 Schlecker, T., Comini, M.A., Melchers, J., Ruppert, T., and Krauth-Siegel, R.L. (2007) Catalytic mechanism of the glutathione peroxidase-type tryparedoxin peroxidase of *Trypanosoma brucei. Biochem. J.*, **405**, 445–454.

21 Melchers, J., Diechtierow, M., Fehér, K., Sinning, I., Tews, I., Krauth-Siegel, R.L., and Muhle-Goll, C. (2008) Structural basis for a distinct catalytic mechanism in *Trypanosoma brucei* tryparedoxin peroxidase. *J. Biol. Chem.*, **283**, 30401–30411.

22 Patel, S., Hussain, S., Harris, R., Sardiwal, S., Kelly, J.M., Wilkinson, S.R., Driscoll, P. C., and Djordjevic, S. (2010) Structural insights into the catalytic mechanism of *Trypanosoma cruzi* GPXI (glutathione peroxidase-like enzyme I). *Biochem. J.*, **425**, 513–522.

23 Piñeyro, M.D., Pizarro, J.C., Lema, F., Pritsch, O., Cayota, A., Bentley, G.A., and Robello, C. (2005) Crystal structure of the tryparedoxin peroxidase from the human parasite *Trypanosoma cruzi. J. Struct. Biol.*, **150**, 11–22.

24 Alphey, M.S., Bond, C.S., Tetaud, E., Fairlamb, A.H., and Hunter, W.N. (2000) The structure of reduced tryparedoxin peroxidase reveals a decamer and insight into reactivity of 2Cys-peroxiredoxins. *J. Mol. Biol.*, **300**, 903–916.

25 Montemartini, M., Kalisz, H.M., Hecht, H. J., Steinert, P., and Flohé, L. (1999) Activation of active-site cysteine residues in the peroxiredoxin-type tryparedoxin peroxidase of *Crithidia fasciculata. Eur. J. Biochem.*, **264**, 516–524.

26 Wilkinson, S.R., Meyer, D.J., Taylor, M.C., Bromley, E.V., Miles, M.A., and Kelly, J.M. (2002) The *Trypanosoma cruzi* enzyme TcGPXI is a glycosomal peroxidase and can be linked to trypanothione reduction by glutathione or tryparedoxin. *J. Biol. Chem.*, **277**, 17062–17071.

27 Alphey, M.S., Leonard, G.A., Gourley, D. G., Tetaud, E., Fairlamb, A.H., and Hunter, W.N. (1999) The high resolution crystal structure of recombinant *Crithidia fasciculata* tryparedoxin-I. *J. Biol. Chem.*, **274**, 25613–25622.

28 Fairlamb, A.H., Blackburn, P., Ulrich, P., Chait, B.T., and Cerami, A. (1985)

Trypanothione: a novel bis(glutathionyl) spermidine cofactor for glutathione reductase in trypanosomatids. *Science*, **227**, 1485–1487.

29 Soito, L., Williamson, C., Knutson, S.T., Fetrow, J.S., Poole, L.B., and Nelson, K.J. (2011) PREX: PeroxiRedoxin classification indEX, a database of subfamily assignments across the diverse peroxiredoxin family. *Nucleic Acids Res.*, **39**, 332–337.

30 Gretes, M.C., Poole, L.B., and Karplus, P.A. (2012) Peroxiredoxins in parasites. *Antioxid. Redox Signal.*, **17**, 608–633.

31 Chae, H.Z., Kim, I.H., Kim, K., and Rhee, S.G. (1993) Cloning, sequencing, and mutation of thiol-specific antioxidant gene of *Saccharomyces cerevisiae*. *J. Biol. Chem.*, **268**, 16815–16821.

32 Park, S.G., Cha, M.K., Jeong, W., and Kim, I.H. (2000) Distinct physiological functions of thiol peroxidase isoenzymes in *Saccharomyces cerevisiae*. *J. Biol. Chem.*, **275**, 5723–5732.

33 Wood, Z.A., Schröder, E., Harris, R.J., and Poole, L.B. (2003) Structure, mechanism and regulation of peroxiredoxins. *Trends Biochem. Sci.*, **28**, 32–40.

34 Wood, Z.A., Poole, L.B., and Karplus, P.A. (2003) Peroxiredoxin evolution and the regulation of hydrogen peroxide signaling. *Science*, **300**, 650–653.

35 Hall, A., Parsonage, D., Poole, L.B., and Karplus, P.A. (2010) Structural evidence that peroxiredoxin catalytic power is based on transition-state stabilization. *J. Mol. Biol.*, **402**, 194–209.

36 Hall, A., Karplus, P.A., and Poole, L.B. (2009) Typical 2-Cys peroxiredoxins: structures, mechanisms and functions. *FEBS J.*, **276**, 2469–2477.

37 Jang, H.H., Lee, K.O., Chi, Y.H., Jung, B.G., Park, S.K., Park, J.H., Lee, J.R., Lee, S.S., Moon, J.C., Yun, J.W. *et al.* (2004) Two enzymes in one; two yeast peroxiredoxins display oxidative stress-dependent switching from a peroxidase to a molecular chaperone function. *Cell*, **117**, 625–635.

38 Piacenza, L., Peluffo, G., Alvarez, M.N., Kelly, J.M., Wilkinson, S.R., and Radi, R. (2008) Peroxiredoxins play a major role in protecting *Trypanosoma cruzi* against

macrophage- and endogenously-derived peroxynitrite. *Biochem. J.*, **410**, 359–368.

39 Acestor, N., Masina, S., Ives, A., Walker, J., Saravia, N.G., and Fasel, N. (2006) Resistance to oxidative stress is associated with metastasis in mucocutaneous leishmaniasis. *J. Infect. Dis.*, **194**, 1160–1167.

40 Castro, H., Teixeira, F., Romao, S., Santos, M., Cruz, T., Flórido, M., Appelberg, R., Oliveira, P., Ferreira-da-Silva, F., and Tomás, A.M. (2011) *Leishmania* mitochondrial peroxiredoxin plays a crucial peroxidase-unrelated role during infection: insight into its novel chaperone activity. *PLoS Pathog.*, **7**, e1002325.

41 Castro, H. and Tomás, A.M. (2008) Peroxidases of trypanosomatids. *Antioxid. Redox Signal.*, **10**, 1593–1606.

42 Brigelius-Flohé, R., Aumann, K.D., Blöcker, H., Gross, G., Kiess, M., Klöppel, K.D., Maiorino, M., Roveri, A., Schuckelt, R., Ursini, F., Wingender, E., and Flohé, L. (1994) Phospholipid-hydroperoxide glutathione peroxidase. Genomic DNA, cDNA, and deduced amino acid sequence. *J. Biol. Chem.*, **269**, 7342–7348.

43 Scheerer, P., Borchert, A., Krauss, N., Wessner, H., Gerth, C., Höhne, W., and Kuhn, H. (2007) Structural basis for catalytic activity and enzyme polymerization of phospholipid hydroperoxide glutathione peroxidase-4 (GPx4). *Biochemistry*, **46**, 9041–9049.

44 Maiorino, M., Ursini, F., Bosello, V., Toppo, S., Tosatto, S.C., Mauri, P., Becker, K., Roveri, A., Bulato, C., Benazzi, L. *et al.* (2007) The thioredoxin specificity of *Drosophila* GPx: a paradigm for a peroxiredoxin-like mechanism of many glutathione peroxidases. *J. Mol. Biol.*, **365**, 1033–1046.

45 Koh, S.C., Didierjean, C., Navrot, N., Panjikar, S., Mulliert, G., Rouhier, N., Jacquot, J.P., Aubry, A., Shawkataly, O., and Corbier, C. (2007) Crystal structures of a poplar thioredoxin peroxidase that exhibits the structure of glutathione peroxidases: insights into redox-driven conformational changes. *J. Mol. Biol.*, **370**, 512–529.

46 Van Assche, T., Deschacht, M., da Luz, R. A., Maes, L., and Cos, P. (2011) *Leishmania*-macrophage interactions: insights into the

redox biology. *Free Radic. Biol. Med.*, **51**, 337–351.

47 Piacenza, L., Alvarez, M.N., Peluffo, G., and Radi, R. (2009) Fighting the oxidative assault: the *Trypanosoma cruzi* journey to infection. *Curr. Opin. Microbiol.*, **12**, 415–421.

48 Goyal, N., Roy, U., and Rastogi, A.K. (1996) Relative resistance of promastigotes of a virulent and an avirulent strain of *Leishmania donovani* to hydrogen peroxide. *Free Radic. Biol. Med.*, **21**, 683–689.

49 Daneshvar, H., Wyllie, S., Phillips, S., Hagan, P., and Burchmore, R. (2012) Comparative proteomics profiling of a gentamicin-attenuated *Leishmania infantum* cell line identifies key changes in parasite thiol-redox metabolism. *J. Proteomics*, **75**, 1463–1471.

50 Pescher, P., Blisnick, T., Bastin, P., and Spath, G.F. (2011) Quantitative proteome profiling informs on phenotypic traits that adapt *Leishmania donovani* for axenic and intracellular proliferation. *Cell Microbiol.*, **13**, 978–991.

51 Piacenza, L., Zago, M.P., Peluffo, G., Alvarez, M.N., Basombrio, M.A., and Radi, R. (2009) Enzymes of the antioxidant network as novel determiners of *Trypanosoma cruzi* virulence. *Int. J. Parasitol.*, **39**, 1455–1464.

52 Walker, J., Acestor, N., Gongora, R., Quadroni, M., Segura, I., Fasel, N., and Saravia, N.G. (2006) Comparative protein profiling identifies elongation factor-1beta and tryparedoxin peroxidase as factors associated with metastasis in *Leishmania guyanensis*. *Mol. Biochem. Parasitol.*, **145**, 254–264.

53 Parodi-Talice, A., Monteiro-Goes, V., Arrambide, N., Avila, A.R., Duran, R., Correa, A., Dallagiovanna, B., Cayota, A., Krieger, M., Goldenberg, S. *et al.* (2007) Proteomic analysis of metacyclic trypomastigotes undergoing *Trypanosoma cruzi* metacyclogenesis. *J. Mass Spectrom.*, **42**, 1422–1432.

54 Barr, S.D. and Gedamu, L. (2003) Role of peroxidoxins in *Leishmania chagasi* survival. Evidence of an enzymatic defense against nitrosative stress. *J. Biol. Chem.*, **278**, 10816–10823.

55 Iyer, J.P., Kaprakkaden, A., Choudhary, M. L., and Shaha, C. (2008) Crucial role of cytosolic tryparedoxin peroxidase in *Leishmania donovani* survival, drug response and virulence. *Mol. Microbiol.*, **68**, 372–391.

56 Piñeyro, M.D., Parodi-Talice, A., Arcari, T., and Robello, C. (2008) Peroxiredoxins from *Trypanosoma cruzi*: virulence factors and drug targets for treatment of Chagas disease? *Gene*, **408**, 45–50.

57 Alvarez, M.N., Peluffo, G., Piacenza, L., and Radi, R. (2011) Intraphagosomal peroxynitrite as a macrophage-derived cytotoxin against internalized *Trypanosoma cruzi*: consequences for oxidative killing and role of microbial peroxiredoxins in infectivity. *J. Biol. Chem.*, **286**, 6627–6640.

58 Wilkinson, S.R., Horn, D., Prathalingam, S.R., and Kelly, J.M. (2003) RNA interference identifies two hydroperoxide metabolizing enzymes that are essential to the bloodstream form of the African trypanosome. *J. Biol. Chem.*, **278**, 31640–31646.

59 Comini, M.A., Krauth-Siegel, R.L., and Flohé, L. (2007) Depletion of the thioredoxin homologue tryparedoxin impairs antioxidative defence in African trypanosomes. *Biochem. J.*, **402**, 43–49.

60 Romao, S., Castro, H., Sousa, C., Carvalho, S., and Tomás, A.M. (2009) The cytosolic tryparedoxin of *Leishmania infantum* is essential for parasite survival. *Int. J. Parasitol.*, **39**, 703–711.

61 Castro, H., Sousa, C., Santos, M., Cordeiro-da-Silva, A., Flohé, L., and Tomás, A.M. (2002) Complementary antioxidant defense by cytoplasmic and mitochondrial peroxiredoxins in *Leishmania infantum*. *Free Radic. Biol. Med.*, **33**, 1552–1562.

62 Wilkinson, S.R., Temperton, N.J., Mondragon, A., and Kelly, J.M. (2000) Distinct mitochondrial and cytosolic enzymes mediate trypanothione-dependent peroxide metabolism in *Trypanosoma cruzi*. *J. Biol. Chem.*, **275**, 8220–8225.

63 Lin, Y.C., Hsu, J.Y., Chiang, S.C., and Lee, S.T. (2005) Distinct overexpression of cytosolic and mitochondrial tryparedoxin peroxidases results in preferential detoxification of different oxidants in

arsenite-resistant *Leishmania amazonensis* with and without DNA amplification. *Mol. Biochem. Parasitol.*, **142**, 66–75.

64 Harder, S., Bente, M., Isermann, K., and Bruchhaus, I. (2006) Expression of a mitochondrial peroxiredoxin prevents programmed cell death in *Leishmania donovani*. *Eukaryot. Cell*, **5**, 861–870.

65 Sela, D., Yaffe, N., and Shlomai, J. (2008) Enzymatic mechanism controls redox-mediated protein–DNA interactions at the replication origin of kinetoplast DNA minicircles. *J. Biol. Chem.*, **283**, 32034–32044.

66 Atwood, J.A.III, Weatherly, D.B., Minning, T.A., Bundy, B., Cavola, C., Opperdoes, F. R., Orlando, R., and Tarleton, R.L. (2005) The *Trypanosoma cruzi* proteome. *Science*, **309**, 473–476.

67 Castro, H., Romao, S., Carvalho, S., Teixeira, F., Sousa, C., and Tomás, A.M. (2010) Mitochondrial redox metabolism in trypanosomatids is independent of tryparedoxin activity. *PLoS ONE*, **5**, e12607.

68 Hsu, J.Y., Lin, Y.C., Chiang, S.C., and Lee, S.T. (2008) Divergence of trypanothione-dependent tryparedoxin cascade into cytosolic and mitochondrial pathways in arsenite-resistant variants of *Leishmania amazonensis*. *Mol. Biochem. Parasitol.*, **157**, 193–204.

69 Andrade, H.M., Murta, S.M., Chapeaurouge, A., Perales, J., Nirde, P., and Romanha, A.J. (2008) Proteomic analysis of *Trypanosoma cruzi* resistance to benznidazole. *J. Proteome. Res.*, **7**, 2357–2367.

70 Nogueira, F.B., Ruiz, J.C., Robello, C., Romanha, A.J., and Murta, S.M. (2009) Molecular characterization of cytosolic and mitochondrial tryparedoxin peroxidase in *Trypanosoma cruzi* populations susceptible and resistant to benznidazole. *Parasitol. Res.*, **104**, 835–844.

71 Wyllie, S., Vickers, T.J., and Fairlamb, A.H. (2008) Roles of trypanothione S-transferase and tryparedoxin peroxidase in resistance to antimonials. *Antimicrob. Agents Chemother.*, **52**, 1359–1365.

72 Wyllie, S., Mandal, G., Singh, N., Sundar, S., Fairlamb, A.H., and Chatterjee, M. (2010) Elevated levels of tryparedoxin peroxidase in antimony unresponsive *Leishmania donovani* field isolates. *Mol. Biochem. Parasitol.*, **173**, 162–164.

73 Mandal, G., Wyllie, S., Singh, N., Sundar, S., Fairlamb, A.H., and Chatterjee, M. (2007) Increased levels of thiols protect antimony unresponsive *Leishmania donovani* field isolates against reactive oxygen species generated by trivalent antimony. *Parasitology*, **134**, 1679–1687.

74 Wyllie, S., Cunningham, M.L., and Fairlamb, A.H. (2004) Dual action of antimonial drugs on thiol redox metabolism in the human pathogen *Leishmania donovani*. *J. Biol. Chem.*, **279**, 39925–39932.

75 Prathalingham, S.R., Wilkinson, S.R., Horn, D., and Kelly, J.M. (2007) Deletion of the *Trypanosoma brucei* superoxide dismutase gene sodb1 increases sensitivity to nifurtimox and benznidazole. *Antimicrob. Agents Chemother.*, **51**, 755–758.

11

Peroxynitrite as a Cytotoxic Effector Against *Trypanosoma cruzi*: Oxidative Killing and Antioxidant Resistance Mechanisms

Madia Trujillo, María Noel Alvarez, Lucía Piacenza, Martín Hugo, Gonzalo Peluffo, and Rafael Radi*

Abstract

Inside the phagosomes of activated macrophages, *Trypanosoma cruzi* is exposed to reactive oxygen species formed by NADPH oxidase, namely the superoxide radical ($O_2^{\bullet-}$) and, through its dismutation, hydrogen peroxide. Moreover, induction of nitric oxide synthase by pro-inflammatory cytokines leads to the production of nitric oxide ($^{\bullet}NO$). Neither $O_2^{\bullet-}$ nor $^{\bullet}NO$ are particularly cytotoxic *per se*, and most of their parasiticidal actions rely on their diffusion-controlled reaction to form peroxynitrite – a potent oxidizing and nitrating species with a higher killing capability towards microorganisms. Thus, the antioxidant mechanisms that allow the parasite to detoxify peroxynitrite and other cytotoxic peroxides constitute an active field of investigation, since they can provide clues for a rationalized drug design. Moreover, although most research has focused on the formation of reactive species and their detoxification during acute infections, Chagas is mostly a chronic disease and no drug is currently available for its treatment at this stage, where the microorganism infects cardiac muscle and other non-phagocytic cells. The role of peroxynitrite in *T. cruzi* infectivity and virulence at the chronic stage of the disease remains to be established.

Introduction

Trypanosoma cruzi is an intracellular parasite that causes Chagas disease, also known as American trypanosomiasis, endemic in 21 Latin American countries, where millions of persons are infected and thousands of people die each year of this illness (http://www.who.int/mediacentre/factsheets/fs340/en/index.html). Macrophage infection plays a key role during the acute phase of the disease. Inside the phagosomes of activated macrophages, the parasites are exposed to reactive oxygen species formed by NADPH oxidase [1,2], namely the superoxide radical ($O_2^{\bullet-}$) and, through its dismutation, hydrogen peroxide (H_2O_2) [3]. Moreover, induction of inducible nitric oxide synthase (iNOS) by pro-inflammatory cytokines leads to the

---

* Corresponding Author

Trypanosomatid Diseases: Molecular Routes to Drug Discovery, First edition. Edited by T. Jäger, O. Koch, and L. Flohé.
© 2013 Wiley-VCH Verlag GmbH & Co. KGaA. Published 2013 by Wiley-VCH Verlag GmbH & Co. KGaA.

production of nitric oxide ($^•$NO) [4–6]. Neither $O_2^{•-}$ nor $^•$NO are particularly cytotoxic, and most of their parasiticidal actions rely on their fast reaction to form peroxynitrite – an oxidizing and nitrating species with a higher capability to kill microorganisms [7–9] (IUPAC recommended names for peroxynitrite anion (ONOO$^-$) and its conjugated acid, peroxynitrous acid (ONOOH), are oxoperoxonitrate (1−) and hydrogen oxoperoxonitrate, respectively. The term peroxynitrite is used to refer to the sum of ONOO$^-$ and ONOOH). Thus, the antioxidant mechanisms that allow the parasite to detoxify peroxynitrite and other cytotoxic peroxides are intensively explored, since they could provide clues for new therapeutic approaches. Moreover, although most research has focused on the formation of reactive species and their detoxification during acute infections, Chagas is mostly a chronic disease and no drug is currently available for its treatment at this stage, where the microorganism infects cardiac muscle and other non-phagocytic cells [10–13]. The roles of reactive oxygen and nitrogen species, in particular peroxynitrite, in *T. cruzi* killing and the antioxidant enzymatic mechanisms that allow parasite survival during chronic infections are only starting to be unraveled.

Peroxynitrite Formation During *T. cruzi*–Mammalian Host Cell Interaction

Once in the mammalian host, metacyclic trypomastigotes infect and replicate intracellularly in different types of cells, macrophages being one of the most important. Phagocytic cells, such as macrophages, have an active role in microbial killing, linking innate and adaptive immune responses. Several molecules on the host cell surface have been described to interact with *T. cruzi*, such as mannose and Toll-like receptors (TLRs) [14,15]. Specifically, TLR2 and TLR4 have been involved in the recognition of *T. cruzi* [16,17], which interact through molecules presents in the trypomastigote membrane. Parasite recognition leads to an upregulation of antimicrobial activity, with the production of pro-inflammatory cytokines and a positive regulation of macrophage oxidative response [18,19].

TLR-mediated phagocytosis is usually accompanied by a "respiratory burst," accomplished by NOX2, a specialized NADPH oxidase enzymatic complex. NOX2 consists of the membrane-bound flavocytochrome *b* gp91^{phox}, which transfers electrons from a cytosolic NADPH to oxygen in the phagocytic vacuole to produce large quantities of $O_2^{•-}$ when activated. Other components of the complex include membrane-bound p22^{phox}, cytosolic proteins p40^{phox}, p47^{phox}, and p67^{phox}, and the small GTPases Rac1 and Rap1; all are translocated to the membrane in a tightly regulated way [20–22]. Some pathogens, among which are some unicellular parasites, manage to evade NOX2 activation in order to survive in the phagosome and efficiently infect the host. It has been debated whether the invasion process of *T. cruzi* activates NOX2 [23–25]. Results from our group and others have shown the formation of $O_2^{•-}$ during *T. cruzi* invasion, which occurs on the luminal side of the phagosome and lasts for around 60–90 min; the magnitude of the respiratory burst is comparable with that elicited by other phagocytic stimuli [26,27].

In the early stage of *T. cruzi* infection, natural killer and helper T (T_h) cells become active when they are presented to peptide antigens exposed on the surface of antigen-presenting cells. Once activated, they secrete cytokines that regulate or assist in the active immune response. Macrophages exposed to TLR agonists and T_h1 cytokines (i.e., interferon (IFN)-γ, tumor necrosis factor (TNF)-α, namely "classically activated macrophages," show alterations in phagocyte physiology with induction of nitric oxide synthase 2 expression, responsible for the prolonged production of large amounts of $^\bullet$NO [4,5] and an enhanced respiratory burst [28,29]. Microbial killing in activated macrophages relies more heavily on the production of reactive oxygen and nitrogen intermediates [30–35]. Under pro-inflammatory conditions, maximal and simultaneous production of $O_2^{\bullet-}$ and $^\bullet$NO will occur. NADPH oxidase assembly in the phagosome membrane results in the formation of $O_2^{\bullet-}$ inside the vacuole, whereas $^\bullet$NO, a hydrophobic radical, diffuses from the cytosol. Inside the phagosome, the diffusion-controlled reaction between $^\bullet$NO and $O_2^{\bullet-}$ yields peroxynitrite, a strong one- and two-electron oxidant, and a precursor of secondary species, which can also lead to one-electron oxidation and nitration reactions, as we will see below [36].

Immunostimulated macrophages are involved in early parasite killing. Many years ago, several investigators demonstrated that the ability of *T. cruzi* to infect and multiply inside mouse macrophages *in vitro* was inhibited by macrophage activation [37–39]. Thereafter, it was suggested that the ability to produce and release H_2O_2 by activated macrophages was related to an enhanced capacity to kill intracellular trypomastigotes [25,40]. Other investigators showed the importance of $^\bullet$NO in infection control [41–44]. In addition, *in vitro* experiments revealed that bolus peroxynitrite addition is effective in compromising *T. cruzi* viability [45]. Moreover, coculture of the non-infective epimastigote form with resting and activated macrophages shows that under conditions of macrophage-derived peroxynitrite formation in the extracellular space, the oxidant was capable of diffusing to parasites causing intracellular probe oxidation and strongly inhibiting *T. cruzi* survival (around 50%) [46].

Macrophage infection studies with *T. cruzi* trypomastigotes were performed to evaluate the role of peroxynitrite during parasite internalization. Experiments using oxidation of 2,7-dichlorodihydrofluorescein diacetate ($DCFH_2$) as a probe for peroxynitrite formation indicated that the oxidant was indeed formed by immunostimulated macrophages (forming simultaneously $O_2^{\bullet-}$ and $^\bullet$NO), but not by naive macrophages (which produce only $O_2^{\bullet-}$) (Figure 11.1a). The amount of peroxynitrite inside the phagosome was sufficient to damage and kill trypomastigotes as evidenced by protein nitroxidative modifications detected in internalized parasites, 60% less amastigote load into macrophages after 24 h, and ultrastructural alterations in parasites visualized in electron microscopy studies (Figure 11.1b). Notably, overexpression of an enzyme with peroxidase and peroxynitrite reductase activity (cytosolic tryparedoxin peroxidase (cTXNPx), see below) significantly diminished cytotoxicity [27]. The progression of Chagas disease to the chronic phase depends on parasite persistence in tissues and on the host immune responses [47,48]. Some parasites can evade the initial assault of the immune system and infect

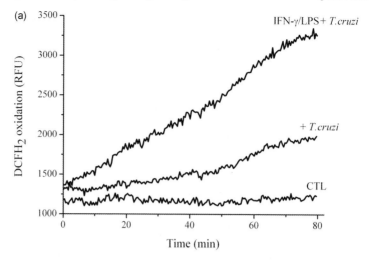

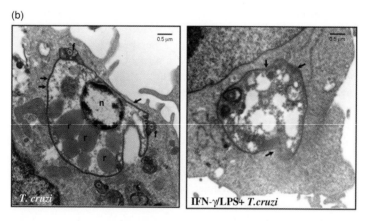

Figure 11.1 Peroxynitrite formation in immunostimulated-infected macrophages: ultrastructural consequences for *T. cruzi* inside the phagosome. (a) Detection of peroxynitrite formed during macrophage infection by *T. cruzi* trypomastigotes. Unstimulated (*T. cruzi*) and immunostimulated (IFN-γ/LPS + *T. cruzi*) macrophages were infected with trypomastigotes (5: 1 parasite/macrophage ratio) in the presence of 30 μM DCFH$_2$. The time course of DCFH$_2$ oxidation was followed in a fluorescence plate reader with filters at $\lambda_{exc} = 485$ nm and $\lambda_{em} = 520$ nm, at pH 7.4 and 37 °C. Control (CTL): uninfected macrophages. (b) Peroxynitrite exposure of phagocytosed *T. cruzi* results in ultrastructural alterations as evidenced by transmission electron microscopy. Micrographs shown unstimulated (*T. cruzi*) and activated (*T. cruzi* + IFN-γ/LPS) infected macrophages at 1 h postinfection; peroxynitrite-producing activated macrophages showed marked damage of *T. cruzi* organelles and membrane disorganization and disappearance. Arrows show normal membrane microtubular structures in phagocytosed trypomastigotes by resting macrophages and reductions of membrane microtubules inside peroxynitrite-producing macrophages. n, *T. cruzi* nucleus; f, flagellum; r, reservosomes.

non-phagocytic cells in organs such as the heart and the digestive tract. Indeed, chagasic cardiomyopathy is characterized by the presence of amastigote nests in the cardiac fiber [49]. *T. cruzi* invasion to cardiomyocytes triggers the production of inflammatory mediators (TNF-α, interleukin (IL)-1β) and the induction of iNOS within the cells [50,51]. They can also be exposed to •NO diffusing from inflammatory cells. Experiments using knockout mice for IFN-γ, IL-12, and NOS isoforms clearly demonstrated a key role of the IL-12/IFN-γ/iNOS axis in the control of *T. cruzi* infection and for the outcome in the disease [52,53]. Moreover, cardiomyocytes and other non-phagocytic cells possess sources of $O_2^{\bullet-}$ such as the mitochondrial electron transport chain or uncoupled nitric oxide synthases [54,55]. The superoxide radical could also be formed inside the parasite from its own electron transport chain or other metabolic processes as well as by redox cycling of anti-chagasic drugs [56–58]. It is therefore tempting to speculate that peroxynitrite could be formed also in infected non-phagocytic cells or even inside the parasite and that it could be implicated in the control of the infection. Host-nitrated proteins have been identified in heart lesions in a mouse model of Chagas disease [59,60]. However, formation of peroxynitrite within or reaching the parasite from external sources and its possible role in controlling proliferation during the chronic stage of the disease is still to be demonstrated.

Peroxynitrite Diffusion and Reactivity with *T. cruzi* Targets

Peroxynitrous acid has a pK_a of 6.5–6.8 [61–63] and therefore the anionic form is more abundant than its conjugated acid at physiological pH. Homolysis of the peroxo bond ($k = 0.9\,s^{-1}$, pH 7.4, 37 °C) makes peroxynitrous acid decay, giving rise to hydroxyl (•OH) and nitrogen dioxide (•NO_2) radicals at approximately 30% yields [64,65]. Both radicals may participate in secondary, indirect reactions, resulting in the oxidation, hydroxylation, or nitration of different targets. In biological systems, however, most peroxynitrite will react directly with different biomolecules before decomposing. Low-molecular-weight and protein thiols, metal centers, and carbon dioxide (CO_2) constitute the main targets for peroxynitrite *in vivo* (for a recent review, see [66]). The direct reaction with thiols involves a two-electron oxidation of the deprotonated form of the thiol by peroxynitrous acid, yielding nitrite and a sulfenic acid intermediate that, in the presence of another accessible thiol group, results in disulfide formation [67,68]. In the case of metal centers, such as those in heme proteins or other metal-containing proteins, mechanisms of reaction with peroxynitrite include one- and two-electron oxidations as well as metal-catalyzed isomerization to nitrate [69–73]. Metal oxidation may result in the formation of strong oxidative species such as compound 1 or 2 of heme peroxidases or other oxo-metal complexes, which may participate in nitro-oxidative target modifications [74]. Moreover, the peroxynitrite anion reacts with CO_2 ($k = 4.6 \times 10^4\,M^{-1}\,s^{-1}$, pH 7.4, 37 °C) forming a transient intermediate that homolyzes to •NO_2 and carbonate radical ($CO_3^{\bullet-}$) in around 35% yields [75–77]; radicals that in turn can participate in indirect oxidation and/or nitration reactions [74].

The main low-molecular-weight thiol in trypanosomatids, trypanothione (the term trypanothione $(T(SH)_2)$ is used for bis(glutathionyl) spermidine and its disulfide is defined as trypanothione disulfide (TS_2) [78]) is oxidized by peroxynitrite with a rate constant of $7200 \, M^{-1} s^{-1}$, pH 7.4, 37 °C [79,80], as expected for a low-molecular-weight dithiol with a pK_a of 7.4 [81,82]. It also reacts with different thiol-containing proteins of the parasite, including the fast-reacting peroxidatic thiols in peroxiredoxins (Prxs) [83] (see below), and with metal-containing proteins such as ascorbate peroxidase and iron-dependent superoxide dismutases (SODs) A and B (Hugo *et al.*, unpublished and Martinez *et al.*, unpublished results). Exposition to peroxynitrite also leads to the nitration of parasite proteins, which is higher when intracellular thiol content decrease [84]. It must be taken into account that, at least during acute infections, most peroxynitrite is formed outside the parasite, inside the phagosome of activated macrophages, and that it must diffuse to and through the parasite plasma membrane to reach intracellular targets and exert its cytotoxic actions. While peroxynitrous acid can passively diffuse through membranes, the anionic species requires the presence of a 4,4'-diisothiocyanodihydrostilbene-2,2'-disulfonic acid (H_2DIDS)-sensitive Cl^-/HCO_3^- exchanger (the presence of a H_2DIDS-sensitive Cl^- channel that contributes to pH homeostasis has been described in *Leishmania major* promastigotes [78]; the Cl^-/HCO_3^- exchanger was also reported to be expressed in different *T. cruzi* stages [85]) [86,87]. Our group has demonstrated that even in the presence of physiological concentrations of CO_2, the diffusion process outcompetes the decay by extracellular reaction with CO_2 if diffusion distances are less than 5 μm [46]. That is particularly so in the case of the intraphagosomal actions of peroxynitrite as diffusion distances are less than 0.1 μm (Figure 11.1b) [27]. Once inside the parasite, the main target for direct peroxynitrite reactivity will be dictated by the rate constants of reactions times target concentrations. Due to the limited capability of diffusion of peroxynitrite anion, and its rapid consumption by intracellular targets, compartmentalization should also be taken into account. Using available data, mostly related to thiols in the parasite, the fractional amount of peroxynitrite that would react with different targets can be estimated. Concerning the cytosol of *T. cruzi* epimastigotes, if only the thiol-containing compounds GSH (the reactivity of peroxynitrite with other relatively abundant low-molecular-weight thiols such as glutathionyl spermidine and ovothiol A has not been investigated so far), $T(SH)_2$, cytosolic tryparedoxin (TXN) I and cTXNPx are considered, and in spite of a much higher rate constant for the reaction with cTXNPx, an important fraction of peroxynitrite is expected to react also with the low-molecular-weight thiols, mostly $T(SH)_2$, due to their much higher concentration. In the presence of physiological concentrations of CO_2, most peroxynitrite is expected to react with it to form $CO_3^{\bullet-}$ and $^\bullet NO_2$, resulting in one-electron oxidation and nitration reactions (Table 11.1). The mitochondria of the parasite can also be exposed to peroxynitrite, either formed endogenously, from the reaction between the diffusible $^\bullet NO$ and respiratory chain-derived $O_2^{\bullet-}$, or diffusing from external sources. The reported mTXNPx concentration inside epimastigote whole homogenates is 1.35 μM, which taking into account that the single mitochondrion occupies 12% of the cell volume in normal epimastigotes [97] would translate into a

Table 11.1 Comparing the reactivity of peroxynitrite with thiol-containing cytosolic targets in *T. cruzi*.

	T(SH)$_2$	GSH	cTXNPx epimastigotes/trypomastigotes	TXNI	CO$_2$
$k^{a)}$ (M^{-1} s^{-1})	7200	1350	$1.5 \pm 0.5 \times 10^6$	3500	4.6×10^4
Concentration (µM)	1100$^{b)}$	700$^{b)}$	5.6$^{c)}$/33.6$^{d)}$	300–500$^{e)}$	1300
$k \times C$ (s^{-1})	7,9	0.95	8.4/50.4	$\sim 10^{-3}$	60

a) pH-dependent rate constants measured at pH 7.4. Note, since normal acidification of the phagosomes is not inhibited by the parasite, the pH of phagosomes harboring *T. cruzi* is acidic, with values in the 5–7 range [88,89] Nevertheless, amastigotes, and trypomastigotes are able to maintain a near-neutral pH over a wide range of external pHs by mechanisms that depend on plasma membrane H$^+$-ATPase [90].

b) Epimastigotes of *T. cruzi* (Silvio strain and Y strain) in the presence of 100 µM putrescine, late logarithmic phase. The concentration of free GSH increases and that of T(SH)$_2$ decreases when epimastigotes are cultured in polyamine-free media [91]. It is also lower in trypomastigotes than in epimastigotes, in Y, and some other strains [92,93].

c) Epimastigotes of *T. cruzi* Dm28-c and Y strain [94]. A value of 2.8 µM was reported for cTXNPx using whole homogenates without taking into account compartmentalization, so we can safely assume that in the cytosol of the parasite the concentration of the enzyme will be at least twice as high.

d) The concentration of cTXNPx was reported to increase (around 6-fold) in trypomastigotes of *T. cruzi* Y strain [95].

e) Estimated from a report indicating that TXNI constitutes around 3% of the total soluble protein content within epimastigotes, late logarithmic phase of growth [96]. Reactivity with CO$_2$ is also shown for comparative purposes.

mitochondrial concentration of 11.3 µM. Thus, the product of reactivity with peroxynitrite (1.8×10^7 M^{-1} s^{-1}, pH 7.4 [83]) times enzyme concentration in the mitochondrion of epimastigotes will be around 20 s^{-1}. The cellular distribution of trypanothione in *T. cruzi* has not been investigated so far, precluding comparisons with low-molecular-weight thiol-mediated peroxynitrite consumption inside the mitochondria. Kinetic considerations indicate that CO$_2$ constitutes a major target for peroxynitrite reactivity also in this compartment. The scenario changes in the infective forms of the parasite (Table 11.1), since during metacyclogenesis the amount of GSH and T(SH)$_2$ decreases [92,93,98], and the expression of both cytosolic and mitochondrial TXNPxs increases in different parasite strains (around 6- and 2-fold for cTXNPx and mTXNPx, respectively, in Y strain [95]), which would allow the peroxidases to compete better for peroxynitrite and limit cytotoxicity [99]. The reactivity of peroxynitrite with other potential targets in *T. cruzi* other than thiol-containing compounds has been less studied. Indeed, the kinetics of the reactions between peroxynitrite and parasitic metal-containing proteins of antioxidant functions, namely ascorbate peroxidase and Fe-SOD A and B, are currently under investigation in our lab.

Exogenous or endogenous exposure of *T. cruzi* to peroxynitrite leads to the disruption of different physiological processes, such as cellular respiration, energetic metabolism and calcium homeostasis, cell motility and growth, and eventually causes parasite death [45,100,101]. The inhibitory effect of peroxynitrite on the energetic metabolism of the parasite depends on the inhibition of succinate dehydrogenase and NADH-fumarate reductase, which play a key role in these parasites since the NADH-dependent segment of the respiratory chain is inactive and electrons from NADH must be transferred to fumarate to produce succinate through fumarate reductase to enter the respiratory chain [102]. Inactivation of both enzymes was reverted by treatment with dithiothreitol, which together with the fact that cysteine residue(s) were critical for activity and the protective actions of competitive inhibitors of the enzymes, indicated that active-site thiol(s) oxidation was involved in peroxynitrite-mediated inactivation of these enzymes [100]. The protective action of methionine 5 mM (a scavenger of peroxynitrite and peroxynitrite-derived species [103]) and uric acid 2 mM (mostly a radical scavenger or repairing agent that reacts quite slowly with peroxynitrite [104,105]), together with the minimal effect of physiological concentrations of CO_2, indicated that most probably the effect of peroxynitrite on critical thiols was at least partially dependent on peroxynitrite-derived radicals, even in the absence of effect of classical hydroxyl radical scavengers [100]. Peroxynitrite dose-dependently inhibited non-mitochondrial Ca^{2+} uptake systems from *T. cruzi* epimastigotes, probably through the inactivation of a P-type Ca^{2+}-ATPase [101]. The oxidant also caused the parasite energetic pool to decrease, but the drop in ATP levels was delayed with respect to the decrease of the ATP-dependent Ca^{2+} transport. Moreover, peroxynitrite inhibited mitochondrial calcium uptake systems of the parasite, an effect that was associated with a decrease in the membrane potential, but was independent of effects on the electron transport chain, and has been proposed to be mediated by lipid and protein oxidation [101], which have been demonstrated to occur when the parasites are exposed to this oxidant [106]. In *T. cruzi*, calcium homeostasis participates in key cellular functions such as multiplication, differentiation, programmed cell death, and host cell invasion [107–109], processes that could therefore be altered by exposition to peroxynitrite.

Peroxynitrite Detoxification Systems

In 2000, Bryk *et al.* reported for the first time the peroxynitrite reductase activity of a thiol-dependent peroxidase of the Prx type [110]. Since then, it has been well established that members of different subgroups of Prxs catalyze the two-electron reduction of peroxynitrite to nitrite [111]. *T. cruzi* expresses a mitochondrial and a cytosolic Prx that have been named TXNPxs since they catalyze the reduction of different peroxides including peroxynitrite using the small protein TXN as reducing substrate [80,83,112,113]. According to the PeroxiRedoxin Classification IndEX (http://csb.wfu.edu/prex/index.php) both mitochondrial and cytosolic TXNPxs (mTXNPx and cTXNPx, respectively) belong to the AhpC/Prx1 subfamily, which is mechanistically classified as typical 2-Cys Prxs and includes TXN peroxidases, *Arabidopsis thaliana* 2-Cys Prx, barley Bas1, *Saccharomyces cerevisiae* TSA1 and TSA2, bacterial alkyl hydroperoxide reductase C (AhpC), and

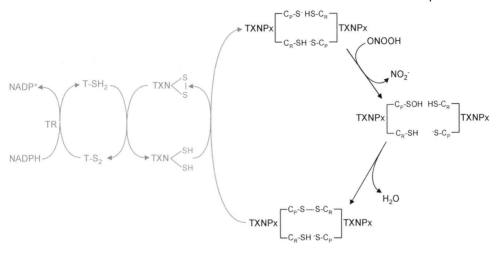

Figure 11.2 Catalytic cycle of *T. cruzi* TXNPxs using peroxynitrite as oxidizing substrate. Both mitochondrial and cytosolic TXNPxs from *T. cruzi* catalyze the two-electron reduction of peroxynitrous acid to nitrite (NO_2^-). These enzymes, which belong to the AhpC/Prx1 subfamily of Prxs, display a ping-pong mechanism of reaction. During the oxidizing part of the catalytic cycle the thiolate in C_P of reduced cytosolic or mitochondrial *Tc*TXNPxs (S_P^-) is oxidized to sulfenic acid (S_POH), with rate constants of $1-2 \times 10^6$ and $1.8 \times 10^7 \, M^{-1} s^{-1}$, respectively, at pH 7.4 and 25 °C. The resulting sulfenic acid reacts with the thiol group of C_R located in another subunit and an intermolecular disulfide is formed. Reduction of the oxidized forms of the enzymes by the sequential action of TXN, trypanothione ($T(SH)_2$), trypanothione reductase (TR), and NADPH has been reported *in vitro*. TXNI has also been proved to be the natural reducing substrate for the cytosolic *Tc*TXNPx *in vivo* (shown in gray). However, the identity of the reducing substrate for the mitochondrial isoform is still a matter of debate. The peroxynitrite reductase activity of *T. cruzi* TXN-dependent peroxidases of the glutathione peroxidase type has not been investigated so far. (Adapted from [115] with kind permission by Elsevier).

mammalian PRDXs 1–4. All Prxs possess a peroxidatic cysteine residue (C_P), which rapidly reduces peroxides such as hydrogen peroxide (H_2O_2), fatty acid hydroperoxides, and other organic hydroperoxides (ROOH) as well as peroxynitrite to water, alcohols, and nitrite, respectively, with different selectivity [114,115]. In the process, C_P gets oxidized to sulfenic acid. In 2-Cys Prxs, which require a second cysteine residue for catalytic activity, this sulfenic acid forms a disulfide bridge with a resolving cysteine (C_R), which in typical 2-Cys Prxs is located in the C-terminus of another subunit to form an intermolecular disulfide bridge. The latter is then reduced by the reducing substrate, which for the AhpC/Prx1 subfamily is usually thioredoxin or a thioredoxin-related protein, such as TXNs in trypanosomatids [114,116] (Figure 11.2). The crystal structure of recombinant cytosolic *Tc*TXNPx (containing a histidine tail) under reduced state has been determined at 2.8-Å resolution (Protein Data Bank ID: 1UUL) [117]. The quaternary structure of *Tcc*TXNPx is an assembly of five symmetric homodimers that associate into a decamer. The C_P (Cys52) is located in a first VCP motif in the N-terminal portion of helix α1, and buried inside the active-site pocket that contains Pro45 and Thr49, residues that are highly conserved among Prxs [118,119]. The thiol in C_P forms a hydrogen bond with O^γ of Thr49 and $N^\epsilon 1$ of Arg128 – interactions that are essential for catalytic activity in the homologous enzyme from *L. donovani* [117,118]. In turn, C_R (Cys173), from the second molecule of the homodimer, is again located in a VCP motif, in a hydrophobic solvent-excluded environment that is also important for activity [117]. Based on the crystal structure of the enzyme, molecular dynamics simulations combined with electrostatics analysis on monomeric and different oligomeric forms of *Tcc*TXNPx were recently performed. The calculations indicate that the pK_a values of C_P are highly dependent on the oligomeric state: a C_P pK_a comparable to that of free cysteine was calculated for the monomer and also for the subunits of the dimer when averaged over time, while all subunits in the decamer show a lowered C_P pK_a. The effect of these C_P pK_a shifts on enzymatic activity of the different oligomeric forms of *Tcc*TXNPx has not been experimentally addressed yet. It is important to note that, even though the mechanism of reaction between peroxides and thiols involves the protonated form of the peroxide and thiolates as reactive species, the fractional amount of thiolate available for a C_P (usually $pK_a < 6.4$ [110,120,121]) compared to free cysteine at physiological pH would only increase by a factor of around 10 and cannot explain the 10^3–10^7 acceleration in rate constants of reaction of C_P in Prxs with respect to the uncatalyzed reaction [122] Therefore, destabilization of the decameric form of these enzymes would be expected to lead to an around 10-fold decrease in enzymatic activity, if only the effects on the pK_a of C_P were considered. Active-site microenvironment factors contributing to the catalytic mechanism of these enzymes are only starting to be identified [122–125], and the relationship between these factors and oligomerization is still unknown.

mTXNPx from *T. cruzi* shows an important sequence similarity with the cytosolic form – it possesses a mitochondrial import sequence at its N-terminus and the C_R is located at a IPC motif. To date, the crystal structure of trypanosomatid mTXNPxs has not been resolved, but light scattering and high-resolution electron microscopy of mTXNPx from *L. infantum* indicated that the mitochondrial enzyme also adopts a decameric, ring-like quaternary structure [126]. Both cytosolic and mitochondrial *Tc*TXNPx rapidly reduced peroxynitrite to nitrite, with rate constants of 1–2 × 10^6 and 1.8 × 10^7 $M^{-1}s^{-1}$, pH 7.4, 25 °C [83] (Figure 11.3). They also reduced other peroxides such as H_2O_2 and artificial organic hydroperoxides such as *tert*-butyl hydroperoxide [83,112,113]. Moreover, the oxidized form of *Tcc*TXNPx is reduced by cytosolic TXNI from *T. brucei* with a rate constant of 1.3 × 10^6 $M^{-1}s^{-1}$ [83]. Although the mitochondrial isoform could also be reduced by cytosolic TXNI from *T. brucei in vitro* [83], it is obviously an artificial situation that does not take into account compartmentalization and the natural reducing substrate for *Tcm*TXNPx *in vivo* is still a matter of debate. A recent report indicated that, according to sequence homology, the second TXN coding sequence in *T. cruzi* (*Tc*TXN2) groups together with TXN3 from *Leishmania*, which is anchored at the mitochondrial outer membrane with the redox-active domain facing the cytosol [127]. The localization of *Tc*TXN2 still requires experimental confirmation. In addition, reduction of TXN by trypanothione requires the latter

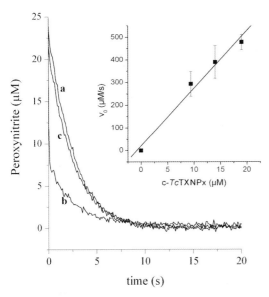

Figure 11.3 Kinetics of peroxynitrite reduction by cTXNPx from *T. cruzi*. The rate constant of peroxynitrite reduction by *Tcc*TXNPx was measured by a direct approach, following peroxynitrite decay at 310 nm ($\varepsilon = 1600\,M^{-1}\,cm^{-1}$). Peroxynitrite in diluted sodium hydroxide was mixed with 100 mM sodium phosphate plus 100 µM dtpa without (a), with wild-type *Tcc*TXNPx (32.2 µM) (b), or with *Tcc*TXNPx mutated at the peroxidatic cysteine residue (37.5 µM) (c). Measured final pH was 7.4. The inset shows a plot of initial rate of peroxynitrite decay versus *Tcc*TXNPx concentration. From this plot a rate constant of peroxynitrite reduction by the enzyme was calculated as $1 \times 10^6\,M^{-1}\,s^{-1}$. The kinetic of the reaction was also measured by two indirect, competition approaches (with horseradish peroxidase oxidation to compound I and with manganese(III)-*meso*-tetrakis)N-methylpyridinium-3-yl) porphyrin oxidation) with similar results. From these experiments, a mean rate constant value of $1.5 \pm 0.5 \times 10^6\,M^{-1}\,s^{-1}$ for peroxynitrite reduction by *Tcc*TXNPx at pH 7.4 was determined. (Adapted from [83] with kind permission by Elsevier).

to be maintained at reduced state by the flavoenzyme trypanothione reductase at the expense of NADPH, but information regarding the occurrence of trypanothione reductase in mitochondria is rather contradictory [128,129]. Alternatively, dihydrolipoamide dehydrogenase/lipoamide was reported to be able to reduce intramitochondrial TXN2 from *L. infantum* [130]. *T. cruzi* expresses other thiol-dependent peroxidases, which show sequence similarity with glutathione peroxidases although TXN is a much more efficient reducing substrate [131]. These enzymes are presented in detail elsewhere in this book. To date, their capacity to catalyze peroxynitrite reduction has not been investigated *in vitro* or in cellular systems. In a recent collaborative work we have demonstrated that a related thiol-dependent glutathione peroxidase from poplar, GPx 5, reduces peroxynitrite with a rate constant of $1.4 \times 10^6\,M^{-1}\,s^{-1}$, pH 7.4, 25 °C [132]. Further studies are required to find out whether thiol-dependent glutathione peroxidase-like enzymes participate in peroxynitrite detoxification in *T. cruzi* and other trypanosomatids.

Likewise, the capacity of the heme-dependent peroxidase ascorbate peroxidase from *T. cruzi* to reduce peroxynitrite *in vitro* remains to be investigated. In any case, the fact that parasites transformed to overexpress this enzyme were more resistant to hydrogen peroxide treatment, but not to peroxynitrite, argues against a role of ascorbate peroxidase in peroxynitrite detoxification [84].

T. cruzi Antioxidant Enzymes as Virulence Mediators

The role of peroxynitrite detoxification by *T. cruzi* antioxidant enzymes in the outcome of the infection has been demonstrated in both cellular and animal models of the disease. At a cellular level, phagocyted wild-type trypomastigotes loaded with dihydrorhodamine showed a much higher probe oxidation than *Tcc*TXNPx-overexpressing trypomastigotes when infecting IFN-γ/lipopolysaccharide (LPS)-activated macrophages, in agreement with the enhanced capacity of these genetically modified cells to detoxify peroxynitrite (Figure 11.4a). Moreover, studies using parasites preloaded with [5,6-^{3}H]uridine as a probe of membrane integrity showed that macrophages activated with IFN-γ and LPS were toxic to wild-type trypomastigotes, while *Tcc*TXNPx-overexpressing cells showed resistance (Figure 11.4b), indicating that the simultaneous generation of $O_2^{\bullet-}$ and $^\bullet$NO is involved in the cytotoxic effect of macrophages on internalized parasites at this time point of the infection (2 h) (Figure 11.4b). Previous reports have shown that the concentration of free thiols (GSH, GSH-Spd, and T(SH)$_2$) varies between the different parasite stages (epimastigotes, trypomastigotes, and amastigotes) and also between different *T. cruzi* strains [93]. Moreover, several proteomic analyses have suggested the upregulation of members of the *T. cruzi* antioxidant network (trypanothione synthetase (TS), mTXNPx; TXN, iron SOD A (FeSODA), and ascorbate peroxidase) in the infective metacyclic trypomastigote compared with the non-infective epimastigote stage [133,134]. Due to the fact that *T. cruzi* is not a clonal population our group has searched for the upregulation of different components of the antioxidant network in several strains belonging to the major phylogenetic groups during the differentiation process to the infective metacyclic trypomastigotes. Our results show for all the analyzed strains, upregulation of cTXNPx, mTXNPx, and TS protein content during metacyclogenesis, making this a general preadaptation process that allows *T. cruzi* to deal with the nitroxidative environment of the vertebrate host found during invasion [95]. Most importantly, a positive association between virulence of different *T. cruzi* strains and cTXNPx, mTXNPx, and TS levels was found, highlighting the interplay between the antioxidant enzyme network and host oxidative defense mechanisms [95]. In accordance, strains of augmented virulence showed an abundant heart inflammatory infiltrate with high parasitemias in the acute phase of Chagas disease. Moreover, overexpression of *Tcc*TXNPx on trypomastigotes increases virulence as evidenced by a 3-fold increase in parasitemia with the presence of severe inflammatory infiltrates in heart and skeletal muscle when compared with the wild strain. These data reinforce the concept that success of infection and progression to the chronic phase depend on parasite antioxidant

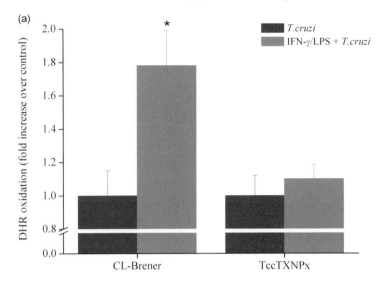

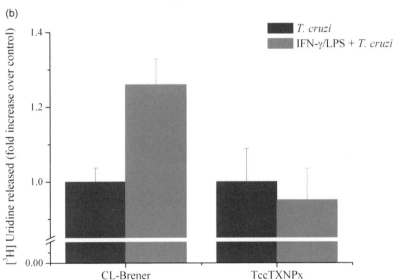

Figure 11.4 *T. cruzi* killing by intraphagosomal peroxynitrite and protective effect of *Tcc*TXNPx. (a) Wild-type (CL-Brener) or *Tcc*TXNPx-overexpressing trypomastigotes preloaded with dihydrorhodamine (DHR) were exposed to unstimulated (*T. cruzi*) or immunostimulated infected (IFN-γ/LPS + *T. cruzi*) macrophages. Dihydrorhodamine oxidation after 2 h of infection was determined in a fluorescence plate reader. (b) Macrophages were infected with wild-type or *Tcc*TXNPx-overexpressing trypomastigotes preloaded with [5,6-³H]uridine. After incubation (2 h) supernatants were collected and radioactivity measured in a liquid scintillation counter. Data are mean ± standard error of three independent experiments. (Taken from [27]).

enzyme levels. *T. cruzi* contains a repertoire of four FeSODs that detoxify $O_2^{\bullet-}$ generated in the cytosol (*Tc*SODB1), glycosomes (*Tc*SODB1-2), and mitochondria (*Tc*SODA and C) [135]. SODs readily eliminate $O_2^{\bullet-}$ at the site of production (e.g., cytosolic redox cycling of drugs, mitochondrial electron transport chain) and may contribute to parasite immune evasion by (i) protecting from direct cytotoxic effects of $O_2^{\bullet-}$, such as aconitase inhibition [136], by its dismutation to H_2O_2, (ii) regulating the $O_2^{\bullet-}$-mediated induction of parasite programmed cell death [137], and (iii) inhibiting the endogenous formation of peroxynitrite. Whether FeSODs constitute virulence factors for infections caused by *T. cruzi* remains to be established.

Conclusions

Macrophages constitute key host cells during the acute infection by *T. cruzi*. Inside the phagosome of immunostimulated macrophages, simultaneous production of $^{\bullet}$NO and $O_2^{\bullet-}$ leads to peroxynitrite formation. Peroxynitrite can diffuse to the parasite where, through oxidation and/or nitration of different targets, it causes the disruption of different physiological processes such as energetic metabolism, calcium homeostasis, cell motility, and growth, and eventually causes parasite death. *T. cruzi* contains a battery of antioxidant enzymes that catalyze the detoxification of the reactive species it encounters. Among them, cytosolic and mitochondrial TXNPxs have been demonstrated to rapidly reduce peroxynitrite as well as other peroxides. Parasites overexpressing these enzymes were more resistant to peroxynitrite-mediated toxicity, either added in bolus or formed by activated macrophages. Interestingly, we tested the content of both cTXNPx and mTXNPx in different *T. cruzi* strains, and found a much higher expression in trypomastigotes compared with epimastigotes, indicating a higher capability of peroxide detoxification. Moreover, when analyzing different naturally occurring *T. cruzi* strains, the content of both enzymes correlated with virulence in an animal model of disease. Also, genetically engineered parasites overexpressing *Tc*cTXNPx recapitulated the high parasitemia and tissue damage observed in the virulent strains [27]. Altogether, these data support that parasitic TXNPxs could constitute drug targets for a rationalized drug development. A potential role of peroxynitrite in controlling *T. cruzi* infection during the chronic stage of Chagas disease, where non-phagocytic cells such as myocytes are the main host cells and can control *T. cruzi* infection by $^{\bullet}$NO-dependent processes [50,51], deserves further investigation.

Acknowledgments

This work was supported by grants from Comisión Sectorial de Investigación Científica, Universidad de la República and National Institutes of Health (2R01Hl063119-05 and 1R01AI095173-01). Financial support was also provided to the authors by the Programa de Desarrollo de Ciencias Básicas (PEDECIBA, Uruguay). M.H. was partially supported by a fellowship from Agencia Nacional de Investigación e Innovación.

References

1 Babior, B.M. (1984) The respiratory burst of phagocytes. *J. Clin. Invest.*, **73**, 599–601.

2 Groemping, Y. and Rittinger, K. (2005) Activation and assembly of the NADPH oxidase: a structural perspective. *Biochem. J.*, **386**, 401–416.

3 De Groote, M.A., Ochsner, U.A., Shiloh, M.U., Nathan, C., McCord, J.M., Dinauer, M.C., Libby, S.J., Vazquez-Torres, A., Xu, Y., and Fang, F.C. (1997) Periplasmic superoxide dismutase protects *Salmonella* from products of phagocyte NADPH-oxidase and nitric oxide synthase. *Proc. Natl. Acad. Sci. USA*, **94**, 13997–14001.

4 Xie, Q.W., Whisnant, R., and Nathan, C. (1993) Promoter of the mouse gene encoding calcium-independent nitric oxide synthase confers inducibility by interferon gamma and bacterial lipopolysaccharide. *J. Exp. Med.*, **177**, 1779–1784.

5 Martin, E., Nathan, C., and Xie, Q.W. (1994) Role of interferon regulatory factor 1 in induction of nitric oxide synthase. *J. Exp. Med.*, **180**, 977–984.

6 MacMicking, J., Xie, Q.W., and Nathan, C. (1997) Nitric oxide and macrophage function. *Annu. Rev. Immunol.*, **15**, 323–350.

7 Ischiropoulos, H., Zhu, L., and Beckman, J.S. (1992) Peroxynitrite formation from macrophage-derived nitric oxide. *Arch. Biochem. Biophys.*, **298**, 446–451.

8 Loumaye, E., Ferrer-Sueta, G., Alvarez, B., Rees, J.F., Clippe, A., Knoops, B., Radi, R., and Trujillo, M. (2011) Kinetic studies of peroxiredoxin 6 from *Arenicola marina*: rapid oxidation by hydrogen peroxide and peroxynitrite but lack of reduction by hydrogen sulfide. *Arch. Biochem. Biophys.*, **514**, 1–7.

9 Nathan, C. and Shiloh, M.U. (2000) Reactive oxygen and nitrogen intermediates in the relationship between mammalian hosts and microbial pathogens. *Proc. Natl. Acad. Sci. USA*, **97**, 8841–8848.

10 de Castro, S.L., Batista, D.G., Batista, M. M., Batista, W., Daliry, A., de Souza, E.M., Menna-Barreto, R.F., Oliveira, G.M., Salomao, K., Silva, C.F., Silva, P.B., and Soeiro Mde, N. (2011) Experimental chemotherapy for Chagas disease: a morphological, biochemical, and proteomic overview of potential *Trypanosoma cruzi* targets of amidines derivatives and naphthoquinones. *Mol. Biol. Int.*, **2011**, 306928.

11 Guedes, P.M., Silva, G.K., Gutierrez, F.R., and Silva, J.S. (2011) Current status of Chagas disease chemotherapy. *Expert Rev. Anti. Infect. Ther.*, **9**, 609–620.

12 Zhang, L. and Tarleton, R.L. (1999) Parasite persistence correlates with disease severity and localization in chronic Chagas' disease. *J. Infect. Dis.*, **180**, 480–486.

13 Nagajyothi, F., Machado, F.S., Burleigh, B.A., Jelicks, L.A., Scherer, P.E., Mukherjee, S., Lisanti, M.P., Weiss, L.M., Garg, N.J., and Tanowitz, H.B. (2012) Mechanisms of *Trypanosoma cruzi* persistence in Chagas disease. *Cell Microbiol.*, **14**, 634–643.

14 Bonay, P. and Fresno, M. (1995) Characterization of carbohydrate binding proteins in *Trypanosoma cruzi*. *J. Biol. Chem.*, **270**, 11062–11070.

15 Campos, M.A. and Gazzinelli, R.T. (2004) *Trypanosoma cruzi* and its components as exogenous mediators of inflammation recognized through Toll-like receptors. *Mediators Inflamm.*, **13**, 139–143.

16 Ropert, C. and Gazzinelli, R.T. (2004) Regulatory role of Toll-like receptor 2 during infection with *Trypanosoma cruzi*. *J. Endotoxin Res.*, **10**, 425–430.

17 Oliveira, A.C., Peixoto, J.R., de Arruda, L. B., Campos, M.A., Gazzinelli, R.T., Golenbock, D.T., Akira, S., Previato, J.O., Mendonca-Previato, L., Nobrega, A., and Bellio, M. (2004) Expression of functional TLR4 confers proinflammatory responsiveness to *Trypanosoma cruzi* glycoinositolphospholipids and higher resistance to infection with *T. cruzi*. *J. Immunol.*, **173**, 5688–5696.

18 Antunez, M.I. and Cardoni, R.L. (2000) IL-12 and IFN-gamma production, and NK cell activity, in acute and chronic experimental *Trypanosoma cruzi* infections. *Immunol. Lett.*, **71**, 103–109.

19 Murray, H.W., Spitalny, G.L., and Nathan, C.F. (1985) Activation of mouse peritoneal macrophages *in vitro* and *in vivo* by interferon-gamma. *J. Immunol.*, **134**, 1619–1622.

20 Ogier-Denis, E., Mkaddem, S.B., and Vandewalle, A. (2008) NOX enzymes and Toll-like receptor signaling. *Semin. Immunopathol.*, **30**, 291–300.

21 Babior, B.M. (2002) The leukocyte NADPH oxidase. *Isr. Med. Assoc. J.*, **4**, 1023–1024.

22 Babior, B.M. (2004) NADPH oxidase. *Curr. Opin. Immunol.*, **16**, 42–47.

23 Cardoni, R.L., Antunez, M.I., Morales, C., and Nantes, I.R. (1997) Release of reactive oxygen species by phagocytic cells in response to live parasites in mice infected with *Trypanosoma cruzi*. *Am. J. Trop. Med. Hyg.*, **56**, 329–334.

24 McCabe, R.E. and Mullins, B.T. (1990) Failure of *Trypanosoma cruzi* to trigger the respiratory burst of activated macrophages. Mechanism for immune evasion and importance of oxygen-independent killing. *J. Immunol.*, **144**, 2384–2388.

25 Tanaka, Y., Tanowitz, H., and Bloom, B.R. (1983) Growth of *Trypanosoma cruzi* in a cloned macrophage cell line and in a variant defective in oxygen metabolism. *Infect. Immun.*, **41**, 1322–1331.

26 de Carvalho, T.U. and de Souza, W. (1987) Cytochemical localization of NADH and NADPH oxidases during interaction of *Trypanosoma cruzi* with activated macrophages. *Parasitol. Res.*, **73**, 213–217.

27 Alvarez, M.N., Peluffo, G., Piacenza, L., and Radi, R. (2011) Intraphagosomal peroxynitrite as a macrophage-derived cytotoxin against internalized *Trypanosoma cruzi*: consequences for oxidative killing and role of microbial peroxiredoxins in infectivity. *J. Biol. Chem.*, **286**, 6627–6640.

28 Cassatella, M.A., Bazzoni, F., Flynn, R.M., Dusi, S., Trinchieri, G., and Rossi, F. (1990) Molecular basis of interferon-gamma and lipopolysaccharide enhancement of phagocyte respiratory burst capability. Studies on the gene expression of several NADPH oxidase components. *J. Biol. Chem.*, **265**, 20241–20246.

29 Green, S.P., Hamilton, J.A., Uhlinger, D.J., and Phillips, W.A. (1994) Expression of p47-phox and p67-phox proteins in murine bone marrow-derived macrophages: enhancement by lipopolysaccharide and tumor necrosis factor alpha but not colony stimulating factor 1. *J. Leukoc. Biol.*, **55**, 530–535.

30 Hickman-Davis, J.M., O'Reilly, P., Davis, I.C., Peti-Peterdi, J., Davis, G., Young, K. R., Devlin, R.B., and Matalon, S. (2002) Killing of Klebsiella pneumoniae by human alveolar macrophages. *Am. J. Physiol.*, **282**, L944–L956.

31 Linares, E., Giorgio, S., Mortara, R.A., Santos, C.X., Yamada, A.T., and Augusto, O. (2001) Role of peroxynitrite in macrophage microbicidal mechanisms *in vivo* revealed by protein nitration and hydroxylation. *Free Radic. Biol. Med.*, **30**, 1234–1242.

32 Vazquez-Torres, A., Jones-Carson, J., Mastroeni, P., Ischiropoulos, H., and Fang, F.C. (2000) Antimicrobial actions of the NADPH phagocyte oxidase and inducible nitric oxide synthase in experimental salmonellosis. I. Effects on microbial killing by activated peritoneal macrophages *in vitro*. *J. Exp. Med.*, **192**, 227–236.

33 Augusto, O., Linares, E., and Giorgio, S. (1996) Possible roles of nitric oxide and peroxynitrite in murine leishmaniasis. *Braz. J. Med. Biol. Res.*, **29**, 853–862.

34 Kane, M.M. and Mosser, D.M. (2000) *Leishmania* parasites and their ploys to disrupt macrophage activation. *Curr. Opin. Hematol.*, **7**, 26–31.

35 Chan, J., Xing, Y., Magliozzo, R.S., and Bloom, B.R. (1992) Killing of virulent *Mycobacterium tuberculosis* by reactive nitrogen intermediates produced by activated murine macrophages. *J. Exp. Med.*, **175**, 1111–1122.

36 Ferrer-Sueta, G. and Radi, R. (2009) Chemical biology of peroxynitrite: kinetics, diffusion, and radicals. *ACS Chem. Biol.*, **4**, 161–177.

37 Hoff, R. (1975) Killing *in vitro* of *Trypanosoma cruzi* by macrophages from mice immunized with *T. cruzi* or BCG,

and absence of cross-immunity on challenge *in vivo. J. Exp. Med.*, **142**, 299–311.

38 Golden, J.M. and Tarleton, R.L. (1991) *Trypanosoma cruzi*: cytokine effects on macrophage trypanocidal activity. *Exp. Parasitol.*, **72**, 391–402.

39 Kress, Y., Tanowitz, H., Bloom, B., and Wittner, M. (1977) *Trypanosoma cruzi*: infection of normal and activated mouse macrophages. *Exp. Parasitol.*, **41**, 385–396.

40 Nathan, C., Nogueira, N., Juangbhanich, C., Ellis, J., and Cohn, Z. (1979) Activation of macrophages *in vivo* and *in vitro*. Correlation between hydrogen peroxide release and killing of *Trypanosoma cruzi*. *J. Exp. Med.*, **149**, 1056–1068.

41 Munoz-Fernandez, M.A., Fernandez, M. A., and Fresno, M. (1992) Synergism between tumor necrosis factor-alpha and interferon-gamma on macrophage activation for the killing of intracellular *Trypanosoma cruzi* through a nitric oxide-dependent mechanism. *Eur. J Immunol.*, **22**, 301–307.

42 Holscher, C., Kohler, G., Muller, U., Mossmann, H., Schaub, G.A., and Brombacher, F. (1998) Defective nitric oxide effector functions lead to extreme susceptibility of *Trypanosoma cruzi*-infected mice deficient in gamma interferon receptor or inducible nitric oxide synthase. *Infect. Immun.*, **66**, 1208–1215.

43 Petray, P., Castanos-Velez, E., Grinstein, S., Orn, A., and Rottenberg, M.E. (1995) Role of nitric oxide in resistance and histopathology during experimental infection with *Trypanosoma cruzi*. *Immunol. Lett.*, **47**, 121–126.

44 Gazzinelli, R.T., Oswald, I.P., Hieny, S., James, S.L., and Sher, A. (1992) The microbicidal activity of interferon-gamma-treated macrophages against *Trypanosoma cruzi* involves an L-arginine-dependent, nitrogen oxide-mediated mechanism inhibitable by interleukin-10 and transforming growth factor-beta. *Eur. J. Immunol.*, **22**, 2501–2506.

45 Denicola, A., Rubbo, H., Rodriguez, D., and Radi, R. (1993) Peroxynitrite-mediated cytotoxicity to *Trypanosoma*

cruzi. Arch. Biochem. Biophys., **304**, 279–286.

46 Alvarez, M.N., Piacenza, L., Irigoin, F., Peluffo, G., and Radi, R. (2004) Macrophage-derived peroxynitrite diffusion and toxicity to *Trypanosoma cruzi. Arch. Biochem. Biophys.*, **432**, 222–232.

47 Rassi, A.Jr., Rassi, A., and Marin-Neto, J.A. (2010) Chagas disease. *Lancet*, **375**, 1388–1402.

48 Girones, N. and Fresno, M. (2003) Etiology of Chagas disease myocarditis: autoimmunity, parasite persistence, or both? *Trends Parasitol.*, **19**, 19–22.

49 Marin-Neto, J.A., Cunha-Neto, E., Maciel, B.C., and Simoes, M.V. (2007) Pathogenesis of chronic Chagas heart disease. *Circulation*, **115**, 1109–1123.

50 Chandrasekar, B., Melby, P.C., Troyer, D. A., Colston, J.T., and Freeman, G.L. (1998) Temporal expression of pro-inflammatory cytokines and inducible nitric oxide synthase in experimental acute Chagasic cardiomyopathy. *Am. J. Pathol.*, **152**, 925–934.

51 Machado, F.S., Martins, G.A., Aliberti, J.C., Mestriner, F.L., Cunha, F.Q., and Silva, J.S. (2000) *Trypanosoma cruzi*-infected cardiomyocytes produce chemokines and cytokines that trigger potent nitric oxide-dependent trypanocidal activity. *Circulation*, **102**, 3003–3008.

52 Durand, J.L., Mukherjee, S., Commodari, F., De Souza, A.P., Zhao, D., Machado, F. S., Tanowitz, H.B., and Jelicks, L.A. (2009) Role of NO synthase in the development of *Trypanosoma cruzi*-induced cardiomyopathy in mice. *Am. J. Trop. Med. Hyg.*, **80**, 782–787.

53 Michailowsky, V., Silva, N.M., Rocha, C. D., Vieira, L.Q., Lannes-Vieira, J., and Gazzinelli, R.T. (2001) Pivotal role of interleukin-12 and interferon-gamma axis in controlling tissue parasitism and inflammation in the heart and central nervous system during *Trypanosoma cruzi* infection. *Am. J. Pathol.*, **159**, 1723–1733.

54 Wen, J.J. and Garg, N.J. (2008) Mitochondrial generation of reactive oxygen species is enhanced at the Q(o) site of the complex III in the myocardium of *Trypanosoma cruzi*-infected mice: beneficial effects of an antioxidant. *J. Bioenerg. Biomembr.*, **40**, 587–598.

55 Silberman, G.A., Fan, T.H., Liu, H., Jiao, Z., Xiao, H.D., Lovelock, J.D., Boulden, B. M., Widder, J., Fredd, S., Bernstein, K.E., Wolska, B.M., Dikalov, S., Harrison, D.G., and Dudley, S.C.Jr. (2010) Uncoupled cardiac nitric oxide synthase mediates diastolic dysfunction. *Circulation*, **121**, 519–528.

56 Docampo, R. and Moreno, S.N. (1986) Free radical metabolism of antiparasitic agents. *Fed. Proc.*, **45**, 2471–2476.

57 Fontecave, M., Graslund, A., and Reichard, P. (1987) The function of superoxide dismutase during the enzymatic formation of the free radical of ribonucleotide reductase. *J. Biol. Chem.*, **262**, 12332–12336.

58 Boveris, A. and Stoppani, A.O. (1977) Hydrogen peroxide generation in *Trypanosoma cruzi*. *Experientia*, **33**, 1306–1308.

59 Dhiman, M., Nakayasu, E.S., Madaiah, Y. H., Reynolds, B.K., Wen, J.J., Almeida, I. C., and Garg, N.J. (2008) Enhanced nitrosative stress during *Trypanosoma cruzi* infection causes nitrotyrosine modification of host proteins: implications in Chagas' disease. *Am. J. Pathol.*, **173**, 728–740.

60 Naviliat, M., Gualco, G., Cayota, A., and Radi, R. (2005) Protein 3-nitrotyrosine formation during *Trypanosoma cruzi* infection in mice. *Braz. J. Med. Biol. Res.*, **38**, 1825–1834.

61 Goldstein, S. and Czapski, G. (1995) The reaction of NO. with $O_2^{\bullet-}$ and HO2$^{\bullet}$: a pulse radiolysis study. *Free Radic. Biol. Med.*, **19**, 505–510.

62 Kissner, R., Nauser, T., Bugnon, P., Lye, P. G., and Koppenol, W.H. (1997) Formation and properties of peroxynitrite as studied by laser flash photolysis, high-pressure stopped-flow technique, and pulse radiolysis. *Chem. Res. Toxicol.*, **10**, 1285–1292.

63 Pryor, W.A. and Squadrito, G.L. (1995) The chemistry of peroxynitrite: a product from the reaction of nitric oxide with superoxide. *Am. J. Physiol.*, **268**, L699–L722.

64 Goldstein, S. and Czapski, G. (1995) Direct and indirect oxidations by peroxynitrite. *Inorg. Chem.*, **34**, 4041–4048.

65 Gerasimov, O.V. and Lymar, S.V. (1999) The yield of hydroxyl radical from the decomposition of peroxynitrous acid. *Inorg. Chem.*, **38**, 4317–4321.

66 Ferrer-Sueta, G. and Radi, R. (2009) Chemical biology of peroxynitrite: kinetics, diffusion, radicals. *ACS Chem. Biol.*, **4**, 161–177.

67 Radi, R., Beckman, J.S., Bush, K.M., and Freeman, B.A. (1991) Peroxynitrite oxidation of sulfhydryls. The cytotoxic potential of superoxide and nitric oxide. *J. Biol. Chem.*, **266**, 4244–4250.

68 Trujillo, M. and Radi, R. (2002) Peroxynitrite reaction with the reduced and the oxidized forms of lipoic acid: new insights into the reaction of peroxynitrite with thiols. *Arch. Biochem. Biophys.*, **397**, 91–98.

69 Thomson, L., Trujillo, M., Telleri, R., and Radi, R. (1995) Kinetics of cytochrome c^{2+} oxidation by peroxynitrite: implications for superoxide measurements in nitric oxide-producing biological systems. *Arch. Biochem. Biophys.*, **319**, 491–497.

70 Ferrer-Sueta, G., Batinic-Haberle, I., Spasojevic, I., Fridovich, I., and Radi, R. (1999) Catalytic scavenging of peroxynitrite by isomeric Mn(III) *N*-methylpyridylporphyrins in the presence of reductants. *Chem. Res. Toxicol.*, **12**, 442–449.

71 Romero, N., Radi, R., Linares, E., Augusto, O., Detweiler, C.D., Mason, R.P., and Denicola, A. (2003) Reaction of human hemoglobin with peroxynitrite. Isomerization to nitrate and secondary formation of protein radicals. *J. Biol. Chem.*, **278**, 44049–44057.

72 Floris, R., Piersma, S.R., Yang, G., Jones, P., and Wever, R. (1993) Interaction of myeloperoxidase with peroxynitrite. A comparison with lactoperoxidase, horseradish peroxidase and catalase. *Eur. J. Biochem.*, **215**, 767–775.

73 Zou, M., Yesilkaya, A., and Ullrich, V. (1999) Peroxynitrite inactivates prostacyclin synthase by heme-thiolate-

catalyzed tyrosine nitration. *Drug Metab. Rev.*, **31**, 343–349.

74 Radi, R. (2004) Nitric oxide, oxidants, and protein tyrosine nitration. *Proc. Natl. Acad. Sci. USA*, **101**, 4003–4008.

75 Denicola, A., Freeman, B.A., Trujillo, M., and Radi, R. (1996) Peroxynitrite reaction with carbon dioxide/bicarbonate: kinetics and influence on peroxynitrite-mediated oxidations. *Arch. Biochem. Biophys.*, **333**, 49–58.

76 Lymar, S.V. and Hurst, J.K. (1995) Rapid reaction between peroxynitrite anion and carbon dioxide: implication for biological activity. *J. Am. Chem. Soc.*, **117**, 8867–8868.

77 Bonini, M.G., Radi, R., Ferrer-Sueta, G., Ferreira, A.M., and Augusto, O. (1999) Direct EPR detection of the carbonate radical anion produced from peroxynitrite and carbon dioxide. *J. Biol. Chem.*, **274**, 10802–10806.

78 Vieira, L., Lavan, A., Dagger, F., and Cabantchik, Z.I. (1994) The role of anions in pH regulation of *Leishmania* major promastigotes. *J. Biol. Chem.*, **269**, 16254–16259.

79 Thomson, L., Denicola, A., and Radi, R. (2003) The trypanothione-thiol system in *Trypanosoma cruzi* as a key antioxidant mechanism against peroxynitrite-mediated cytotoxicity. *Arch. Biochem. Biophys.*, **412**, 55–64.

80 Trujillo, M., Budde, H., Pineyro, M.D., Stehr, M., Robello, C., Flohe, L., and Radi, R. (2004) *Trypanosoma brucei* and *Trypanosoma cruzi* tryparedoxin peroxidases catalytically detoxify peroxynitrite via oxidation of fast reacting thiols. *J. Biol. Chem.*, **279**, 34175–34182.

81 Moutiez, M., Meziene-Cherif, D., Aumercier, M., Sergheraert, C., and Tartar, A. (1994) Compared reactivities of trypanothione and glutathione in conjugation reactions. *Chem. Pharm. Bull.*, **42**, 2641–2644.

82 Trujillo, M., Alvarez, B., Souza, J.M., Romero, N., Castro, L., Thomson, L., and Radi, R. (2010) Mechanisms and biological consequences of peroxynitrite-dependent protein oxidation and nitration, in *Nitric Oxide Biology and Pathobiology* (ed. L.J. Ignarro), Elsevier, Los Angeles, CA, pp. 61–102.

83 Pineyro, M.D., Arcari, T., Robello, C., Radi, R., and Trujillo, M. (2011) Tryparedoxin peroxidases from *Trypanosoma cruzi*: high efficiency in the catalytic elimination of hydrogen peroxide and peroxynitrite. *Arch. Biochem. Biophys.*, **507**, 287–295.

84 Piacenza, L., Peluffo, G., Alvarez, M.N., Kelly, J.M., Wilkinson, S.R., and Radi, R. (2008) Peroxiredoxins play a major role in protecting *Trypanosoma cruzi* against macrophage- and endogenously-derived peroxynitrite. *Biochem. J.*, **410**, 359–368.

85 Gil, J.R., Soler, A., Azzouz, S., and Osuna, A. (2003) Ion regulation in the different life stages of *Trypanosoma cruzi*. *Parasitol. Res.*, **90**, 268–272.

86 Denicola, A., Souza, J.M., and Radi, R. (1998) Diffusion of peroxynitrite across erythrocyte membranes. *Proc. Natl. Acad. Sci. USA*, **95**, 3566–3571.

87 Marla, S.S., Lee, J., and Groves, J.T. (1997) Peroxynitrite rapidly permeates phospholipid membranes. *Proc. Natl. Acad. Sci. USA*, **94**, 14243–14248.

88 Ley, V., Robbins, E.S., Nussenzweig, V., and Andrews, N.W. (1990) The exit of *Trypanosoma cruzi* from the phagosome is inhibited by raising the pH of acidic compartments. *J. Exp. Med.*, **171**, 401–413.

89 Murphy, R.F., Powers, S., and Cantor, C.R. (1984) Endosome pH measured in single cells by dual fluorescence flow cytometry: rapid acidification of insulin to pH 6. *J. Cell Biol.*, **98**, 1757–1762.

90 Van Der Heyden, N. and Docampo, R. (2000) Intracellular pH in mammalian stages of *Trypanosoma cruzi* is K^+-dependent and regulated by H^+-ATPases. *Mol. Biochem. Parasitol.*, **105**, 237–251.

91 Ariyanayagam, M.R. and Fairlamb, A.H. (2001) Ovothiol and trypanothione as antioxidants in trypanosomatids. *Mol. Biochem. Parasitol.*, **115**, 189–198.

92 Krauth-Siegel, R.L. and Comini, M.A. (2008) Redox control in trypanosomatids, parasitic protozoa with trypanothione-based thiol metabolism. *Biochim. Biophys. Acta*, **1780**, 1236–1248.

93 Maya, J.D., Repetto, Y., Agosin, M., Ojeda, J.M., Tellez, R., Gaule, C., and Morello, A. (1997) Effects of nifurtimox and benznidazole upon glutathione and trypanothione content in epimastigote, trypomastigote and amastigote forms of *Trypanosoma cruzi*. *Mol. Biochem. Parasitol.*, **86**, 101–106.

94 Pineyro, M.D., Parodi-Talice, A., Arcari, T., and Robello, C. (2008) Peroxiredoxins from *Trypanosoma cruzi*: virulence factors and drug targets for treatment of Chagas disease? *Gene.*, **408**, 45–50.

95 Piacenza, L., Zago, M.P., Peluffo, G., Alvarez, M.N., Basombrio, M.A., and Radi, R. (2009) Enzymes of the antioxidant network as novel determiners of *Trypanosoma cruzi* virulence. *Int. J. Parasitol.*, **39**, 1455–1464.

96 Wilkinson, S.R., Meyer, D.J., Taylor, M.C., Bromley, E.V., Miles, M.A., and Kelly, J.M. (2002) The *Trypanosoma cruzi* enzyme TcGPXI is a glycosomal peroxidase and can be linked to trypanothione reduction by glutathione or tryparedoxin. *J. Biol. Chem.*, **277**, 17062–17071.

97 de Souza, W. (1984) Cell biology of *Trypanosoma cruzi*. *Int. Rev. Cytol.*, **86**, 197–283.

98 Ariyanayagam, M.R., Oza, S.L., Mehlert, A., and Fairlamb, A.H. (2003) Bis (glutathionyl)spermine and other novel trypanothione analogues in *Trypanosoma cruzi*. *J. Biol. Chem.*, **278**, 27612–27619.

99 Piacenza, L., Alvarez, M.N., Peluffo, G., and Radi, R. (2009) Fighting the oxidative assault: the *Trypanosoma cruzi* journey to infection. *Curr. Opin. Microbiol.*, **12**, 415–421.

100 Rubbo, H., Denicola, A., and Radi, R. (1994) Peroxynitrite inactivates thiol-containing enzymes of *Trypanosoma cruzi* energetic metabolism and inhibits cell respiration. *Arch. Biochem. Biophys.*, **308**, 96–102.

101 Thomson, L., Gadelha, F.R., Peluffo, G., Vercesi, A.E., and Radi, R. (1999) Peroxynitrite affects Ca^{2+} transport in *Trypanosoma cruzi*. *Mol. Biochem. Parasitol.*, **98**, 81–91.

102 Denicola, A., Rubbo, H., Haden, L., and Turrens, J.F. (2002) Extramitochondrial localization of NADH-fumarate reductase

in trypanosomatids. *Comp. Biochem. Physiol. B*, **133**, 23–27.

103 Pryor, W.A., Jin, X., and Squadrito, G.L. (1994) One- and two-electron oxidations of methionine by peroxynitrite. *Proc. Natl. Acad. Sci. USA*, **91**, 11173–11177.

104 Santos, C.X., Anjos, E.I., and Augusto, O. (1999) Uric acid oxidation by peroxynitrite: multiple reactions, free radical formation, and amplification of lipid oxidation. *Arch. Biochem. Biophys.*, **372**, 285–294.

105 Squadrito, G.L., Cueto, R., Splenser, A.E., Valavanidis, A., Zhang, H., Uppu, R.M., and Pryor, W.A. (2000) Reaction of uric acid with peroxynitrite and implications for the mechanism of neuroprotection by uric acid. *Arch. Biochem. Biophys.*, **376**, 333–337.

106 Gadelha, F.R., Thomson, L., Fagian, M.M., Costa, A.D., Radi, R., and Vercesi, A.E. (1997) Ca^{2+}-independent permeabilization of the inner mitochondrial membrane by peroxynitrite is mediated by membrane protein thiol cross-linking and lipid peroxidation. *Arch. Biochem. Biophys.*, **345**, 243–250.

107 Moreno, S.N., Silva, J., Vercesi, A.E., and Docampo, R. (1994) Cytosolic-free calcium elevation in *Trypanosoma cruzi* is required for cell invasion. *J. Exp. Med.*, **180**, 1535–1540.

108 Lammel, E.M., Barbieri, M.A., Wilkowsky, S.E., Bertini, F., and Isola, E.L. (1996) *Trypanosoma cruzi*: involvement of intracellular calcium in multiplication and differentiation. *Exp. Parasitol.*, **83**, 240–249.

109 Irigoin, F., Inada, N.M., Fernandes, M.P., Piacenza, L., Gadelha, F.R., Vercesi, A.E., and Radi, R. (2009) Mitochondrial calcium overload triggers complement-dependent superoxide-mediated programmed cell death in *Trypanosoma cruzi*. *Biochem. J.*, **418**, 595–604.

110 Bryk, R., Griffin, P., and Nathan, C. (2000) Peroxynitrite reductase activity of bacterial peroxiredoxins. *Nature*, **407**, 211–215.

111 Trujillo, M., Ferrer-Sueta, G., and Radi, R. (2008) Peroxynitrite detoxification and its biologic implications. *Antioxid. Redox Signal*, **10**, 1607–1620.

112 Guerrero, S.A., Lopez, J.A., Steinert, P., Montemartini, M., Kalisz, H.M., Colli, W., Singh, M., Alves, M.J., and Flohe, L. (2000) His-tagged tryparedoxin peroxidase of *Trypanosoma cruzi* as a tool for drug screening. *Appl. Microbiol. Biotechnol.*, **53**, 410–414.

113 Wilkinson, S.R., Temperton, N.J., Mondragon, A., and Kelly, J.M. (2000) Distinct mitochondrial and cytosolic enzymes mediate trypanothione-dependent peroxide metabolism in *Trypanosoma cruzi*. *J. Biol. Chem.*, **275**, 8220–8225.

114 Hofmann, B., Hecht, H.J., and Flohe, L. (2002) Peroxiredoxins. *Biol. Chem.*, **383**, 347–364.

115 Trujillo, M., Ferrer-Sueta, G., and Radi, R. (2008) Kinetic studies on peroxynitrite reduction by peroxiredoxins. *Methods Enzymol.*, **441**, 173–196.

116 Poole, L.B. (2007) The catalytic mechanism of peroxiredoxins. *Subcell. Biochem.*, **44**, 61–81.

117 Pineyro, M.D., Pizarro, J.C., Lema, F., Pritsch, O., Cayota, A., Bentley, G.A., and Robello, C. (2005) Crystal structure of the tryparedoxin peroxidase from the human parasite *Trypanosoma cruzi*. *J. Struct. Biol.*, **150**, 11–22.

118 Flohe, L., Budde, H., Bruns, K., Castro, H., Clos, J., Hofmann, B., Kansal-Kalavar, S., Krumme, D., Menge, U., Plank-Schumacher, K., Sztajer, H., Wissing, J., Wylegalla, C., and Hecht, H.J. (2002) Tryparedoxin peroxidase of *Leishmania donovani*: molecular cloning, heterologous expression, specificity, and catalytic mechanism. *Arch. Biochem. Biophys.*, **397**, 324–335.

119 Nelson, K.J., Knutson, S.T., Soito, L., Klomsiri, C., Poole, L.B., and Fetrow, J.S. (2011) Analysis of the peroxiredoxin family: active-site structure and sequence information for global classification and residue analysis. *Proteins*, **79**, 947–964.

120 Trujillo, M., Clippe, A., Manta, B., Ferrer-Sueta, G., Smeets, A., Declercq, J.P., Knoops, B., and Radi, R. (2007) Pre-steady state kinetic characterization of human peroxiredoxin 5: taking advantage of Trp84 fluorescence increase upon oxidation. *Arch. Biochem. Biophys.*, **467**, 95–106.

121 Ogusucu, R., Rettori, D., Munhoz, D.C., Netto, L.E., and Augusto, O. (2007) Reactions of yeast thioredoxin peroxidases I and II with hydrogen peroxide and peroxynitrite: rate constants by competitive kinetics. *Free Radic. Biol. Med.*, **42**, 326–334.

122 Ferrer-Sueta, G., Manta, B., Botti, H., Radi, R., Trujillo, M., and Denicola, A. (2011) Factors affecting protein thiol reactivity and specificity in peroxide reduction. *Chem. Res. Toxicol.*, **24**, 434–450.

123 Hall, A., Parsonage, D., Poole, L.B., and Karplus, P.A. (2010) Structural evidence that peroxiredoxin catalytic power is based on transition-state stabilization. *J. Mol. Biol.*, **402**, 194–209.

124 Nagy, P., Karton, A., Betz, A., Peskin, A.V., Pace, P., O'Reilly, R.J., Hampton, M.B., Radom, L., and Winterbourn, C.C. (2011) Model for the exceptional reactivity of peroxiredoxins 2 and 3 with hydrogen peroxide: a kinetic and computational study. *J. Biol. Chem.*, **286**, 18048–18055.

125 Billiet, L., Geerlings, P., Messens, J., and Roos, G. (2012) The thermodynamics of thiol sulfenylation. *Free Radic. Biol. Med.*, **52**, 1473–1485.

126 Castro, H., Budde, H., Flohe, L., Hofmann, B., Lunsdorf, H., Wissing, J., and Tomas, A.M. (2002) Specificity and kinetics of a mitochondrial peroxiredoxin of *Leishmania infantum*. *Free Radic. Biol. Med.*, **33**, 1563–1574.

127 Castro, H., Romao, S., Carvalho, S., Teixeira, F., Sousa, C., and Tomas, A.M. (2010) Mitochondrial redox metabolism in trypanosomatids is independent of tryparedoxin activity. *PLoS ONE*, **5**, e12607.

128 Meziane-Cherif, D., Aumercier, M., Kora, I., Sergheraert, C., Tartar, A., Dubremetz, J.F., and Ouaissi, M.A. (1994) *Trypanosoma cruzi*: immunolocalization of trypanothione reductase. *Exp. Parasitol.*, **79**, 536–541.

129 Smith, K., Opperdoes, F.R., and Fairlamb, A.H. (1991) Subcellular distribution of trypanothione reductase in bloodstream and procyclic forms of *Trypanosoma* *brucei. Mol. Biochem. Parasitol.*, **48**, 109–112.

130 Castro, H., Romao, S., Gadelha, F.R., and Tomas, A.M. (2008) *Leishmania infantum*: provision of reducing equivalents to the mitochondrial tryparedoxin/tryparedoxin peroxidase system. *Exp. Parasitol.*, **120**, 421–423.

131 Wilkinson, S.R. and Kelly, J.M. (2003) The role of glutathione peroxidases in trypanosomatids. *Biol. Chem.*, **384**, 517–525.

132 Selles, B., Hugo, M., Trujillo, M., Srivastava, V., Wingsle, G., Jacquot, J.P., Radi, R., and Rouhier, N. (2012) Hydroperoxide and peroxynitrite reductase activity of poplar thioredoxin-dependent glutathione peroxidase 5: kinetics, catalytic mechanism and oxidative inactivation. *Biochem. J.*, **442**, 369–380.

133 Atwood, J.A.3rd, Weatherly, D.B., Minning, T.A., Bundy, B., Cavola, C., Opperdoes, F.R., Orlando, R., and Tarleton, R.L. (2005) The *Trypanosoma cruzi* proteome. *Science*, **309**, 473–476.

134 Parodi-Talice, A., Monteiro-Goes, V., Arrambide, N., Avila, A.R., Duran, R., Correa, A., Dallagiovanna, B., Cayota, A., Krieger, M., Goldenberg, S., and Robello, C. (2007) Proteomic analysis of metacyclic trypomastigotes undergoing *Trypanosoma cruzi* metacyclogenesis. *J. Mass. Spectrom.*, **42**, 1422–1432.

135 Mateo, H., Marin, C., Perez-Cordon, G., and Sanchez-Moreno, M. (2008) Purification and biochemical characterization of four iron superoxide dismutases in *Trypanosoma cruzi. Mem. Inst. Oswaldo. Cruz.*, **103**, 271–276.

136 Gardner, P.R. (2002) Aconitase: sensitive target and measure of superoxide. *Methods Enzymol.*, **349**, 9–23.

137 Piacenza, L., Irigoin, F., Alvarez, M.N., Peluffo, G., Taylor, M.C., Kelly, J.M., Wilkinson, S.R., and Radi, R. (2007) Mitochondrial superoxide radicals mediate programmed cell death in *Trypanosoma cruzi*: cytoprotective action of mitochondrial iron superoxide dismutase overexpression. *Biochem. J.*, **403**, 323–334.

12
Selenoproteome of Kinetoplastids

*Alexei V. Lobanov and Vadim N. Gladyshev**

Abstract

Selenocysteine (Sec) is a naturally occurring twenty first amino acid that is present in the active sites of several oxidoreductases. Proteins containing Sec, selenoproteins, occur in all three domains of life; however, the use of Sec in lower eukaryotes, and in particular in parasitic protists, is variable, because many organisms have lost the ability to utilize Sec. The genomes of flagellated protozoa *Trypanosoma* and *Leishmania* encode three selenoproteins. Two of these proteins are distant homologs of mammalian SelK and SelT. The third selenoprotein is a novel multidomain selenoprotein designated SelTryp. This protein appears to be a Kinetoplastida-specific protein and has neither Sec- nor cysteine-containing homologs in the human host. In all three selenoproteins, Sec is present within predicted redox motifs. The use of selenium for protein synthesis was verified by metabolically labeling *Trypanosoma* cells with [75]Se. In addition, a complete set of genes coding for components of the Sec insertion machinery was identified in the Kinetoplastida genomes. Further studies revealed that the selenoproteome of *Trypanosoma* is dispensable, but relevant for long-term protection. Finally, it was found that *T. b. brucei* cells are sensitive to auranofin, the drug that targets selenoproteins.

Introduction

Several years ago, the genomes of the kinetoplastids *Trypanosoma* and *Leishmania* were sequenced and annotated [1–3]. Correct genome annotation and understanding of functions of proteins encoded in kinetoplastid genomes are crucial for drug development and disease prevention [4,5]. One of the challenges with proper genome annotation is that the existing annotation tools could not recognize genes coding for selenocysteine (Sec)-containing proteins. This is because Sec (the twenty first naturally occurring amino acid in the genetic code) is encoded by UGA, which is recognized as one of three signals that terminate protein synthesis [6,7].

* Corresponding Author

Trypanosomatid Diseases: Molecular Routes to Drug Discovery, First edition. Edited by T. Jäger, O. Koch, and L. Flohé.
© 2013 Wiley-VCH Verlag GmbH & Co. KGaA. Published 2013 by Wiley-VCH Verlag GmbH & Co. KGaA.

Earlier studies revealed that *L. major*, *T. cruzi*, and *T. brucei* contain a gene coding for a homolog of selenophosphate synthetase. This enzyme generates selenophosphate – a selenium donor compound used for biosynthesis of Sec [8]. However, selenophosphate synthetase may also be involved in the pathways other than Sec biosynthesis [9], so the question whether *Leishmania* and other Kinetoplastida utilize Sec remained unanswered.

Whether UGA is treated as a stop codon or used for incorporation of Sec into nascent polypeptides depends on the presence of the Sec insertion sequence (SECIS) element in the 3'-untranslated regions of translated mRNAs [6]. Several computational tools have been developed for the identification of SECIS elements. Also, it was reported that SECIS elements in closely related species show significant homology [10]. This allows application of evolutionary criteria that reduce the number of candidates during genome searches. In the case of Kinetoplastida, the availability of multiple completely sequenced genomes allowed simultaneous analysis of several of these genomes to be performed to identify selenoprotein genes present in these organisms.

Identification of selenoprotein genes in Kinetoplastida was carried out by searching available genomic sequences for SECIS element candidates that satisfy eukaryotic consensus SECIS structure, have reasonable similarity to known SECIS elements, and have at least one homolog in other Kinetoplastida. As a result, three putative selenoprotein genes were identified in these organisms. Two of them belonged to protein families found in many other eukaryotic species. The third selenoprotein showed no homology to known proteins and was concluded to represent a new selenoprotein family.

Kinetoplastid Selenoproteome

Trypanosoma and *Leishmania* were examined by searching available sequenced genomes of these organisms for the occurrence of homologs of known selenoprotein genes with TBLASTN. This approach detected two selenoprotein families, homologous to human SelK and SelT. SECIS elements in the SelK family satisfied the default pattern of SECISearch, but the SECIS elements in SelT genes differed from the typical SECIS structure and their identification posed a challenge, as they could not be detected even with the loose pattern of SECISearch [11]. A modified version of SECISearch was then developed, and the analysis of entire genomes and genome survey sequences of *T. congolense*, *T. cruzi*, *T. vivax*, *T. gambiense*, *T. b. brucei*, *L. major*, *L. infantum*, and *L. braziliensis* was carried out. An additional requirement was the presence of SECIS homologs in other Kinetoplastida. During this analysis, six homologous groups of candidates were identified. All selenoprotein-coding genes that were found in *Leishmania* and *Trypanosoma* lacked introns. The candidates included homologs of SelK and SelT, as well as a new selenoprotein family designated SelTryp (Figure 12.1). The remaining candidates could be filtered out because they lacked predicted open reading frames with suitable in-frame TGA codons upstream of SECIS elements.

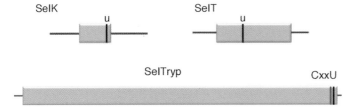

Figure 12.1 Selenoproteome of kinetoplastids. Three selenoprotein families are present in *Trypanosoma* and *Leishmania* cells. SelT and SelK have distant homologs in mammals, and SelTryp is unique for kinetoplastids. Location of Sec in selenoproteins is indicated by vertical lines and a one-letter designation for Sec, U. SelTryp has a conserved CxxU motif in the C-terminal tail (Cys and Sec separated by two other residues). Boxes indicate coding sequences and horizontal lines indicate untranslated sequences.

Analysis of SelTryp sequences revealed distant homology to rhodanese-like proteins and the presence of conserved cysteines in the rhodanese domains within a six-amino-acid active-site loop (CxGGxR) suggested that this protein belonged to the YceA subfamily [12]. The N-terminal sequences of SelTryp belonged to a metallo-β-lactamase superfamily of proteins. The lack of secondary structures in the C-terminal region of SelTryp suggested the presence of a flexible C-terminal Sec-containing tail. Subcellular localization prediction tools suggested a mitochondrial localization of SelTryp. In SelTryp, Sec is present within a CxxU motif, which suggests a redox function for this motif.

To verify selenium insertion into *Trypanosoma* proteins, *Trypanosoma* cells were metabolically labeled with ^{75}Se. This analysis showed that selenoproteins were expressed in *Trypanosoma* cells at low levels. In addition, the necessary components of the Sec insertion machinery (selenophosphate synthetase, Sec tRNA-specific elongation factor, Sec-tRNA) were identified [8,11].

Since gold compounds (such as auranofin) were shown to inhibit eukaryotic selenoenzymes, the impact of auranofin on the growth of *T. b. brucei* was studied. It was shown that this compound was toxic for bloodstream and procyclic stages of the parasite, making auranofin an interesting drug candidate [11].

Selenoproteome is Dispensable

Based on the results discussed above, it was proposed that selenoproteins, especially the trypanosomatid-specific SelTryp, might represent promising novel targets for the development of anti-parasitic drugs. To check whether targeting selenoproteins is a valid strategy for drug discovery against kinetoplastids, a study was conducted with *T. brucei* [13]. Unlike other amino acids, Sec is formed by a tRNA$^{[Ser]Sec}$-dependent conversion of serine [14,15]. The use of *T. brucei* knockout cell lines deficient for phosphoseryl-tRNA kinase (PSTK) and SecS genes revealed that these two proteins were required for Sec-tRNA formation [16], suggesting the occurrence of the pathway of Sec-tRNA synthesis that requires phosphoserine-tRNA as an intermediate, as was previously suggested for other eukaryotes that utilize selenoproteins. As such, *T. brucei* could also be used as a model to elucidate the *in vivo* pathway of Sec-tRNA formation in eukaryotes [16].

Surprisingly, it was found that neither PSTK nor SecS were essential for normal growth [16]. However, since these studies were conducted using procyclic cells, it was possible that selenoproteins may still have an essential role in the bloodstream form of *T. brucei*. To test this hypothesis, two alleles of the SecS gene in the bloodstream *T. brucei* NYSM cells were replaced by homologous recombination. Further analysis by acid urea polyacrylamide electrophoresis [17] confirmed accumulation of Sec-tRNA. However, the mean generation times for the *T. brucei* NYSM strain and SecS knockout grown in the standard bloodstream medium HMI-9 [18] were the same.

These results were unexpected because of the earlier report that showed that *T. brucei* is sensitive to nanomolar concentrations of auranofin [11]. Additional experiments showed that the sensitivity of the procyclic and bloodstream SecS knockout cell lines to auranofin was the same, and thus the role of selenoproteins and their relationship to auranofin toxicity remains unclear. Further studies are needed to address these issues. It should be noted that the growth of the procyclic and bloodstream parental cell lines, and the corresponding knockout cell lines, was reduced with increasing concentrations of H_2O_2.

Selenoproteome is Relevant for Long-Term Protection

Another study examined whether selenoproteins may be required for cells growing under suboptimal conditions by analyzing the effects of RNA interference of *T. brucei* selenophosphate synthetase SPS2 [19]. This study showed that SPS2 is involved in oxidative stress protection of the parasite and that its absence had a drastic effect on parasite survival under conditions of an oxidizing environment, leading to an apoptotic-like phenotype and cell death. Therefore, the Sec pathway in *Trypanosoma* did play a relevant role for parasite survival.

The authors demonstrated that, if the medium was replaced every day, there was no effect of SPS2 deficiency on cell growth. However, if the medium was replaced every fourth day, then SPS2 knockdown led to severe growth inhibition. The analysis of cell morphology of *T. brucei* cells showed that the knockdown cells had no nuclei (or they were fragmented), while the non-induced cells appeared normal. Also, an almost 4-fold increase in the degraded DNA peak corresponding to dead parasites was observed, which was consistent with an apoptotic-like phenotype [20]. Taken together, these results suggested that SPS2 was required for the cells growing in suboptimal conditions.

Conclusions

An *in silico* analysis of available sequenced Kinetoplastida genomes revealed the presence of three selenoprotein families. Two of them, SelT and SelK, were distant homologs of previously identified mammalian selenoproteins, and a third selenoprotein, SelTryp, appears to be unique to Kinetoplastida. This selenoprotein has two rhodanese and one rubredoxin:oxygen oxidoreductase domains, in addition to the Sec-containing C-terminal tail, and its function is unknown. The presence of selenoproteins was confirmed by metabolic labeling of *Trypanosoma* cells with ^{75}Se. These findings, as well as the presence of the Sec-incorporating machinery in Kinetoplastida genomes, demonstrated that these organisms utilize selenium. However, further experiments proved that normal growth of procyclic and bloodstream *T. brucei* in cell culture did not require selenoproteins. Selenoproteins also did not confer protection against short-term exposure to H_2O_2; however, Sec synthesis was involved in the long-term protection against oxidative stress. Thus, while Sec biosynthesis in kinetoplastids may be relevant for long-term protection against certain forms of stress, the exact roles of selenoproteins require further investigation.

References

1 Berriman, M., Ghedin, E., Hertz-Fowler, C., Blandin, G., Renauld, H., Bartholomeu, D.C., Lennard, N.J., Caler, E., Hamlin, N.E., and Haas, B. (2005) The genome of the African trypanosome *Trypanosoma brucei*. *Science*, **309**, 416–422.

2 El-Sayed, N.M., Myler, P.J., Blandin, G., Berriman, M., Crabtree, J., Aggarwal, G., Caler, E., Renauld, H., Worthey, E.A., and Hertz-Fowler, C. (2005) Comparative genomics of trypanosomatid parasitic protozoa. *Science*, **309**, 404–409.

3 Ivens, A.C. (2005) The genome of the kinetoplastid parasite, *Leishmania major*. *Science*, **309**, 436–442.

4 Krauth-Siegel, R.L., Bauer, H., and Schirmer, R.H. (2005) Dithiol proteins as guardians of the intracellular redox milieu in parasites: old and new drug targets in trypanosomes and malaria-causing plasmodia. *Angew. Chem. Int. Ed.*, **44**, 690–715.

5 Bhatia, V., Sinha, M., Luxon, B., and Garg, N. (2004) Utility of the *Trypanosoma cruzi* Sequence database for identification of potential vaccine candidates by *in silico* and *in vitro* screening. *Infect. Immun.*, **72**, 6245–6254.

6 Low, S.C. and Berry, M.J. (1996) Knowing when not to stop: selenocysteine incorporation in eukaryotes. *Trends Biochem. Sci.*, **21**, 203–208.

7 Tujebajeva, R.M., Copeland, P.R., Xu, X.M., Carlson, B.A., Harney, J.W., Driscoll, D.M., Hatfield, D.L., and Berry, M.J. (2000) Decoding apparatus for eukaryotic selenocysteine insertion. *EMBO Rep.*, **1**, 158–163.

8 Jayakumar, P.C., Musande, V.V., Shouche, Y.S., and Patole, M.S. (2004) The selenophosphate synthetase gene from *Leishmania major*. *DNA Seq.*, **15**, 66–70.

9 Romero, H., Zhang, Y., Gladyshev, V.N., and Salinas, G. (2005) Evolution of selenium utilization traits. *Genome Biol.*, **6**, R66.

10 Kryukov, G.V., Castellano, S., Novoselov, S.V., Lobanov, A.V., Zehtab, O., Guigo, R., and Gladyshev, V.N. (2003) Characterization of mammalian selenoproteomes. *Science*, **300**, 1439–1443.

11 Lobanov, A.V., Gromer, S., Salinas, G., and Gladyshev, V.N. (2006) Selenium metabolism in *Trypanosoma*: characterization of selenoproteomes and identification of a Kinetoplastida-specific selenoprotein. *Nucleic Acids Res.*, **34**, 4012–4024.

12 Bordo, D. and Bork, P. (2002) The rhodanese/Cdc25 phosphatase superfamily. Sequence–structure–function relations. *EMBO Rep.*, **3**, 741–746.

13 Aeby, E., Seidel, V., and Schneider, A. (2009) The selenoproteome is dispensable in blood-stream forms of *Trypanosoma brucei*. *Mol. Biochem. Parasit.*, **168**, 191–193.

14 Commans, S. and Böck, A. (1999) Selenocysteine inserting tRNAs: an

overview. *FEMS Microbiol. Rev.*, **23**, 335–351.

15 Hatfield, D.L., Carlson, B.A., Xu, X.M., Mix, H., and Gladyshev, V.N. (2006) Selenocysteine incorporation machinery and the role of selenoproteins in development and health. *Prog. Nucleic Acid Res. Mol. Biol*, **81**, 97–142.

16 Aeby, E., Palioura, S., Pusnik, M. *et al.* (2009) The canonical pathway for selenocysteine insertion is dispensable in Trypanosomes. *Proc. Natl. Acad. Sci. USA*, **106**, 5088–5092.

17 Varshney, U., Lee, C.-P., and RajBhandary, U.L. (1991) Direct analysis of aminoacylation levels of tRNAs *in vivo. J. Biol. Chem.*, **266**, 24712–24718.

18 Hesse, F., Selzer, P.M., Mühlstadt, K., and Duszenko, M. (1995) A novel cultivation technique for long-term maintenance of bloodstream form trypanosomes *in vitro. Mol. Biochem. Parasitol*, **70**, 157–166.

19 Costa, F.C., Oliva, M.A., de Jesus, T.C., Schenkman, S., and Thiemann, O.H. (2011) Oxidative stress protection of Trypanosomes requires selenophosphate synthase. *Mol. Biochem. Parasitol.*, **180**, 47–50.

20 Casanova, M., Portales, P., Blaineau, C., Crobu, L., Bastien, P., and Pages, M. (2008) Inhibition of active nuclear transport is an intrinsic trigger of programmed cell death in trypanosomatids. *Cell Death Differ.*, **15**, 1910–1920.

13
Replication Machinery of Kinetoplast DNA

*Rachel Bezalel-Buch, Nurit Yaffe, and Joseph Shlomai**

Abstract

Kinetoplast DNA (kDNA) is a unique DNA network found in the single mitochondrion of trypanosomatids. It consists of several thousand duplex DNA minicircles and a few dozen DNA maxicircles, which are interlocked in a giant topological catenane. Replication of kDNA includes the duplication of free minicircles and catenated maxicircles, followed by the splitting and segregation of the progeny networks upon cell division. The remarkable machinery that carries out the replication process of this unusual mitochondrial genome is described here. Recent advances in the identification and characterization of replication proteins and in the regulation of kDNA replication, as well as the re-evaluation of the potential use of kDNA replication proteins as targets for the development of anti-trypanosomal drugs are discussed.

Introduction: kDNA Network and its Monomeric Subunits

Kinetoplast DNA (kDNA) is the mitochondrial genome of flagellated protozoa of the order Kinetoplastida. Our current understanding of this remarkable DNA structure and its unique replication machinery is based mainly on the study of the non-pathogenic species of the family Trypanosomatidae, especially *Crithidia fasciculata* and *Leishmania tarentolae*, as well as several pathogenic species of this family, such as *Trypanosoma brucei*, *T. cruzi*, *Leishmania* spp., and *Phytomonas* spp. Studies in these species yielded the "classical" view of kDNA, as a two-dimensional, fishnet-like network consisting of several thousand duplex DNA minicircles (0.5–10 kb in the different species) and several dozen maxicircles (20–40 kb), which are linked topologically into a catenane structure (reviewed in [1,2]). The network is condensed in the mitochondrial matrix, forming a disk-shaped structure. Histone H1-like proteins, known as the kinetoplast-associated proteins (KAPs), were implicated in the process of kDNA condensation [3,4]. While this chapter focuses solely on the structure and replication of the "classical" kDNA network, other forms of

---

* Corresponding Author

Trypanosomatid Diseases: Molecular Routes to Drug Discovery, First edition. Edited by T. Jäger, O. Koch, and L. Flohé.
© 2013 Wiley-VCH Verlag GmbH & Co. KGaA. Published 2013 by Wiley-VCH Verlag GmbH & Co. KGaA.

"non-classical" kDNA, consisting of topologically unlinked DNA minicircles, have been described in free-living, as well as parasitic species, of this group (reviewed in [5]).

Maxicircles encode for mitochondrial products, such as ribosomal RNA and protein subunits of the respiratory chain. Their mRNA transcripts undergo a post-transcriptional editing process, to create translatable open reading frames. The guide RNA (gRNA) molecules, which participate in the editing of maxicircles transcripts, are encoded mainly by the kDNA minicircles (recently reviewed in [6]). Minicircles are topologically relaxed and singly-interlocked to each other [7], while maxicircles form a topological catenane, which is threaded within the minicircles network, forming a "network within a network" [8,9].

Here, we present an overview of recent advances (last 5–6 years) in the understanding of the control of kDNA replication in trypanosomatids. Recent studies have focused on the enzyme components of the kDNA replication machinery. These included proteins that bind the kDNA replication origins [10–15], as well as enzymes that catalyze the priming of kDNA synthesis [16,17], kDNA chain elongation [18–20], repair of kDNA replicating intermediates [21,22], unwinding of the kDNA double helix [23–25], and the topological reactions required during kDNA replication [26,27]. Other recent studies have focused on the identification of the regulatory mechanisms that trigger and control the action of the kDNA replication machinery, yielding new insights into the regulation of minicircle and maxicircle replication [10–13,15,23–25]. Yet other studies were aimed at the structural dynamics of the replicating networks, and the regulation of their replication and segregation [13,27–29]. Earlier studies on the kDNA replication machinery were discussed in previous reviews (e.g., [1,2]).

Replication of kDNA Minicircles, Maxicircles, and Networks

kDNA networks replicate in a discrete kinetoplast S phase during the S phase of the cell cycle [28,30]. The current model (Figure 13.1) describing the replication of kDNA networks [1,2] suggests that during S phase covalently closed (CC) minicircles are decatenated from the network by a DNA topoisomerase II (TopoII; yet to be identified). They are released into the kinetoflagellar zone (KFZ), located near the network surface closer to the basal body [31], where they replicate as free DNA circles, through theta (θ) structure intermediates. Two conserved minicircle sequence blocks (CSBs), a 12mer (CSB-3), known as the universal minicircle sequence (UMS), and the 10mer CSB-1, overlap with the 5′-termini of the newly synthesized minicircle H- and L-strands, and hence were proposed as the replication origins of the minicircle L- and H-strands, respectively [32,33]. The UMS sequence GGGGTTGGTGTA and the hexamer sequence ACGCCC (in CSB-1) were conserved in all trypanosomatid species studied [1]. Initiation of the continuous L-strand synthesis, which starts minicircle replication, is by the synthesis of an RNA primer at the UMS. Discontinuous H-strand synthesis was suggested to initiate opposite the conserved hexamer sequence, using the displaced parental L-strand as a template (reviewed in [1,2]). The minicircle replication initiator UMSBP [13] and

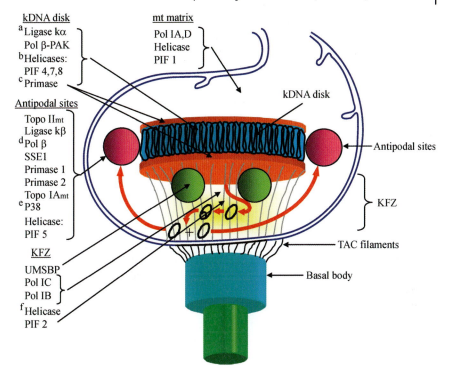

kDNA disk
[a]Ligase kα
Pol β-PAK
[b]Helicases:
PIF 4,7,8
[c]Primase

mt matrix
Pol IA,D
Helicase
PIF 1

kDNA disk

Antipodal sites
Topo IImt
Ligase kβ
[d]Pol β
SSE1
Primase 1
Primase 2
Topo IAmt
[e]P38
Helicase:
PIF 5

Antipodal sites

KFZ

KFZ
UMSBP
Pol IC
Pol IB
[f]Helicase
PIF 2

TAC filaments

Basal body

Figure 13.1 kDNA replication proteins and the kDNA replication model. The model is based mainly on studies in *C. fasciculata* and *T. brucei*. During replication, CC minicircles are released from the network into the KFZ by a DNA TopoII. They initiate their replication at the KFZ, forming theta (θ) structure intermediates. Free progeny minicircles then migrate to the antipodal sites, where repair of most discontinuities in Okazaki fragments occurs. The minicircles are then reattached to the network periphery by a DNA TopoII (TopoII$_{mt}$). Repair enzymes then complete the repair of the remaining discontinuities in the reattached minicircles just prior to the division and segregation of the network. The TAC filaments system, linking the kDNA to the flagellar basal body, is shown. Replication proteins are grouped according to their intramitochondrial localization to four regions on the kDNA disk or surrounding it, as follows: (i) in the two antipodal sites, at the edge of the kDNA disk; (ii) in the KFZ; (iii) throughout the kDNA disk; and (iv) throughout the mitochondrial matrix (mt matrix). A cell cycle-dependent localization of kDNA replication proteins was observed with several replication proteins (e.g., DNA Pol β, TopoII, SSE1, UMSBP, LIG kα, TopoIA$_{mt}$, and PIF8). [a]LIG kα was localized to both faces of the kDNA disk and the KFZ in *C. fasciculata*, and throughout the kDNA disk in *T. brucei* [21,50]. [b]PIF8 was localized to the face of the disk, distal to the basal body and its clustering at this location changes at different stages of kDNA replication [48]. [c]Primase refers to the DNA primase described in [43]. [d]LIG kβ was localized at the two antipodal sites and at the two faces of the kDNA disk in *C. fasciculata* and showed a discrete localization to the antipodal sites in *T. brucei* [21]. [e]p38 was localized throughout the mitochondrion and was enriched at the antipodal sites [15]. [f]Cells with an increased *Tb*PIF2 level, due to knockdown of *Tb*HslU1U2 were examined. *Tb*PIF2 is positioned as an elongated zone or two distinct foci in the KFZ [25]. (Reprinted and modified with permission from [2]. © 2005, Elsevier.)

protein p38 [15], as well as DNA primase 2 (PRI2) [16], DNA polymerases POLIB–D [18] and DNA TopoIA$_{mt}$ [26], where proposed to function in this process. The resulting progeny minicircles contain nicks and gaps, since unlike in other replication systems, repair of replicating minicircles occurs only after the completion of DNA strand synthesis. DNA helicase PIF1 [23], as well as the mitochondrial DNA TopoII$_{mt}$ [23,34], were implicated in the process of progeny minicircle segregation. Minicircles are then transferred, by a yet unknown mechanism, onto two antipodal reattachment sites, at the edge of the network. At these sites, primer-excision, gap-filling, and nick-sealing activities were proposed to occur, through the action of repair enzymes, including the structure-specific endonuclease 1 (SSE1) and DNA polymerase β (Pol β) (reviewed in [1]), as well as the recently described DNA ligase kβ (LIG kβ) [21] and DNA helicase *Tb*PIF5 [24], which are located at these sites. Then, minicircles, still containing discontinuities, are reattached to the network by TopoII$_{mt}$. The reattached minicircles undergo final gap-filling and nick-sealing, suggested to be catalyzed by Pol β–PAK (reviewed in [1,2]) and the recently described LIG kα [21], both located throughout the network.

Maxicircles undergo replication while topologically interlocked with minicircles and other maxicircles in the network. The maxicircle genome consists of a region encoding typical mitochondrial products and a non-coding variable region, containing repeated sequences, which also contains the replication origin. Catenated maxicircles replicate via theta (θ) structure intermediates (reviewed in [1]). It has been recently reported that the *T. brucei* DNA primase 1 (*Tb*PRI1) [17], as well as the DNA helicase *Tb*PIF2 [25], function in maxicircle replication. It had been earlier suggested that mitochondrial RNA polymerase also plays a role in maxicircle replication (reviewed in [1]). It has been shown, in both earlier and recent studies [28,35,36], that during kDNA replication, maxicircles accumulate gradually in the middle of the network [9,28]. They are stretched out between the segregating progeny networks and, hence, maxicircle segregation is the final event during the process of the network division [28].

The inheritance of a complete repertoire of gRNA molecules in each of the progeny kDNA networks is vital to mitochondrial function and cell survival. Hence, progeny minicircles have to duplicate once per generation and be distributed throughout the replicating network, in a pattern that would enable the equal distribution of the genetic information upon the network division and segregation of the progeny networks. The mechanism of book-keeping, which controls a single replication initiation per each individual minicircle, is yet unknown (for further discussion, see [1]).

Early experiments have shown that in both *C. fasciculata* and *T. brucei* newly replicated progeny minicircles reattach to the replicating network at two antipodal sites. However, in *C. fasciculata* they are uniformly distributed around the network periphery, whereas in *T. brucei* they accumulate near the two polar attachment sites [9]. These observations revealed two strategies that are applied in trypanosomatids for the reattachment of minicircles to replicating kDNA networks. The first, known as the "annular rotating disk" mechanism, is based mainly on studies in the species *C. fasciculata*. Here, the uniform distribution of newly replicated minicircles throughout the network periphery is due to the relative movement of the two antipodal sites and the kinetoplast disk [37]. The second, known as the "polar replication model," was extensively studied in *T. brucei*, revealing the accumulation of minicircles near the two polar attachment sites [9].

kDNA replication is tightly linked with cell morphogenesis during the trypanosome cell cycle (recently reviewed in [38]). The proximal end of the basal body is linked to the kDNA disk via the filaments of the tripartite attachment complex (TAC) [39], and the basal body movement drives the segregation and positioning of daughter kinetoplasts [38]. Perturbation of TAC proteins p166 [29] and AEP-1 [40] resulted in defects in kDNA segregation. In a recent study, Gluenz *et al.* [28] have found that kDNA S phase and the repositioning of the new basal body from the anterior to the posterior side of the old basal body occur at the same time. Based on the temporal correlation between basal body positioning and kDNA rotation, these investigators suggested that the rotational movements of the two structures are causally linked [28].

Components of the kDNA Replication Machinery: Replication Proteins and Complexes

Currently, many of the proteins anticipated in the replication of kDNA have been identified and characterized (Figure 13.1). This was achieved in earlier work, mainly by protein purification and intramitochondrial localization by fluorescence microscopy. Recent studies have used, in addition, genomics and proteomics approaches and molecular genetics techniques.

Recognition of the Replication Origin: UMS-Binding Protein (UMSBP) and p38

The UMS-binding protein (UMSBP) [41] is a sequence-specific single-stranded DNA-binding protein that interacts with the 12mer UMS and the hexamer sequence (in the context of 14mer sequence) at the origin region. It was first purified from *C. fasciculata* and orthologs of the *UMSBP* gene have been found in the genomes of other trypanosomatids species [13]. In the species *C. fasciculata*, UMSBP is a 13.7-kDa polypeptide, containing five CCHC-type zinc-finger motifs, which was immunolocalized to two distinct foci at the KFZ [1].

Binding of UMSBP to kDNA in the trypanosomatid cell was shown in *C. fasciculata*, using *in vivo* protein–DNA cross-linking analysis [14] and its functional role, as a minicircle replication initiator, was examined in *T. brucei* using RNA interference (RNAi) analysis [13]. The *T. brucei* genome contains two distinct *UMSBP* orthologs, named *TbUMSBP1* and *TbUMSBP2*, whose simultaneous silencing resulted in cell growth arrest [13]. Analysis of minicircle replication intermediates in the RNAi-induced cells revealed a significant increase in the abundance of free, CC prereplicated minicircles, with a concomitant decrease in the abundance of nicked and gapped (N/G) replication intermediates. These observations indicated that in the RNAi-induced cells, minicircles were released from the network, but failed to initiate their replication, supporting the function of UMSBP in minicircle replication initiation [13]. Fluorescence microscopy of DAPI-stained cells revealed that the *TbUMSBPs* knocked-down cells developed large nuclei and kinetoplasts (around 2- and 5-fold larger than in the uninduced cells, respectively), with the accumulation of high amounts of DNA in both organelles. Biochemical analyses of isolated kDNA networks from the *TbUMSBPs* knocked-down cells, as well as electron microscopy of thin sections of cells, indicated their content of unsegregated kDNA networks [13]. Immunofluorescence analyses revealed that the block of kDNA segregation, observed in the knocked-down cells, is accompanied by impairment of the flagellar basal bodies segregation, as well as of the flagella separation.

In a recent study, Kapeller *et al.* [10] have found that UMSBP interacts with two of the mitochondrial histone H1-like proteins, KAP3 and KAP4 [3,4]. This study has shown that protein–protein interactions between UMSBP and the KAP proteins resulted in the decondensation of the KAP-condensed kDNA network. It further demonstrated that UMSBP-mediated decondensation of kDNA *in vitro* enhanced the network accessibility to DNA-interacting proteins, enabling the topological decatenation of kDNA by DNA TopoII, to yield free minicircle monomers. Based on these observations, it was speculated that UMSBP may function *in vivo* in the remodeling of kDNA, enabling the prereplication release of minicircles from the network and, consequently, promoting their replication initiation.

Liu *et al.* [15] have identified a mitochondrial DNA-binding protein in *T. brucei* that binds specifically the conserved minicircle origin sequences. This protein, named p38, was described previously (as RBP38) in trypanosomatids (e.g., [42]), and was associated with expression of nuclear genes and binding to GT-rich sequences. p38 was localized throughout the mitochondrion and was specifically enriched at or near the antipodal sites flanking the kDNA disk. Silencing of the *P38* gene by RNAi resulted in the loss of kDNA minicircles and maxicircles, as well as of free minicircle replication intermediates, indicating a role for this protein in kDNA replication. Knockdown of *P38* also resulted in the accumulation of a novel, extremely underwound, free minicircle species (Fraction S), which generates a Z-DNA region. It was found that p38 binds an oligonucleotide containing the UMS and an oligonucleotide containing the conserved hexamer sequence. Based on these observations, p38 was suggested to affect kDNA replication through its capacity to bind the replication origin.

Priming of DNA Synthesis: DNA Primases

Li and Englund [43] have reported on the purification and characterization of a mitochondrial DNA primase from *C. fasciculata*, whose encoding gene has not yet been identified. It was immunolocalized to two specific zones above and below the kDNA disk (reviewed in [1]).

Recently, Hines and Ray [16,17] have identified two mitochondrial DNA primases from *T. brucei*, PRI1 and PRI2, which are essential for kDNA replication. These primases contain an RNA recognition motif (RRM) and a primase motif (PriCT-2) [44]. Fluorescence microscopy localized both PRI1 and PRI2 to the antipodal sites flanking the kDNA disk. The *PRI1* gene contains two sequence elements, similar to the conserved octamer sequence involved in the cyclic expression of several S-phase-expressed genes in *C. fasciculata* [45]. Expression of *PRI1* mRNA is cyclic and reaches maximal levels during S phase. Recombinant PRI1 and PRI2 display DNA primase activity, yielding oligoribonucleotide products on a poly(dT) template. Silencing of *PRI1* by RNAi resulted in cell growth arrest and shrinkage of the network accompanied by preferential decrease of maxicircles abundance, leading to the loss of kDNA. Analysis of minicircle and maxicircle replication intermediates revealed that, whereas minicircle replication was not affected during the first 2 days post-RNAi induction, maxicircle replication was significantly and rapidly inhibited, suggesting that PRI1 functions in priming of maxicircle replication [17]. Silencing of *PRI2* by RNAi resulted in a significant loss of both minicircles and maxicircles at similar rates. Analysis of the minicircle replication intermediates in the *PRI2* knocked-down cells revealed a significant increase in the abundance of CC mini-circles with concomitant decrease in abundance of the N/G species upon RNAi induction. In contrast, analysis of maxicircle replication intermediates revealed that both the CC and N/G species were rapidly lost at the same rate [16], suggesting the function of PRI2 in minicircle replication.

kDNA Chain Elongation: DNA Polymerases

Early studies (reviewed in [1]) led to the identification of four genes, designated *TbPOLIA–D*, which encode DNA polymerases that are related to the bacterial DNA Pol I family. *Tb*POLIA and *Tb*POLID were found to be distributed uniformly throughout the mitochondrial matrix, while *Tb*POLIB and *Tb*POLIC were confined to one or two spots at the KFZ [46]. RNAi analyses have shown [46] that silencing of *TbPOLIB* and *TbPOLIC* resulted in the shrinking of the kDNA network. Silencing of *TbPOLIC* resulted in a decrease in the copy number of minicircles and maxicircles. In addition, two DNA polymerases β (Pol β and Pol β-PAK) were identified and localized at the antipodal sites and throughout the replicated network, respectively. They were implicated in gap-filling repair activities at these sites [1].

In a recent study, Bruhn *et al.* [19] reported that silencing of *POLIB* resulted in growth inhibition and progressive loss of kDNA networks. They observed a significant increase in the relative abundance of unreplicated CC minicircles, as minicircle copy number declines. A decrease in abundance of both leading and lagging strand minicircle progeny was observed, indicating that *Tb*POLIB partici-pates in both leading and lagging strand synthesis. Interestingly, two-dimensional gel electrophoresis analysis of minicircle replication intermediates in *TbPOLIB*-silenced cells revealed the accumulation of a novel population of free minicircles. Its partial characterization suggested that it is similar to the fraction of multiply interlocked CC minicircle dimers (fraction U), previously reported in DNA TopoII$_{mt}$ and *Tb*PIF1 helicase-depleted cells [23]. Chandler *et al.* [20] have recently found that knockdown of *Tb*POLID resulted in cell growth arrest and a rapid decline in minicircle and maxicircle abundance, along with the transient accumulation of minicircle replication intermediates and progressive loss of the kDNA network. With the exception of *Tb*POLIA, which seems not to be essential under normal growth conditions, replication of the kDNA network requires the three other Pol I-type DNA polymerases, *Tb*POLIB, *Tb*POLIC, and *Tb*POLID, suggesting their non-redundant roles during kDNA replication [20]. A recent report [18] demonstrated that these three mitochondrial DNA polymerases are also essential for survival of bloodstream-form *T. brucei*, providing a direct evidence that kDNA replication is essential for viability of bloodstream-form trypanosomes.

Unwinding of Duplex kDNA Circles and More: Kinetoplast DNA Helicases

The *T. brucei* genome contains eight genes, named *TbPIF1–8*, encoding for DNA helicases, which are related to the yeast gene encoding *Sc*Pif1p mitochondrial helicase. Six of these helicases are mitochondrial, but differ in their intramitochondrial localization. While *Tb*PIF1 localizes throughout the mitochondrion, *Tb*PIF4, 7, and 8 are predominantly in the kDNA disk, *Tb*PIF2 in the KFZ, and *Tb*PIF5 is enriched in the antipodal sites [25].

*Tb*PIF1 DNA helicase [23] is proposed to play a role in minicircle replication. A recombinant *Tb*PIF1 protein displayed an ATP-dependent DNA helicase activity in a DNA unwinding assay *in vitro*. RNAi silencing of *Tb*PIF1 blocked free minicircle replication, resulting in kDNA loss. Minicircle replication intermediates decrease following RNAi induction, along with the accumulation of multiply interlocked, CC minicircle dimers (fraction U) – a species found to accumulate also during silencing of the *TOPOIIMT* [23] or *POLIB* [19] by RNAi. Analysis of minicircle replication intermediates revealed a significant decrease in the abundance of the N/G species, which are replaced by fraction U, indicating that fraction U is likely to be derived from unsegregated dimeric replication intermediates. Hence, it was proposed that *Tb*PIF1 DNA helicase participates together with the DNA TopoII$_{mt}$ in the segregation of progeny minicircles [23,34].

*Tb*PIF2 DNA helicase [25] was found to be essential for maxicircle, but not for minicircle, replication. A recombinant *Tb*PIF2 protein displayed an ATP-dependent DNA unwinding activity *in vitro*. Silencing of *Tb*PIF2 by RNAi resulted in the loss of maxicircles with no effect on the replication of minicircles, while its overexpression caused several fold increase in the number of maxicircles. These observations indicated that maxicircle abundance is controlled by the level of *Tb*PIF2. It was also found that *Tb*PIF2 level increased following RNAi of the *Tb*HslVU protease [47], indicating that it is a *Tb*HslVU substrate (see below).

Recombinant *Tb*PIF5 DNA helicase [24] was found to display DNA helicase activity in a DNA unwinding assay *in vitro*. However, silencing of *Tb*PIF5 by RNAi, as well as knockout of one *TbPIF5* allele, showed no change in the cell phenotype, while knockout of both alleles was apparently lethal. Overexpression of *TbPIF5* resulted in a decrease in both CC and G/N minicircle replication intermediates and shrinkage of the network, with only a mild effect on the level of maxicircles abundance. Overexpression of *Tb*PIF5 caused an accumulation of fraction H minicircle species consisting of replication intermediates in which elongation of the lagging strand is blocked, while the leading strand is completed. These observations indicated that *Tb*PIF5 plays a role in the maturation of Okazaki fragments.

Among the eight PIF1-like proteins in *T. brucei*, *Tb*PIF8 is the most divergent [48]. It is the smallest member of the family, lacking at least two of the seven conserved helicase motifs [49]. Since it lacks essential residues in its Walker A motif, it is plausible that *Tb*PIF8 does not have ATPase or helicase activity. *Tb*PIF8 clusters on the face of the kDNA disk, which is distal to the basal body. The pattern of *Tb*PIF8 localization varies during the different stages of kDNA replication. During pre-replication of kDNA, it resides mainly in the central part of the distal face of the kDNA disk. During early kDNA replication, it spreads and covers nearly the entire distal face. After replication is completed, it covers the entire distal face of the disk with two diffused zones and then, at a later stage, it caps the whole distal face of the replicated kDNA. Finally, it clusters predominantly on one corner of the daughter kinetoplasts. Silencing of *Tb*PIF8 by stem–loop RNAi arrests cell growth and causes defects in kDNA segregation. The most common segregation defect was asymmetric division, where the two sister kinetoplasts differ in size. *Tb*PIF8 knockdown causes only limited kDNA shrinkage, but results in disorganization of the networks [48]. Although the function of *Tb*PIF8 has not yet been defined, it was suggested that it is essential for cell viability and is important for the maintenance of kDNA.

kDNA Repair Enzymes: Mitochondrial DNA Ligases

Repair activities in kDNA replication, including primer-excision, gap-filling, and nick-sealing of both the lagging and leading strand, occur only after the completion of the minicircle DNA strand synthesis. These activities take place at two different sites and during two distinct stages of kDNA replication. The first kDNA repair process occurs at the two antipodal sites prior to reattachment of minicircles to the network, where primer-excision is proposed to be catalyzed by SSE1 and RNase H1, and gap-filling is by Pol β (reviewed in [1]). Covalent sealing of the nicks was suggested to be catalyzed at this stage by the recently identified LIG kβ [21,22,50]. The second kDNA repair process occurs while minicircles are reattached to the network. Final closure of the remaining discontinuities is proposed to be catalyzed by Pol β-PAK and the recently identified DNA LIG kα [21,22,50], just prior to the network division [13]. Here, we discuss only the recently described mitochondrial DNA ligases [21,22,50]. Earlier work on kDNA repair is discussed elsewhere [1,2].

The presence of the two mitochondrial DNA ligases, distinct in both their location and time of function during kDNA replication, was recently reported in a series of studies by Dan Ray's group [21,22,50]. Sinha *et al.* [22] detected the gene *LIG kβ* encoding a mitochondrial DNA ligase in *C. fasciculata*. The encoded LIG kβ contains both the ligase consensus pattern and the ligase active-site motif [22]. The protein was localized at the two antipodal sites and also at the two faces of the kDNA disk in *C. fasciculata*, but showed a discrete localization to the antipodal sites in analysis of the *T. brucei* LIG kβ ortholog [21]. As LIG kβ coimmunoprecipitated with Pol β, it was proposed to function with Pol β in the joining of Okazaki fragments in nascent minicircles at the antipodal sites.

Shortly after the identification of LIG kβ, the presence of a second mitochondrial DNA ligase, LIG kα, was reported in *T. brucei* and *C. fasciculata* [21,50]. It was localized to both faces of the kDNA disk and to the KFZ in *C. fasciculata*, while a *T. brucei* LIG kα ortholog was localized throughout the kDNA disk. In *C. fasciculata* LIG kα was detected in dividing or newly divided kinetoplasts. In synchronized cell cultures, specific mRNA transcripts of *LIG kβ* reach their maximal level during S phase, whereas the level of *LIG kα* mRNA is maximal later in the cell cycle, during mitosis and subsequent cell division. LIG kα protein was also found to be unstable and to decay with a half-life of 100 min. Considering the localization of LIG kα to the network during kDNA division and segregation, it was suggested that LIG kα may play a role in the final closure of discontinuities in minicircles, just prior to the networks division [50].

Knockdown of *LIG kβ* expression by RNAi had no detectable effect on cell growth and morphology. On the other hand, knockdown of *LIG kα* expression resulted in cell growth arrest. *LIG kα* RNAi induction resulted in depletion of the pool of free CC minicircles and the accumulation of N/G minicircles within the network. The inhibition of ligation of discontinuities in the minicircles was followed by the loss of kDNA [21].

Topological Reactions During kDNA Replication: DNA Topoisomerases

Considering the complex topological structure of kDNA, it is anticipated that its replication and segregation would require an extensive involvement of topoisomerases. Action of topoisomerases is anticipated in the replication of minicircles and maxicircles, as well as in catalyzing the topological interconversions of minicircle monomers and catenane networks, the segregation of progeny minicircles, the remodeling of the replicating network, and finally the scission and segregation of the replicated networks. Earlier studies on the role of topoisomerases in kDNA replication were discussed in [1,2]. The following is an update of recent reports on the role of DNA topoisomerases in kDNA replication.

Lindsay *et al.* [27] have recently described a new function of the *Tb*TopoII$_{mt}$ during kDNA replication, showing that, in addition to its previously observed function in the post-replication reattachment of minicircles to the network, it also mends holes in the network, created by minicircle prereplication release. Silencing of *TbTOPOII$_{MT}$* by RNAi resulted in enlarging holes in the kDNA network with the progress in minicircle release, leading to network fragmentation. Knockdown of *TbTOPOII$_{MT}$* does not appear to affect minicircle release [27,51], raising the long-standing question of the identity of the type II DNA topoisomerase that catalyzes the prereplication release of minicircles from the network.

Socca and Shapiro [26] have recently reported on the presence of three type IA DNA topoisomerases in African trypanosomes. They designated one of these topoisomerases, which is phylogenetically distinct, TopoIA$_{mt}$. Its intramitochondrial localization varies with the progress in kDNA replication – a feature shared by several other kDNA replication proteins (e.g., [50,52]). In non-replicating cells no signal of TopoIA$_{mt}$ could be detected, and as kDNA replication progresses, it first forms capping on one side of the network and then, gradually, it is localized to the antipodal sites. Silencing of *TopoIA$_{mt}$* by RNAi resulted in significant accumulation of kDNA late theta structure replication intermediates, leading to kDNA loss and cell growth arrest. This report has provided evidence for the essential role of a type IA topoisomerase in the resolution of late theta structures *in vivo*.

Regulation of kDNA Replication

Our understanding of the mechanisms that regulate the replication of kDNA and their linkage to cell cycle control is still poor. However, a recent report by Gluenz *et al.* [28] has significantly contributed to the understanding of kDNA replication in the context of global cellular processes. These investigators described the intimate linkage between the process of replication of kDNA minicircles and maxicircles and the processes of cytoskeletal remodeling and cell morphogenesis. Their observations indicate that cytoskeleton-mediated morphogenesis orchestrates the whole cycle of kDNA replication. In this section, we discuss recent reports describing the regulation of several kDNA replication proteins through redox signaling, cyclic expression, and specific protein degradation.

Replication Initiation: Redox Regulation of UMSBP Binding to the Replication Origin

Regulation of the priming events at replication origins plays a key role in the control of genomes replication. It is mediated through the interactions of specific *cis*-element(s) at replication origins with their counterpart *trans*-acting proteins, the origin-binding proteins or origin recognition complexes (ORCs) (recently reviewed in [53]). Hence, the regulation of the minicircle origin-binding protein UMSBP was anticipated to significantly affect the initiation of kDNA replication. Early studies in synchronized *C. fasciculata* cell cultures have shown that the steady-state levels of UMSBP mRNA and protein are apparently constant throughout the entire cell cycle [52], suggesting that regulation of UMSBP activity *in vivo* may be of a post-translational nature. Further studies revealed that UMSBP binding to the conserved origin sequences is dependent on the protein redox state and that the protein binds to DNA only in its reduced monomeric form (reviewed in [1,54]).

In a recent study, Sela *et al.* [12] have used synchronized *C. fasciculata* cell cultures to monitor, independently, UMSBP's DNA-binding activity and its redox state throughout the entire cell cycle. These analyses revealed that both UMSBP activity and its redox state fluctuate in correlation, in a cell cycle-dependent manner, displaying maximal levels of DNA-binding activity and UMSBP reduction during S and M/G_1 phases. These observations suggested that UMSBP activity is regulated *in vivo* through a cell cycle-dependent control of the protein's redox state.

The hypothesis that regulation of UMSBP is mediated in the trypanosomatid cell by redox signaling [54] was examined *in vitro* by coupling the UMSBP–UMS DNA binding reaction to a reconstituted multienzyme reaction of the trypanothione (TS_2)-based redox cascade pathway. In this pathway, using NADPH as the primary source of electrons, trypanothione reductase (TR) reduces TS_2 to yield $T(SH)_2$, which reduces tryparedoxin (TXN), which in turn reduces tryparedoxin peroxidase (TXNPx) and glutathione peroxidase (GPx), that can then reduce hydroperoxides (recently reviewed in [55,56]). These studies have demonstrated that the trypanothione-based pathway, coupled to the UMSBP–DNA binding reaction, has the capacity to reversibly activate the binding of UMSBP to the origin sequence [12]. This is through the opposing effects of TXN and TXNPx on the redox state of UMSBP, functioning as a redox-mediated molecular switch.

A recent surface plasmon resonance (SPR) analysis of UMSBP–UMS DNA interactions [11] revealed that redox affects the association of UMSBP with DNA, but has little or no effect on the dissociation of UMSBP from the nucleoprotein complex. These observations suggested that redox signaling may control the binding of UMSBP to the replication origin and hence, the triggering of minicircle replication initiation. However, the release of UMSBP from the nucleoprotein complex may be regulated by a distinct mechanism [11].

Periodic Expression of kDNA Replication Genes

Earlier studies in *C. fasciculata* showed [57] that the levels of mRNA transcripts of genes encoding for several nuclear and mitochondrial DNA replication proteins, such as *LIG1, RPA1, DHFR-TS, TOPOII$_{MT}$*, and *KAP3*, cycle in parallel during the cell cycle. Their mRNAs levels were maximal just prior to S phase and then declined sharply with the completion of DNA replication. It was found that two or more copies of the consensus (C/A)AUAGAA(G/A) octamer are required in the 5′- and/or 3′-flanking regions of the transcripts for S-phase expression of these genes (reviewed in [1]).

Recently, Li *et al.* [58] have searched the *L. major* genome for S-phase-expressed genes, based on their content of the post-transcriptional cycling control elements [59]. Using this approach, an *L. major* gene, *LmP105*, was identified, which encodes a protein that was localized to the antipodal sites flanking the kinetoplast disk in a cell cycle-dependent manner. mRNA transcripts of *Lmp105* were found to cycle, displaying maximal levels during S phase. Silencing of the *T. brucei* ortholog, *TbP93*, by RNAi resulted in cell growth arrest and the shrinkage and loss of kDNA. N/G forms of minicircle replication intermediates were preferentially lost during RNAi induction, suggesting the involvement of *Tb*P93 in minicircle replication.

Examination of the novel mitochondrial DNA primases [16,17] revealed that the *T. brucei PRI1* gene contains two sequence elements that are similar to the conserved octamer consensus sequence described above. Monitoring the levels of *PRI1* mRNA transcripts in a synchronized *T. brucei* culture showed that *PRI1* mRNA displays cyclic expression, reaching a maximal level shortly before doubling of the number of kinetoplasts [17].

A recent report, describing the variation in transcript levels of the *LIG kα* and *LIG kβ* genes during the cell cycle, revealed that regulation by the conserved cycling elements may be more complex than was initially anticipated. Studies in synchronized *C. fasciculata* cell cultures [50] revealed that the variation in the transcript levels of *LIG kα* and *LIG kβ* are out of phase with one another. The level of *LIG kβ* transcript was maximal during S phase and minimal during cell division, whereas the level of *LIG kα* transcript was maximal during mitosis and subsequent cell division. In this case, although sequences flanking *LIG kβ* do not contain the consensus octamer sequence (related sequences are present at this site), the *LIG kβ* transcripts cycle reaching their maximal level at S phase. In contrast, the *LIG kα* transcripts, do not cycle in the same manner as the S phase expressing proteins, despite the presence of two 5'-flanking copies of the conserved hexamer sequence and a related 3'-flaking sequence [50].

Role of a Mitochondrial HslVU Protease in the Regulation of kDNA Replication

Li *et al.* [47] have recently reported on a bacterial-like HslVU protease in the *T. brucei* mitochondrion. Silencing of *TbHslVU* by RNAi resulted in a selective increase of kDNA minicircles and an increase in the size of the kDNA network, revealing a kDNA segregation defect. Measurement of total minicircles revealed a 20-fold increase during *TbHslVU* RNAi, while the increase of maxicircles was only 2.8-fold. Analysis of free minicircle replication intermediates showed that the levels of CC and G/N free minicircles increased by 5- to 6-fold, implying that silencing of *TbHslVU* enhanced the rate of minicircle replication. These observations indicated that the *Tb*HslVU complex plays a role in the regulation of kDNA replication. It has been speculated [47] that *Tb*HslVU could degrade a protein that may function as a master positive regulator of minicircle replication.

The first direct support for such a novel mechanism in regulation of kDNA replication has been demonstrated in the case of maxicircle replication [25]. As described above, *Tb*PIF2 DNA helicase functions in maxicircle replication. Analyses of cells, in which *TbPIF2* was either silenced by RNAi or alternatively overexpressed in the cell, demonstrated that the level of maxicircle synthesis is roughly proportional to the abundance of the *Tb*PIF2 DNA helicase [25]. These observations suggested that *Tb*PIF2 helicase may function as a regulator of maxicircle synthesis. Silencing of *TbHslVU* by RNAi resulted in ~5 fold increase in the level of *Tb*PIF2 protein. There was no change in the levels of the *TbPIF2* mRNA transcripts or in the level of another replication enzyme, Pol β, under these conditions, providing evidence that this mitochondrial proteasome-like protease controls maxicircle replication.

Conclusion: kDNA Replication Machinery as an Anti-Trypanosomal Drug Target

With the recent discoveries of major kDNA replication proteins, such as the origin-binding proteins, DNA primases, helicases, polymerases, and ligases, most of the proteins anticipated to function in the kDNA replication machinery have now been identified and characterized (Figure 13.1). However, despite the recent advances in the study of the regulation of kDNA replication, our understanding of the control of kDNA replication initiation and segregation, as well as the mechanisms that link these processes to the cell cycle, still pose major challenges to researchers in the field.

A long-standing question in the study of pathogenic species of trypanosomatids has been whether mitochondrial functions, including kDNA replication machinery, are promising targets for the development of anti-trypanosomal drugs. Considering that the kDNA system is found exclusively in trypanosomatids, it could be anticipated that the kDNA replication machinery would provide attractive targets for anti-trypanosomal drugs. However, early observations [60,61] demonstrating that dyskinetoplastid bloodstream-form trypanosomes survive and retain their infectivity, led to the conclusion that kDNA is dispensable for bloodstream-form trypanosomes. Consequently, mitochondrial functions have not been evaluated as promising targets for anti-trypanosomal drugs (reviewed in [62]).

A decade ago, this view was challenged by several studies that revealed the requirement for RNA editing in bloodstream-form parasites [63], the need for maxicircle-encoded subunit A6 of the ATP synthase complex for generation of the mitochondrial membrane potential [64], and the requirement for the kinetoplast for the differentiation of bloodstream-form to procyclic-form parasites [65]. Cristodero *et al.* [66] have shown that editing of the imported tRNA$_{\text{Trp}}$ occurs in both procyclic and bloodstream forms of trypanosomes. These investigators have also found that two mitochondria-specific translation factors are essential for the bloodstream form, indicating that mitochondrial translation is essential in this stage of the parasite life cycle.

A recent series of reports strongly corroborate these earlier studies, providing direct evidence that kDNA replication is essential for the survival of bloodstream-form parasites. Chowdhury *et al.* [67] have recently provided the first evidence indicating that inhibition of kDNA replication is lethal to bloodstream-form trypanosomes, demonstrating that the trypanocidal effect of ethidium bromide on bloodstream-form trypanosomes results mainly from its inhibitory effect on the initiation of minicircle replication. RNAi silencing of the *TbTOPOII*$_{MT}$ gene in bloodstream-form *T. brucei* suggested the requirement for a kDNA replication protein in bloodstream-form trypanosome. These studies revealed the reduction of cell growth rate in the *TbTOPOII*$_{MT}$ knocked-down cells and a modest loss of kDNA networks relative to that observed in procyclic-form trypanosomes [51]. Clear evidence for the dependence of bloodstream-form trypanosomes on kDNA replication proteins for their survival has recently been provided by Michelle

Klingbeil's group [18], revealing that the function of each of the three mitochondrial DNA polymerases, POLIB, POLIC, and POLID, is crucial for bloodstream-form parasite viability.

The accumulating data demonstrating that kDNA replication is indispensable in bloodstream-form parasites and the recent advances in our understanding of the kDNA replication machinery should raise again interest in mitochondrial functions, including the kDNA replication proteins, as promising targets for the development of drugs against pathogenic trypanosomatids.

Acknowledgments

This research was supported by The Israel Science Foundation (grant 1127/10). R.B.-B. and N.Y. contributed equally to this chapter.

References

1 Shlomai, J. (2004) The structure and replication of kinetoplast DNA. *Curr. Mol. Med.*, **4**, 623–647.

2 Liu, B., Liu, Y., Motyka, S.A., Agbo, E.E., and Englund, P.T. (2005) Fellowship of the rings: the replication of kinetoplast DNA. *Trends Parasitol.*, **21**, 363–369.

3 Xu, C.W., Hines, J.C., Engel, M.L., Russell, D.G., and Ray, D.S. (1996) Nucleus-encoded histone H1-like proteins are associated with kinetoplast DNA in the trypanosomatid *Crithidia fasciculata*. *Mol. Cell. Biol.*, **16**, 564–576.

4 Xu, C. and Ray, D.S. (1993) Isolation of proteins associated with kinetoplast DNA networks *in vivo*. *Proc. Natl. Acad. Sci. USA*, **90**, 1786–1789.

5 Lukes, J., Guilbride, D.L., Votypka, J., Zikova, A., Benne, R., and Englund, P.T. (2002) Kinetoplast DNA network: evolution of an improbable structure. *Eukaryot. Cell*, **1**, 495–502.

6 Aphasizhev, R. and Aphasizheva, I. (2011) Uridine insertion/deletion editing in trypanosomes: a playground for RNA-guided information transfer. *Wiley Interdiscip. Rev. RNA*, **2**, 669–685.

7 Chen, J., Rauch, C.A., White, J.H., Englund, P.T., and Cozzarelli, N.R. (1995) The topology of the kinetoplast DNA network. *Cell*, **80**, 61–69.

8 Shapiro, T.A. (1993) Kinetoplast DNA maxicircles: networks within networks. *Proc. Natl. Acad. Sci. USA*, **90**, 7809–7813.

9 Ferguson, M.L., Torri, A.F., Perez-Morga, D., Ward, D.C., and Englund, P.T. (1994) Kinetoplast DNA replication: mechanistic differences between *Trypanosoma brucei* and *Crithidia fasciculata*. *J. Cell Biol.*, **126**, 631–639.

10 Kapeller, I., Milman, N., Yaffe, N., and Shlomai, J. (2011) Interactions of a replication initiator with histone H1-like proteins remodels the condensed mitochondrial genome. *J. Biol. Chem.*, **286**, 40566–40574.

11 Sela, D. and Shlomai, J. (2009) Regulation of UMSBP activities through redox-sensitive protein domains. *Nucleic Acids Res.*, **37**, 279–288.

12 Sela, D., Yaffe, N., and Shlomai, J. (2008) Enzymatic mechanism controls redox-mediated protein–DNA interactions at the replication origin of kinetoplast DNA minicircles. *J. Biol. Chem.*, **283**, 32034–32044.

13 Milman, N., Motyka, S.A., Englund, P.T., Robinson, D., and Shlomai, J. (2007) Mitochondrial origin-binding protein UMSBP mediates DNA replication and segregation in trypanosomes. *Proc. Natl. Acad. Sci. USA*, **104**, 19250–19255.

14 Onn, I., Kapeller, I., Abu-Elneel, K., and Shlomai, J. (2006) Binding of the universal minicircle sequence binding protein at the kinetoplast DNA replication origin. *J. Biol. Chem.*, **281**, 37468–37476.

15 Liu, B., Molina, H., Kalume, D., Pandey, A., Griffith, J.D., and Englund, P.T. (2006) Role of p38 in replication of *Trypanosoma brucei* kinetoplast DNA. *Mol. Cell. Biol.*, **26**, 5382–5393.

16 Hines, J.C. and Ray, D.S. (2011) A second mitochondrial DNA primase is essential for cell growth and kinetoplast minicircle DNA replication in *Trypanosoma brucei*. *Eukaryot. Cell*, **10**, 445–454.

17 Hines, J.C. and Ray, D.S. (2010) A mitochondrial DNA primase is essential for cell growth and kinetoplast DNA replication in *Trypanosoma brucei*. *Mol. Cell. Biol.*, **30**, 1319–1328.

18 Bruhn, D.F., Sammartino, M.P., and Klingbeil, M.M. (2011) Three mitochondrial DNA polymerases are essential for kinetoplast DNA replication and survival of bloodstream form *Trypanosoma brucei*. *Eukaryot. Cell*, **10**, 734–743.

19 Bruhn, D.F., Mozeleski, B., Falkin, L., and Klingbeil, M.M. (2010) Mitochondrial DNA polymerase POLIB is essential for minicircle DNA replication in African trypanosomes. *Mol. Microbiol.*, **75**, 1414–1425.

20 Chandler, J., Vandoros, A.V., Mozeleski, B., and Klingbeil, M.M. (2008) Stem-loop silencing reveals that a third mitochondrial DNA polymerase, POLID, is required for kinetoplast DNA replication in trypanosomes. *Eukaryot. Cell*, **7**, 2141–2146.

21 Downey, N., Hines, J.C., Sinha, K.M., and Ray, D.S. (2005) Mitochondrial DNA ligases of *Trypanosoma brucei*. *Eukaryot. Cell*, **4**, 765–774.

22 Sinha, K.M., Hines, J.C., Downey, N., and Ray, D.S. (2004) Mitochondrial DNA ligase in *Crithidia fasciculata*. *Proc. Natl. Acad. Sci. USA*, **101**, 4361–4366.

23 Liu, B., Yildirir, G., Wang, J., Tolun, G., Griffith, J.D., and Englund, P.T. (2010) TbPIF1, a *Trypanosoma brucei* mitochondrial DNA helicase, is essential for kinetoplast minicircle replication. *J. Biol. Chem.*, **285**, 7056–7066.

24 Liu, B., Wang, J., Yildirir, G., and Englund, P.T. (2009) TbPIF5 is a *Trypanosoma brucei* mitochondrial DNA helicase involved in processing of minicircle Okazaki fragments. *PLoS Pathog.*, **5**, e1000589.

25 Liu, B., Wang, J., Yaffe, N., Lindsay, M.E., Zhao, Z., Zick, A., Shlomai, J., and Englund, P.T. (2009) Trypanosomes have six mitochondrial DNA helicases with one controlling kinetoplast maxicircle replication. *Mol. Cell*, **35**, 490–501.

26 Scocca, J.R. and Shapiro, T.A. (2008) A mitochondrial topoisomerase IA essential for late theta structure resolution in African trypanosomes. *Mol. Microbiol.*, **67**, 820–829.

27 Lindsay, M.E., Gluenz, E., Gull, K., and Englund, P.T. (2008) A new function of *Trypanosoma brucei* mitochondrial topoisomerase II is to maintain kinetoplast DNA network topology. *Mol. Microbiol.*, **70**, 1465–1476.

28 Gluenz, E., Povelones, M.L., Englund, P.T., and Gull, K. (2011) The kinetoplast duplication cycle in *Trypanosoma brucei* is orchestrated by cytoskeleton-mediated cell morphogenesis. *Mol. Cell. Biol.*, **31**, 1012–1021.

29 Zhao, Z., Lindsay, M.E., Roy Chowdhury, A., Robinson, D.R., and Englund, P.T. (2008) p166, a link between the trypanosome mitochondrial DNA and flagellum, mediates genome segregation. *EMBO J.*, **27**, 143–154.

30 Woodward, R. and Gull, K. (1990) Timing of nuclear and kinetoplast DNA replication and early morphological events in the cell cycle of *Trypanosoma brucei*. *J. Cell Sci.*, **95**, 49–57.

31 Drew, M.E. and Englund, P.T. (2001) Intramitochondrial location and dynamics of *Crithidia fasciculata* kinetoplast minicircle replication intermediates. *J. Cell Biol.*, **153**, 735–744.

32 Birkenmeyer, L., Sugisaki, H., and Ray, D. S. (1987) Structural characterization of site-specific discontinuities associated with replication origins of minicircle DNA from *Crithidia fasciculata*. *J. Biol. Chem.*, **262**, 2384–2392.

33 Hines, J.C. and Ray, D.S. (2008) Structure of discontinuities in kinetoplast DNA-

associated minicircles during S phase in *Crithidia fasciculata*. *Nucleic Acids Res.*, **36**, 444–450.

34 Shapiro, T.A. (1994) Mitochondrial topoisomerase II activity is essential for kinetoplast DNA minicircle segregation. *Mol. Cell. Biol.*, **14**, 3660–3667.

35 Fairlamb, A.H., Weislogel, P.O., Hoeijmakers, J.H., and Borst, P. (1978) Isolation and characterization of kinetoplast DNA from bloodstream form of *Trypanosoma brucei*. *J. Cell Biol.*, **76**, 293–309.

36 Hoeijmakers, J.H. and Weijers, P.J. (1980) The segregation of kinetoplast DNA networks in *Trypanosoma brucei*. *Plasmid*, **4**, 97–116.

37 Perez-Morga, D.L. and Englund, P.T. (1993) The attachment of minicircles to kinetoplast DNA networks during replication. *Cell*, **74**, 703–711.

38 Vaughan, S. (2010) Assembly of the flagellum and its role in cell morphogenesis in *Trypanosoma brucei*. *Curr. Opin. Microbiol.*, **13**, 453–458.

39 Ogbadoyi, E.O., Robinson, D.R., and Gull, K. (2003) A high-order trans-membrane structural linkage is responsible for mitochondrial genome positioning and segregation by flagellar Basal bodies in trypanosomes. *Mol. Biol. Cell*, **14**, 1769–1779.

40 Ochsenreiter, T., Anderson, S., Wood, Z.A., and Hajduk, S.L. (2008) Alternative RNA editing produces a novel protein involved in mitochondrial DNA maintenance in trypanosomes. *Mol. Cell. Biol.*, **28**, 5595–5604.

41 Tzfati, Y., Abeliovich, H., Kapeller, I., and Shlomai, J. (1992) A single-stranded DNA-binding protein from *Crithidia fasciculata* recognizes the nucleotide sequence at the origin of replication of kinetoplast DNA minicircles. *Proc. Natl. Acad. Sci. USA*, **89**, 6891–6895.

42 Sbicego, S., Alfonzo, J.D., Estevez, A.M., Rubio, M.A., Kang, X., Turck, C.W., Peris, M., and Simpson, L. (2003) RBP38, a novel RNA-binding protein from trypanosomatid mitochondria, modulates RNA stability. *Eukaryot. Cell*, **2**, 560–568.

43 Li, C. and Englund, P.T. (1997) A mitochondrial DNA primase from the trypanosomatid *Crithidia fasciculata*. *J. Biol. Chem.*, **272**, 20787–20792.

44 Iyer, L.M., Koonin, E.V., Leipe, D.D., and Aravind, L. (2005) Origin and evolution of the archaeo-eukaryotic primase superfamily and related palm-domain proteins: structural insights and new members. *Nucleic Acids Res.*, **33**, 3875–3896.

45 Mahmood, R., Hines, J.C., and Ray, D.S. (1999) Identification of *cis* and *trans* elements involved in the cell cycle regulation of multiple genes in *Crithidia fasciculata*. *Mol. Cell. Biol.*, **19**, 6174–6182.

46 Klingbeil, M.M., Motyka, S.A., and Englund, P.T. (2002) Multiple mitochondrial DNA polymerases in *Trypanosoma brucei*. *Mol. Cell*, **10**, 175–186.

47 Li, Z., Lindsay, M.E., Motyka, S.A., Englund, P.T., and Wang, C.C. (2008) Identification of a bacterial-like HslVU protease in the mitochondria of *Trypanosoma brucei* and its role in mitochondrial DNA replication. *PLoS Pathog.*, **4**, e1000048.

48 Wang, J., Englund, P.T., and Jensen, R.E. (2012) TbPIF8, a *Trypanosoma brucei* protein related to the yeast Pif1 helicase, is essential for cell viability and mitochondrial genome maintenance. *Mol. Microbiol.*, **83**, 471–485.

49 Bochman, M.L., Sabouri, N., and Zakian, V.A. (2010) Unwinding the functions of the Pif1 family helicases. *DNA Repair*, **9**, 237–249.

50 Sinha, K.M., Hines, J.C., and Ray, D.S. (2006) Cell cycle-dependent localization and properties of a second mitochondrial DNA ligase in *Crithidia fasciculata*. *Eukaryot. Cell*, **5**, 54–61.

51 Wang, Z. and Englund, P.T. (2001) RNA interference of a trypanosome topoisomerase II causes progressive loss of mitochondrial DNA. *EMBO J.*, **20**, 4674–4683.

52 Abu-Elneel, K., Robinson, D.R., Drew, M.E., Englund, P.T., and Shlomai, J. (2001) Intramitochondrial localization of universal minicircle sequence-binding protein, a trypanosomatid protein that binds kinetoplast minicircle replication origins. *J. Cell Biol.*, **153**, 725–734.

53 Mechali, M. (2010) Eukaryotic DNA replication origins: many choices for appropriate answers. *Nat. Rev. Mol. Cell. Biol.*, **11**, 728–738.

54 Shlomai, J. (2010) Redox control of protein-DNA interactions: from molecular mechanisms to significance in signal transduction, gene expression, and DNA replication. *Antioxid. Redox Signal.*, **13**, 1429–1476.

55 Flohe, L. (2012) The trypanothione system and the opportunities it offers to create drugs for the neglected kinetoplast diseases. *Biotechnol. Adv.*, **30**, 294–301.

56 Krauth-Siegel, R.L. and Comini, M.A. (2008) Redox control in trypanosomatids, parasitic protozoa with trypanothione-based thiol metabolism. *Biochim. Biophys. Acta.*, **1780**, 1236–1248.

57 Pasion, S.G., Brown, G.W., Brown, L.M., and Ray, D.S. (1994) Periodic expression of nuclear and mitochondrial DNA replication genes during the trypanosomatid cell cycle. *J. Cell Sci.*, **107**, 3515–3520.

58 Li, Y., Sun, Y., Hines, J.C., and Ray, D.S. (2007) Identification of new kinetoplast DNA replication proteins in trypanosomatids based on predicted S-phase expression and mitochondrial targeting. *Eukaryot. Cell*, **6**, 2303–2310.

59 Zick, A., Onn, I., Bezalel, R., Margalit, H., and Shlomai, J. (2005) Assigning functions to genes: identification of S-phase expressed genes in *Leishmania major* based on post-transcriptional control elements. *Nucleic Acids Res.*, **33**, 4235–4242.

60 Stuart, K.D. (1971) Evidence for the retention of kinetoplast DNA in an acriflavine-induced dyskinetoplastic strain of *Trypanosoma brucei* which replicates the altered central element of the kinetoplast. *J. Cell Biol.*, **49**, 189–195.

61 Riou, G.F., Belnat, P., and Benard, J. (1980) Complete loss of kinetoplast DNA sequences induced by ethidium bromide or by acriflavine in *Trypanosoma equiperdum. J. Biol. Chem.*, **255**, 5141–5144.

62 Schnaufer, A., Domingo, G.J., and Stuart, K. (2002) Natural and induced dyskinetoplastic trypanosomatids: how to live without mitochondrial DNA. *Int. J. Parasitol.*, **32**, 1071–1084.

63 Schnaufer, A., Panigrahi, A.K., Panicucci, B., Igo, R.P.Jr., Wirtz, E., Salavati, R., and Stuart, K. (2001) An RNA ligase essential for RNA editing and survival of the bloodstream form of *Trypanosoma brucei. Science*, **291**, 2159–2162.

64 Schnaufer, A., Clark-Walker, G.D., Steinberg, A.G., and Stuart, K. (2005) The F1-ATP synthase complex in bloodstream stage trypanosomes has an unusual and essential function. *EMBO J.*, **24**, 4029–4040.

65 Timms, M.W., van Deursen, F.J., Hendriks, E.F., and Matthews, K.R. (2002) Mitochondrial development during life cycle differentiation of African trypanosomes: evidence for a kinetoplast-dependent differentiation control point. *Mol. Biol. Cell*, **13**, 3747–3759.

66 Cristodero, M., Seebeck, T., and Schneider, A. (2010) Mitochondrial translation is essential in bloodstream forms of *Trypanosoma brucei. Mol. Microbiol.*, **78**, 757–769.

67 Roy Chowdhury, A., Bakshi, R., Wang, J., Yildirir, G., Liu, B., Pappas-Brown, V., Tolun, G., Griffith, J.D., Shapiro, T.A., Jensen, R.E., and Englund, P.T. (2010) The killing of African trypanosomes by ethidium bromide. *PLoS Pathog.*, **6**, e1001226.

14

Life and Death of *Trypanosoma brucei*: New Perspectives for Drug Development

Torsten Barth, Jasmin Stein, Stefan Mogk, Caroline Schönfeld,
Bruno K. Kubata, and Michael Duszenko[*]

Abstract

Cell death is a life-long companion for any cell and molecular processes evolved in order to deal with life-threatening situations like starvation or poisoning. It is also known that in metazoa different pathways exist by which a cell undergoes suicide for the benefit of the whole organism, collectively known as apoptosis. Although protozoa generally lack caspases, a formerly thought indispensable prerequisite for apoptosis, an inducible caspase-independent form of apoptosis as a mechanism of cell density regulation has been described in African trypanosomes. Here, we review the current status of cell death mechanisms in *Trypanosoma brucei* including necrosis, autophagy, and apoptosis. We will discuss which of these events are necessary to cope with stressful situations, and which are probably needed to ensure continuance of infection and transmittance to the insect vector. Since autophagy and apoptosis are essential for the parasite's survival, we will also discuss possible pathway junctions suitable for drug development.

Necrosis

Any cell will undergo necrosis if changes of the environmental conditions are contradictory to cell integrity. This might be extensive temperature shifts, high pressure, non-isotonic conditions, or the appearance of substances that either dissolve the membrane integrity or lead to a breakdown of the energy metabolism. In any case, this is an accidental cell death and mostly a rather rapid process. Detection of necrosis is usually performed by light or electron microscopy, or by uptake of specific dyes that are unable to cross intact membranes. Propidium iodide is often used in this respect, because it is excluded from viable cells, but penetrates damaged membranes, intercalates into DNA (one molecule of dye binds to about 5 bp), and is then readily detectable by fluorescence-activated cell sorting measurements (Figure 14.1). However, if conditional changes appear gradually, a cell would react accordingly to cope with the respective stress

[*] Corresponding Author

Trypanosomatid Diseases: Molecular Routes to Drug Discovery, First edition. Edited by T. Jäger, O. Koch, and L. Flohé.
© 2013 Wiley-VCH Verlag GmbH & Co. KGaA. Published 2013 by Wiley-VCH Verlag GmbH & Co. KGaA.

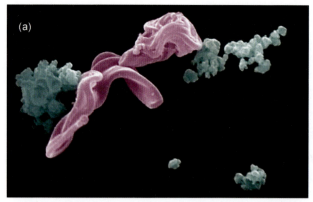

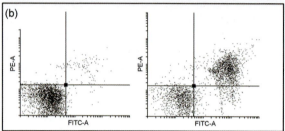

Figure 14.1 Necrosis in African trypanosomes after H$_2$O$_2$ treatment. (a) Scanning electron micrograph of trypanosomes incubated for 3 h in culture medium containing 40 μM H$_2$O$_2$. (b) Flow cytometry double staining with propidium iodide (PE-A) and Annexin-V-FLUOS (FITC-A) to detect necrosis and apoptosis. Left panel: control trypanosomes incubated in culture medium; right panel: trypanosomes incubated for 3 h in culture medium containing 40 μM H$_2$O$_2$. Quadrants: dots in the lower-left quadrant represent viable cells; dots in the lower-right quadrant represent apoptotic cells (Annexin positive); dots in the upper-right quadrant represent necrotic cells (Annexin and propidium iodide positive).

condition. In this case, signs of autophagic cell death or apoptosis may also be detected as a consequence of the cellular response [1].

Necrosis in bloodstream-form trypanosomes is easily detected by incubating the parasites in, for example, glucose-free media or using sufficient concentrations of trypanocidal drugs (Figure 14.1). Although induction of necrosis in trypanosomes might appear as a perfect alternative to remove parasites from the host, severe side-effects may appear during this process that could threaten the host's life. First, drugs intervening with the parasites metabolism in a way to cause necrosis will probably also interact with at least some of the host's cells. For example, depletion of glucose would kill the trypanosomes, but would also lead to anemia, to coma, and finally to death caused by a hypoglycemic shock. The reason is that most, if not all, of the central metabolic pathways are evolutionarily highly conserved. Here again, glycolysis is a very good example: trypanosomes as well as the other flagellates of the order Kinetoplastida possess an organelle called a glycosome that contains most of the glycolytic enzymes [2,3]. Thus, although the organization of this pathway as well as the structure of several glycolytic enzymes show differences and peculiarities as compared with their mammalian counterpart, so far no specific inhibition of glycolysis in trypanosomes could be established, although crystal structures of many glycolytic enzymes exist of both mammalian and trypanosomal origin [4–6]. Secondly, mass destruction of parasites would lead to a massive inflammation reaction that, especially in local areas like the meningeal compartment, may have deleterious effects.

Autophagic Cell Death

Autophagy in general is a survival mechanism of a cell to cope with different stress situations. The most plausible and best-analyzed scenario is starvation. In this case part of the cytosol including organelles is engulfed by a double membrane that is formed elsewhere within the cell and delivered to the lysosome for degradation. Following fusion of the outer membrane of the autophagosome with the lysosome, the inner autophagosomal membrane as well as its contents are degraded by lysosomal hydrolases and the remaining substrates (e.g., nucleosides, amino acids, carbohydrates, and lipids) are released into the cytosol for biosynthesis of essential biopolymers (nucleic acids, proteins, etc.). In this way, a cell can survive for some time by eating its less important constituents to form urgently needed molecules. If nutrition does not return to a normal supply, the cell will enter autophagic cell death, most obviously characterized by a massive increase of lysosomes and vacuolization. In contrast to the constitutively occurring engulfment of parts of the cytosol by the lysosome itself (microautophagy), the process has been called macroautophagy. Interestingly, this is not the only cellular event where macroautophagy is involved. In fact, it became increasingly clear during the last decade that autophagy is also involved during cell differentiation and generally during cellular remodeling as an adaptation to environmental changes [7]. In addition, it plays significant roles in disease [8] and infection [9]. We will briefly describe the general molecular machinery involved in the autophagic process, before we concentrate on trypanosomes. Macroautophagy (further referred to as autophagy) starts with the formation of a phagophore (also called an isolation membrane) at a certain place within the cell that has been called the "phagophore assembly site" or "pre-autophagosomal structure" (PAS). It is a long-standing question where the PAS originates. Data have been presented that, on the one hand, it is formed as an elongation of the endoplasmic reticulum [10] or, on the other hand, that the outer mitochondrial membrane contributes to PAS formation [11]. Although autophagy occurs constitutively at a low basal level, the PAS is massively formed in response to a defined signal (e.g., in the absence of amino acids). The central regulator is the serine/-threonine kinase TOR, an enzyme that was named due to its inhibition by rapamycin, hence its name "target of rapamycin." Rapamycin, a macrolide, was originally isolated from *Streptomyces hygroscopicus* and used as an anti-fungal drug, before it was discovered that it has a pronounced immunosuppressive effect by inhibiting the intracellular response of B- and T-cells to interleukin-2 [12]. As we know now, rapamycin associates with the soluble protein FK-binding protein 12 (FKBP12) before it directly binds to the TOR complex 1 (TORC1) to inhibit its kinase activity. TORC1 and TORC2 are two distinct cytosolic complexes consisting of several proteins with TOR as the catalytic center of both complexes [13]. TORC1 senses many different cellular signals like the amino acid concentration, the availability of growth factors, the energy status of the cell, and stress. Sufficient supply of these signals and the absence of stress lead the cell to an anabolic rather than catabolic metabolism, inducing cell growth, cell cycle progression, and cell proliferation. On the contrary, deficiency of these signals, an increase in stress, or binding of rapamycin–FKBP12 leads to the opposite effects and induces autophagy (Figure 14.2a) [13]. Usually, TORC2 does not bind rapamycin–FKBP12 and does not induce autophagy, but is involved in cytoskeleton organization and cell volume control [14]. Inhibition of TORC1 blocks phosphorylation of the downstream signal

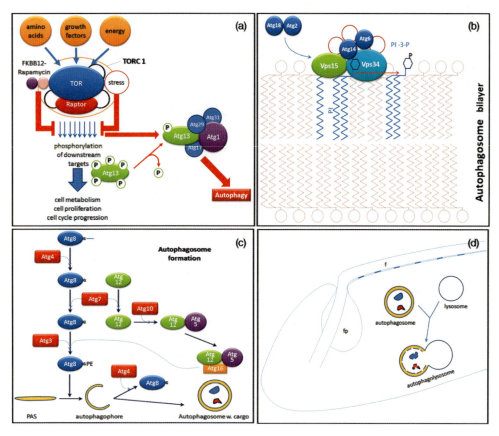

Figure 14.2 Schematic description of autophagy. (a) Regulation of the induction of autophagy; (b) vesicle nucleation and generation of membranes; (c) autophagosome formation by the Atg8 and Atg12 ubiquitin-like pathways; and (d) fusion of a lysosome and autophagosome to an autophagolysosome and vesicle breakdown. (See text for more details.).

molecules and induces autophagy. Key players in autophagy induction are autophagy-related proteins (Atg) which are encoded in autophagy-related genes (*ATG*). TORC1 phosphorylates Atg13 to inhibit autophagy. Under starvation conditions, TORC1 becomes inactive and Atg13 is readily dephosphorylated, forming a complex with Atg1 and Atg17. The activated complex induces formation of the PAS by activating a protein complex consisting beside others (e.g., Atg6, Atg14, Vps15) of class III phosphatidylinositol-3 kinase (Vps34). This Vps34 (Vps = vacuolar protein sorting) leads to formation of phosphatidylinositol-3-phosphate that is enriched in the inner bilayer of the autophagosome membrane thereby attracting additional Atg proteins like the Atg18–Atg2 complex to increase the membrane's size (Figure 14.2b). The next step (i.e., formation of a vesicular structure) includes bending of the double membrane, which is induced by binding of Atg8 to phosphatidylethanolamine (PE). Atg8, a ubiquitin-like protein, reacts with the cysteine protease Atg4, which removes amino acids until a glycine residue is exposed at the C-terminus. It is then conjugated to PE by the E1-like activating enzyme Atg7 and the E2-like conjugating enzyme Atg3. Conjugation of Atg8 is supported by Atg12, Atg5, and Atg16 – a protein complex that works as an E3-like enzyme and needs activity of Atg7 and Atg10 for its own formation. Finally, Atg8 is released from PE by Atg4 (Figure 14.2c) [15]. The newly formed autophagosomes carry a cargo of engulfed cytoplasmic materials including cytosol with all solutes, macromolecules like ribosomes, and organelles. The outer membrane of the autophagosome fuses with a lysosome, thereby forming an autophagolysosome. Now the lysosomal hydrolases will degrade the inner autophagosomal membrane and all constituents of the cargo to release the degradation products (amino acids, nucleosides, sugars, lipids) into the cytosol (Figure 14.2d).

We will now describe differences in the autophagy mechanisms in trypanosomes in order to discuss possible drug targets. There is no doubt that trypanosomes undergo autophagy, which is clearly visible in electron micrographs (Figure 14.3). Obviously, autophagy is already visible under control conditions (Figure 14.3a), but is especially induced during starvation or incubation with nanoparticles (Figure 14.3b and c). Since a bioinformatics survey had revealed that a considerably lower number of *ATG* genes seem to be present in Kinetoplastida, it was speculated that autophagy in these parasites may be more simply organized than in higher eukaryotes [16]. However, as we know now, the major principles are very much comparable, although some peculiarities exist that could indeed serve as targets for drug development. It already starts with the TORC complexes. As described above, TORC1 is usually the target of rapamycin and its inhibition leads to the induction of autophagy. In African trypanosomes, both TORC1 and TORC2 are present and build from two different TOR kinases (*Tb*TOR1 and *Tb*TOR2) and different adapter proteins, including *Tb*TOR-like 1 and *Tb*TOR-like 2 [17]. As in the mammalian system, both complexes are involved in cell cycle progression and cell division, but in contrast, TORC1 is not affected by rapamycin in the nanomolar range in trypanosomes. Instead, rapamycin inhibits TORC2, leading to a disruption of cytokinesis and subsequently cell death [17]. Since TOR and TOR-like proteins are considerably different to their mammalian counterparts and rapamycin inhibits

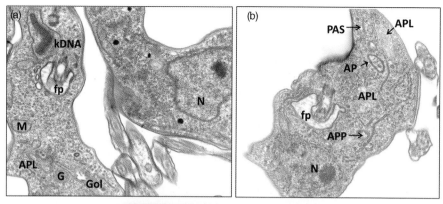

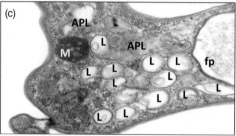

Figure 14.3 Electron micrographs showing the development of autophagy in *T. brucei*. (a) Untreated control cells showing a very low but visible rate of autophagy; (b) autophagy induced by nanoparticles labeled with bovine serum albumin (BSA) for uptake by trypanosomes; and (c) final stage of autophagy close to autophagic cell death induced by amino acid starvation for 24 h. AP, autophagosome; APL, autophagolysosome; APP, autophagophore; fp, flagellar pocket; G, glycosome; Gol, Golgi apparatus; kDNA, kinetoplast DNA; L, lysosome; M, mitochondrion; PAS, phagophore assembling site; N, nucleus.

specifically TORC2 instead of TORC1 as in the host's system, the parasitic TOR and TOR-like proteins could indeed be valuable targets for drug development, especially as they are involved in cell cycle control and progression. This is further supported by the finding that the TOR-like 1 kinase seems specifically involved in formation of acidocalcisomes – unique and essential organelles in Kinetoplastida [18]. The next step, namely formation of the autophagosome bilayer, depends primarily on Vps34. The respective ortholog of this protein has been investigated in trypanosomes, and seems especially involved in Golgi segregation as well as in receptor-mediated endocytosis and in exocytosis [19]. Its involvement in autophagy was not explored in this study, but RNA interference-induced knockdown mutants showed severe growth defects, indicating that *Tb*Vps34 is needed for a correct cytokinesis. It might thus be advisable to investigate more about PAS membrane formation in trypanosomes in order to gain more information about this step and to analyze its suitability for drug development. Finally, autophagosome formation and progress of autophagy has been investigated in several laboratories [9].

Trypanosomes contain all orthologs for the Atg8 pathway and possess three possible *ATG8* genes, named *ATG8.1*, *ATG8.2*, and *ATG8.3* [9]. The respective protein Atg8.3 contains an insertion of 16 amino acids and seems not to be involved in autophagosome formation. The function of Atg8.1 is confusing. Since it is one amino acid shorter and ends with a glycine residue on its C-terminal end, it will not be processed by Atg4. It is, however, expressed (as judged from our unpublished reverse transcription-polymerase chain reaction data) and is probably responsible for the constitutively occurring basal autophagy observed at any time in this parasite independent of autophagy induction (see control cells, Figure 14.3a). In contrast, Atg8.2 contains a single amino acid extension on the C-terminal end. We have solved the three-dimensional structure of *Tb*Atg8.1/2 and could show by homology modeling with Atg4 from rats that it fits perfectly with its ubiquitin fold to this protease, extending its C-terminus into the catalytic site (Figure 14.4) [20]. Obviously, Atg8.2 represents the true ortholog of LC3, the human counterpart, and is responsible for execution of induced autophagy. In this case it is activated upon limited proteolysis by Atg4 and binds to PE. Accordingly, immunofluorescence images of trypanosomes starved by amino acid removal from the media show a punctuated (i.e., membrane-bound) localization of this protein, while it has a clear cytosolic distribution in non-starved control cells [21]. So far it remains to be demonstrated that *T. brucei* contains a functioning Atg12–Atg5 conjugation system. While a bioinformatics survey did not reveal clear homologs in trypanosomes, experimental evidence was presented showing that the respective proteins are active in *Leishmania* [22].

There are several ways to induce autophagy in trypanosomes, even though the use of rapamycin is critical because it inhibits TORC2 rather than TORC1. The most obvious way is amino acid starvation. In this case, we see at the level of electron microscopy clear morphological signs of autophagy, including formation of PASs,

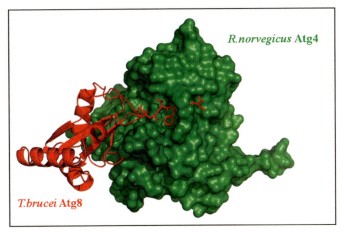

Figure 14.4 Homology modeling docking the crystal structure of *Tb*Atg8 to Atg4 from rat. Note: the C-terminal amino acid (cysteine) of Atg8 fits perfectly into the active center of Atg4.

autophagosomes, and autophagolysosomes. If starvation proceeds, trypanosomes show an increasing number of lysosomes, vacuolization of the cell, and eventually cell death (Figure 14.3c).

Interestingly, we see the same signs of autophagy when we treat trypanosomes with different nanoparticles. Owing to their small size, in the range of 1–1000 nm, they offer new properties and new functions as compared to larger particles. They can be subdivided into different classes, such as liposomes, emulsions, ceramic nanoparticles, metallic nanoparticles, gold shell nanoparticles, and quantum dots [23,24]. These particles can be made up of different materials like TiO_2, ZnO_2, SiO_2, semiconductor material with unique fluorescent properties, or supermagnetic iron oxide [23]. Beyond their size, one main advantage of these particles is the surface variability, which allows a wide range of use. Different coats can be attached to the surface of the particles. These coats can be fluorophores to trace the routes the particles take within the cell and to study the mode of action, but also proteins or antibodies to target specific cells. In addition, nanoparticles can be filled with different drugs to utilize them as a drug carrier system. In our study we used either human transferrin (Tf)- or bovine serum albumin (BSA)-coated Fe_2O_3 nanoparticles, both of a size of around 10 nm. The latter coat is known to be taken up by fluid-phase endocytosis [25,26], while transferrin is incorporated due to receptor-mediated endocytosis by trypanosomes [25]. Treatment of bloodstream-form *T. brucei* with these two nanoparticle formulations causes massive endocytosis and readily induced autophagy detectable via electron microscopy. We detected PASs, autophagosomes, and autophagolysosomes after nanoparticle treatment (Figure 14.3b).

Apoptosis in Protozoan Parasites

Apoptosis, formerly called programmed cell death, was originally described as a way for metazoan organisms to get rid of unwanted cells that are either no longer necessary, like in embryology [27,28], or even perilous for the survival of the whole organism [29]. Two mechanisms have been described: (i) the respective cell gets a signal from the organism via so-called death receptors to kill itself [30] or (ii) vital cell functions are damaged (e.g., by radiation or viral infection) forcing this cell to disappear [31,32]. In both cases, caspases, a defined class of cysteine proteases, are activated by limited proteolysis to induce a controlled cell death avoiding inflammation [33]. The necessity of this form of cell death is most obvious in the case of immune cells, where myriads of "wrong" cells (i.e., cells expressing an antibody or a T-cell receptor with deleterious effects on the organism itself) have to die in a silent way. Either way of classical apoptosis is characterized by three indispensable prerequisites: the function of caspases as starting points of self-destruction, the avoidance of inflammatory reactions, and the benefit of the organism as a driving force during evolution of this induced cell death. Cellular self-destruction induces a set of morphological and biochemical changes that are used to define apoptosis on a molecular basis, and to separate it from necrosis and autophagic cell death. Among others, the most prominent changes are: shrinkage of the cell, blebbing, segmentation of the nucleus, single-strand DNA breaks, exposure of phosphatidylserine in the outer leaflet of the plasma membrane, and loss of potential of the inner mitochondrial membrane [34,35]. To detect these changes, usually light or electron microscopic techniques together with FACS analyses are used. The former include the TUNEL test (terminal deoxynucleotidyl transferase dUTP nick endlabeling) to detect DNA strand breaks, the latter Annexin staining (to measure phosphatidylserine exposure) and tetramethylrhodamine ethyl ester staining to measure loss of the inner membrane potential ($\Delta\Psi$).

Considering apoptosis in trypanosomes poses two serious problems: (i) protozoa do not possess caspases and (ii) is it hard to believe that a single-cell organism may develop a molecular mechanism for its own death during evolution. Nevertheless, investigating cell death in protozoa showed that at least some of the hallmarks of apoptosis (see above) can also be found in single-cell organisms [36,37], including trypanosomes [38,39].

In this situation, the discovery of metacaspases in plants, fungi, and protists as a class of proteins closely related to caspases in animals seemed like the missing link. However, although metacaspases seem to be involved in cell death in plants and fungi, there is no conclusive evidence for their participation in protozoa apoptosis. In fact, *T. brucei* contains five metacaspases, but they are not involved in apoptosis here, as we [40] and others [41] could show. This is also true for *Leishmania* [42,43]. The next step to solve the dilemma of apoptosis in protozoan parasites was the observation that a caspase-independent apoptosis exists in metazoa [44]. In this case, a small redox enzyme located in the intermembrane space of mitochondria, the so-called apoptosis-inducing factor (AIF), is released and translocates to the nucleus to induce chromatin condensation and DNA degradation [45,46]. Unfortunately, no ortholog of AIF has so far been detected in protozoan parasites, but endonuclease G (Endo G) seems to perform the same sort of action if released from the intermembrane space during induction of cell death [47]. We have analyzed cell death in trypanosomes upon prostaglandin (PG) D_2 (PGD$_2$) application (Figure 14.5). The reason to investigate PGD$_2$ effects on the parasite was based on our discovery that trypanosomes produce prostaglandins [48], which was especially interesting because the PGD$_2$ concentration is remarkably high in the cerebrospinal fluid (CSF) of late-stage sleeping sickness patients [49]. We originally considered that PGD$_2$ may induce differentiation from slender to stumpy parasites, but readily observed cell death of the stumpy population. Interestingly, we detected nearly all classical hallmarks of apoptosis, but found no indication of necrosis or autophagic cell death [50,51]. These results clearly show the parallel appearance of different populations that respond differently to signaling molecules. In terms of parasite survival within the host this seems to have major consequences. Cell density regulation is a major problem for a parasite to survive. Considering continuous proliferation with a generation doubling time of about 8 h (as in trypanosomes), parasite density would exceed an acceptable level in blood, thus killing a human in less than 2 weeks. Trypanosomes deal with this problem by expressing a dense surface coat consisting of 10^7 identical protein molecules, the so-called variant surface

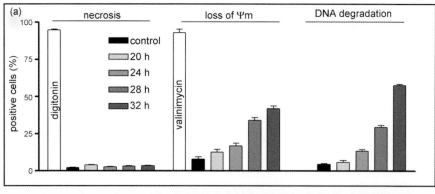

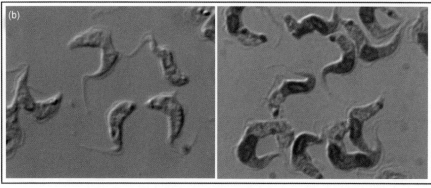

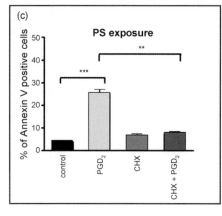
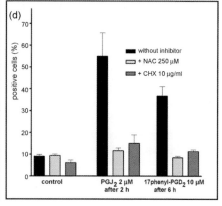

Figure 14.5 Hallmarks of apoptosis in *T. brucei*. (a) Treatment of trypanosomes between 20 and 30 h with PGD_2 in axenic culture: left panel, negative test of necrosis; middle panel, loss of potential ($\Delta\Psi$) for the inner mitochondrial membrane; right panel, DNA degradation. (b) Left panel, untreated and thus TUNEL-negative control cells; right panel, positive TUNEL test in PGD_2-treated cells after 24 h. (c) Annexin-V staining for phosphatidylserine in the outer leaflet of the plasma membrane. (d) Measurement of ROS production due to PGD_2 induced apoptosis, Note: ROS formation is inhibited by preincubation of trypanosomes with *N*-acetylcysteine (NAC, reducing agent) or cycloheximide (CHX, inhibition of protein biosynthesis); in the latter panel either one of the metabolic degradation products of PGD_2, namely PHJ_2, or the non-degraded PGD_2 analog 17-phenyl-PG_2 was used. (Results are taken from [50,51].)

glycoprotein (VSG). This coat protects the parasite from the cellular immune response as well as from complement. It is, however, immunogenic and leads to formation of specific antibodies. All parasites carrying the same coat are then opsonized and killed by the immune system. Due to antigenic variation, new populations appear spontaneously carrying a different coat [52–54]. A trypanosomal infection is thus characterized by an oscillating population density in blood. In addition to this host-induced density regulation, trypanosomes differentiate in blood from a dividing slender to a non-dividing stumpy form that is preadapted to survive in the insect vector [55–57]. This differentiation depends on the slender population density [58] and is induced by a secreted low-molecular-weight factor (stumpy inducing factor (SIF) [58]) of so far unknown chemical identity that enriches in conditioned culture media [59]. Most likely SIF works like an autocrine mediator that is released from slender cells and induces slender cells to differentiate to the stumpy form.

The presence of two different populations offers the basis for a parasite-induced density regulation. In fact, trypanosomes do not behave like single self-contained individual organisms, but as members of populations, talking to each other via quorum sensing [9,60]. In this way, the dividing slender population grows until the local population density reaches a point where the concentration of the secreted SIF is high enough to induce cell differentiation in its neighbor cells. Consequently, the number of slender cells decreases while the stumpy population increases. Stumpy trypanosomes do not divide anymore and do not undergo antigenic variation [61]. In addition, they are vulnerable to PGD_2 that induces formation of reactive oxygen species (ROS) which then leads to changes of the mitochondrion membrane integrity and the release of Endo G [50,51]. Endo G translocates to the nucleus and leads by activation of its nuclease activity to the onset of this caspase-independent form of apoptosis [62]. Considering this concept, it seems like a mechanistic strategy of the parasite to control its cell density during the course of infection (Figure 14.6). The advantages are: (i) the parasitemia will usually not reach a density that would kill the host just by the pure number of parasites (e.g., because of its high glucose consumption), (ii) the slender population cannot become completely extinct, since the SIF concentration would decrease with a decrease of the slender population and the movement of the parasite, (iii) an apoptotic cell death of the stumpy population would not induce inflammation, and (iv) this mechanism is independent of VSG-specific antibodies and works also in immunologically privileged organs like the brain. The latter point seems especially important during the late stage of sleeping sickness. Taken together, apoptosis of the stumpy population has indeed an altruistic quality as it enables the dividing slender form to keep the infection going and increases the chances of the parasite to be transmitted to the insect vector.

Analyzing the brain stage of sleeping sickness, two possible entry gates exists: the blood–brain barrier and the blood–CSF barrier. In the literature, data have been presented to support either the first way [63,64] or the second way [65]. We have investigated the early brain infection stage in rodents (i.e., between 20 and 35 days post-infection) using electron microscopy, and detected parasites within the stroma

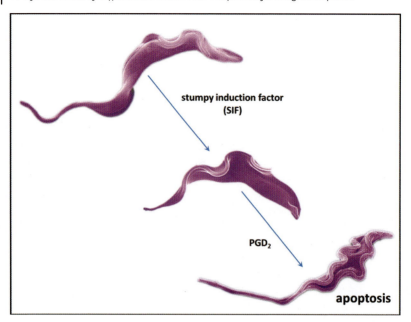

Figure 14.6 Mechanism of cell density regulation in *T. brucei*. Schematic representation of SIF-induced differentiation from slender to stumpy parasites and PGD$_2$-induced apoptosis that leads to cell-cycle-arrested trypanosomes and finally cell death. Scanning electron micrographs of cells obtained from infected rats or from PGD$_2$-treated parasites in cell culture.

of the choroid plexus, in the ventricles, and in the meningeal space, especially in a pial and subpial location outside the glia limitans [66]. This space just outside the brain parenchyma seems an ideal area for the parasite to reside. Here they are not attacked by immune cells or VSG-specific antibodies and they can move back into lymph (via the nasal lymphatic vessels [67]) or blood (via the arachnoid villi) to produce the observed relapses after killing of the blood parasites, such as by suramin – a drug that does not penetrate into the brain. On the other hand, PGD$_2$ of parasite origin would be needed to control parasite density in this very limited space and could also be distributed via CSF to induce the well-known sleep disturbances [68]. Thus, apoptosis of stumpy cells seems to be an inevitable prerequisite to allow the survival of trypanosomes for a prolonged time in the mammalian host.

Considering apoptosis in trypanosomes as a possible drug target, it seems obvious that neither induction of apoptosis or inhibition of apoptosis would offer a suitable strategy. In the first case, only non-dividing stumpy forms would disappear with little effect on the ongoing infection, while in the latter case an unhampered parasitemia would result with a disastrous effect on the host. However, the addition of the stumpy induction factor would be very effective. From our study we know that this factor is fairly small (molecular weight below 500 Da), hydrophilic, and relatively unstable. Especially the latter point renders handling during preparation difficult and thus the chemical identity of SIF is still elusive. However, due to its expected functionality, isolation and chemical identification is an ongoing project in our group. Another big problem to deal with in sleeping sickness is caused by the infiltration of the brain during the late stage. As mentioned above, trypanosomes enter the choroid plexus and travel via CSF to the meningeal space to settle within the pia mater [66]. In order to reach the CSF, parasites have to cross two barriers – the fenestrated endothelium to enter the stroma of the plexus and finally the epithelium cell wall to enter the ventricle. Both cell layers are placed on a basal membrane, which has also to be opened by the parasite. So far, the molecular mechanism of how trypanosomes open the gates is not well understood. We have observed that at least some parasites within the stroma lost their VSG coat prior to their uptake and digestion by phagocytes. We consider it most likely that trypanosomes, similar to cancer cell migration, need the action of secreted metalloproteases to gain access through the cell barrier. Trypanosomes encode a zinc-dependent protease (MSP-B) that is especially expressed and secreted during trans-formation from blood forms to the procyclic insect form to remove the VSG coat [69]. This protease seems also to be a very good candidate to facilitate entry into the stroma and maybe furthermore into the ventricle. In order to block the parasite's entry into CSF, one may consider developing inhibitors for this pathway, such as an effective protease inhibitor. However, this would only work prior to the late stage as a preventive drug. Instead, it seems more promising to treat late-stage disease by administering trypanocidal drugs intrathecally by lumbar injection. In this case it does not have to cross the blood–brain barrier or the blood–CSF barrier and should have access to trypanosomes in the pial compartment. It should be noted that this form of application is used in brain cancer chemotherapy with considerable success [70]. In this case, the drug should be soluble and stable in CSF, and be able to move between the pial cell layers. At the moment it seems worthwhile to explore this route of drug administration in more detail, because it could probably be performed under field conditions.

Outlook

Trypanosomes, as any other cell, possess a spectrum of measures to resist cell death. The most obvious scenario is autophagy, but this is also true for the onset of necrosis. In addition, the stumpy form undergoes PGD_2-induced apoptosis and other forms of apoptosis may exist [38]. It is certainly too early to announce drug candidates that interfere with the parasite's ability to induce and control cell death mechanisms. However, induction of an irrepressible autophagy (e.g., by nano-particles) seems possible and should be explored in detail. This would be especially promising using nanoparticles that carry trypanocidal drugs inside to be released after uptake by the parasite. Another promising aspect seems to us to be the intrathecal application of trypanocidal drugs to attack trypanosomes residing within the pia mater. Apart from that, the ability of trypanosomes to handle life-threatening situations and their disposition to use cell death mechanisms for epidemiologically effective infections should be analyzed in molecular detail to explore addition toeholds to fight trypanosomiasis.

References

1 Maiuri, M.C., Zalckvar, E., Kimchi, A., and Kroemer, G. (2007) Self-eating and self-killing: crosstalk between autophagy and apoptosis. *Nat. Rev. Mol. Cell Biol.*, **8**, 741–752.

2 Opperdoes, F.R. and Borst, P. (1977) Localization of nine glycolytic enzymes in a microbody-like organelle in *Trypanosoma brucei*: the glycosome. *FEBS Lett.*, **80**, 360–364.

3 Coley, A.F., Dodson, H.C., Morris, M.T., and Morris, J.C. (2011) Glycolysis in the African trypanosome: targeting enzymes and their subcellular compartments for therapeutic development. *Mol. Biol. Int.*, **2011**, 123702.

4 Verlinde, C.L., Hannaert, V., Blonski, C., Willson, M., Perie, J.J. *et al.* (2001) Glycolysis as a target for the design of new anti-trypanosome drugs. *Drug Resist. Updat.*, **4**, 50–65.

5 Wierenga, R.K., Noble, M.E., Postma, J.P., Groendijk, H., Kalk, K.H. *et al.* (1991) The crystal structure of the "open" and the "closed" conformation of the flexible loop of trypanosomal triosephosphate isomerase. *Proteins*, **10**, 33–49.

6 Sirover, M.A. (1999) New insights into an old protein: the functional diversity of mammalian glyceraldehyde-3-phosphate dehydrogenase. *Biochim. Biophys. Acta*, **1432**, 159–184.

7 He, C. and Klionsky, D.J. (2009) Regulation mechanisms and signaling pathways of autophagy. *Annu. Rev. Genet.*, **43**, 67–93.

8 Mehrpour, M., Esclatine, A., Beau, I., and Codogno, P. (2010) Autophagy in health and disease. 1. Regulation and significance of autophagy: an overview. *Am. J. Physiol.*, **298**, C776–C785.

9 Duszenko, M., Ginger, M.L., Brennand, A., Gualdron-Lopez, M., Colombo, M.I. *et al.* (2011) Autophagy in protists. *Autophagy*, **7**, 127–158.

10 Hayashi-Nishino, M., Fujita, N., Noda, T., Yamaguchi, A., Yoshimori, T. *et al.* (2010) Electron tomography reveals the endoplasmic reticulum as a membrane source for autophagosome formation. *Autophagy*, **6**, 301–303.

11 Hailey, D.W., Rambold, A.S., Satpute-Krishnan, P., Mitra, K., Sougrat, R. *et al.* (2010) Mitochondria supply membranes for autophagosome biogenesis during starvation. *Cell*, **141**, 656–667.

12 Calne, R.Y., Collier, D.S., Lim, S., Pollard, S.G., Samaan, A. *et al.* (1989) Rapamycin for immunosuppression in organ allografting. *Lancet*, **2**, 227.

13 Foster, K.G. and Fingar, D.C. (2010) Mammalian target of rapamycin (mTOR): conducting the cellular signaling symphony. *J. Biol. Chem.*, **285**, 14071–14077.

14 Sarbassov, D.D., Ali, S.M., Kim, D.H., Guertin, D.A., Latek, R.R. *et al.* (2004) Rictor, a novel binding partner of mTOR, defines a rapamycin-insensitive and raptor-independent pathway that regulates the cytoskeleton. *Curr. Biol.*, **14**, 1296–1302.

15 Geng, J. and Klionsky, D.J. (2008) The Atg8 and Atg12 ubiquitin-like conjugation systems in macroautophagy. 'Protein modifications: beyond the usual suspects' review series. *EMBO Rep.*, **9**, 859–864.

16 Herman, M., Gillies, S., Michels, P.A., and Rigden, D.J. (2006) Autophagy and related processes in trypanosomatids: insights from genomic and bioinformatic analyses. *Autophagy*, **2**, 107–118.

17 Barquilla, A., Crespo, J.L., and Navarro, M. (2008) Rapamycin inhibits trypanosome cell growth by preventing TOR complex 2 formation. *Proc. Natl. Acad. Sci. USA*, **105**, 14579–14584.

18 de Jesus, T.C.L., Tonelli, R.R., Nardelli, S.C., Augusto, L.D., Motta, M.C.M. *et al.* (2010) Target of rapamycin (TOR)-like 1 kinase is involved in the control of polyphosphate levels and acidocalcisome maintenance in *Trypanosoma brucei*. *J. Biol. Chem.*, **285**, 24131–24140.

19 Hall, B.S., Gabernet-Castello, C., Voak, A., Goulding, D., Natesan, S.K. *et al.* (2006) *Tb*Vps34, the trypanosome orthologue of Vps34, is required for Golgi complex segregation. *J. Biol. Chem.*, **281**, 27600–27612.

20 Koopmann, R., Muhammad, K., Perbandt, M., Betzel, C., and Duszenko, M. (2009)

Trypanosoma brucei ATG8: structural insights into autophagic-like mechanisms in protozoa. *Autophagy*, **5**, 1085–1091.

21 Alvarez, V.E., Kosec, G., Anna, C.S., Turk, V., Cazzulo, J.J. *et al.* (2008) Autophagy is involved in nutritional stress response and differentiation in *Trypanosoma cruzi. J. Biol. Chem.*, **283**, 3454–3464.

22 Williams, R.A.M., Woods, K.L., Juliano, L., Mottram, J.C., and Coombs, G.H. (2009) Characterization of unusual families of ATG8-like proteins and ATG12 in the protozoan parasite *Leishmania major. Autophagy*, **5**, 159–172.

23 Medina, C., Santos-Martinez, M.J., Radomski, A., Corrigan, O.I., and Radomski, M.W. (2007) Nanoparticles: pharmacological and toxicological significance. *Br. J. Pharmacol.*, **150**, 552–558.

24 McNeil, S.E. (2005) Nanotechnology for the biologist. *J. Leukoc. Biol.*, **78**, 585–594.

25 Coppens, I., Opperdoes, F.R., Courtoy, P.J., and Baudhuin, P. (1987) Receptor-mediated endocytosis in the bloodstream form of *Trypanosoma brucei. J. Protozool.*, **34**, 465–473.

26 Webster, P. (1989) Endocytosis by African trypanosomes. I. Three-dimensional structure of the endocytic organelles in *Trypanosoma brucei* and *T. congolense. Eur. J. Cell Biol.*, **49**, 295–302.

27 Vogt, C. (1842) *Untersuchungen uber die Entwicklungsgeschichte der Geburtshelferkroete (Alytes obstetricans)*, Jent & Gassmann, Solothurn.

28 Jacobson, M.D., Weil, M., and Raff, M.C. (1997) Programmed cell death in animal development. *Cell*, **88**, 347–354.

29 Saunders, J.W.Jr. (1966) Death in embryonic systems. *Science*, **154**, 604–612.

30 Denecker, G., Vercammen, D., Declercq, W., and Vandenabeele, P. (2001) Apoptotic and necrotic cell death induced by death domain receptors. *Cell Mol. Life Sci.*, **58**, 356–370.

31 Cosulich, S. and Clarke, P. (1996) Apoptosis: does stress kill? *Curr. Biol.*, **6**, 1586–1588.

32 Basu, S. and Kolesnick, R. (1998) Stress signals for apoptosis: ceramide and c-Jun kinase. *Oncogene*, **17**, 3277–3285.

33 Hotchkiss, R.S. and Nicholson, D.W. (2006) Apoptosis and caspases regulate death and inflammation in sepsis. *Nat. Rev. Immunol.*, **6**, 813–822.

34 Van Cruchten, S. and Van den Broeck, W. (2002) Morphological and biochemical aspects of apoptosis, oncosis and necrosis. *Anat. Histol. Embryol.*, **31**, 214–223.

35 Welburn, S.C., Macleod, E., Figarella, K., and Duzensko, M. (2006) Programmed cell death in African trypanosomes. *Parasitology*, **132** (Suppl.), S7–S18.

36 Madeo, F., Engelhardt, S., Herker, E., Lehmann, N., Maldener, C. *et al.* (2002) Apoptosis in yeast: a new model system with applications in cell biology and medicine. *Curr. Genet.*, **41**, 208–216.

37 Madeo, F., Herker, E., Maldener, C., Wissing, S., Lachelt, S. *et al.* (2002) A caspase-related protease regulates apoptosis in yeast. *Mol. Cell*, **9**, 911–917.

38 Welburn, S.C., Dale, C., Ellis, D., Beecroft, R., and Pearson, T.W. (1996) Apoptosis in procyclic *Trypanosoma brucei rhodesiense in vitro. Cell Death Differ.*, **3**, 229–236.

39 Welburn, S.C., Lillico, S., and Murphy, N.B. (1999) Programmed cell death in procyclic form *Trypanosoma brucei rhodesiense* – identification of differentially expressed genes during con A induced death. *Mem. Inst. Oswaldo Cruz*, **94**, 229–234.

40 Szallies, A., Kubata, B.K., and Duzenko, M. (2002) A metacaspase of *Trypanosoma brucei* causes loss of respiration competence and clonal death in the yeast *Saccharomyces cerevisiae. FEBS Lett.*, **517**, 144–150.

41 Mottram, J.C., Helms, M.J., Coombs, G.H., and Sajid, M. (2003) Clan CD cysteine peptidases of parasitic protozoa. *Trends Parasitol.*, **19**, 182–187.

42 Zangger, H., Mottram, J.C., and Fasel, N. (2002) Cell death in Leishmania induced by stress and differentiation: programmed cell death or necrosis? *Cell Death Differ.*, **9**, 1126–1139.

43 Ambit, A., Fasel, N., Coombs, G.H., and Mottram, J.C. (2008) An essential role for the *Leishmania major* metacaspase in cell cycle progression. *Cell Death Differ.*, **15**, 113–122.

44 Susin, S.A., Lorenzo, H.K., Zamzami, N., Marzo, I., Snow, B.E. *et al.* (1999) Molecular characterization of mitochondrial apoptosis-inducing factor. *Nature*, **397**, 441–446.

45 Cande, C., Cecconi, F., Dessen, P., and Kroemer, G. (2002) Apoptosis-inducing factor (AIF): key to the conserved caspase-independent pathways of cell death? *J. Cell Sci.*, **115**, 4727–4734.

46 Joza, N., Pospisilik, J.A., Hangen, E., Hanada, T., Modjtahedi, N. *et al.* (2009) AIF: Not just an apoptosis-inducing factor. *Ann. NY Acad. Sci.*, **1171**, 2–11.

47 Li, L.Y., Luo, L., and Wang, X.D. (2001) Endonuclease G is an apoptotic DNase when released from mitochondria. *Nature*, **412**, 95–99.

48 Kubata, B.K., Duszenko, M., Kabututu, Z., Rawer, M., Szallies, A. *et al.* (2000) Identification of a novel prostaglandin f (2alpha) synthase in Trypanosoma brucei. *J. Exp. Med.*, **192**, 1327–1338.

49 Pentreath, V.W., Rees, K., Owolabi, O.A., Philip, K.A., and Doua, F. (1990) The somnogenic T lymphocyte suppressor prostaglandin D2 is selectively elevated in cerebrospinal fluid of advanced sleeping sickness patients. *Trans. R. Soc. Trop. Med. Hyg.*, **84**, 795–799.

50 Figarella, K., Rawer, M., Uzcategui, N.L., Kubata, B.K., Lauber, K. *et al.* (2005) Prostaglandin D2 induces programmed cell death in Trypanosoma brucei bloodstream form. *Cell Death Differ.*, **12**, 335–346.

51 Figarella, K., Uzcategui, N.L., Beck, A., Schoenfeld, C., Kubata, B.K. *et al.* (2006) Prostaglandin-induced programmed cell death in Trypanosoma brucei involves oxidative stress. *Cell Death Differ.*, **13**, 1802–1814.

52 Vickerman, K. (1969) On the surface coat and flagellar adhesion in trypanosomes. *J. Cell Sci.*, **5**, 163–193.

53 Vickerman, K. (1978) Antigenic variation in trypanosomes. *Nature*, **273**, 613–617.

54 Cross, G.A. (1978) Antigenic variation in trypanosomes. *Proc. R. Soc. Lond. B*, **202**, 55–72.

55 Matthews, K.R. (1999) Developments in the differentiation of Trypanosoma brucei. *Parasitol. Today*, **15**, 76–80.

56 Brown, R.C., Evans, D.A., and Vickerman, K. (1973) Changes in oxidative metabolism and ultrastructure accompanying differentiation of the mitochondrion in Trypanosoma brucei. *Int. J. Parasitol.*, **3**, 691–704.

57 Feagin, J.E., Jasmer, D.P., and Stuart, K. (1986) Differential mitochondrial gene expression between slender and stumpy bloodforms of Trypanosoma brucei. *Mol. Biochem. Parasitol.*, **20**, 207–214.

58 Vassella, E., Reuner, B., Yutzy, B., and Boshart, M. (1997) Differentiation of African trypanosomes is controlled by a density sensing mechanism which signals cell cycle arrest via the cAMP pathway. *J. Cell Sci.*, **110**, 2661–2671.

59 Hamm, B., Schindler, A., Mecke, D., and Duszenko, M. (1990) Differentiation of Trypanosoma brucei bloodstream trypomastigotes from long slender to short stumpy-like forms in axenic culture. *Mol. Biochem. Parasitol.*, **40**, 13–22.

60 van Zandbergen, G., Luder, C.G., Heussler, V., and Duszenko, M. (2010) Programmed cell death in unicellular parasites: a prerequisite for sustained infection? *Trends Parasitol.*, **26**, 477–483.

61 Black, S.J., Hewett, R.S., and Sendashonga, C.N. (1982) *Trypanosoma brucei* variable surface antigen is released by degenerating parasites but not by actively dividing parasites. *Parasite Immunol.*, **4**, 233–244.

62 Gannavaram, S., Vedvyas, C., and Debrabant, A. (2008) Conservation of the pro-apoptotic nuclease activity of endonuclease G in unicellular trypanosomatid parasites. *J. Cell Sci.*, **121**, 99–109.

63 Mulenga, C., Mhlanga, J.D., Kristensson, K., and Robertson, B. (2001) *Trypanosoma brucei brucei* crosses the blood–brain barrier while tight junction proteins are preserved in a rat chronic disease model. *Neuropathol. Appl. Neurobiol.*, **27**, 77–85.

64 Grab, D.J. and Kennedy, P.G. (2008) Traversal of human and animal trypanosomes across the blood–brain barrier. *J. Neurovirol.*, **14**, 344–351.

65 Schmidt, H. (1983) The pathogenesis of trypanosomiasis of the CNS. Studies on

parasitological and neurohistological findings in *Trypanosoma rhodesiense* infected vervet monkeys. *Virchows Arch. A,* **399**, 333–343.

66 Wolburg, H., Mogk, S., Acker, S., Frey, C., Meinert, M. *et al.* (2012) Late stage infection in sleeping sickness. *PLoS ONE,* **7**, e34304.

67 Johnston, M., Zakharov, A., Papaiconomou, C., Salmasi, G., and Armstrong, D. (2004) Evidence of connections between cerebrospinal fluid and nasal lymphatic vessels in humans, non-human primates and other mammalian species. *Cerebrospinal Fluid Res.,* **1**, 2.

68 Hayaishi, O., Urade, Y., Eguchi, N., and Huang, Z.L. (2004) Genes for prostaglandin d synthase and receptor as well as adenosine A2A receptor are involved in the homeostatic regulation of NREM sleep. *Arch. Ital. Biol.,* **142**, 533–539.

69 de Sousa, K.P., Atouguia, J., and Silva, M.S. (2010) Partial biochemical characterization of a metalloproteinase from the bloodstream forms of *Trypanosoma brucei brucei* parasites. *Protein J.,* **29**, 283–289.

70 Cradock, J.C., Kleinman, L.M., and Davignon, J.P. (1977) Intrathecal injections – a review of pharmaceutical factors. *Bull. Parent. Drug Assoc.,* **31**, 237–247.

Part Three
Validation and Selection of Drug Targets in Kinetoplasts

Trypanosomatid Diseases: Molecular Routes to Drug Discovery, First edition. Edited by T. Jäger, O. Koch, and L. Flohé.
© 2013 Wiley-VCH Verlag GmbH & Co. KGaA. Published 2013 by Wiley-VCH Verlag GmbH & Co. KGaA.

15

Rational Selection of Anti-Microbial Drug Targets: Unique or Conserved?

*Boris Rodenko and Harry P. de Koning**

Abstract

When contemplating a strategy for drug development against an infectious agent such as a bacterium or parasite, there are obvious advantages to choosing a "unique" target in the pathogen. Clearly, inhibition of a pathogen-specific enzyme or pathway that is absent in the mammalian host may be expected to result in fewer adverse effects than inhibition of a highly conserved protein. Yet, through the very definition of a "novel target," significant practical challenges must be overcome in the drug development process that would likely be less challenging for a pharmacologically well-explored target. The novel target requires much fundamental research before and during the initial screening right through to lead optimization and preclinical toxicity testing. This undoubtedly increases costs substantially, discouraging the involvement of pharmaceutical companies. The alternative paradigm, which we discuss here, is for a well-explored target for which a large body of functional and structural data exists, as well as targeted compound libraries and ADME/Tox data on target modulators. This chapter gives a number of specific examples of anti-parasite drugs in (preclinical) studies that act on conserved targets, and makes the case that this approach may lead to faster development of desperately needed novel and safe anti-parasite therapy.

Introduction

When contemplating a strategy for drug development against an infectious agent such as a bacterium or parasite, there are obvious advantages to choosing a "unique" target in the pathogen. Clearly, inhibition of a pathogen-specific enzyme or pathway that is absent in the mammalian host may be expected to result in fewer adverse effects than inhibition of a highly conserved protein. Certainly, the identification of unique targets has become almost routine given the ease of comparative genomics and, for many pathogens, well-developed reverse genetics techniques for target validation exist, such as gene knockout, RNA interference (RNAi), overexpression, and site-directed mutagenesis. Yet, through the very

---

* Corresponding Author

Trypanosomatid Diseases: Molecular Routes to Drug Discovery, First edition. Edited by T. Jäger, O. Koch, and L. Flohé.
© 2013 Wiley-VCH Verlag GmbH & Co. KGaA. Published 2013 by Wiley-VCH Verlag GmbH & Co. KGaA.

definition of a "novel target," significant practical challenges must be overcome in the drug development process that would be less challenging for a pharmacologically well-explored target. For instance, functional assays suitable for high-throughput screening are unlikely to have been developed; structural information about the protein or its active site is probably limited or absent; inhibitors that could form the basis for structural optimization or a targeted compound library are unknown; and there is unlikely to be extensive pharmacological knowledge about the class of inhibitors that will emerge from hit-to-lead optimization. Thus, the novel target requires a great deal of fundamental research before and during the initial screening right through to lead optimization and preclinical toxicity testing. This undoubtedly increases costs substantially, discouraging the involvement of pharmaceutical companies. The alternative paradigm is for a well-explored target for which a large body of functional and structural data exists, as well as targeted compound libraries and ADME/Tox (absorption, distribution, metabolism, elimination, and toxicity) data on target modulators. Private companies with an existing drug development program for such a target may be more inclined to enroll a similar pathogen target in an existing screening and lead optimization protocol than to initiate such an effort *de novo*. In this chapter, we discuss this paradigm alluding to a number of specific examples of anti-parasitic drugs that act on conserved targets.

Phosphodiesterases

Cyclic nucleotide specific phosphodiesterases (PDEs) play a central role in cyclic nucleotide signaling events. PDEs convert the signaling molecules $5',3'$-cyclic adenosine and/or guanosine monophosphate (cAMP or cGMP) into the corresponding $5'$-monophosphates ($5'$- AMP or $5'$-GMP). All human PDEs are actively pursued as drug targets, and are under investigation both in industrial and academic laboratories. A number of PDE inhibitors are on the market for the treatment of a variety of clinical conditions, including the PDE3 inhibitor cilostazol (Pletal®; Otsuka Pharma) for intermittent claudication, the PDE4 inhibitor roflumilast (Daxas®; Nycomed Pharma) for chronic obstructive pulmonary disease, and the PDE5 inhibitors tadalafil (Cialis®; Lilly), vardenafil (Levitra®; Bayer), and sildenafil (Viagra®; Pfizer) for erectile dysfunction.

Eleven PDE families are encoded by the human genome and, due to differential splicing mechanisms, an estimated total of approximately 100 different PDEs are synthesized and function in different human tissues [1]. Despite the great variety in the human PDE families, their catalytic domains all show high structural homology. Nevertheless, PDE-inhibiting drugs currently on the market are highly family-selective, proving that through chemical optimization PDE inhibitors can be developed that show minimal interaction with the catalytic domains of related PDE family members. Many protozoan parasites including *Toxoplasma*, *Plasmodium*, and the kinetoplastids *Trypanosoma brucei* and *Leishmania major* have one or more genes encoding class 1 PDEs. The genomes of Kinetoplastida encode four different class 1 PDEs (PDEs A–D) but no other PDE classes are encoded [2–4], similar to the situation in humans. All kinetoplastid genomes sequenced to date reveal the same set of PDE genes and the encoded PDEs are highly conserved between the species (reviewed in [5]). In *T. brucei* the two PDEs of the B family have been explored as drug targets [3]. Despite their high similarity, their subcellular localization is distinct; whereas *Tb*PDEB1 is localized primarily in the flagellum, *Tb*PDEB2 is predominantly located within the cell body, although it is also present in the flagellum [6,7]. *Tb*PDEB1 and *Tb*PDEB2 are the major factors controlling intracellular cAMP levels, and abrogating their activity by RNAi dramatically increases the intracellular cAMP concentration and induces complete trypanosome cell lysis, both in culture and in a mouse model [7]. A sequence comparison of the catalytic domains of *Tb*PDEB1 and *Tb*PDEB2 demonstrated that not only are they closely related to each other, but also to the human PDEs. X-ray crystallography has further revealed an extensive degree of structural conservation between human and kinetoplastid PDEs over large evolutionary distances [8,9]. Nevertheless, the crystal structures of *Lmj*PDEB1 and of the catalytic domain of *Tc*PDEC1 revealed a parasite-specific subpocket, termed the P-pocket, connected to the substrate-binding pocket, which neighbors the active site of human PDEs [8,9]. Structural and sequence homology data revealed that the gate to the P-pocket in all kinetoplastid PDEs is sterically open and accessible, while this pocket is blocked by two large gating residues in human PDEs [9]. This feature is currently under exploration for the design of parasite-selective PDE inhibitors. For example, based on the catechol scaffold of the human PDE4 inhibitor rolipram the group of Ke rationally designed small molecules, such as 1-(3-(4-hydroxybutoxy)-4-methoxyphenyl)-3-methylbutan-1-one (Figure 15.1), that specifically extend into the parasite-specific subpocket [5]. Furthermore, the group of Docampo synthesized and tested a range of compounds, initially designed as potential PDE4 inhibitors or obtained by virtual screening, as inhibitors of PDEC of *T. cruzi* [10]. *Tc*PDEC is a dual-substrate PDE, accepting both cAMP and cGMP as substrates. Several molecules, such as ZL-N-68 (Figure 15.1 and Table 15.1), displayed favorable selectivity for *Tc*PDEC over human PDE4D2, and a clear correlation between inhibition of *Tc*PDEC activity (and hence increased levels of intracellular cAMP) and anti-parasite potency was established.

At Nycomed Pharma, the company marketing the PDE4 inhibitor roflumilast for chronic obstructive pulmonary disease, high-throughput screening of a 400 000-membered proprietary compound library revealed several compound classes with high inhibitory activity against *T. brucei* PDEB1 [11]. One lead compound, a tetrahydrophthalazinone termed Cpd A (Figure 15.1 and Table 15.1), displayed high inhibitory activity against *Tb*PDEB1 (IC$_{50}$ ~10 nM). Cpd A appeared to be a 200-fold more potent *Tb*PDEB1 inhibitor than dipyridamole, which had until then been the most potent inhibitor of *Tb*PDEB1 and *Tb*PDEB2 known. Cpd A inhibited *T. brucei* proliferation with an EC$_{50}$ of 30–70 nM *in vitro* and, importantly, displayed identical activity against cell lines resistant to the drugs currently used in the field. The correlation between inhibition of *T. brucei* PDE activity, the resulting highly increased cAMP levels, and cell death provided pharmacological validation of

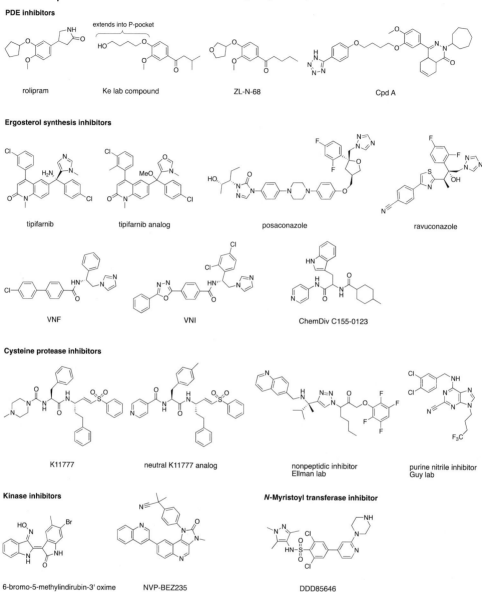

Figure 15.1 Selected inhibitors targeting conserved proteins; most of the inhibitors shown are currently in (preclinical) development for the treatment of parasite infections.

T. brucei PDEBs as drug targets. Currently, the TI Pharma T4-302 consortium have undertaken the hit-to-lead development of compound scaffolds identified in this screening campaign to render compounds more specific for parasite PDEs, making full use of the knowhow and experience of developing inhibitors against individual human PDEs.

Table 15.1 Conserved targets and promising lead compounds.

Target enzyme	Function	Inhibitor	References
*Tb*PDEB1 and *Tb*PDEB2	*T. brucei* phosphodiesterases: control of intracellular cAMP levels	Cpd A	[11]
*Tc*PDEC	*T. cruzi* phosphodiesterase: control of intracellular cAMP and cGMP levels	ZL-N-68	[10]
*Tc*CYP51	*T. cruzi* lanosterol 14α-demethylase: ergosterol biosynthesis	tipifarnib derivatives	[16]
		posaconazole	[19]
		ravuconazole	[19]
		VNF	[22]
*Tb*NMT	*T. brucei* N-myristoyltransferase: myristoylation of proteins for stabilization and targeting to membranes	DDD85646	[31,32]
Cruzain	*T. cruzi* cathepsin L ortholog: involved in differentiation, nutrient processing, and immune evasion	K11777	[38]
		tetrafluorophenoxymethyl ketone derivative	[40,41]
PI3K	*T. brucei* phosphoinositide 3-kinases: maintenance of Golgi structure, protein trafficking and cytokinesis	NVP-BEZ235	[59]
*Lm*CRK3	*Leishmania* sp. Cdc2-related kinase 3: cell cycle control	indirubin 3'-oxime derivatives	[60]
*Ld*GSK-3	*Leishmania* spp. glycogen synthase kinase: multifunctional kinase (e.g., involved in transcription, cell cycle control, and differentiation)	indirubin 3'-oxime derivatives	[61]

Ergosterol Synthesis

Farnesylation is essential for the membrane anchoring and thus correct functioning of important oncogenes such as Ras and Rheb [12], and inhibition of this process, mediated by protein farnesyl transferase (PFT), is a validated and well-explored anti-cancer strategy [13,14]. In a drug repositioning approach, aimed at exploiting *T. cruzi* PFT as a drug target, researchers at the University of Washington in Seattle screened several inhibitors against human PFT for inhibitory activity against *Tc*PFT. Surprisingly, they found that the Johnson & Johnson Pharmaceuticals anti-cancer drug candidate tipifarnib, while displaying an IC_{50} of around 75 nM against the *T. cruzi* PFT enzyme, had an EC_{50} of only 4 nM against *T. cruzi* amastigotes in culture [15], suggesting a mode of action distinct from PFT inhibition. Given the structural similarity (the presence of an imidazole pharmacophore) between tipifarnib and known inhibitors of the *T. cruzi* cytochrome P450 enzyme, lanosterol 14α-demethylase (*Tc*CYP51), an enzyme in the ergosterol biosynthesis pathway, the researchers rightly suspected that tipifarnib was in fact inhibiting *Tc*CYP51. *T. cruzi* amastigotes are dependent on *de novo* sterol biosynthesis and cannot rely on host cell-derived cholesterol, making them highly sensitive to inhibitors of enzymes in ergosterol biosynthesis. Using the anti-cancer drug tipifarnib as a lead for anti-Chagas drug development has obvious advantages: the drug is orally available, has a long half-life (16 h), displays little inhibitory activity against mammalian cytochrome P450 enzymes, is well tolerated in humans, and can readily be synthesized using inexpensive starting materials. In an attempt to develop the lead compound away from inhibiting human PFT and human cytochrome P450, while maintaining *Tc*CYP51 affinity, the researchers used rational design based on the cocrystal structure of tipifarnib occupying the active site of human PFT and a model of tipifarnib docked into the active site of *Tc*CYP51. Several rounds of optimization yielded tipifarnib analogs (Figure 15.1 and Table 15.1) with subnanomolar trypanocidal potency against *T. cruzi*, but practically devoid of mammalian PFT affinity [16]. Importantly, the leads displayed much lower potency for inhibition of human cytochrome P450 (3A4) than the azole-based CYP51 inhibitors discussed next and efficacy studies in mice are ongoing.

As fungi also are highly dependent on CYP51 for the production of ergosterol, a critical component of the fungal cellular membrane, the pharmaceutical industry has put considerable effort in developing inhibitors of fungal CYP51 to treat fungal infections in humans. A number of azole-based anti-fungal drugs are now on the market and several groups have shown that some of these, including the recently developed anti-fungal drugs posaconazole and ravuconazole (Figure 15.1 and Table 15.1), are also potent inhibitors of *T. cruzi* CYP51 [17,18], and show a curative effect in mouse models of acute and chronic Chagas disease (reviewed in [19]). Posaconazole (Noxafil[®]; Merck) is now under evaluation in phase II clinical trials for the treatment of Chagas disease, as is a prodrug of ravuconazole (E12-24; Eisai), another azole anti-fungal [20]. While being highly active *in vitro* against *T. cruzi*, in animal models ravuconazole has a suppressive, rather than curative activity. This has been ascribed to the relatively short terminal plasma half-life of ravuconazole in mice (4.5 h) [18] and dogs (8.8 h) [21]. Nevertheless, this drug is an interesting anti-Chagas drug candidate, as the longer half-life in humans (4–8 days), combined with a large volume of distribution, would allow for sufficient tissue exposure levels to have a curative effect. Moreover, ravuconazole requires a much less cumbersome synthetic route than posaconazole, making it a more affordable drug for the economically less powerful.

Other groups have also embarked on the development of inhibitors against the kinetoplastid CYP51. In a high-throughput screening campaign the group of Lepesheva and Waterman screened a collection of azole derivatives of the Novartis

Research Institute, revealing two imidazole containing structures, VNF and VNI (Figure 15.1 and Table 15.1), which both irreversibly inhibit *T. cruzi* and *T. brucei* CYP51 at a 1: 1 stoichiometry, while affecting the human enzyme only slightly at a 100-fold excess [22]. In another approach this group also identified a tryptophanyl containing dipeptide-like compound, ChemDiv C155-0123 (Figure 15.1), as a potent, reversible inhibitor of *Tc*CYP51 [23]. This compound was found independently as a strong inhibitor of *Tc*CYP51 at the Sandler Center (UCSF), although initially resulting from a screen against *Mycobacterium tuberculosis* CYP51 [24]. ChemDiv C155-0123 was found to inhibit endogenous sterol synthesis in *T. cruzi* epimastigotes and showed partial curative effects in a mouse model of acute Chagas disease [25]. The recently solved crystal structures of *T. cruzi* CYP51 bound with inhibitors, including posaconazole and VNF, may help to increase the potency of these molecules, while optimizing selectivity [17].

N-Myristoyl Transferase

The enzyme *N*-myristoyltransferase (NMT) catalyzes the cotranslational transfer of myristate from myristoyl-CoA to the N-terminal glycine of a subset of eukaryotic proteins. This is a post-translational modification that has been implicated in subcellular targeting to membrane locations and/or activation and stabilization of the substrate protein [26]. NMT has been pursued as a promising drug target, since its essentiality has been demonstrated in many organisms. For example, several pharmaceutical companies have aimed campaigns at targeting NMT from the yeast *Candida albicans*, resulting in the development of peptidomimetic inhibitors and small-molecule inhibitors containing, for example, a benzofuran or benzothiazole scaffold (reviewed in [27]). In kinetoplastid parasites NMT also plays an essential role in *Leishmania* and *Trypanosoma* species [28], and RNAi knockdown of NMT expression in *T. brucei* was shown to prevent parasitemia in infected mice [29].

A number of compounds targeting fungal NMT were screened for inhibitory activity on *Tb*NMT but none were found to display sufficient inhibitory activity on purified recombinant orthologs from *T. brucei* or *L. major* ($IC_{50} \geq 0.25 \, \mu M$) and their whole-cell anti-parasitic effects were disappointing [30]. In the absence of clear structural leads, yet convinced of the druggability of this conserved enzyme, researchers at the Dundee Drug Discovery Unit initiated a high-throughput screening campaign using a greater than 63 000 compound diversity library against *Tb*NMT. They identified a hit that was further optimized by several rounds of medicinal chemistry to lead compound DDD85646 (Figure 15.1 and Table 15.1) [31,32]. While this lead displayed high potency against *Tb*NMT ($IC_{50} = 2 \, nM$), it showed little specificity, as it also strongly inhibited the human ortholog (*Hs*NMT $IC_{50} = 4 \, nM$) and NMT of other species, including *L. major* (*Lm*NMT $IC_{50} = 2 \, nM$) and *T. cruzi* (*Tc*NMT $IC_{50} = 2 \, nM$). Nevertheless, bloodstream-form trypanosomes (*T. brucei* $EC_{50} = 2 \, nM$) were found to be much more susceptible to the drug than human cells (MRC5 $EC_{50} = 400 \, nM$). Moreover, the compound showed curative effects in a *T. brucei* acute mouse model after oral administration and was well tolerated at efficacious doses *in vivo* [31].

As a clear correlation between NMT inhibition and trypanocidal activity had been established, the enhanced susceptibility of trypanosomes for NMT inhibition must arise from differential downstream effects between host and parasite cells or from differential cellular pharmacokinetic behavior. Over 60 potential substrates of *Tb*NMT have been predicted by bioinformatics, two of which (ADP-ribosylation factor-1 protein (ARF-1) and ADP-ribosylation factor-like protein (ARL-1)) have been characterized and shown to be essential for bloodstream parasite viability [27,33,34]. Accordingly, inhibition of *Tb*NMT would be expected to have pleiotropic effects by affecting multiple downstream pathways. Exposure of bloodstream-form *T. brucei* to DDD85646 resulted in a morphological phenotype that closely resembled an expanded flagellar pocket phenotype observed when endocytosis was disrupted by knockdown of clathrin heavy chain, *Tb*RAB5 or *Tb*ARF1 [31]. Bloodstream-form *T. brucei* maintain an extremely high endocytic rate (9 times faster than fibroblasts and 2.6 times faster than macrophages [26,35]) in order to remove antibody from the cell surface and to continuously replace its variant surface glycoprotein (VSG) coat. The endocytic rate is the more phenomenal when one realizes that all this is performed exclusively in the flagellar pocket (i.e., 5% of the cell surface area). The basis for the apparent selectivity of DDD85646 against *T. brucei* likely lies in its effect on endocytosis, which, when disturbed, rapidly causes gross cellular defects because of the imbalance in membrane recycling. This explains why the same compound, inhibiting *Hs*NMT with very similar affinity, had hardly any effect on human cell lines. Thus, the selectivity of DDD85646 for trypanosome over human NMT is rooted in the basic cell biology of the parasite rather than in differences in the respective enzymes. Clearly, the importance of a solid understanding of fundamental cell biology and biochemistry in these parasites cannot be underestimated when targeting conserved proteins.

Proteases

Proteases have been investigated and used as drug targets for the treatment of diseases such as diabetes, osteoporosis, various cancers, and infectious diseases. Several cysteine protease inhibitors have reached the market or are in advanced clinical trials. One example is IDN-6556 (Pfizer), a selective pan-caspase inhibitor used for treating pathologies where liver damage can occur due to enhanced apoptosis, such as hepatic dysfunction, liver transplantations, and hepatitis B or C infections. Another example is the use of cathepsin K inhibitors including odanacatib (Merck) and relacatib (GlaxoSmithKline) for the treatment of osteoporosis. Numerous protease inhibitors, including saquinavir (Roche) and atazanavir (Bristol Myers) have been developed and approved for the treatment of AIDS [36]. Most of the protease inhibitors, be it probe compounds to study protease function or drug leads, are molecules containing a peptide-based recognition motif equipped with an electrophilic trapping moiety, which reacts with the active site cysteine (or serine/threonine in the case of other proteases) forming a reversible or irreversible covalent bond.

Kinetoplastid parasites produce cathepsins that are highly homologous to their human counterparts. *T. cruzi* cruzain is a close ortholog of human cathepsin L and is expressed in all life cycle stages. The enzyme has been shown to play a role in a range of processes including differentiation, nutrient processing, and immune evasion (reviewed in [37]). When testing a focused library of cathepsin inhibitors, initially developed by Khepri Pharmaceuticals in San Francisco for the treatment of chronic conditions such as osteoporosis or psoriasis, researchers at UCSF found that these compounds had promising activity against *T. cruzi*. Further studies showed that these inhibitors selectively targeted the *T. cruzi* cathepsin L ortholog cruzain. A drug lead resulting from this effort is the vinylsulfone K11777 (Figure 15.1 and Table 15.1), which has proved to have a curative effect in acute and non-acute models of infection in mice, and to ameliorate cardiac damage in dogs. Moreover, K11777 has shown efficacy against a range of *T. cruzi* strains, including benznidazole- or nifurtimox-resistant isolates from different geographic locations [38].

Preclinical development of K11777 as an anti-Chagas drug in collaboration with the Institute for One World Health was put on hold in 2005 due to apparent liver toxicity indicated by elevated alanine aminotransferase levels, when the drug was found to inhibit isolated liver enzymes *in vitro*. Further investigation into the apparent liver toxicity revealed that K11777 was in fact not toxic to hepatocytes at therapeutic concentrations and the team at UCSF have taken up preclinical investigation again in collaboration with the National Institute of Allergy and Infectious Diseases (National Institutes of Health). The US Food and Drug Administration has now approved K11777 to enter a phase I safety trial in the United States [39].

The sequences of cruzain and human cathepsins display remarkable homology, while the active sites are virtually identical [40,41]. Yet, *T. cruzi* parasites are particularly vulnerable to inhibition of cruzain, which is primarily due to the lack of redundancy of this enzyme. While the highly homologous human papain superfamily consists of a variety of cathepsins (i.e., cathepsins B, L, K, S, F, and V), the parasite is dependent on only a single cathepsin, cruzain. In humans, cathepsins are primarily found in lysosomes, being responsible for the degradation of endocytosed material including extracellular antigens. Localization of cruzain in the epimastigote stage is also predominantly in the lysosome. In the intracellular amastigote stage, however (relevant for drug targeting in infection), cruzain is additionally present in the flagellar pocket and on the surface of the parasite, directly in contact with the host cell cytoplasm [37]. Consistent with the varied location, cruzain has an unusually broad pH profile, between 4.5 and 9.0 [42].

The likely trypanocidal mode of action of K11777 is through targeting unprocessed cruzain as it is leaving the endoplasmic reticulum, leading to accumulation of the inactive enzyme in the Golgi and subsequently cell death [43]. For a selective anti-trypanosomal drug, it is desirable that the compound does not accumulate in the acidic lysosomal compartment – be it of host cells or the parasite itself – through the presence of a basic moiety in the drug (a process called lysosomotropism). Not only would such sequestration of the drug in acidic compartments lead to a lower cytoplasmic concentration, it might also lead to a selective inhibition of lysosomal host cathepsins, which would enhance the likelihood of unwanted side-effects. For this reason, recent efforts were directed at replacing basic groups by neutral moieties in these cathepsin inhibitors, which has resulted in highly trypanocidal "neutral" analogs of K11777, that displayed improved trypanocidal activity despite a reduced affinity for cruzain in a biochemical assay [44,45]. The recent structures of human and parasite cathepsins cocrystallized with inhibitors revealed sites for modification in the inhibitor to enhance selectivity for the parasite protease over its human ortholog [46]. Such structure-based design has now afforded a series of novel drug leads against *T. cruzi* [40,41]. A similar structure-based optimization strategy resulted in a series of inhibitors [47] targeting essential *T. brucei* cathepsins such as rhodesain, a cathepsin L-like protease, and *Tb*CatB, the *T. brucei* cathepsin B ortholog, shown to facilitate iron acquisition by lysosomal degradation of host transferrin and essential for parasite survival both *in vitro* and *in vivo* [48].

A drawback of peptide-based drugs, such as K11777, is that they are vulnerable to degradation by proteases, which not only limits their oral bioavailability, but also makes them relatively unstable in blood where they are prone to serum proteases. These processes considerably reduce their half-life in the body and give the drug less chance to reach the target site, limiting its efficacy. Synthetic efforts to overcome this problem have been directed at the development of non-peptidic protease inhibitors. Replacement of hydrolysis-sensitive moieties (amide/peptide bonds) from the lead structure was reported by Ellman *et al.*, which led to non-peptidic, mechanism-based cruzain inhibitors with high stability in plasma, such as the tetrafluorophenoxymethyl ketone shown in the Figure 15.1 [40,41]. Other scaffold-hopping strategies include aryl thio semicarbazones [49–51] and macrocyclic vinyl sulfones [52]. Aiming at the development of inhibitors for *Tb*CatB, the team of Guy focused on structure-based optimization of pharmacophoric regions connected via a purine scaffold [47,53]. Optimization of these purine-nitrile protease inhibitors improved selectivity for *Tb*CatB over human cathepsins B and L, and resulted in a metabolically stable and orally available lead compound shown in the Figure 15.1 [54].

While the most active trypanocidal inhibitors known to date are irreversible, recent efforts are addressed at the development of reversible inhibitors of parasite cysteine proteases. For chronic indications or at least for a prolonged course of treatment, as expected for anti-Chagas therapy, inhibition of the target protease by an irreversible mechanism may be undesirable, due to risks of reduced selectivity and immunogenic potential. Efforts at the development of reversible parasite cathepsin inhibitors include the screening of a focused cathepsin inhibitor library, which has revealed drug-like lead structures bearing a nitrile or ketone-based warhead [55].

Kinases

Initially, kinases were not considered as suitable drug targets by the pharmaceutical industry, primarily because the development of selective inhibitors for this enzyme class was seen as virtually impossible. The best hope for acceptable selectivity is through targeting of the substrate-binding pocket with small molecules; however, this is uncommonly difficult as this pocket is usually shallow and not well defined. Therefore, the small ATP-binding pocket seems more suitable for targeting, although the notion that it is highly conserved throughout diverse families of kinases appears to almost preclude the development of sufficiently selective inhibitors. Moreover, formidable competition must be overcome by ATP-mimetic competitive inhibitors given the high cellular ATP concentrations. Mindful of the critical role protein kinases play in signaling cascades and cell division, researchers nevertheless attempted to overcome these hurdles and embarked on the development of anti-cancer kinase inhibitors through structure-based design (see [56,57] for recent reviews). A number of ATP-competitive kinase inhibitors with reasonable selectivity have now been approved, mostly for oncological use, of which imatinib (Gleevec®), targeting the Bcr–Abl kinase in chronic myeloid leukemia patients, is probably the most famous example. Vast investments by the pharmaceutical industry have since led to kinase inhibitors with picomolar selectivity, isoform selectivity, and allosteric binding modes that circumvent the ATP-binding pocket. Overall, an important lesson learned from the kinase field was that exclusive selectivity for the biological target was not an essential requirement for effective and safe clinical application. Rather, targeting cell cycle regulation protein kinases, such as cyclin-dependent kinases (CDKs), would mostly affect rapidly dividing cells, such as cancer cells, while normal cells, most of which do not divide, would be much less affected. It is precisely this reason that makes cell cycle kinases also attractive targets in protozoan parasites, many of which depend on rapid cell division.

In kinetoplastids, genetic knockdown or knockout strategies have validated several kinases as drug targets, including glycogen synthase kinase-3 (GSK-3) [58], target of rapamycin (TOR), phosphoinositide 3-kinase (PI3K) [59], and the CDK CRK3 (Table 15.1) [60]. These kinases have in addition been probed by small molecules. Screening of libraries containing several classes of kinase inhibitors revealed indirubins, known to inhibit mammalian CDK and GSK-3 kinases, also as potent inhibitors of *L. mexicana* CRK-3 [60] and *L. donovani* GSK-3 [61]. The indirubins displayed anti-leishmanial activity in a macrophage infection model *in vitro*, and arrested both promastigote and axenic amastigote growth in culture. *L. mexicana* promastigotes exposed to indirubin-3'-oxime showed aberrant morphology and an altered DNA content, consistent with disruption of the cell cycle through inhibition of a CDK [60]. Structural data and a docking study on the mammalian and leishmanial GSK-3 showed differences in indirubin binding that could be exploited for making inhibitors more selective for leishmanial GSK-3, leading to 6-bromo-5-methylindirubin-3'-oxime (Figure 15.1) [61].

Several inhibitors of human PI3K and the kinase domain of mammalian TOR, in various stages of clinical and preclinical development, were evaluated for anti-kinetoplastid activity *in vitro* against *T. brucei*, *T. cruzi*, *L. major*, and *L. donovani*, and in mouse models of kinetoplastid infection [59]. An advanced clinical candidate against solid tumors, the Novartis compound NVP-BEZ235 (Figure 15.1 and

Table 15.1), was shown to display subnanomolar potency against *T. b. rhodesiense* growth and cleared parasitemia in an acute mouse model of *T. b. rhodesiense* infection.

Instead of repurposing existing kinase inhibitors, researchers at the Sandler Center (UCSF) are investigating the *T. brucei* kinome as their starting point for *ab initio* drug discovery. Their strategy combines the systematic use of RNAi to identify essential kinases with a chemical biology approach in which small-molecule probes are used that covalently modify active-site residues in a subset of the *T. brucei* kinome [45]. Similar target kinases were found by either method, showing the validity of their approach. Whole-cell and biochemical screens using kinase-targeted small-molecule libraries to yield drug-like inhibitors, and subsequent hit optimization, are currently ongoing [45]. The emergence of kinase inhibitors as a drug strategy for the treatment of kinetoplastid infections is a further example of (a class of) conserved proteins as promising targets for anti-protozoal therapy.

Concluding Remarks

The examples given in this chapter clearly demonstrate that not only is it possible to target conserved drug targets in protozoa, it is a very promising route to accelerated drug development, aided by partnerships with industry and the extensive pharmacological and medicinal chemistry knowledge about such targets from other branches of human medicine. The examples also show that many of the most promising (pre)-clinical developments of anti-kinetoplastid agents are using this approach, even to the point of repurposing existing anti-cancer drugs, which self-evidently act on human targets. A successful example of such repurposing of an agent developed against cancer has been in use since 1990: α-difluoromethylornithine (eflornithine), an inhibitor of ornithine decarboxylase (ODC) in the polyamine biosynthesis pathway. Despite having a higher affinity for the human enzyme than for the corresponding *T. b. brucei* enzyme, it failed as an anti-cancer drug while being the only wholly new drug to be introduced for advanced sleeping sickness since melarsoprol in the 1930s. The basis of its selectivity lie in its rapid clearance form circulation, combined with a very high turnover rate of human ODC; in contrast *Tb*ODC is very stable (reviewed in [62]).

All this is not to diminish the value of high-throughput screening against live parasites, which have led to some very good results in recent years, including the discovery of fexinidazole [63] and the promising series of oxaboroles [64], both for the treatment of sleeping sickness. While this approach may yield a faster route to compounds with potent anti-protozoal activity than target-based drug design, the trade-off is that hit optimization can be more difficult due to lack of understanding of the mechanism of its anti-parasitic actions.

In conclusion, it is encouraging to see that over the past years several research teams have realized that aiming at conserved rather than unique targets may lead to faster anti-parasite drug development.

References

1 Conti, M. and Beavo, J. (2007) Biochemistry and physiology of cyclic nucleotide phosphodiesterases: essential components in cyclic nucleotide signaling. *Annu. Rev. Biochem.*, **76**, 481–511.

2 Gould, M.K. and de Koning, H.P. (2011) Cyclic-nucleotide signalling in protozoa. *FEMS Microbiol. Rev.*, **35**, 515–541.

3 Shakur, Y., de Koning, H.P., Ke, H., Kambayashi, J., and Seebeck, T. (2011) Therapeutic potential of phosphodiesterase inhibitors in parasitic diseases. *Handb. Exp. Pharmacol.*, **204**, 487–510.

4 Kunz, S., Beavo, J.A., D'Angelo, M.A., Flawia, M.M., Francis, S.H., Johner, A., Laxman, S. *et al.* (2006) Cyclic nucleotide specific phosphodiesterases of the kinetoplastida: a unified nomenclature. *Mol. Biochem. Parasitol.*, **145**, 133–135.

5 Seebeck, T., Sterk, G.J., and Ke, H. (2011) Phosphodiesterase inhibitors as a new generation of antiprotozoan drugs: exploiting the benefit of enzymes that are highly conserved between host and parasite. *Future Med. Chem.*, **3**, 1289–1306.

6 Luginbuehl, E., Ryter, D., Schranz-Zumkehr, J., Oberholzer, M., Kunz, S., and Seebeck, T. (2010) The N terminus of phosphodiesterase *Tbr*PDEB1 of *Trypanosoma brucei* contains the signal for integration into the flagellar skeleton. *Eukaryot. Cell*, **9**, 1466–1475.

7 Oberholzer, M., Marti, G., Baresic, M., Kunz, S., Hemphill, A., and Seebeck, T. (2007) The *Trypanosoma brucei* cAMP phosphodiesterases *Tbr*PDEB1 and *Tbr*PDEB2: flagellar enzymes that are essential for parasite virulence. *FASEB J.*, **21**, 720–731.

8 Wang, H., Yan, Z., Geng, J., Kunz, S., Seebeck, T., and Ke, H. (2007) Crystal structure of the *Leishmania major* phosphodiesterase *Lmj*PDEB1 and insight into the design of the parasite-selective inhibitors. *Mol. Microbiol.*, **66**, 1029–1038.

9 Wang, H., Kunz, S., Chen, G., Seebeck, T., Wan, Y., Robinson, H., Martinelli, S. *et al.* (2012) Biological and structural characterization of *Trypanosoma cruzi* phosphodiesterase C and implications for the design of parasite selective inhibitors. *J. Biol. Chem.*, **287**, 11788–11797.

10 King-Keller, S., Li, M., Smith, A., Zheng, S., Kaur, G., Yang, X., Wang, B. *et al.* (2010) Chemical validation of phosphodiesterase C as a chemotherapeutic target in *Trypanosoma cruzi*, the etiological agent of Chagas' disease. *Antimicrob. Agents Chemother.*, **54**, 3738–3745.

11 de Koning, H.P., Gould, M.K., Sterk, G.J., Tenor, H., Kunz, S., Luginbuehl, E., and Seebeck, T. (2012) Pharmacological validation of *Trypanosoma brucei* phosphodiesterases as novel drug targets. *J. Infect. Dis.*, **206**, 229–237.

12 Casey, P.J., Solski, P.A., Der, C.J., and Buss, J.E. (1989) p21ras is modified by a farnesyl isoprenoid. *Proc. Natl. Acad. Sci. USA*, **86**, 8323–8327.

13 Kohl, N.E., Mosser, S.D., deSolms, S.J., Giuliani, E.A., Pompliano, D.L., Graham, S.L., Smith, R.L. *et al.* (1993) Selective inhibition of ras-dependent transformation by a farnesyltransferase inhibitor. *Science*, **260**, 1934–1937.

14 Mesa, R.A. (2006) Tipifarnib: farnesyl transferase inhibition at a crossroads. *Expert Rev. Anticancer Ther.*, **6**, 313–319.

15 Hucke, O., Gelb, M.H., Verlinde, C.L., and Buckner, F.S. (2005) The protein farnesyltransferase inhibitor Tipifarnib as a new lead for the development of drugs against Chagas disease. *J. Med. Chem.*, **48**, 5415–5418.

16 Kraus, J.M., Tatipaka, H.B., McGuffin, S.A., Chennamaneni, N.K., Karimi, M., Arif, J., Verlinde, C.L. *et al.* (2010) Second generation analogues of the cancer drug clinical candidate tipifarnib for anti-Chagas disease drug discovery. *J. Med. Chem.*, **53**, 3887–3898.

17 Lepesheva, G.I., Hargrove, T.Y., Anderson, S., Kleshchenko, Y., Furtak, V., Wawrzak, Z., Villalta, F. *et al.* (2010) Structural insights into inhibition of sterol 14alpha-demethylase in the human pathogen *Trypanosoma cruzi*. *J. Biol. Chem.*, **285**, 25582–25590.

18 Urbina, J.A., Payares, G., Sanoja, C., Lira, R., and Romanha, A.J. (2003) In vitro and in vivo activities of ravuconazole on

Trypanosoma cruzi, the causative agent of Chagas disease. *Int. J. Antimicrob. Agents*, **21**, 27–38.

19 Buckner, F.S. and Urbina, J.A. (2012) Recent developments in sterol 14-demethylase inhibitors for Chagas disease. *Int. J. Parasitol. Drugs Drug Resist.*, **2**, 236–242.

20 Clayton, J. (2010) Chagas disease: pushing through the pipeline. *Nature*, **465**, S12–15.

21 Diniz Lde, F., Caldas, I.S., Guedes, P.M., Crepalde, G., de Lana, M., Carneiro, C.M., Talvani, A. *et al.* (2010) Effects of ravuconazole treatment on parasite load and immune response in dogs experimentally infected with *Trypanosoma cruzi*. *Antimicrob. Agents Chemother.*, **54**, 2979–2986.

22 Lepesheva, G.I., Villalta, F., and Waterman, M.R. (2011) Targeting *Trypanosoma cruzi* sterol 14-alpha-demethylase (CYP51). *Adv. Parasitol.*, **75**, 65–87.

23 Lepesheva, G.I., Hargrove, T.Y., Kleshchenko, Y., Nes, W.D., Villalta, F., and Waterman, M.R. (2008) CYP51: a major drug target in the cytochrome P450 superfamily. *Lipids*, **43**, 1117–1125.

24 Chen, C.K., Doyle, P.S., Yermalitskaya, L.V., Mackey, Z.B., Ang, K.K., McKerrow, J.H., and Podust, L.M. (2009) *Trypanosoma cruzi* CYP51 inhibitor derived from a *Mycobacterium tuberculosis* screen hit. *PLoS Negl. Trop. Dis.*, **3**, e372.

25 Doyle, P.S., Chen, C.K., Johnston, J.B., Hopkins, S.D., Leung, S.S., Jacobson, M.P., Engel, J.C. *et al.* (2010) A nonazole CYP51 inhibitor cures Chagas' disease in a mouse model of acute infection. *Antimicrob. Agents Chemother.*, **54**, 2480–2488.

26 Thilo, L. (1985) Quantification of endocytosis-derived membrane traffic. *Biochim. Biophys. Acta*, **822**, 243–266.

27 Bowyer, P.W., Tate, E.W., Leatherbarrow, R.J., Holder, A.A., Smith, D.F., and Brown, K.A. (2008) N-myristoyltransferase: a prospective drug target for protozoan parasites. *ChemMedChem*, **3**, 402–408.

28 Price, H.P., Menon, M.R., Panethymitaki, C., Goulding, D., McKean, P.G., and Smith, D.F. (2003) Myristoyl-CoA:protein N-myristoyltransferase, an essential

enzyme and potential drug target in kinetoplastid parasites. *J. Biol. Chem.*, **278**, 7206–7214.

29 Price, H.P., Guther, M.L., Ferguson, M.A., and Smith, D.F. (2010) Myristoyl-CoA: protein N-myristoyltransferase depletion in trypanosomes causes avirulence and endocytic defects. *Mol. Biochem. Parasitol.*, **169**, 55–58.

30 Panethymitaki, C., Bowyer, P.W., Price, H.P., Leatherbarrow, R.J., Brown, K.A., and Smith, D.F. (2006) Characterization and selective inhibition of myristoyl-CoA: protein N-myristoyltransferase from *Trypanosoma brucei* and *Leishmania major*. *Biochem. J.*, **396**, 277–285.

31 Frearson, J.A., Brand, S., McElroy, S.P., Cleghorn, L.A., Smid, O., Stojanovski, L., Price, H.P. *et al.* (2010) N-Myristoyltransferase inhibitors as new leads to treat sleeping sickness. *Nature*, **464**, 728–732.

32 Brand, S., Cleghorn, L.A., McElroy, S.P., Robinson, D.A., Smith, V.C., Hallyburton, I., Harrison, J.R. *et al.* (2012) Discovery of a novel class of orally active trypanocidal N-myristoyltransferase inhibitors. *J. Med. Chem.*, **55**, 140–152.

33 Price, H.P., Goulding, D., and Smith, D.F. (2005) ARL1 has an essential role in *Trypanosoma brucei*. *Biochem. Soc. Trans.*, **33**, 643–645.

34 Price, H.P., Stark, M., and Smith, D.F. (2007) *Trypanosoma brucei* ARF1 plays a central role in endocytosis and Golgi–lysosome trafficking. *Mol. Biol. Cell*, **18**, 864–873.

35 Overath, P. and Engstler, M. (2004) Endocytosis, membrane recycling and sorting of GPI-anchored proteins: *Trypanosoma brucei* as a model system. *Mol. Microbiol.*, **53**, 735–744.

36 Qiu, X. and Liu, Z.P. (2011) Recent developments of peptidomimetic HIV-1 protease inhibitors. *Curr. Med. Chem.*, **18**, 4513–4537.

37 Sajid, M., Robertson, S.A., Brinen, L.S., and McKerrow, J.H. (2011) Cruzain: the path from target validation to the clinic. *Adv. Exp. Med. Biol.*, **712**, 100–115.

38 McKerrow, J.H., Doyle, P.S., Engel, J.C., Podust, L.M., Robertson, S.A., Ferreira, R., Saxton, T. *et al.* (2009) Two approaches to

discovering and developing new drugs for Chagas disease. *Mem. Inst. Oswaldo Cruz*, **104** (Suppl 1), 263–269.

39 Leslie, M. (2011) Infectious diseases. Drug developers finally take aim at a neglected disease. *Science*, **333**, 933–935.

40 Brak, K., Kerr, I.D., Barrett, K.T., Fuchi, N., Debnath, M., Ang, K., Engel, J.C. *et al.* (2010) Nonpeptidic tetrafluorophenoxymethyl ketone cruzain inhibitors as promising new leads for Chagas disease chemotherapy. *J. Med. Chem.*, **53**, 1763–1773.

41 Brak, K., Doyle, P.S., McKerrow, J.H., and Ellman, J.A. (2008) Identification of a new class of nonpeptidic inhibitors of cruzain. *J. Am. Chem. Soc.*, **130**, 6404–6410.

42 Judice, W.A., Puzer, L., Cotrin, S.S., Carmona, A.K., Coombs, G.H., Juliano, L., and Juliano, M.A. (2004) Carboxydipeptidase activities of recombinant cysteine peptidases. Cruzain of *Trypanosoma cruzi* and CPB of *Leishmania mexicana*. *Eur. J. Biochem.*, **271**, 1046–1053.

43 Engel, J.C., Torres, C., Hsieh, I., Doyle, P. S., and McKerrow, J.H. (2000) Upregulation of the secretory pathway in cysteine protease inhibitor-resistant *Trypanosoma cruzi*. *J. Cell Sci.*, **113**, 1345–1354.

44 Jaishankar, P., Hansell, E., Zhao, D.M., Doyle, P.S., McKerrow, J.H., and Renslo, A.R. (2008) Potency and selectivity of P2/P3-modified inhibitors of cysteine proteases from trypanosomes. *Bioorg. Med. Chem. Lett.*, **18**, 624–628.

45 Robertson, S.A. and Renslo, A.R. (2011) Drug discovery for neglected tropical diseases at the Sandler Center. *Future Med. Chem.*, **3**, 1279–1288.

46 Brinen, L.S., Hansell, E., Cheng, J., Roush, W.R., McKerrow, J.H., and Fletterick, R.J. (2000) A target within the target: probing cruzain's P1′ site to define structural determinants for the Chagas' disease protease. *Structure*, **8**, 831–840.

47 Mallari, J.P., Shelat, A.A., Kosinski, A., Caffrey, C.R., Connelly, M., Zhu, F., McKerrow, J.H. *et al.* (2009) Structure-guided development of selective *Tb*catB inhibitors. *J. Med. Chem.*, **52**, 6489–6493.

48 Abdulla, M.H., O'Brien, T., Mackey, Z.B., Sajid, M., Grab, D.J., and McKerrow, J.H. (2008) RNA interference of *Trypanosoma brucei* cathepsin B and L affects disease progression in a mouse model. *PLoS Negl. Trop. Dis.*, **2**, e298.

49 Fujii, N., Mallari, J.P., Hansell, E.J., Mackey, Z., Doyle, P., Zhou, Y.M., Gut, J. *et al.* (2005) Discovery of potent thiosemicarbazone inhibitors of rhodesain and cruzain. *Bioorg. Med. Chem. Lett.*, **15**, 121–123.

50 Du, X., Guo, C., Hansell, E., Doyle, P.S., Caffrey, C.R., Holler, T.P., McKerrow, J.H. *et al.* (2002) Synthesis and structure-activity relationship study of potent trypanocidal thio semicarbazone inhibitors of the trypanosomal cysteine protease cruzain. *J. Med. Chem*, **45**, 2695–2707.

51 Greenbaum, D.C., Mackey, Z., Hansell, E., Doyle, P., Gut, J., Caffrey, C.R., Lehrman, J. *et al.* (2004) Synthesis and structure–activity relationships of parasiticidal thiosemicarbazone cysteine protease inhibitors against *Plasmodium falciparum*, *Trypanosoma brucei*, and *Trypanosoma cruzi*. *J. Med. Chem.*, **47**, 3212–3219.

52 Chen, Y.T., Lira, R., Hansell, E., McKerrow, J.H., and Roush, W.R. (2008) Synthesis of macrocyclic trypanosomal cysteine protease inhibitors. *Bioorg. Med. Chem. Lett.*, **18**, 5860–5863.

53 Mallari, J.P., Shelat, A.A., Obrien, T., Caffrey, C.R., Kosinski, A., Connelly, M., Harbut, M. *et al.* (2008) Development of potent purine-derived nitrile inhibitors of the trypanosomal protease *Tb*catB. *J. Med. Chem.*, **51**, 545–552.

54 Mallari, J.P., Zhu, F., Lemoff, A., Kaiser, M., Lu, M., Brun, R., and Guy, R.K. (2010) Optimization of purine-nitrile *Tb*catB inhibitors for use *in vivo* and evaluation of efficacy in murine models. *Bioorg. Med. Chem.*, **18**, 8302–8309.

55 Ang, K.K., Ratnam, J., Gut, J., Legac, J., Hansell, E., Mackey, Z.B., Skrzypczynska, K.M. *et al.* (2011) Mining a cathepsin inhibitor library for new anti-parasitic drug leads. *PLoS Negl. Trop. Dis.*, **5**, e1023.

56 Crawford, J.J., Hoeflich, K.P., and Rudolph, J. (2012) p21-Activated kinase inhibitors: a patent review. *Expert. Opin. Ther. Pat.*, **22**, 293–310.

57 Chahrour, O., Cairns, D., and Omran, Z. (2012) Small molecule kinase inhibitors as anti-cancer therapeutics. *Mini Rev. Med. Chem.*, **12**, 399–411.

58 Ojo, K.K., Gillespie, J.R., Riechers, A.J., Napuli, A.J., Verlinde, C.L., Buckner, F.S., Gelb, M.H. *et al.* (2008) Glycogen synthase kinase 3 is a potential drug target for African trypanosomiasis therapy. *Antimicrob. Agents Chemother.*, **52**, 3710–3717.

59 Diaz-Gonzalez, R., Kuhlmann, F.M., Galan-Rodriguez, C., Madeira da Silva, L., Saldivia, M., Karver, C.E., Rodriguez, A. *et al.* (2011) The susceptibility of trypanosomatid pathogens to PI3/mTOR kinase inhibitors affords a new opportunity for drug repurposing. *PLoS Negl. Trop. Dis.*, **5**, e1297.

60 Grant, K.M., Dunion, M.H., Yardley, V., Skaltsounis, A.L., Marko, D., Eisenbrand, G., Croft, S.L. *et al.* (2004) Inhibitors of *Leishmania mexicana* CRK3 cyclin-dependent kinase: chemical library screen and antileishmanial activity. *Antimicrob. Agents Chemother.*, **48**, 3033–3042.

61 Xingi, E., Smirlis, D., Myrianthopoulos, V., Magiatis, P., Grant, K.M., Meijer, L.,

Mikros, E. *et al.* (2009) 6-Br-5methylindirubin-3′oxime (5-Me-6-BIO) targeting the leishmanial glycogen synthase kinase-3 (GSK-3) short form affects cell-cycle progression and induces apoptosis-like death: exploitation of GSK-3 for treating leishmaniasis. *Int. J. Parasitol.*, **39**, 1289–1303.

62 Delespaux, V. and de Koning, H.P. (2007) Drugs and drug resistance in African trypanosomiasis. *Drug Resist. Updates*, **10**, 30–50.

63 Kaiser, M., Bray, M.A., Cal, M., Bourdin Trunz, B., Torreele, E., and Brun, R. (2011) Antitrypanosomal activity of fexinidazole, a new oral nitroimidazole drug candidate for treatment of sleeping sickness. *Antimicrob. Agents Chemother.*, **55**, 5602–5608.

64 Nare, B., Wring, S., Bacchi, C., Beaudet, B., Bowling, T., Brun, R., Chen, D. *et al.* (2010) Discovery of novel orally bioavailable oxaborole 6-carboxamides that demonstrate cure in a murine model of late-stage central nervous system African trypanosomiasis. *Antimicrob. Agents Chemother.*, **54**, 4379–4388.

16
Drug Targets in Trypanosomal and Leishmanial Pentose Phosphate Pathway

Marcelo A. Comini*, Cecilia Ortíz, and Juan José Cazzulo

Abstract

Trypanosomatids utilize glucose to sustain critical cellular functions. A key metabolic pathway that relies on glucose is the pentose phosphate pathway (PPP), which comprises reactions oxidizing substrates (oxidative phase) and interconversions to phosphorylated saccharides (non-oxidative phase). The products (ribose-5-phosphate), intermediates (glyceraldehyde-3-phosphate, fructose-6-phosphate), and cofactor (NADPH) of this metabolism are used in the synthesis of nucleic acids and lipids, and for the maintenance of redox homeostasis. Enzymes from the oxidative branch (i.e., glucose-6-phosphate dehydrogenase (G6PDH), 6-phosphogluconolactonase (6PGL), and 6-phosphogluconate dehydrogenase (6PGDH)) are phylogenetically related to their cyanobacterial and plant counterparts, and play an essential house-keeping role in the parasites. The components of the non-oxidative branch (i.e., ribose-phosphate isomerase (RPI), ribose-phosphate epimerase (RPE), transketolase (TKT), and transaldolase (TAL) are more heterogeneous, with a member that has no orthologous sequence in mammals (RPI) and others (RPE and TKT) that are developmentally regulated and species-specific dispensable. Except for 6PGDH, no systematic drug discovery studies have been performed on PPP enzymes. Only few chemical entities have been identified as inhibitors of G6PDH, and there are no investigations addressing this issue for 6PGL, RPI, RPE, TKT, and TAL. Thus, the search for inhibitors against PPP enzymes from trypanosomatids does not keep pace with the substantial information available on their biochemical and structural properties. The aim of this chapter is to attract attention towards PPP enzymes that qualify as trypanosomatid drug targets.

Pentose Phosphate Pathway in Trypanosomatids: General Considerations and Biological Relevance

Trypanosomiasis and leishmaniasis are life-threatening diseases of mammals for which an effective, safe, and affordable chemotherapy and/or immunoprophylaxis (vaccine) remain major and challenging goals for the scientific and public health

* Corresponding Author

Trypanosomatid Diseases: Molecular Routes to Drug Discovery, First edition. Edited by T. Jäger, O. Koch, and L. Flohé.
© 2013 Wiley-VCH Verlag GmbH & Co. KGaA. Published 2013 by Wiley-VCH Verlag GmbH & Co. KGaA.

domain. Over the last decades, this situation has prompted the search for suitable drug target candidates – an enterprise that requires a detailed biochemical, biological, and structural analysis of the metabolic pathways and their components [1]. The glucose-based metabolism of trypanosomatids is among those critical pathways that have been investigated thoroughly but not completely. In most organisms glucose is metabolized through two major pathways: the glycolytic, or Embden–Meyerhof, pathway, and the pentose phosphate pathway (PPP). Both pathways start from glucose-6-phosphate (G6P), but have different functions, which all are important for survival. Whereas glycolysis is the chief pathway to catabolize glucose gaining energy in the form of ATP, the PPP is involved in the production of ribose-5-phosphate (R5P), required for nucleotide and nucleic acid synthesis, and for sustaining reducing power in the form of NADPH, which is essential for a number of biosynthetic processes and for the protection of the cell against oxidative stress (see below and Chapter 9 of this volume). The pathway consists of two branches, an oxidative branch, involving glucose-6-phosphate dehydrogenase (G6PDH), 6-phosphogluconolactonase (6PGL), and 6-phosphogluconate dehydrogenase (6PGDH), and a non-oxidative, or sugar interconversion, branch, involving ribose-5-phosphate isomerase (RPI), ribulose-5-phosphate epimerase (RPE), transaldolase (TAL), and transketolase (TKT) (Figure 16.1). The PPP has also been known as the pentose phosphate cycle, since, when functioning as a whole, the fructose-6-phosphate (F6P) and glyceraldehyde-3-phosphate (Gly3P) formed can be converted back to G6P, entering the oxidative branch again. However, the PPP does not need to act as a cycle and the different enzymatic reactions will be operative according to the cell needs [2].

As opposed to the glycolytic pathway, which has been thoroughly studied in trypanosomatids over the last three decades, the PPP received much less attention up to the late 1990s. At present, is known that all seven enzymes of the pathway are expressed in the four major stages of the life cycle of *Trypanosoma cruzi* (epimastigote and metacyclic trypomastigote in the insect vector, amastigote and bloodstream trypomastigote in the mammal) [3] and in promastigotes of *Leishmania mexicana* [4], whereas the pathway is developmentally regulated in *T. brucei*, with expression of all components in the procyclic (insect dwelling) form and the oxidative branch enzymes in the bloodstream form [5]. The functionality of the pathway has been demonstrated in *T. cruzi* epimastigotes [3], and in *L. braziliensis* [6] and *L. mexicana* promastigotes [4] by determining the amount of [^{14}C]CO$_2$ released from glucose labeled in C1 or C6. A similar study has not been conducted on *T. brucei*, although several lines of evidence point that this pathway is fully active at least in the procyclic stage. At this point it is worth noting that trypanosomatids contain an organelle called the glycosome, which has a peroxisomal origin and evolved to host several components or steps of key pathways such as glycolysis, gluconeogenesis, PPP, lipid biosynthesis, purine salvage, and pyrimidine biogenesis ([7] and Chapter 7 of this volume). Accordingly, several enzymes of the PPP are localized in the glycosomes, although not exclusively, as discussed below for each enzymatic entity [8]. Another interesting aspect of the trypanosomatids

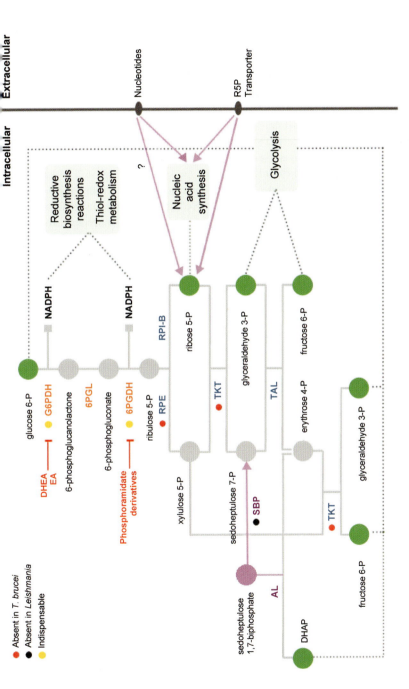

Figure 16.1 Scheme of the PPP in trypanosomatids: components, biological relevance, and inhibitors. The substrates and products of the PPP that are shared with other metabolic pathways labeled with a green dot. Characterized enzyme inhibitors are shown in red. The enzymes of the oxidative and non-oxidative phase of the PPP are in orange and light blue, respectively: G6PDH, glucose-6-phosphate dehydrogenase; 6PGL, 6-phosphogluconolactonase; 6PGDH, 6-phosphogluconate dehydrogenase; RPI-B, type B ribose phosphate isomerase; RPE, ribose phosphate epimerase; TKT, transketolase; TAL, transaldolase; AL, aldolase. Salvage pathways for R5P are depicted in magenta, and include: (i) membrane transporters for R5P and/or nucleotides, (ii) the phosphorylation of ribose by ribose kinase (question mark, ?), and (iii) the riboneogenesis pathway where by the concerted action of aldolase (AL) and sedoheptulose bisphosphatase (SBP), dihydroxyacetone phosphate (DHAP), and glyceraldehyde-3-phosphate are converted into sedoheptulose-7-phosphate. Enzymes absent in infective T. brucei and Leishmania spp. are marked with a red and black dot, respectively. Enzymes of proved indispensability are indicated with yellow dot. Promising enzyme inhibitors are shown in red.

enzymes from the oxidative branch (G6PDH, 6PGL, and 6PGDH) is their evolutionary link to cyanobacteria and plant orthologs – a phylogenetic relationship that supports the endosymbiotic theory of a photosynthetic plastid harbored by a Kinetoplastid ancestor [9,10].

G6PDH, which catalyzes the oxidation of G6P to 6-phosphogluconolactone with the concomitant reduction of NADP to NADPH, is the first and, probably, rate-limiting enzyme of the PPP. The number of genes encoding for G6PDH differs between trypanosomatids, with *T. brucei* and *L. mexicana* harboring a single-copy sequence [11,12], and *T. cruzi* containing five different putative sequences, two of them being pseudogenes [13]. The enzyme is predominantly distributed in the cytosol, with a minor fraction compartmentalized in glycosomes, although a typical peroxisomal targeting sequence (PTS) is absent [3,8,11,14]. The production of NADPH in this organelle likely serves to support the biosynthesis of lipids and sterols, and the antioxidant defense [12,15–19]. The indispensability of G6PDH has been confirmed for the infective form of African trypanosomes by means of RNA interference [20]. The deleterious phenotype observed (growth arrest and reduced tolerance to H_2O_2) is likely a consequence of a depletion in the nucleotide and NADPH pools. A critical role of G6PDH in the defense against oxidative stress has also been demonstrated in *T. cruzi* [13]. The enzyme activity increased about 45-fold in trypomastigotes subjected to H_2O_2 challenge and, under non-stress conditions, G6PDH levels were markedly elevated in the infective stages (trypomastigote and amastigote) [13]. Also, other studies revealed that G6PDH is more abundant in *T. cruzi* strains of higher virulence [21,22]. However, chemical validation of G6PDH remains controversial (see the "Inhibitor Discovery Against PPP Enzymes" section).

6PGL, the second enzyme of the oxidative phase, is responsible for decreasing the lifetime of the highly reactive 6-phosphogluconolactone by hydrolytic cleavage to 6-phosphogluconate [11]. In *T. brucei*, a single-copy gene encodes a putative 6PGL that displays a dual subcellular localization – about 85% being in the cytosol and 15% in the glycosomes [23]. A PTS-1 targets the protein to the glycosomes [11]. In promastigotes of different strains from *L. mexicana*, 6PGL was by far the most prominent enzymatic activity of the PPP [4]. The essentiality of 6PGL has not yet been addressed for any trypanosomatid; however, although the lactone can hydrolyze spontaneously, it is tempting to speculate that under certain conditions, (i.e., high NADPH demand) 6-phosphogluconolactone may accumulate to toxic levels that require catalytic elimination. Such function for 6PGL may be critical inside the glycosomes, where a high concentration of the electrophilic 6-phosphogluconolactone [24] may lead to the irreversible inactivation of key metabolic enzymes.

6PGDH is the best-studied enzyme of the PPP in *T. brucei*, and, to a lesser extent, in *T. cruzi* and *L. mexicana*. It catalyzes, in the presence of NADP, the reversible oxidative decarboxylation of 6-phosphogluconate to ribulose-5-phosphate (Ru5P) with concomitant production of NADPH and carbonic anhydride [25]. 6PGDH activity is predominantly cytosolic, with a small glycosomal component in procyclic *T. brucei* [14]. The biological importance of 6PGD for bloodstream *T. b. rhodesiense* and intracellular amastigotes of *T. cruzi* was first revealed by cytotoxicity studies performed with specific enzyme inhibitors [26] (see the "Inhibitor Discovery Against PPP Enzymes" section). Unpublished observations of Barrett *et al.* indicate that the enzyme is indispensable for bloodstream *T. brucei* [27,28]. Taking into account that the infective stage of African trypanosomes depends exclusively on glycolysis for energy production and glucose-6-phosphate isomerase has been shown to be extremely sensitive to 6-phosphogluconate [29], the deleterious phenotype of 6PGDH-depleted *T. brucei* was suggested to be caused by accumulation of phosphorylated gluconate with concomitant inhibition of glycolysis [28]. This effect is likely amplified *in vivo* by an increment in the flux of G6P through the PPP and the consequent increased formation of the phosphorylated intermediate [30]. Whether a shortage in R5P also contributes to this phenotype remains to be investigated.

RPI catalyzes the isomerization of R5P and Ru5P that will proceed in either direction depending on the relative substrate and product concentrations. If R5P is abundant, the phosphorylated sugar will be diverted to the production of precursors for aromatic vitamins (not yet fully documented for trypanosomatids) and glycolytic intermediates, whereas a decline in R5P will stimulate the reverse reaction leading to its own synthesis and that of nucleotides and cofactors. According to their distribution among the phylogenetic scale, RPIs are classified into type A (with representatives in all three kingdoms of life) or type B (restricted to some bacteria and protozoa) [31]. Trypanosomatids lack type A RPI but are endowed with type B RPI [32], whose activity was detected in different life stages of *T. brucei* [5], *L. tropica* and *L. major* [33], and *T. cruzi* [34]. Although the essentiality of RPI for trypano-somatids remains to be demonstrated, the adverse phenotype observed in phyloge-netically distant organisms, namely *Escherichia coli* [31] and human [35], deficient in this enzyme points to an evolutionary conserved critical function for this protein. The absence of type B RPIs in mammalian genomes and the significant structural divergence between both enzyme classes (see below) have raised trypanosomal RPIs to the level of attractive drug target candidates [34,36].

RPE is responsible for catalyzing the interconversion of R5P and xylulose-5-phosphate (X5P). The genome of the CL Brener clone of *T. cruzi* harbors two genes encoding RPEs with one of them containing a PTS-1 at the C-terminus. The enzyme is expressed in all four biological stages of this parasite and, in contrast to other PPP enzymes, is not upregulated in metacyclic trypomastigotes. It is present in membrane-bound vesicles [3] – a behavior of unknown biological relevance. The genome of *Leishmania* encodes for two isoenzymes that differ in the presence and absence of a glycosomal targeting sequence [37]. In promastigotes of different strains of *L. mexicana*, the activity of RPE was almost 3-fold higher than that of the competing enzyme, RPI [4]. In *T. brucei*, RPE, and also TKT, activity is detected in the procyclic form, but not in parasites isolated from mice [5], indicating that the non-oxidative segment of the PPP is dispensable for the latter. A possible explanation for this exceptional metabolic adaptation is to constrain sugar metabolization to the production of R5P and NADPH via the oxidative phase of the PPP in order to meet the remarkably high proliferation rate of bloodstream parasites. In summary, RPE does not qualify as potential drug target against African trypanosomes, but the biological importance of this enzyme for the intracellular parasites *Leishmania* spp. and *T. cruzi* remains to be investigated.

TAL transfers a dihydroxyacetone unit from F6P to erythrose-4-phosphate (E4P) to synthesize sedoheptulose-7-phosphate and, as byproduct, Gly3P. The backward reaction is also catalyzed by the enzyme. TAL activity was detected in the cytosol of bloodstream *T. brucei* [5]. The presence of this enzyme was also identified in the four developmental stages of *T. cruzi* with a 3- to 5-fold higher activity in the highly infective metacyclic trypomastigotes [3]. Unpublished data propose the presence of four TAL isoforms in *T. cruzi* epimastigotes [38]. Promastigotes of *L. mexicana* also display TAL activity [4]. The role of TAL in trypanosomatids has not yet been addressed. In higher eukaryotes the enzyme plays an important function as a regulator of the metabolic fluxes through the PPP [39] – a function that can be shared by the New World trypanosomes (*T. cruzi* and *Leishmania* spp.), which present a fully active PPP, but likely not by *T. brucei*, because the infective form presents a defective non-oxidative branch (see above) and deletion of TKT gene, whose product will synthesize the substrates for TAL, in the procyclic stage went phenotypically unnoticed (see below) [40]. Thus, TAL can be disregarded as drug target candidate for African trypanosomes, and its role in *T. cruzi* and *Leishmania* spp. deserves further research to draw final conclusions in this respect.

TKT is a thiamine diphosphate-dependent enzyme capable of catalyzing two reversible reactions that involve the transfer of two carbons from: (i) X5P to R5P to produce sedoheptulose-7-phosphate and Gly3P, and (ii) from X5P to E4P to generate F6P and Gly3P. The four developmental stages of *T. cruzi* express TKT activity that in epimastigotes is distributed among the cytosol (around 80%) and the small granule fraction (around 20%) representing the glycosomes [3]. TKT activity was reported to occur in several species of *Leishmania* [41], and a dual cytosolic and glycosomal localization of the protein has been unambiguously demonstrated in *L. mexicana* promastigotes [42]. In *T. brucei*, TKT is encoded by a single-copy gene containing a PTS-1 [42], which is actively expressed and repressed in the procyclic and bloodstream stage, respectively [5,40]. The biological relevance of TKT has only been addressed for African trypanosomes [40], whereby, at least under *in vitro* growth conditions, TKT-null mutants of the procyclic form did not exhibit any growth or morphologic phenotype despite a remarkable alteration in the metabolic profile (i.e., accumulation of TKT substrates and lack of sedoheptulose-7-phosphate). A role for TKT in *T. cruzi* and *Leishmania* has yet to be determined, but since they harbor a fully operative PPP, the enzyme may function in preventing the accumulation of toxic phosphorylated carbohydrate intermediates of the pathway in the glycosome and/or in modulating NADPH production by redirecting sugar phosphates towards the oxidative branch of the cycle [40].

In other organisms such as yeast, an NADP-independent salvage pathway for the synthesis of R5P from glycolytic intermediates is operative. This is the so-called riboneogenesis pathway that *via* the combined action of TKT and aldolase, glycolytic intermediates are transformed into sedoheptulose-1,7-bisphosphate, which is further hydrolyzed by the enzyme sedoheptulose-1,7-bisphosphatase to sedoheptulose-7-phosphate. This product can be transformed into R5P by TKT (Figure 16.1).

Candidate genes encoding for this protein are present in the genome of *T. brucei* and *T. cruzi*, but are absent in *Leishmania* [37]. Whether riboneogenesis is functional in these parasites and to what extent it contributes to the intracellular pool of R5P should be investigated.

Biochemical and Structural Hallmarks of Trypanosomatids PPP Enzymes

To assess the possibility of one or more of the PPP enzymes being suitable targets for chemotherapy, a detailed comparison of their structure and properties with those of the corresponding mammalian enzymes is required. The most relevant biochemical and structural features from the components of the trypanosomal and leishmanial PPP that can provide a basis for the development of specific inhibitors are summarized below.

G6PDHs from the TriTryps share about 64–69% amino acid identity between each other and about 50% identity with the human ortholog. The kinetic constants for substrate (K_m for G6P ~60–200 μM) and coenzyme (K_m for NADP ~4–12 μM) reported for G6PDH from *T. cruzi* [13], *T. brucei* [14], and *L. mexicana* [20] were of the same order of magnitude, suggesting an overall conservation of the major catalytic and ligand-binding residues. The k_{cat} reported for *T. brucei* and *L. mexicana* G6PDH is noteworthy (k_{cat} of 16–22 s^{-1} [20]) almost one order of magnitude lower than those observed for the *T. cruzi* and human enzymes (k_{cat} of 130–190 s^{-1}) [13,43], and indicates a lower catalytic efficiency of the former enzymes. Also striking is the significant sensitiveness of *T. cruzi* G6PDH to inhibition by NADPH (K_i for NADPH of 0.76 versus 9 μM for the *T. cruzi* and human enzyme, respectively) [13,44], suggesting a tight control of the enzyme activity by the intracelular NADPH/NADP ratio. Other major molecular and structural features that distinguish the *T. cruzi* enzyme from the human counterpart are: (i) the trypanosomal protein forms highly stable tetramers ([45]; Ortíz *et al.*, unpublished) whereas the human enzyme exists in a rapid equilibrium between monomeric, dimeric, and tetrameric species [46], and (ii) *T. cruzi* G6PDH, but not the enzymes from *T. brucei* and *L. mexicana* and neither the human counterpart, contains an N-terminal extension with non-conserved cysteines, some of them engaged in the formation of disulfide bridges that stabilize a more active conformation of the enzyme ([13]; Ortíz *et al.*, unpublished). Crystals of the protein in the apo-state (Protein Data Bank (PDB) ID: 4E9I) and with bound G6P (PDB ID 3EM5) have recently been obtained, and diffracted at 2.9- and 3.4-Å resolution, respectively [45]. The refined structures are currently being subjected to a thorough comparative analysis with the human ortholog in order to explore molecular differences that can be exploited for the design or optimization of specific drugs.

The *T. brucei* and *T. cruzi* representatives for 6PGL have been expressed in recombinant soluble forms exhibiting a monomeric conformation (Beluardi and Cazzulo, unpublished; [47]) similar to that reported for the enzyme from bovine erythrocytes [48]. Kinetic studies on 6PGL are very difficult, because its substrate is very unstable and must be generated *in situ*. Nevertheless, a K_m value of 50 μM has been determined for the *T. cruzi* enzyme [38], which is close to one of the values reported for the rat liver enzyme (80 μM) [49]. The crystal structure of *T. brucei* 6PGL has recently been solved at about 2 Å in the absence (PDB ID: 2J0E) [47] and presence of ligands (PDB ID: 3E7F, 3EB9) [23], which facilitates a detailed mechanistic and dynamic characterization of the enzyme [23,50]. The atomic coordinates for the crystal structure of 6PGL from *L. braziliensis* (PDB ID: 3CH7; Arakati and Merrit, unpublished) and *L. guyanensis* (PDB ID: 3CSS; Painter and Merrit, unpublished) have also been deposited. Although the structure of the human ortholog remains to be elucidated, its low amino acid identity (below 20%) with the plastid-like parasite proteins (below 20%) predicts important structural differences.

6PGDH from kinetoplastids exhibits low amino acid sequence identity (below 35%) with its mammalian counterpart that translates into distinct affinities for ligands [51]. The reported K_m values for NADP are 1.5, 5.9, and 3–30 μM, for the *T. brucei*, *T. cruzi*, and human enzymes, respectively, and the corresponding values for 6PG are 3.5, 22.2, and 20–32 μM, respectively [30,52,53]. The apparent K_m values for 6PG and NADP for the *L. mexicana* enzyme were 6.9 and 5.2 μM, respectively [54]. The K_i for NADPH and Ru5P was 0.6 and 30 μM, respectively, for the *T. brucei* enzyme. These differences in kinetic parameters originate in subtle structural differences (see below) and are particularly noteworthy for *T. brucei* 6PGDH, since they can, at least in part, explain the remarkable sensitivity of the enzyme to a number of inhibitors (see the "Inhibitor Discovery Against PPP Enzymes" section).

The three-dimensional structure of *T. brucei* 6PGDH has been determined at 2.8-Å resolution (PDB ID: 1PGJ [55]) and thoroughly compared against the sheep liver enzyme [56]. Despite the low protein sequence identity between both enzymes, a high conservation was observed in the overall structure and for residues directly engaged in substrate and coenzyme binding. However, several secondary residues surrounding the substrate binding site (i.e., either making direct contact with the substrate or shaping the active site at the interface between subunits), and others bridging the C-terminal tail on the coenzyme binding site, differed significantly in identity or structural arrangement and were proposed to account for the different affinities for substrate/coenzyme and inhibitors [56]. The analysis of this structural data [57] has facilitated a rational design of inhibitors (see the "Inhibitor Discovery Against PPP Enzymes" section). Homology modeling of the *L. mexicana* and *T. cruzi* 6GPDH suggests a limited structural divergence among kinetoplastid proteins, raising the possibility for designing inhibitors equally effective against the enzymes from these species [54]. The atomic coordinates of human 6PGDH have recently been deposited (PDB ID: 2JKV; Ng *et al.*, unpublished). Comparison with the structure of the parasite protein should contribute to the improvement of inhibitor specificity (see the "Inhibitor Discovery Against PPP Enzymes" section).

RPI from trypanosomatids can be considered as an ideal drug target, because it belongs to the B-type RPI group that is absent in mammalian genomes, and lacks structural similarity with the A-type enzymes. The protein from *T. cruzi*, the only representative from a trypanosomatid that has been characterized, is a homodimer [32,34]. *T. cruzi* RPI presented K_m values in the millimolar range (K_m for R5P and Ru5P of 4 and 1.4 mM, respectively), similar to those reported for the enzyme from human erythrocytes (e.g., K_m for R5P of 2.2 mM) [58], despite the significant differences at the active-site motif. The three-dimensional structure of *T. cruzi* RPI-B has been determined at 2.2-Å resolution in the apo-form or in complex with D-R5P or the inhibitors 4-phospho-D-erythronohydroxamic acid and D-allose-6-phosphate (PDB ID: 3K7O, 3K7P, 3K7S, 3K8C, and 3M1P) [34]. This study further revealed the occurrence of small conformational changes upon substrate binding, the critical role of a phosphate-binding loop close to the active site, both contributing to substrate and inhibitor binding, and the identity of residues responsible for catalysis.

In the case of *T. cruzi* TKT, the apparent K_m values determined for R5P, E4P, and X5P were 1.34, 0.1, and 0.07 mM, respectively [38]. For the leishmanial enzyme, only the apparent K_m for R5P, 2.75 mM, was determined [42], whereas the homolog from *T. brucei* showed apparent K_m values for R5P and X5P of 0.8 and 0.2 mM, respectively [40]. The K_m values for the recombinant human enzyme, recently reported by Mitschke *et al.* [59], were 0.48 and 0.25 mM for R5P and X5P, respectively. As previously proposed for the *T. brucei* enzyme [40], a regulatory role in the PPP may also be envisaged for *T. cruzi* and *L. mexicana* TKT because of the low R5P concentration in steady-state and the high K_m values of these enzymes for this substrate. The crystal structure of *L. mexicana* TKT has been solved at 2.22 Å (PDB ID: 1R9J), and comparison with the structures of eukaryote orthologs (i.e., yeast and maize) revealed a high degree of similarity at the active site, cofactor, and ion-binding regions [42]. A high-resolution structure of the human enzyme has been recently determined at 1.75 Å (PDB ID: 3MOS [59]), but not yet compared to the leishmanial protein. At least two residues that are important for cofactor and substrate binding in the mammal enzyme (Gln189 and Lys260 in human TKT) [59] are not conserved in the trypanosomatid's proteins.

Inhibitor Discovery Against PPP Enzymes

Only a handful of compounds have been investigated as potential inhibitors of kinetoplastid G6PDH, most of them previously identified as inhibitors of the human enzyme. The steroids dehydroepiandrosterone (DHEA) and epiandrosterone (EA) inhibited the *T. brucei* enzyme with K_i values about 6-fold lower than those reported for the human enzyme [20]. Strikingly, *L. mexicana* G6PDH was not affected by similar concentrations of the drugs [20]. The same inhibitors also were active against the enzyme from *T. cruzi*, but the K_i values obtained, close to 22 μM for DHEA and to 4.8 μM for EA [60], were higher than those for the human enzyme (8.9–6.2 μM for DHEA and 3–3.4 μM for EA [20]). The 16α-bromated (16Br) derivatives of both drugs were more active than the parental precursors, with IC_{50} values about 5-fold lower for 16BrDHEA and 2.5-fold lower for 16BrEA (Figure 16.2) [60]. All these compounds were uncompetitive inhibitors for both substrates – a very rare mechanism where the inhibitor exerts its activity by binding to the ternary enzyme–coenzyme–substrate complex. The recent elucidation of the *T. cruzi* G6PDH structure (46) may disclose the so far unknown binding site of these drugs. The bromated derivatives were toxic for *T. cruzi* epimastigotes with LD_{50} values ranging from 12 to 20 μM [60], similar to the

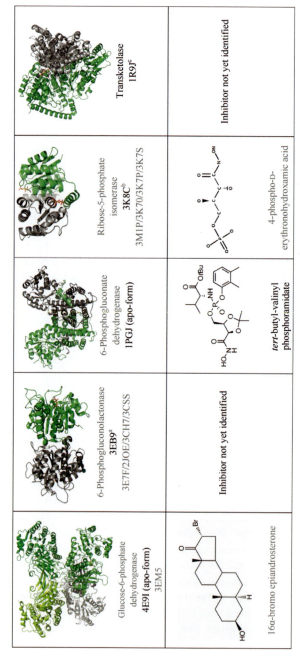

Figure 16.2 Three-dimensional structure and best inhibitors identified for PPP enzymes of trypanosomatids. Bold IDs indicate the PDB ID corresponding to the structure shown. The protein subunits are shown in different colors; dark brown depicts the following ligands: [a]citrate, [b]4-deoxy-4-phospho-D-erythronohydroxamic acid, and [c]thiamine diphosphate.

values obtained for DHEA and EA against the bloodstream form of *T. brucei* [20]. For both microorganisms the *in vivo* potency of the steroids was more than 10-fold lower than the inhibitory activity displayed against the recombinant enzymes. On the other hand, metacyclic promastigotes of *L. mexicana* were not affected by similar concentrations of both steroids [20]. The specific action of steroids against G6PDH from different trypanosomatids has been confirmed using trangenic cell lines [22]. At the *in vivo* level, DHEA administered subcutaneously to male rats infected with *T. cruzi* led to a significant reduction in parasitemia, which was associated with enhanced lymphoproliferative (thymocyte and macrophage proliferation) and pro-inflammatory (interleukin-12, nitric oxide production) responses [61,62]. The contribution of trypanosomal G6PDH inhibition by DHEA to the trypanostatic effect exerted by the drug *in vivo* has not yet been addressed. A new class of inhibitors, namely the molecular tweezers or clips, has been recently developed against G6PDH [63]. They consist of two naphthalene or anthracene molecules linked by a benzene moiety with phosphate groups as inorganic substituent. A representative of the benzene–naphthalene family proved to inhibit *T. cruzi* G6PDH with an IC_{50} of $3\,\mu M$ (Ortíz *et al.*, unpublished), which is 2-fold lower than that reported for the yeast enzyme ($7\,\mu M$) [63]. The compound did not exhibit a significant toxicity against *T. cruzi* epimastigotes ($LD_{50} \sim 100\,\mu M$), which may be due to poor drug uptake and/or metabolization (i.e., low permeability and dephosphorylation).

As part of an ongoing target-based drug discovery program, Barrett and coworkers performed a systematic search for 6PGDH inhibitors of the *T. brucei* enzyme. Large differences between the trypanosomal and sheep enzymes in the affinity for substrate analogs (e.g., the K_i value for 6-P-2-deoxygluconate *versus* 6-phosphogluconate was 200-fold lower for *T. brucei* 6PGDH than for the sheep enzyme) [30] has prompted the design of substrate-based inhibitors [28]. Several phosphonated monosaccharides showed acceptable selectivity against the parasite enzyme with K_i values in the micro- to submicromolar range [64]. Based on molecular modeling and structural analysis [55,57], new substrate-based analogs were synthesized and tested [65]. One of the first series ((2*R*)-2-methyl-4,5-dideoxy-6-phosphogluconate) and six of the second ((2*R*)-2-methyl-4-deoxy-6-phosphogluconate) were able to inhibit competitively both enzymes, one of them showing some selectivity towards the enzyme from the parasite. Compounds of the third series (2,4-dideoxy-6-phosphogluconate) were completely inactive. The major conclusion arising from this work indicates that substituents at positions 2 and 4, but not at 6 (the phosphate moiety), are critical for effective inhibitor binding. Three of the compounds showed a moderate activity against *T. b. rhodesiense* trypomastigotes (below $12\,\mu M$) and two had a moderate toxicity against *T. cruzi* amastigotes (below $10\,\mu M$), but none of them had any significant anti-leishmanial activity [65]. Taking into account that suramin, a polysulfonated benzyl-rich drug used to treat African trypanosomiasis, inhibited *T. brucei* 6PGDH, several related triphenylmethane derivatives were assayed [57]. In general, the compounds exhibited a moderate activity and selectivity towards the parasite enzyme that opens the possibility to use the most active molecules as drug scaffolds. Some hydroxamate derivatives of D-erythronic acid, analogs of the high-energy intermediate from the 6PGDH reaction, were potent and selective inhibitors of the *T. brucei* enzyme, with K_i values in the nanomolar range [26]. However, the poor drug-like characteristic of these molecules (e.g., low permeability and instability) will hamper their clinical use. In an attempt to improve these features, Ruda *et al.* [66] synthesized a number of phosphate pro-drugs of the inhibitor 4-phospho-D-erythronohydroxamic acid, which was a more selective inhibitor of the *T. brucei* enzyme than of the sheep liver enzyme (K_i values 0.035 and 1.1 μM, respectively). Most of the compounds were toxic for *T. brucei*. More recently Ruda *et al.* [67] have developed new pro-drugs, aryl-phosphoramidates of 2,3-*O*-isopropylidene-4-erythronohydroxamate that increased by four order of magnitude the killing potency of the compound (e.g., EC_{50} of 330 μM and 0.008 μM for the drug and the best pro-drug, respectively) (Figure 16.2). Moreover, rational modifications of satellite alkyl groups (i.e., amino acid side-chain, amino acid, and aryl ester groups) entailed a significant increase in the stability of the compounds. So far, no experiment has been conducted on an animal model to scrutinize the potential of the most potent compounds. In the search for novel molecules that may serve as future drug scaffolds, a novel "virtual fragment screening" approach was implemented [68]. In this strategy, the structure of *Lactococcus lactis* 6PGDH was used as docking template because atomic coordinates for ligand binding to the active site were available and this region is almost identical to that of *T. brucei* 6PGDH. The initial selection of compounds was restricted according to their molecular weight (molecules less than 320 Da) and the presence of functional groups resembling phosphate. Nearly 10% of the 64 000 preselected compounds could be docked into the structure and only 71 (0.1%) qualified as promising candidates for testing. Finally, 10 compounds displayed $IC_{50} < 50$ μM against *T. brucei* 6PGDH and encouraging physicochemical and pharmacological properties.

So far, there is no information available on inhibitors of RPI (most of the compounds tested as potential inhibitors of *T. cruzi* type B RPI were inactive or poorly active, with the exception of 4-phospho-D-erythronohydroxamic acid (Figure 16.2), a competitive inhibitor of R5P with a K_i value of 1.2 mM [32,34]), RPE, 6PGL, TAL, and TKT from trypanosomatids. A recent high-throughput screening against human TKT detected a couple of compounds displaying a reasonable IC_{50} (around 4 μM) and a potent growth-inhibitory effect against tumor cells (EC_{50} 0.4–10 μM) [69]. It will be interesting to test the activity of these new molecules towards TKT from trypanosomatids, since a positive hit may serve as potential scaffold for further development of more selective versions.

Conclusions

Although the general organization and relevance of the PPP is similar in trypanosomatids and mammals, some of the enzymes present marked differences, either in structure or in kinetics, or in both, which makes them suitable candidates as targets for specific chemotherapy. In this respect, several of the trypanosomal and leishmanial PPP enzymes appear to be ideal, since they fulfill important prerequisites for entering in a fast-track drug discovery program: (i) indispensability for parasite survival or virulence and/or functional/structural divergence with mammal counterparts, (ii) suitable expression in recombinant active forms, (iii) availability of assays to test enzyme activity, and (iv) availability of structural data. The particular oligomeric arrangement and/or allosteric properties exhibited by the parasite enzymes offer additional structural niches for the design of specific inhibitors.

Acknowledgments

We thank the following: Drs Frank Gerrit and Thomas Schrader (Universität Duisburg-Essen) for providing G6PDH clip inhibitor; Drs Horacio Botti and Alejandro Buschiazzo (Protein Crystallography Unit, Institut Pasteur de Montevideo) for providing PDB codes for *T. cruzi* G6PDH; and The Agencia Nacional de Investigación e Innovación (grant Innova Uruguay, agreement DCI-ALA/2007/ 19.040 between Uruguay and the European Commission) and Comisión Intersectorial de Investigaciones Científicas, Universidad de la República, Uruguay, for financial support to M.A.C. and C.O.

References

1 Fairlamb, A.H., Ridley, R.G., and Vial, H.J. (2003) *Drugs Against Parasitic Diseases R&D Methodologies and Issues*, WHO, Geneva.

2 Stryer, L. (1999) *Biochemistry*, 4th edn, Freeman, New York, pp. 559–565.

3 Maugeri, D. and Cazzulo, J.J. (2004) The pentose phosphate pathway in *Trypanosoma cruzi. FEMS Microbiol. Lett.*, **234**, 117–123.

4 Maugeri, D.A., Cazzulo, J.J., Burchmore, R.J., Barrett, M.P., and Ogbunude, P.O. (2003) Pentose phosphate metabolism in *Leishmania mexicana. Mol. Biochem. Parasitol.*, **130**, 117–125.

5 Cronin, C.N., Nolan, D.P., and Voorheis, H.P. (1989) The enzymes of the classical pentose phosphate pathway display differential activities in procyclic and bloodstream forms of *Trypanosoma brucei. FEBS Lett.*, **244**, 26–30.

6 Keegan, F.P., Sansone, L., and Blum, J.J. (1987) Oxidation of glucose, ribose, alanine and glutamate by *Leishmania braziliensis panamensis. J. Protozool.*, **34**, 174–179.

7 Michels, P.A., Bringaud, F., Herman, M., and Hannaert, V. (2006) Metabolic functions of glycosomes in trypanosomatids. *Biochim. Biophys. Acta.*, **1763**, 1463–1477.

8 Opperdoes, F.R. and Szikora, J.P. (2006) *In silico* prediction of the glycosomal enzymes of *Leishmania major* and trypanosomes. *Mol. Biochem. Parasitol.*, **147**, 193–206.

9 Krepinsky, K., Plaumann, M., Martin, W., and Schnarrenberger, C. (2001) Purification and cloning of chloroplast 6-phosphogluconate dehydrogenase from spinach. Cyanobacterial genes for chloroplast and cytosolic isoenzymes encoded in eukaryotic chromosomes. *Eur. J. Biochem.*, **268**, 2678–2686.

10 Hannaert, V., Bringaud, F., Opperdoes, F.R., and Michels, P.A. (2003) Evolution of energy metabolism and its compartmentation in Kinetoplastida. *J. Mol. Biol.*, **331**, 653–665.

11 Duffieux, F., Van Roy, J., Michels, P.A., and Opperdoes, F.R. (2000) Molecular characterization of the first two enzymes of the pentose phosphate pathway of *Trypanosoma brucei. J. Biol. Chem.*, **275**, 27559–27565.

12 Hannaert, V., Saavedra, E., Duffieux, F., Szikora, J.P., Rigden, D.J., Michels, P.A., and Opperdoes, F.R. (2003) Plant-like traits associated with metabolism of *Trypanosoma* parasites. *Proc. Natl. Acad. Sci. USA*, **100**, 1067–1071.

13 Igoillo-Esteve, M. and Cazzulo, J.J. (2006) The glucose-6-phosphate dehydrogenase from *Trypanosoma cruzi*: its role in the defense of the parasite against oxidative stress. *Mol. Biochem. Parasitol.*, **149**, 170–181.

14 Heise, N. and Opperdoes, F.R. (1999) Purification, localization and characterization of glucose-6-phosphate dehydrogenase of *Trypanosoma brucei*. *Mol. Biochem. Parasitol.*, **99**, 21–32.

15 Dufernez, F., Yernaux, C., Gerbod, D., Noël, C., Chauvenet, M., Wintjens, R., Edgcomb, V.P., Capron, M., Opperdoes, F.R., and Viscogliosi, E. (2006) The presence of four iron-containing superoxide dismutase isozymes in trypanosomatidae: characterization, subcellular localization, and phylogenetic origin in *Trypanosoma brucei*. *Free Radic. Biol. Med.*, **40**, 210–225.

16 Wilkinson, S.R., Prathalingam, S.R., Taylor, M.C., Ahmed, A., Horn, D., and Kelly, J.M. (2006) Functional characterisation of the iron superoxide dismutase gene repertoire in *Trypanosoma brucei*. *Free Radic. Biol. Med.*, **40**, 198–209.

17 Plewes, K.A., Barr, S.D., and Gedamu, L. (2003) Iron superoxide dismutases targeted to the glycosomes of *Leishmania chagasi* are important for survival. *Infect. Immun.*, **71**, 5910–5920.

18 Schlecker, T., Schmidt, A., Dirdjaja, N., Voncken, F., Clayton, C., and Krauth-Siegel, R.L. (2005) Substrate specificity, localization, and essential role of the glutathione peroxidase-type tryparedoxin peroxidases in *Trypanosoma brucei*. *J. Biol. Chem.*, **280**, 14385–14389.

19 Colasante, C., Robles, A., Li, C.H., Schwede, A., Benz, C., Voncken, F., Guilbride, D.L., and Clayton, C. (2007) Regulated expression of glycosomal phosphoglycerate kinase in *Trypanosoma brucei*. *Mol. Biochem. Parasitol.*, **151**, 193–204.

20 Cordeiro, A.T., Thiemann, O.H., and Michels, P.A. (2009) Inhibition of *Trypanosoma brucei* glucose-6-phosphate dehydrogenase by human steroids and their effects on the viability of cultured parasites. *Bioorg. Med. Chem.*, **17**, 2483–2489.

21 Mielniczki-Pereira, A.A., Chiavegatto, C.M., López, J.A., Colli, W., Alves, M.J., and Gadelha, F.R. (2006) *Trypanosoma cruzi* strains, Tulahuen 2 and Y, besides the difference in resistance to oxidative stress, display differential glucose-6-phosphate and 6-phosphogluconate dehydrogenases activities. *Acta Trop.*, **101**, 54–60.

22 Gupta, S., Igoillo-Esteve, M., Michels, P.A., and Cordeiro, A.T. (2011) Glucose-6-phosphate dehydrogenase of trypanosomatids: characterization, target validation, and drug discovery. *Mol. Biol. Int.*, **2011**, 135701.

23 Duclert-Savatier, N., Poggi, L., Miclet, E., Lopes, P., Ouazzani, J., Chevalier, N., Nilges, M., Delarue, M., and Stoven, V. (2009) Insights into the enzymatic mechanism of 6-phosphogluconolactonase from *Trypanosoma brucei* using structural data and molecular dynamics simulation. *J. Mol. Biol.*, **388**, 1009–1021.

24 Rakitzis, E.T. and Papandreou, P. (1998) Reactivity of 6-phosphogluconolactone with hydroxylamine: the possible involvement of glucose-6-phosphate dehydrogenase in endogenous glycation reactions. *Chem. Biol. Interact.*, **113**, 205–216.

25 Hanau, S., Montin, K., Cervellati, C., Magnani, M., and Dallocchio, F. (2010) 6-phosphogluconate dehydrogenase mechanism evidence for allosteric modulation by substrate. *J. Biol. Chem.*, **285**, 21366–21371.

26 Dardonville, C., Rinaldi, E., Barrett, M.P., Brun, R., Gilbert, I.H., and Hanau, S. (2004) Selective inhibition of *Trypanosoma brucei* 6-phosphogluconate dehydrogenase by high-energy intermediate and transition-state analogues. *J. Med. Chem.*, **47**, 3427–3437.

27 Barrett, M.P. and Gilbert, I.H. (2002) Perspectives for new drugs against trypanosomiasis and leishmaniasis. *Curr. Top. Med. Chem.*, **2**, 471–482.

28 Hanau, S., Rinaldi, E., Dallocchio, F., Gilbert, I.H., Dardonville, C., Adams, M.J., Gover, S., and Barrett, M.P. (2004) 6-phosphogluconate dehydrogenase: a target for drugs in African trypanosomes. *Curr. Med. Chem.*, **11**, 1345–1359.

29 Marchand, M., Kooystra, U., Wierenga, R.K., Lambeir, A.M., Van Beeumen, J., Opperdoes, F.R., and Michels, P.A. (1989) Glucosephosphate isomerase from *Trypanosoma brucei*. Cloning and characterization of the gene and analysis of the enzyme. *Eur. J. Biochem.*, **184**, 455–464.

30 Hanau, S., Rippa, M., Bertelli, M., Dallocchio, F., and Barrett, M.P. (1996) 6-Phosphogluconate dehydrogenase from *Trypanosoma brucei*. Kinetic analysis and inhibition by trypanocidal drugs. *Eur. J. Biochem.*, **240**, 592–599.

31 Sørensen, K.I. and Hove-Jensen, B. (1996) Ribose catabolism of *Escherichia coli*: characterization of the RpiB gene encoding ribose phosphate isomerase B and of the *rpiR* gene, which is involved in regulation of RpiB expression. *J. Bacteriol.*, **178**, 1003–1011.

32 Stern, A.L., Burgos, E., Salmon, L., and Cazzulo, J.J. (2007) Ribose 5-phosphate type B from *Trypanosoma cruzi*: kinetic properties and site-directed mutagenesis reveal information about the reaction mechanism. *Biochem. J.*, **401**, 279–285.

33 Al-Mulla Hummadi, Y.M., Al-Bashir, N.M., and Najim, R.A. (2006) *Leishmania major* and *Leishmania tropica*: II. Effect of an immunomodulator, S(2) complex on the enzymes of the parasites. *Exp. Parasitol.*, **112**, 85–91.

34 Stern, A.L., Naworyta, A., Cazzulo, J.J., and Mowbray, S.L. (2011) Structures of type B ribose 5-phosphate isomerase from *Trypanosoma cruzi* shed light on the determinants of sugar specificity in the structural family. *FEBS J.*, **278**, 793–808.

35 Huck, J.H., Verhoeven, N.M., Struys, E.A., Salomons, G.S., Jakobs, C., and van der Knaap, M.S. (2004) Ribose-5-phosphate isomerase deficiency: new inborn error in the pentose phosphate pathway associated with a slowly progressive leukoencephalopathy. *Am. J. Hum. Genet.*, **74**, 745–751.

36 Zhang, R.G., Andersson, C.E., Skarina, T., Evdokimova, E., Edwards, A.M., Joachimiak, A., Savchenko, A., and Mowbray, S.L. (2003) The 2.2 A resolution structure of RpiB/AlsB from *Escherichia coli* illustrates a new approach to the ribose-5-phosphate isomerase reaction. *J. Mol. Biol.*, **332**, 1083–1094.

37 Opperdoes, F.R. and Coombs, G.H. (2007) Metabolism of *Leishmania*: proven and predicted. *Trends Parasitol.*, **23**, 149–158.

38 Igoillo-Esteve, M., Maugeri, D., Stern, A.L., Beluardi, P., and Cazzulo, J.J. (2007) The pentose phosphate pathway in *Trypanosoma cruzi*: a potential target for the chemotherapy of Chagas disease. *An. Acad. Bras. Cienc.*, **79**, 649–663.

39 Perl, A. (2007) The pathogenesis of transaldolase deficiency. *IUBMB Life*, **59**, 365–373.

40 Stoffel, S.A., Alibub, V.P., Hubert, J., Ebikeme, C., Portais, J.C., Bringaud, F., Schweingrubere, M.E., and Barrett, M.P. (2011) Transketolase in *Trypanosoma brucei*. *Mol. Biochem. Parasitol.*, **179**, 1–7.

41 Martin, E., Simon, M.W., Schaefer, F.W., and Mukkada, A.J. (1976) Enzymes of carbohydrate metabolism in four human species of *Leishmania*: a comparative study. *J. Protozool.*, **23**, 600–607.

42 Veitch, N.J., Maugeri, D.A., Cazzulo, J.J., Lindqvist, Y., and Barrett, M.P. (2004) Transketolase from *Leishmania mexicana* has a dual subcellular localisation. *Biochem. J.*, **382**, 759–767.

43 Cohen, P. and Rosemeyer, M.A. (1975) Glucose-6-phosphate dehydrogenase from human erythrocytes. *Methods Enzymol.*, **41**, 208–214.

44 Wang, X.T., Au, S.W., Lam, V.M., and Engel, P.C. (2002) Recombinant human glucose-6-phosphate dehydrogenase. Evidence for a rapid-equilibrium random-order mechanism. *Eur. J. Biochem.*, **269**, 3417–3424.

45 Ortíz, C., Larrieux, N., Medeiros, A., Botti, H., Comini, M., and Buschiazzo, A. (2011) Expression, crystallization and preliminary X-ray crystallographic analysis of glucose-6-phosphate dehydrogenase from the human pathogen *Trypanosoma cruzi* in complex with substrate. *Acta. Crystallogr. F*, **67**, 1457–1461.

46 Wrigley, N.G., Heather, J.V., Bonsignore, A., and De Flora, A. (1972) Human erythrocyte glucose 6-phosphate dehydrogenase: electron microscope studies on structure and interconversion of

tetramers, dimers and monomers. *J. Mol. Biol.*, **68**, 483–499.

47 Delarue, M., Duclert-Savatier, N., Miclet, E., Haouz, A., Giganti, D., Ouazzani, J., Lopez, P., Nilges, M., and Stoven, V. (2007) Three dimensional structure and implications for the catalytic mechanism of 6-phosphogluconolactonase from *Trypanosoma brucei. J. Mol. Biol.*, **366**, 868–881.

48 Bauer, H.P., Srihari, T., Jochims, J.C., and Hofer, H.W. (1983) 1.6-phosphogluconolactonase. Purification, properties and activities in various tissues. *Eur. J. Biochem.*, **133**, 163–168.

49 Schofield, P.J. and Sols, A. (1976) Rat liver 6-phosphogluconolactonase: a low K_m enzyme. *Biochem. Biophys. Res. Commun.*, **71**, 1313–1318.

50 Calligari, P.A., Salgado, G.F., Pelupessy, P., Lopes, P., Ouazzani, J., Bodenhausen, G., and Abergel, D. (2012) Insights into internal dynamics of 6-phosphogluconolactonase from *Trypanosoma brucei* studied by nuclear magnetic resonance and molecular dynamics. *Proteins*, **80**, 1196–1210.

51 Barrett, M.P. (1997) The pentose phosphate pathway and parasitic protozoa. *Parasitol. Today*, **13**, 11–16.

52 Igoillo-Esteve, M. and Cazzulo, J.J. (2004) The 6-phosphogluconate dehydrogenase from *Trypanosoma cruzi*: the absence of two inter-subunit salt bridges as a reason for enzyme instability. *Mol. Biochem. Parasitol.*, **133**, 197–207.

53 Pearse, B.M. and Rosemeyer, M.A. (1974) Human 6-phosphogluconate dehydrogenase purification of the erythrocyte enzyme and the influence of ions and NADPH on its activity. *Eur. J. Biochem.*, **42**, 213–223.

54 González, D., Pérez, J.L., Serrano, M.L., Igoillo-Esteve, M., Cazzulo, J.J., Barrett, M. P., Bubis, J., and Mendoza-León, A. (2010) The 6-phosphogluconate dehydrogenase of *Leishmania* (*Leishmania Mexicana*): gene characterisation and protein structure prediction. *J. Mol. Microbiol. Biotechnol.*, **19**, 213–223.

55 Phillips, C., Dohnalek, J., Gover, S., Barrett, M.P., and Adams, M.J. (1998) A 2.8 Å resolution structure of

6-phosphogluconate dehydrogenase from the Protozoan parasite *Trypanosoma brucei*: comparison with the sheep enzyme accounts for differences in activity with coenzyme and substrate analogues. *J. Mol. Biol.*, **282**, 667–681.

56 Adams, M.J., Ellis, G.H., Gover, S., Naylor, C.E., and Phillips, C. (1994) Crystallographic study of coenzyme, coenzyme analogue and substrate binding in 6-phosphogluconate dehydrogenase: implications for NADP specificity and the enzyme mechanism. *Structure*, **2**, 651–668.

57 Bertelli, M., El-Bastawissy, E., Knaggs, M. H., Barrett, M.P., Hanau, S., and Gilbert, I. H. (2001) Selective inhibition of 6-phosphogluconate dehydrogenase from *Trypanosoma brucei. J. Comput. Aided Mol. Des.*, **15**, 465–475.

58 Moltmann, E.A. (1972) Aldose–ketose isomerases, in *The Enzymes*, 3rd edn (ed. P.D. Boyer), Academic Press, New York, vol. **6**, pp. 271–354.

59 Mitschke, L., Parthier, C., Schroder-Tittmann, K., Coy, J., Ludtke, S., and Tittmann, K. (2010) The crystal structure of human transketolase and new insights into its mode of action. *J. Biol. Chem.*, **285**, 31559–31570.

60 Cordeiro, A.T. and Thiemann, O.H. (2010) 16-bromoepiandrosterone, an activator of the mammalian immune system, inhibits glucose 6-phosphate dehydrogenase from *Trypanosoma cruzi* and is toxic to these parasites grown in culture. *Bioorg. Med. Chem.*, **18**, 4762–4768.

61 Dos Santos, C.D., Toldo, M.P., and do Prado, J.C. (2005) *Trypanosoma cruzi*: The effects of dehydroepiandrosterone (DHEA) treatment during experimental infection. *Acta Trop.*, **95**, 109–115.

62 Filipin, M., del, V., Caetano, L.C., Brazão, V., Santello, F.H., Toldo, M.P., and do Prado, J. (2010) DHEA and testosterone therapies in *Trypanosoma cruzi*-infected rats are associated with thymic changes. *Res. Vet. Sc.*, **89**, 98–103.

63 Kirsch, M., Talbiersky, P., Polkowska, J., Bastkowski, F., Schaller, T., de Groot, H., Klärner, F.G., and Schrader, T. (2009)

A mechanism of efficient G6PD inhibition by a molecular clip. *Angew. Chem. Int. Ed. Engl.*, **48**, 2886–2890.

64 Pasti, C., Rinaldi, E., Cervellati, C., Dallocchio, F., Hardré, R., Salmon, L., and Hanau, S. (2003) Sugar derivatives as new 6-phosphogluconate dehydrogenase inhibitors selective for the parasite *Trypanosoma brucei*. *Bioorg. Med. Chem.*, **11**, 1207–1214.

65 Dardonville, C., Rinaldi, E., Hanau, S., Barrett, M.P., Brun, R., and Gilbert, I.H. (2003) Synthesis and biological evaluation of substrate-based inhibitors of 6-phosphogluconate dehydrogenase as potential drugs against African trypanosomiasis. *Bioorg. Med. Chem.*, **11**, 3205–3214.

66 Ruda, G.F., Alibu, V.P., Mitsos, C., Bidet, O., Kaiser, M., Brun, R., Barrett, M.P., and Gilbert, I.H. (2007) Synthesis and biological evaluation of phosphate prodrugs of 4-phospho-D-erythronohydroxamic acid, an inhibitor of

6-phosphogluconate dehydrogenase. *Chem. Med. Chem.*, **2**, 1169–1180.

67 Ruda, G.F., Wong, P.E., Alibu, V.P., Norval, S., Read, K.D., Barrett, M.P., and Gilbert, I.H. (2010) Aryl phosphoramidates of 5-phospho erythronohydroxamic acid, a new class of potent trypanocidal compounds. *J. Med. Chem.*, **53**, 6071–6078.

68 Ruda, G.F., Campbell, G., Alibu, V.P., Barrett, M.P., Brenk, R., and Gilbert, I.H. (2010) Virtual fragment screening for novel inhibitors of 6-phosphogluconate dehydrogenase. *Bioorg. Med. Chem.*, **18**, 5056–5062.

69 Hammes, H.P., Du, X., Edelstein, D., Taguchi, T., Matsumura, T., Ju, Q., Lin, J., Bierhaus, A., Nawroth, P., Hannak, D., Neumaier, M., Bergfeld, R., Giardino, I., and Brownlee, M. (2003) Benfotiamine blocks three major pathways of hyperglycemic damage and prevents experimental diabetic retinopathy. *Nat. Med.*, **9**, 294–299.

17

GDP-Mannose: A Key Point for Target Identification and Drug Design in Kinetoplastids

Sébastien Pomel and *Philippe M. Loiseau*

Abstract

In kinetoplastids, the glycoconjugate precursor GDP-mannose appears to be a metabolic key-point in host–parasite interactions. GDP-mannose metabolism includes transport systems and a part of the glycolysis pathway that have been extensively studied as therapeutic targets and possible sources of inhibitors. This chapter focuses on the enzyme systems currently considered as real or potential targets for the development of new drugs based on GDP-mannose metabolism. Thus, some biochemical reactions of the mannosylation pathway are critical for parasite survival, providing potential therapeutic targets worthy of further investigations. Although the main enzyme systems involved in GDP-mannose metabolism have been identified, few of them are validated as interesting targets. GDP-mannose pyrophosphorylase (GDP-MP) is currently the most deeply studied protein with the identification of substrate analogs as specific inhibitors of kinetoplastid GDP-MP. Others are worthy of further studies to assess their potential as drug targets, mainly phosphomannomutase, GDP-mannose-dependent mannosyltransferases, and mannosyl phosphate transferases. Conversely, dolichol-phosphate mannose synthase, phosphomannose isomerase, and the GDP-mannose transporter (LPG2) are either not clearly essential for parasite survival and/or virulence, or their validation is species-dependent. Thus, new chemical series could emerge from the design of specific inhibitors of kinetoplastid proteins. However, well-known anti-parasitic chemical scaffolds should not be discarded for drug design in order to potentially combine inhibition of two mechanisms of action for killing the parasites, giving these inhibitors a multitarget action. Thus, drug design should integrate drug access to the target considering drug metabolism and pharmacokinetics. Moreover, the cost of drug synthesis and its stability in formulation should be considered.

Introduction

Eukaryotic glycosylation involves many types of mannose-containing glycoconjugates, like *N*-glycosylated proteins, glycolipids, or glycosylphosphatidylinositol (GPI)

* Corresponding Author

Trypanosomatid Diseases: Molecular Routes to Drug Discovery, First edition. Edited by T. Jäger, O. Koch, and L. Flohé.
© 2013 Wiley-VCH Verlag GmbH & Co. KGaA. Published 2013 by Wiley-VCH Verlag GmbH & Co. KGaA.

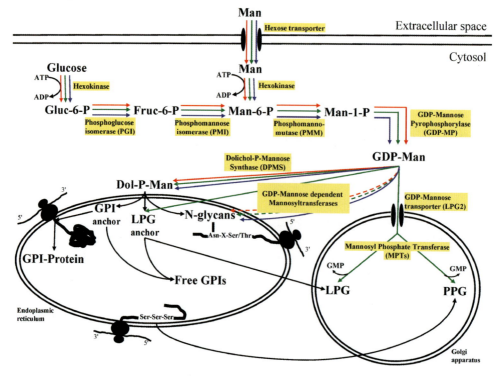

Figure 17.1 Comparison of GDP-mannose biosynthesis and consumption in human and kinetoplastids. GDP-mannose is synthesized by the same pathway in both human and kinetoplastids. In these organisms, this sugar-nucleotide is used as an activated mannose donor on the cytosolic side of the ER for N-glycosylation, GPI, or LPG biosynthesis: GDP-mannose can either be transferred to dolichol-phosphate via the DPMS or to glycan precursors for N-glycosylation via some GDP-mannose-dependent mannosyltransferases. GPIs can either be used as anchors for some proteins or secreted as free GPIs (GIPLs in *Leishmania*). Specifically in *Leishmania*, a GDP-mannose transporter (LPG2) allows the entry in the Golgi apparatus of the sugar-nucleotide, which is then used for phosphoglycan biosynthesis (present in LPG and PPG) via MPTs. Lines in blue, red, and green represent human, trypanosomal, and leishmanial enzymes, respectively. Dashed lines represent putative enzymes, whose expression has been predicted from genome sequences.

protein membrane anchors, which have important functions in a broad range of biological processes including protein folding, intercellular interactions such as cell–cell recognition, cell–matrix binding or host–pathogen adhesion, and signaling pathways [1]. For instance, N-glycan structures have been described to dictate protein folding in the endoplasmic reticulum (ER) and several glycoconjugate-mediated host–parasite interactions can subvert some host cell signaling pathways [2–4]. In kinetoplastid organisms, glycoconjugates are diverse in composition, and constitute a protective surface coat involved in parasite survival, infectivity, and virulence [5,6]. The parasite *Leishmania* produces large amounts of unusual mannosylated cell-surface associated glycoconjugates such as GPI-anchored glycoproteins, lipophosphoglycans (LPGs), glycosylinositolphospholipids (GIPLs), or proteophosphoglycans (PPGs). Free GPIs (also named GIPLs in *Leishmania*) are the major cellular glycolipids in kinetoplastids. Three groups of GIPLs have been characterized based on the composition of their glycan moiety: type I (analogous to GPI anchors with the structure mannose-α1,6-mannose-α1,4-*N*-acetylglucosamine-α1,6-PI, also referred as Man-α1,6-Man-α1,4-GlcN-α1,6-PI), type II (analogous to LPG anchors with the structure Man-α1,3-Man-α1,4-GlcN-α1,6-PI) or hybrid of type I and type II (containing features of both GPI and LPG anchors with the Man-α1,6(Man-α1,3)-Man-α1,4-GlcN-α1,6-PI motif) [7]. These GIPLs are differentially expressed depending on the leishmanial species or developmental stages. Both LPGs and PPGs are constituted of mannose oligomers, called β-mannans, which have been shown to play an important role in parasite virulence [8]. Since mannose is present in every kinetoplastid glycoconjugate, except for the *O*-linked mucins in *Trypanosoma cruzi*, biosynthesis of GDP-mannose, the activated mannose donor, is a promising pathway to identify new therapeutic targets for drug design. This chapter focuses on enzymes and transporters used in the biosynthetic pathway of GDP-mannose and on its utilization in the ER or Golgi apparatus for glycoconjugate mannosylation. All the potential targets analyzed in this chapter are mentioned in Figure 17.1 and illustrated by a colored arrow. A comparison of these pathways in both mammals and kinetoplastids is essential to define new targets for drug design (Figure 17.1).

Comparison of Mannosylation Pathways between Mammals and Kinetoplastids

In eukaryotes, the production of GDP-mannose depends on the synthesis of mannose-6-phosphate (M6P), which can be generated either after mannose internalization from the extracellular medium by means of hexose transporters and further phosphorylation by hexokinase or by the action of phosphomannose isomerase (PMI) on fructose-6-phosphate (F6P) (Figure 17.1). Sharma and Freeze have recently shown that 95% of the incoming mannose in mammals blood is catabolized by hexokinase while the mannose released by intracellular glycan processing of protein-bound oligosaccharides is preferentially released from cells as free mannose and could account for most of the mannose found in blood (50–100 μM) [9]. Since mannose is not a common sugar in the diet, M6P synthesis seems to mainly depend on PMI activity in mammals [1]. F6P can be produced from the first two reactions of glycolysis catalyzed by hexokinase and phosphoglucose isomerase (PGI). Once synthesized, M6P is converted by the phosphomannomutase (PMM) in mannose-1-phosphate (M1P), which is transformed by the GDP-mannose pyrophosphorylase (GDP-MP) to generate GDP-mannose. In the kinetoplastid *Leishmania major*, GDP-mannose turnover is very rapid in promastigote forms (around 30 s) and may be even more acute in intracellular amastigotes, where glucose is at a low concentration [6]. This sugar-nucleotide is then used as a mannose donor for all mannosylation reactions either directly via

GDP-mannose-dependent mannosyltransferase or indirectly via dolichol-phosphate mannose synthase (DPMS).

All the enzymes cited above are present in both pluricellular and unicellular eukaryotic organisms. In addition to these enzymes, the kinetoplastid protozoan parasite *Leishmania* spp. has developed a pathway where GDP-mannose can be directly internalized in the Golgi apparatus via the GDP-mannose transporter LPG2 to produce phosphoglycan-containing glycoconjugates, such as LPG or PPG, by the action of mannosyl phosphate transferases (MPTs) [10].

Enzymes and Transporters Involved in Mannosylation in Mammals and Kinetoplastids

In this section, the enzymes needed for GDP-mannose biosynthesis and utilization in kinetoplastids and mammals are presented, and their targetability for drug design are discussed. All potential targets, as well as their cellular localization, structure, validation, and inhibitors, are summarized in Table 17.1.

Hexose Transporter

In mammals, mannose can either be internalized by an energy-dependent transporter (SGLT4) or by energy-independent facilitated diffusion transporters (GLUT1, GLUT2, and GLUT3) [48,49]. SGLT4 has been described to transport mannose with a higher affinity than glucose [50]. Structural modeling of both GLUT1 and GLUT3 allowed the identification of the substrate binding sites and revealed the presence of 12 trans-membrane domains in these transporters [51,52]. Moreover, using freeze-fracture microscopy and biochemical analyses, Carruthers *et al.* suggest that GLUT1 is a tetramer [51]. While GLUT1 has a widespread tissue distribution, GLUT2 and GLUT3 are more specifically expressed in hepatocytes and neurons, respectively. GLUT1 deficiency syndrome is associated with infantile seizure, delayed development, and microcephaly, while a disorder in GLUT2 expression leads to Fanconi–Bickel syndrome characterized by hepatomegaly, renal tubular dysfunction, and dwarfism. A classic inhibitor of SGLTs is phlorizin, which can inhibit GLUTs as well [48,49]. GLUTs can also be inhibited by phloretin and cytochalasin B, while forskolin is active on both GLUT1 and GLUT3 [49,52,53]. Putative binding sites of cytochalasin B and forskolin were identified on the three-dimensional structure of GLUT3 [52].

In kinetoplastids, mannose can be transported by two proteins in *T. brucei* (*Tb*HT1 and *Tb*HT2), one in *T. cruzi* (*Tc*HT1), and three in *L. mexicana* (*Lm*GT1, *Lm*GT2, and *Lm*GT3) [11]. In *T. brucei*, *Tb*HT1 is expressed almost exclusively in the bloodstream form, while *Tb*HT2 is primarily expressed in the procyclic form. In *Leishmania*, *Lm*GT1 and *Lm*GT3 are expressed in both promastigote and amastigote stages, while *Lm*GT2 is downregulated in amastigotes. The null mutant of the *Lm*GT gene cluster in *Leishmania* grows more slowly than wild-type parasites in the promastigote form and shows a dramatic reduced viability in intracellular

Table 17.1 Enzymes and transporters involved in GDP-mannose biosynthesis and consumption for mannosylation in human and kinetoplastids: summary of mutant phenotypes and current inhibitors of these potential targets.

Potential targets	Species	Isoforms	Localization	Mutant phenotypes	Inhibitors[a),b)]	References
Hexose transporter	Leishmania spp.	LmGT1	flagellar membrane	reduced intracellular viability of ΔLmGT null mutant	FCCP,[b)] DCCD,[b)] monensin,[b)] and KCN[b)]	[11,12]
		LmGT2	pellicular plasma membrane			
		LmGT3	pellicular plasma membrane			
	T. brucei	TbHT1	?	?	FCCP[b)] and KCN[b)] active in procyclic but not bloodstream forms	[11]
		TbHT2	?			
	T. cruzi	TcHT1	?	?		
Hexokinase	Leishmania spp.	hexokinase glucokinase	glycosome glycosome	?	pyrophoshate[a)] ?	[13,14] [13]
	T. brucei	TbHK1	glycosome	switch to an unglycosylated form of procyclin (RNA interference)	lonidamine,[a),b)] quercetin,[a),b)] ebselen,[a),b)] and m-bromophenyl glucosamide[a),b)]	[15–19]
		TbHK2 Glucokinase	glycosome ?	? ?	pyrophoshate[a)] ?	[20]
	T. cruzi	Hexokinase	glycosome (mainly) and cytosol	? ?	pyrophosphate[a)]	[13,21]
		Glucokinase	glycosome	? ?	bisphosphonate[a),b)]	[13,22]

(continued)

Table 17.1 (Continued)

Potential targets	Species	Isoforms	Localization	Mutant phenotypes	Inhibitors[a),b)]	References
PGI	*Leishmania* spp.	PGI	cytosol and glycosome in the same proportions	?	5PAH[a)] and 5PAA[a)]	[23,24]
	T. brucei	PGI	glycosome	?	5PAH[a)] and 5PAA[a)]	[24,25]
	T. cruzi	PGI	cytosol and glycosome in the same proportions	?	erythrose-4-phosphate,[a)] 6-phosphogluconate,[a)] and mannose-6-phosphate[a)]	[24]
PMI	*Leishmania* spp.	PMI	cytosol	attenuated infection of Δ*lmpmi* mutants in vitro and in vivo	?	[26]
	T. brucei	PMI	?	?	?	
	T. cruzi	PMI	?	?	?	
PMM	*Leishmania* spp.	PMM	cytosol	inability of Δ*lmpmm* mutants to infect macrophages *in vitro* or mice *in vivo*	?	[27,28]
	T. brucei	PMM	?	?	?	
	T. cruzi	PMM	?	?	?	
GDP-MP	*Leishmania* spp.	GDP-MP	cytosol	essential for amastigote virulence and survival *in vitro* and *in vivo* (knockout)	piperazinyl-aryl-quinoline[a),b)]	[29–32]
	T. brucei	GDP-MP	cytosol	essential for bloodstream-form survival *in vitro* (RNA interference)	GDP-6-deoxymannose[a)]	[33]
	T. cruzi	?	?	?	?	

			ER subcompartment			[27,34]
DPMS	*Leishmania* spp.	DPMS		Δ*dpms* mutants remain infectious *in vitro* and *in vitro*	?	
	T. brucei	DPMS	ER	?	squaryldiamide-derived sugar-nucleotides[a),b] and thiazolidinone[a),b]	[35–37]
GDP-mannose-dependent mannosyltransferase	*T. cruzi*	?	?	?	?	
	Leishmania spp.	putative ALG2	?	?	?	
		putative ALG11	?			
	T. brucei	putative ALG2	?	?	?	
		putative ALG11	?			
	T. cruzi	putative ALG2	?	?	?	
		putative ALG11	?			
GDP-mannose transporter	*L. mexicana*	LPG2	Golgi apparatus	Δ*lpg2* mutants remain infectious	?	[38]
	L. donovani		Golgi apparatus	Δ*lpg2* mutants present an attenuated virulence *in vitro* and *in vivo*	?	[39,40]
	L. major		Golgi apparatus	Δ*lpg2* mutants are unable to survive in the sandfly vector and macrophages but persist indefinitely in mice and induce immunity	?	[41,42]
Mannosylphosphate transferase	*Leishmania* spp.	i-MPT	Golgi apparatus?	?	?	[10,43]
	Leishmania spp.	e-MPT	Golgi apparatus?	accumulation of truncated form of LPG in viable JEDI mutant lacking e-MPT activity	donor and acceptor substrate analogs[a]	[10,43–47]

See text for abbreviations.
a) Inhibitors active on the purified enzyme.
b) Inhibitors active on parasites *in vitro*.

amastigotes, indicating that these gene products could be interesting targets for drug design. None of the kinetoplastid transporters are sensitive to the classical inhibitors cytochalasin B or phloretin [12]. However, in *T. brucei* procyclic form, and in both promastigote and amastigote stages of *Leishmania*, hexose transport is sensitive to the protonophore FCCP (carbonyl cyanide-4-(trifluoromethoxy)-phenyl-hydrazone) or KCN (potassium cyanide), suggesting a proton-coupled ATPase dependence. Hexose uptake in amastigote is also inhibited by DCCD (N',N'-dicyclohexylcarbo-di-imide), an inhibitor of H^+-ATPase, and by the ionophore monensin [12]. This sensitivity to H^+-ATPase inhibitors was, however, not observed in both the *T. cruzi* and *T. brucei* bloodstream forms, showing that hexose transport in these parasites is only mediated by facilitated diffusion.

Hexokinase

In humans, four hexokinase isozymes have been identified, which differ in their catalytic and regulatory properties. Hexokinases I, II, and III have a dimeric structure of about 100 kDa, while hexokinase IV (also called glucokinase) is a single chain of 50 kDa. Hexokinases are allosterically inhibited by reaction product accumulation (glucose-6-phosphate (G6P)), whereas glucokinase is not. Several hexokinase inhibitors are currently in preclinical or clinical phase trials for anti-cancer treatment, in particular 2-deoxyglucose, 3-bromopyruvate, and lonidamine [54]. The mechanism of regulation of hexokinase I by G6P has been inferred from its crystal structure [55,56]. This enzyme, as well as the hexokinase II, is either free in the cytosol or associated with the outer membrane of mitochondria, conferring direct access to ATP generated by this organelle [57,58]. At the concentration of 0.2 mM, G6P was reported to favor dissociation of hexokinase I from the mitochondrial membrane. Conversely, hexokinase III is preferentially localized at the nuclear periphery, and glucokinase can shuttle between cytoplasm and nucleus [59]. Glucokinase has an important role in the regulation of glucose metabolism and represents a novel therapeutic target in type 2 diabetes [60]. A crystal structure of this enzyme revealed that its kinetic properties can be modulated through an allosteric site by synthetic thiobenzamide-derived activators [61]. The knowledge of this allosteric binding site allowed the design of new activators, such as sulfonamides, benzimidazoles, or 2-methylbenzofurans, and improvement of their structures for type 2 diabetes treatment [62–64]. In human, hexokinases can phosphorylate glucose as well as other hexoses like mannose. In contrast to what is observed in bacteria or kinetoplastids, glucokinase of vertebrates is not specific to glucose, but can phosphorylate other hexoses as well [13,65].

Using crystallographic analysis, Cordeiro *et al.* showed that glucokinase in *T. cruzi* is a loose tetrameric assembly of monomers of 42 kDa [66]. *T. cruzi* hexokinase is highly selective for glucose, in opposition to mammalian hexokinases, but also to its *T. brucei* and *Leishmania* spp. homologs [13,21]. In these kinetoplastid organisms, both glucokinase and hexokinase are located in the glycosome, an organelle that contains the first seven steps of glycolysis as well as enzymes of the oxidative branch of the pentose phosphate pathway, enabling these organisms to maintain a high glycolytic flux in this cell compartment. Glycolytic enzyme mislocalization in the cytosol of these parasites produces glucose toxicity and cell death, indicating that location of these proteins into the glycosome is required for parasite survival [14,67]. This phenomenon of glycolytic enzyme compartmentalization has also been observed during the life cycle of another protozoan parasite, *Toxoplasma*, allowing an optimization of energy delivery to cellular processes that are critical for parasite survival such as active transporter mechanisms on the plasma membrane or parasite motility [68]. The genome of *T. brucei* encodes for two hexokinases that are 98% identical: the active isoform *Tb*HK1, and *Tb*HK2 which was initially identified as inactive. Chambers *et al.* have shown, however, that *T. brucei* hexokinase activity can be generated from a homohexamer of *Tb*HK1 as well as from a heterohexamer of *Tb*HK1 and *Tb*HK2 [20]. Furthermore, no inhibition was observed on trypano-somatid hexokinases as well as on *T. cruzi* or *L. major* glucokinases, by using the reaction product G6P [13,20,21]. In *T. brucei*, hexokinase 1 can be inhibited by classical hexokinase inhibitors, such as lonidamine [15], but also by the biflavonoid quercetin [16], or, much more potently, by novel inhibitors identified by high-throughput screening (HTS), such as 2-phenyl-1,2-benzisoselenazol-3(2H)-one, also named ebselen [17]. Unlike *Tb*HK1, *Tb*HK2 can be inhibited by pyrophosphates [20]. Bisphosphonates can also be used as hexokinase inhibitors in *T. cruzi* [22]. A three-dimensional homology model of *Tb*HK1 has recently allowed the selection of a compound among glucosamine derivatives that specifically inhibits the parasite enzyme *in vitro*: *m*-bromophenyl glucosamide [18]. Silencing of *Tb*HK1 leads to a switch of expression from a glycosylated to an unglycosylated form of procyclin (glycoproteins expressed in the procyclic form of *Trypanosoma*) suggesting that procyclin (un)glycosylated form expression depends on glucose metabolism [19].

Phosphoglucose Isomerase (PGI)

PGI, also known as G6P isomerase,, is a dimeric enzyme that catalyzes the reversible interconversion of G6P to F6P. Two distinct PGI expression products are encoded by the human genome: type A (63.2 kDa) and B (69.8 kDa) [69]. The two major PGI isoforms are homodimers of type A, whereas the less-represented isoforms 3 and 4 are heterodimers of type A and B or homodimers of type B, respectively. The crystal of human PGI (type A) has allowed analyzing the catalytic mechanism of this enzyme [70]. Hereditary PGI deficiency is the second most erythroenzymopathy in glycolysis, which is associated with non-spherotic hemolytic anemia. Experimental compounds that can be considered as potent PGI inhibitors are D-F6P, 6-phosphogluconate, and *N*-bromoacetyl-aminoethyl phosphate [54].

Although *T. brucei* and *L. mexicana* PGIs share 56 and 47% identity, respectively, with the human homolog, comparative analysis of their crystal structures shows that the overall fold and substrate-binding residues are conserved in these three enzymes [25,71]. Compared to human, a larger active site was observed in *Leishmania* – a property that could be further used for rational drug design strategies. However, this difference was not observed in *T. brucei* PGI. A competitive inhibitor known to be active on rabbit muscle PGI, the 5-phosphoarabinonohydroxamic acid (5PAH), was found to have a 4-fold affinity for *T. brucei* PGI over the mammalian homolog ($K_i = 0.05$ μM for *T. brucei* PGI and $K_i = 0.2$ μM for rabbit PGI). Thus, structural knowledge of the inhibition mechanism of the *T. brucei* PGI by 5PAH could help in the future for the development of inhibitors with improved specificity. Both 5PAH and the derivative 5-phospho-D-arabinonate (5PAA) are active, but do not show a significant selectivity for the leishmanial PGI [23]. In *T. cruzi*, PGI can be inhibited either by erythrose-4-phosphate, 6-phosphogluconate, or M6P [24]. In contrast to all other PGIs, which are dimeric, PGI from *T. cruzi* is trimeric. Moreover, in this kinetoplastid organism as well as in *Leishmania*, PGI is localized in the same proportions in the glycosome and in the cytosol, whereas the enzyme is essentially restricted in the glycosome in *T. brucei*.

Apart from these classical glycolytic targets that have been extensively studied in kinetoplastids in recent years, GDP-mannose metabolism includes enzymes and transporters that are predominantly involved in the mannosylation process. Some of them have been identified as promising targets for drug design.

Phosphomannose Isomerase (PMI)

This enzyme catalyzes the reversible isomerization of F6P to M6P. A PMI deficiency leads to congenital disorder of glycosylation type Ib (CDG-Ib) in human, character-ized by hypoglycemia, coagulopathy, protein-losing enteropathy, and liver fibrosis [72]. Despite the fact that hexokinase provides an alternative pathway for M6P synthesis from mannose, the dietary uptake of this sugar is minor and not sufficient for normal glycosylation. However, oral mannose supplementation has been reported to be successful in treating this disease [73]. The compound 5PAH has been shown to inhibit competitively human PMI with the lowest K_i value (41 nM) ever reported for PMI inhibitors [74]. Moreover, benzoisothiazolone and dithiazo-limine scaffolds have been recently identified by HTS as specific non-competitive PMI inhibitors [75,76]. A three-dimensional homology model of human PMI has also allowed us to understand the catalytic mechanism of this enzyme and, especially, to identify the key residues involved in ligand binding [77].

Leishmanial and trypanosomal PMIs have low identity with the human homologous enzyme (from 30 to 33%), suggesting that this protein may be an attractive target for anti-leishmanial drug development. However, a functional analysis of PMI in *Leishmania* revealed that Δ*lmpmi* knockout mutants are able to grow in media deficient for free mannose, and present an attenuated but not completely blocked infection rate *in vitro* and *in vivo* [26]. No functional study has been performed so far on trypanosomal PMIs. PMI seems therefore not to be an ideal target for drug design.

Phosphomannomutase (PMM)

PMM, which catalyzes the conversion of M6P to M1P, is encoded by two isoforms in human: PMM2 is expressed in all tissues, whereas PMM1 expression is restricted to the brain and lungs. Inherited deficiency of PMM leads to CDG-Ia – the most frequent type of CDG characterized by severe psychomotor and mental retardation, dysmorphy, coagulation abnormalities, and dysfunction of several organs [78]. In contrast to CDG-Ib, mannose supplementation is ineffective in CDG-Ia patients. Two major therapeutic approaches have nevertheless been used to increase M1P levels in these patients: treatment by membrane-permeable molecules increasing the availability and/or metabolic flux of M1P precursors, a method which is not currently satisfactory enough due to the low stability and/or high toxicity of compounds, or PMM replacement or enhancement, which seems to be more promising. Crystal structure analysis of human PMM1 bound to M1P revealed the catalytic mechanism of this homodimeric enzyme [79]. Since the active-site structure and kinetic properties are conserved in both PMM1 and PMM2, it seems likely that PMM2 substrate binding mode and catalysis is similar to PMM1.

In *Leishmania*, Δ*lmpmm* mutants are unable to infect macrophages *in vitro* and mice *in vivo*, and gene replacement with human PMM2 does not restore parasite virulence, suggesting that this enzyme could be a promising drug target for the development of anti-leishmanial inhibitors [27,28]. However, a comparative analysis of crystals of human PMM2 with the leishmanial homolog shows that both enzymes have high degrees of similarities in both primary (55% of identity) and tertiary structures [28]. This result indicates that the development of *Leishmania*-selective PMM inhibitors will be laborious. In trypanosomes, PMMs may be more easily targeted since they have a slightly lower identity to human homologs (from 46 to 51%), compared with the leishmanial enzyme. However, no functional data are currently available concerning these trypanosomal enzymes.

Guanosine-Diphospho-D-mannose Pyrophosphorylase (GDP-MP)

In mammalian organisms, GDP-MP was mainly studied in the pig [80,81]. The swine native enzyme appears to be a complex of about 450 kDa with an α-subunit (43 kDa) and a β-subunit (37 kDa), the latter having the GDP-MP activity. In human, no data are currently available concerning the properties of GDP-MP. Nonetheless, two homologs of the porcine β-subunit have been characterized in the human genome. Sequence alignments revealed that the porcine β-subunit of GDP-MP presents 90% and 97% identity with its human homologs β1 and β2, respectively. In addition, the human β2 isoform shows a slightly better homology with *L. mexicana* GDP-MP (49%), compared to β1 (46%).

Deletion of the gene encoding GDP-MP in *L. mexicana* is critical for amastigote survival *in vitro* and leads to a total loss of virulence *in vivo* [29,30]. At the promastigote stage, these deletion mutants present an abnormal morphology and cytokinesis, and completely lack mannose-containing glycoproteins and glycolipids. Likewise, GDP-MP silencing by RNA interference is lethal for the *T. brucei* bloodstream form, showing that this enzyme is also essential for survival of these parasites [33]. Among several GDP-mannose analogs that have been tested as potential GDP-MP inhibitors in this study, only GDP-6-deoxymannose showed a significant enzyme inhibition with an IC_{50} of 13 μM. A HTS assay set up to select GDP-MP inhibitors in *Leishmania major* allowed to identify a quinoline derivative that demonstrated an *in vitro* activity on *Leishmania* GDP-MP and on intracellular parasite proliferation with IC_{50} values of 0.58 μM and 21.9 μM, respectively [31]. A subsequent structure–activity relationship study revealed piperazinyl-aryl-quinolines as potent GDP-MP inhibitors. A biochemical analysis of leishmanial GDP-MP has shown that this enzyme self-associates to form an enzymatically active and stable hexamer of about 240 kDa, while the monomer does not display any catalytic activity *in vitro* [32]. Based on the *L. mexicana* GDP-MP structural homology with the uridyltransferase from *Streptococcus pneumoniae* (Glmu) and thymidylyltransferase from *Pseudomonas aeruginosa* (RmlA), a three-dimensional model of the GDP-MP from *L. mexicana* has been generated [82]. The top-ranking structural model of this enzyme suggests the GDP-MP hexamerization is established by head-to-head interactions. However, no data was reported in this work concerning the region of the catalytic site in the enzyme quaternary structure. A recent *in silico* analysis of both human and *L. infantum* GDP-MPs allowed the delineation of both enzyme catalytic sites and the identification of a motif of amino acids specific to the parasite protein [83]. This specific motif could then be used as a target to design compounds that selectively inhibit the leishmanial GDP-MP, but not the human homolog.

Dolichol-Phosphate Mannose Synthase (DPMS)

Owing to the lack of GDP-mannose transporter in the ER, eukaryotic cells developed a typical strategy to transfer mannose in this organelle for mannosylation reactions [1]. In this way, DPMS transfers mannose from GDP-mannose to dolichol-phosphate, a derivative of polyprenols, and synthesizes dolichol-phosphate mannose (DPM) on the cytosolic side of the ER. DPM is subsequently translocated to the luminal side of the ER, presumably by a putative flippase, and then used as a mannosyl donor for *N*-glycosylation or GPI biosynthesis. Mammalian DPMS contains a catalytic DPM1 and DPM2/DPM3 regulatory subunits [84]. A deficiency in DPM1 in human leads to CDG-Ie, a disease which causes essentially the same symptoms as CDG-Ia [85,86].

In spite of the relatively weak identity between both trypanosomal and leishmanial DPMS with their human counterpart (30%), a structural analysis of the three-dimensional model of DPM1 in the yeast *Saccharomyces cerevisiae* has revealed that the tertiary structure of this protein is well conserved among species [87]. In particular, residues of the enzyme active-site cleft are highly conserved. Furthermore, DPMS from *T. brucei* can be functionally expressed both in yeast and in *E. coli* [88]. As for human, DPMS is localized to the ER in trypanosomatids [34,35]. This enzyme is associated particularly with a subcompartment in the ER of *L. mexicana* that is involved in GPI biosynthesis. Despite the fact that some inhibitors, such as squaryldiamide-derived sugar-nucleotides or thiazolidinones, have been reported to be active on *T. brucei* DPMS, no analysis was realized with these compounds on the human homologous enzyme [36,37]. Some 8-substitued fluorescent analogs of GDP-mannose synthesized by Collier and Wagner are also of great interest as DPMS inhibitor candidates [89]. Thiazolidinones possess a trypanocidal activity, suggesting that DPMS could be essential for *T. brucei* survival. However, a functional analysis of DPMS by knockout in *L. mexicana* revealed that Δ*dpms* mutants remain infectious to both macrophages and mice [27].

GDP-Mannose-Dependent Mannosyltransferases

In mammalian cells, three GDP-mannose-dependent mannosyltransferases (ALG1, ALG2, and ALG11) are sequentially involved in early steps of N-glycosylation by adding mannose from GDP-mannose on dolichol-P-P-glycan on the cytosolic side of the ER [1]. These precursors are then flipped on the luminal side of the ER to be further glycosylated using DPM as a mannose donor (see above). Defects in ALG1, ALG2, or ALG11 lead to CDG-Ik, CDG-Ii, or CDG-Ip, respectively [90–92]. CDG-Ik and CDG-Ip patients develop a severe disease engendering recurrent seizures and developmental retardation with death in early infancy, while CDG-Ii patients are normal at birth, but in their first year of life develop mental retardation, seizures, coloboma of the iris, hypomyelination, hepatomegaly, and coagulation abnormalities. Putative ALG2 and ALG11 exist in the genomes of *T. brucei*, *T. cruzi*, and *Leishmania* spp., and have a relatively low identity with their human homolog (from 37 to 38% and from 33 to 35% identity with hALG2 and hALG11, respectively), suggesting a potential targetability of these enzymes in kinetoplastids to design new drugs.

Moreover, LPG anchors in *Leishmania* as well as some GIPLs are assembled on the same alkylacyl-PI as the GPI anchor precursors, except that the second mannose is linked in α-1,3 rather than in α-1,6 [1,5]. Several complementary works indicate that this linkage is catalyzed on the cytosolic face of the ER by a GDP-mannose-dependent mannosyltransferase [93,94]. This α-1,3-mannosyltransferase could also be used as a target to rationally design new anti-kinetoplastid agents.

GDP-Mannose Transporter (LPG2)

In *Leishmania*, different mutants lacking LPG or phosphoglycan biosynthetic genes have been generated [41,95]. Among them, the *lpg2⁻* mutant lacks the *lpg2* gene encoding for a Golgi GDP-mannose transporter absent in mammalian cells. However, homologs of this sugar-nucleotide transporter have been identified in fungi and plants [96]. In addition to GDP-mannose, LPG2 is able to transport two other sugar-nucleotides, GDP-D-arabinose and GDP-L-fucose, which have been detected in *L. major* cell extracts [6,39]. Using several biochemical approaches, Hong *et al.* showed that GDP-mannose transporter consists of a hexameric complex composed exclusively of LPG2 subunits. The role of LPG2 has been studied in several leishmanial species. While *L. mexicana* Δ*lpg2* mutants remain infectious, a deficiency in this transporter in *L. donovani* leads to an attenuation of virulence in mammalian host both *in vitro* and *in vivo* [38,40]. In *L. major, lpg2*⁻ null mutants are unable to survive in the sandfly vector and macrophages, but persist indefinitely at a low level and induce immunity in mice [41,42]. Nonetheless, the loss of amastigote virulence in *L. major lpg2*⁻ null mutants is probably not due to the absence of phosphoglycans [97]. Neither structural studies nor inhibitor design have been performed on LPG2 to date.

Mannosyl Phosphate Transferases (MPTs)

In *Leishmania*, phosphoglycans are polymers synthesized in the Golgi apparatus composed of (Gal-β1,4-Man-α1-PO$_4$⁻) repeat units (around 4–40 repeats in pro-mastigote forms and only around 10 repeats in amastigote forms) and a small oligosaccharide cap. Functional analysis of a viable *lpg*⁻ mutant in *L. donovani*, called JEDI, revealed that phosphoglycans are synthesized by sequential action of an initiating-MPT (i-MPT) and an elongating-MPT (e-MPT), followed by a galactosyl-transferase [43]. The MPTs, which belong to a unique class of enzymes non-existent in human biology, have not been purified or cloned. These enzymes transfer α-D-mannose phosphate from the GDP-mannose donor either to the GPI anchor (i-MPT) or to the (Gal-β1,4-Man-α1-PO$_4$⁻) acceptor substrate (e-MPT), with the release of GMP. In mammalian cells, mannose-containing glycoconjugates are rather synthesized by the transfer of mannose from GDP-mannose with the release of GDP. A biochemical analysis of e-MPT in the three leishmanial species *L. donovani*, *L. major*, and *L. mexicana* using synthetic acceptor substrate analogs allowed the characterization of the enzyme substrate specificities in these parasites [44]. These analogs were created by replacing the mannose moiety by another sugar, or the phosphate moiety by a thiophosphate, a boranophosphate, or a methylphosphonate. Other substrate analogs of e-MPT have been further characterized: the acceptor derivative β-D-Gal-1,4-α-D-Man methanephosphonate, or the bisubstrate inhibitor comprising the acceptor substrate bound to a guanosine subunit through a non-hydrolyzable methylene-biphosphonate that mimics the pyrophosphate moiety of the GDP-mannose donor [45,46]. Moreover, some imino sugar molecules have been shown to have some promising inhibitory properties on *L. donovani* e-MPT [47].

Conclusion

The first therapeutic targets identified in kinetoplastids were from energy metabolism, such as glycolysis and mitochondrial enzymes. As soon as new proteins were identified in other pathways (proteinases, lipid metabolism, redox enzyme system, etc.), they were evaluated as potential drug targets with mixed success regarding parasite specificity in inhibitor design. More recently, the deciphering of the cellular and biochemical host–parasite relationships has provided new parasite proteins responsible for the synthesis of glycosylated ligands that are recognized by host cells. In this way, GDP-mannose, a glycoconjugate precursor, is considered as a metabolic key-point in host–parasite interactions in kinetoplastids since some biochemical reactions of the mannosylation pathway are critical for parasite survival, providing potential therapeutic targets. From GDP-mannose metabolism, a few enzymes have been validated as interesting targets. Among them, GDP-MP appears to be presently the most promising one with the design of specific inhibitors. PMM, GDP-mannose-dependent mannosyltransferases, and MPTs are worthy of further studies for their potential as drug targets. Moreover, the glycolytic pathway includes two proteins involved in GDP-mannose metabolism. Inhibition of these enzymes or hexose transporters would impact on both energy metabolism and biosynthesis of glyco-conjugates involved in host cell recognition. Nevertheless, DPMS, PMI, and GDP-mannose transporter (LPG2) do not seem to be essential for parasite survival and virulence or their validation is species-dependent.

Three-dimensional modeling studies of the relevant parasite enzyme systems comparative to their human counterparts, if they exist, are the key tools for drug design. From the studies carried out on the GDP-mannose pathway, only a few inhibitors active on enzyme systems and *in vitro* against parasites have been evaluated *in vivo*. Thus, drug design should integrate its access to the target considering drug metabolism and pharmacokinetics. Moreover, the cost of drug synthesis and its stability in formulation should be considered.

References

1 Varki, A.,Cummings, R.D.,Esko, J.D., Freeze, H.H.,Stanley, P.,Bertozzi, C.R., Hart, G.W., and Etzler, M.E. (eds) (2009) *Essentials of Glycobiology*, 2nd edn, Cold Spring Harbor Laboratory Press, Cold Spring Harbor, NY.

2 Molinari, M. (2007) *N*-Glycan structure dictates extension of protein folding or onset of disposal. *Nat. Chem. Biol.*, 3, 313–320.

3 Tachado, S.D., Mazhari-Tabrizi, R., and Schofield, L. (1999) Specificity in signal transduction among glycosylphosphatidylinositols of *Plasmodium falciparum, Trypanosoma brucei, Trypanosoma cruzi* and *Leishmania* spp. *Parasite Immunol.*, 21, 609–617.

4 Das, P., Lahiri, A., Lahiri, A., and Chakravortty, D. (2010) Modulation of the arginase pathway in the context of microbial pathogenesis: a metabolic enzyme moonlighting as an immune modulator. *PLoS Pathog.*, 6, e1000899.

5 McConville, M.J., Mullin, K.A., Ilgoutz, S. C., and Teasdale, R.D. (2002) Secretory pathway of trypanosomatid parasites. *Microbiol. Mol. Biol. Rev.*, 66, 122–154.

6 Turnock, D.C. and Ferguson, M.A. (2007) Sugar nucleotide pools of *Trypanosoma brucei, Trypanosoma cruzi*, and *Leishmania major. Eukaryot. Cell*, 6, 1450–1463.

7 Mukhopadhyay, S. and Mandal, C. (2006) Glycobiology of *Leishmania donovani. Indian J. Med. Res.*, 123, 203–220.

8 Ralton, J.E., Naderer, T., Piraino, H.L., Bashtannyk, T.A., Callaghan, J.M., and McConville, M.J. (2003) Evidence that intracellular β1-2 mannan is a virulence factor in *Leishmania* parasites. *J. Biol. Chem.*, 278, 40757–40763.

9 Sharma, V. and Freeze, H.H. (2011) Mannose efflux from the cells: a potential source of mannose in blood. *J. Biol. Chem.*, 286, 10193–10200.

10 Chandra, S., Ruhela, D., Deb, A., and Vishwakarma, R.A. (2010) Glycobiology of the *Leishmania* parasite and emerging targets for antileishmanial drug discovery. *Expert Opin. Ther. Targets*, 14, 739–757.

11 Landfear, S.M. (2011) Nutrient transport and pathogenesis in selected

parasite protozoa. *Eukaryot. Cell*, **10**, 483–493.

12 Tetaud, E., Barrett, M.P., Bringaud, F. and Baltz, T. (1997) Kinetoplastid glucose transporters. *Biochem. J.*, **325**, 569–580.

13 Caceres, A.J., Quinones, W., Gualdron, M., Cordeiro, A., Avilan, L., Michels, P.A.M., and Concepcion, J.L. (2007) Molecular and biochemical characterization of novel glucokinases from *Trypanosoma cruzi* and *Leishmania* spp. *Mol. Biochem. Parasitol.*, **156**, 235–245.

14 Kumar, R., Gupta, S., Srivastava, R., Sahasrabuddhe, A.A., and Gupta, C.M. (2010) Expression of a PTS2-truncated hexokinase produces glucose toxicity in *Leishmania donovani*. *Mol. Biochem. Parasitol.*, **170**, 41–44.

15 Chambers, J.W., Fowler, M.L., Morris, M.T., and Morris, J.C. (2008) The anti-trypanosomal agent lonidamine inhibits *Trypanosoma brucei* hexokinase 1. *Mol. Biochem. Parasitol.*, **158**, 202–207.

16 Dodson, H.C., Lyda, T.A., Chambers, J.W., Morris, M.T., Christensen, K.A., and Morris, J.C. (2011) Quercetin, a fluorescent biflavonoid, inhibits *Trypanosoma brucei* hexokinase 1. *Exp. Parasitol.*, **127**, 423–428.

17 Sharlow, E.R., Lyda, T.A., Dodson, H.C., Mustata, G., Morris, M.T., Leimgruber, S. S., Lee, K.H. *et al.* (2010) A target-based high throughput screen yields *Trypanosoma brucei* hexokinase small molecules inhibitors with antiparasitic activity. *PLoS Negl. Trop. Dis.*, **4**, e659.

18 Willson, M., Sanejouand, Y.H., Perie, J., Hannaert, V., and Opperdoes, F. (2002) Sequencing, modeling, and selective inhibition of *Trypanosoma brucei* hexokinase. *Chem. Biol.*, **9**, 839–847.

19 Morris, J.C., Wang, Z., Drew, M.E., and Englund, P.T. (2002) Glycolysis modulates trypanosome glycoprotein expression as revealed by an RNAi library. *EMBO J.*, **21**, 4429–4438.

20 Chambers, J.W., Kearns, M.T., Morris, M. T., and Morris, J.C. (2008) Assembly of heterohexameric trypanosome hexokinases reveals that hexokinase 2 is a regulable enzyme. *J. Biol. Chem.*, **283**, 14963–14970.

21 Caceres, A.J., Portillo, R., Acosta, H., Rosales, D., Quinones, W., Avilan, L.,

Salazar, L. *et al.* (2003) Molecular and biochemical characterization of hexokinase from *Trypanosoma cruzi*. *Mol. Biochem. Parasitol.*, **126**, 251–262.

22 Sanz-Rodriguez, C.E., Concepcion, J.L., Pekerar, S., Oldfield, E., and Urbina, J.A. (2007) Bisphosphonates as inhibitors of *Trypanosoma cruzi* hexokinase: kinetic and metabolic studies. *J. Biol. Chem.*, **282**, 12377–12387.

23 Cordeiro, A.T., Hardré, R., Michels, P.A. M., Salmon, L., Delboni, L.F., and Thiemann, O.H. (2004) *Leishmania mexicana mexicana* glucose-6-phosphate isomerase: crystallization, molecular-replacement solution and inhibition. *Acta Crystallogr. D*, **60**, 915–919.

24 Concepcion, J.L., Chataing, B., and Dubourdieu, M. (1999) Purification and properties of phosphoglucose isomerase of *Trypanosoma cruzi*. *Comp. Biochem. Physiol. B*, **122**, 211–222.

25 Arsenieva, D., Appavu, B.L., Mazock, G.H., and Jeffery, C.J. (2008) Crystal of phosphoglucose isomerase from *Trypanosoma brucei* complexed with glucose-6-phosphate at 1.6 Å resolution. *Proteins*, **74**, 72–80.

26 Garami, A. and Ilg, T. (2001) The role of phosphomannose isomerase in *Leishmania mexicana* glycoconjugate synthesis and virulence. *J. Biol. Chem.*, **276**, 6566–6575.

27 Garami, A., Mehlert, A., and Ilg, T. (2001) Glycosylation defects and virulence phenotypes of *Leishmania mexicana* phosphomannomutase and dolicholphosphate-mannose synthase gene deletion mutants. *Mol. Cell. Biol.*, **21**, 8168–8183.

28 Kedzierski, L., Malby, R.L., Smith, B.J., Perugini, M.A., Hodder, A.N., Ilg, T., Colman, P.M., and Handman, E. (2006) Structure of *Leishmania mexicana* phosphomannomutase highlights similarities with human isoforms. *J. Mol. Biol.*, **363**, 215–227.

29 Garami, A. and Ilg, T. (2001) Disruption of mannose activation in *Leishmania mexicana*: GDP-mannose pyrophosphorylase is required for virulence, but not for viability. *EMBO J.*, **20**, 3657–3666.

30 Stewart, J., Curtis, J., Spurck, T.P., Ilg, T., Garami, A., Baldwin, T., Courret, N. *et al.* (2005) Characterization of a *Leishmania mexicana* knockout lacking guanosine-diphosphate mannose pyrophosphorylase. *Int. J. Parasitol.*, **35**, 861–873.

31 Lackovic, K., Parisot, J.P., Sleebs, N., Baell, J.B., Debien, L., Watson, K.G., Curtis, J.M. *et al.* (2010) Inhibitors of *Leishmania* GDP-mannose pyrophosphorylase identified by high-throughput screening of small-molecule chemical library. *Antimicrob. Agents Chemother.*, **54**, 1712–1719.

32 Davis, A.J., Perugini, M.A., Smith, B.J., Stewart, J.D., Ilg, T., Hodder, A.N., and Handman, E. (2004) Properties of GDP-mannose pyrophosphorylase, a critical enzyme and drug target in *Leishmania mexicana. J. Biol. Chem.*, **279**, 12462–12468.

33 Denton, H., Fyffe, S., and Smith, T.K. (2010) GDP-mannose pyrophosphorylase is essential in the bloodstream form of *Trypanosoma brucei. Biochem. J.*, **425**, 603–614.

34 Ilgoutz, S.C., Mullin, K.A., Southwell, B.R., and McConville, M.J. (1999) Glycosylphosphatidylinositol biosynthetic enzymes are localized to a stable tubular subcompartment of the endoplasmic reticulum in *Leishmania mexicana. EMBO J.*, **18**, 3643–3654.

35 Prado-Figueroa, M., Raper, J. and Opperdoes, F.R. (1994) Possible localization of dolichol-dependent mannosyltransferase of *Trypanosoma brucei* to the rough endoplasmic reticulum. *Mol. Biochem. Parasitol.*, **63**, 255–264.

36 Niewiadomski, S., Beebeejaun, Z., Denton, H., Smith, T.K., Morris, R.J., and Wagner, G.K. (2010) Rationally designed squaryldiamides – a novel class of sugar-nucleotide mimics? *Org. Biomol. Chem.*, **8**, 3488–3499.

37 Smith, T.K., Young, B.L., Denton, H., Hughes, D.L., and Wagner, G.K. (2009) First small molecular inhibitors of *T. brucei* dolicholphosphate mannose synthase (DMPS), a validated drug in African sleeping sickness. *Bioorg. Med. Chem. Lett.*, **19**, 1749–1752.

38 Ilg, T., Demar, M., and Harbecke, D. (2001) Phosphoglycan repeat-deficient *Leishmania mexicana* parasites remain infectious to macrophages and mice. *J. Biol. Chem.*, **276**, 4988–4997.

39 Hong, K., Ma, D., Beverley, S.M., and Turco, S.J. (2000) The *Leishmania* GDP-mannose transporter is an autonomous, multi-specific, hexameric complex of LPG2 subunits. *Biochemistry*, **39**, 2013–2022.

40 Gaur, U., Showalter, M., Hickerson, S., Dalvi, R., Turco, S.J., Wilson, M.E., and Beverley, S.M. (2009) *Leishmania donovani* lacking the Golgi GDP-man transporter LPG2 exhibit attenuated virulence in mammalian hosts. *Exp. Parasitol.*, **122**, 182–191.

41 Späth, G.F., Lye, L.F., Segawa, H., Sacks, D.L., Turco, S.J., and Beverley, S.M. (2003) Persistence without pathology in phosphoglycan-deficient *Leishmania major. Science*, **301**, 1241–1243.

42 Kébaïer, C., Uzonna, J.E., Beverley, S.M. and Scott, P. (2006) Immunization with persistent attenuated Δ*lpg2 Leishmania major* parasites requires adjuvant to provide protective immunity in C57BL/6 mice. *Infect. Immun.*, **74**, 777–780.

43 Descoteaux, A., Mengeling, B.J., Beverley, S.M., and Turco, S.J. (1998) *Leishmania donovani* has distinct mannosylphosphoryl-transferases for the initiation and elongation phases of lipophosphoglycan repeating unit biosynthesis. *Mol. Biochem. Parasitol.*, **94**, 27–40.

44 Routier, F.H., Higson, A.P., Ivanova, I.A., Ross, A.J., Tsvetkov, Y.E., Yashunsky, D.V., Bates, P.A. *et al.* (2000) Characterization of the elongating α-D-mannosyl phosphate transferase from three species of *Leishmania* using synthetic acceptor substrate analogues. *Biochemistry*, **39**, 8017–8025.

45 Borodkin, V.S., Ferguson, M.A.J., and Nikolaev, A.V. (2001) Synthesis of β-D-Galp-(1 → 4)-α-D-Manp methanephosphonate, a substrate analogue for the elongating α-D-mannosyl phosphate transferase in the *Leishmania. Tetrahedron Lett.*, **42**, 5305–5308.

46 Borodkin, V.S., Ferguson, M.A.J., and Nikolaev, A.V. (2004) Synthesis of potential bisubstrate inhibitors of *Leishmania* elongating α-D-mannosyl phosphate transferase. *Tetrahedron Lett.*, **45**, 857–862.

47 Ruhela, D., Chatterjee, P., and Vishwakarma, R.A. (2005) 1-Oxabicyclic β-lactams as new inhibitors of elongating MPT – a key enzyme responsible for assembly of cell surface phosphoglycans of *Leishmania* parasites. *Org. Biomol. Chem.*, **3**, 1043–1048.

48 Wright, E.M., Loo, D.D., and Hirayama, B.A. (2011) Biology of human sodium glucose transporters. *Physiol. Rev.*, **91**, 733–794.

49 Augustin, R. (2010) The protein family of glucose transport facilitators: it's not only about glucose after all. *IUBMB Life*, **62**, 315–333.

50 Tazawa, S., Yamato, T., Fujikura, H., Hiratochi, M., Itoh, F., Tomae, M., Takemura, Y. *et al.* (2005) SLC5A9/SGLT4, a new Na$^+$-dependent glucose transporter, is an essential transporter for mannose, 1,5-anhydro-D-glucitol, and fructose. *Life Sci.*, **76**, 1039–1050.

51 Carruthers, A., DeZutter, J., Ganguly, A. and Devaskar, S.U. (2009) Will the original glucose transporter isoform please stand up! *Am. J. Physiol. Endocrinol. Metab.*, **297**, E836–E848.

52 Dwyer, D.S. (2001) Model of the 3-D structure of the GLUT3 glucose transporter and molecular dynamics simulation of glucose transport. *Proteins*, **42**, 531–541.

53 Uldry, M. and Thorens, B. (2004) The SCL2 family of facilitated hexose and polyol transporters. *Pflugers Arch.*, **447**, 480–489.

54 Scatena, R., Bottoni, P., Pontoglio, A., Mastrototaro, L., and Giardina, B. (2008) Glycolytic enzyme inhibitors in cancer treatment. *Expert Opin. Investig. Drugs*, **17**, 1533–1545.

55 Aleshin, A.E., Zeng, C., Bartunik, H.D., Fromm, H.J., and Honzatko, R.B. (1998) Regulation of hexokinase I: crystal structure of recombinant human brain hexokinase complexed with glucose and phosphate. *J. Mol. Biol.*, **282**, 345–357.

56 Aleshin, A.E., Zeng, C., Bourenkov, G.B., Bartunik, H.D., Fromm, H.J., and Honzatko, R.B. (1998) The mechanism of regulation of hexokinase: new insights from the crystal structure of recombinant human brain hexokinase complexed with glucose and glucose-6-phosphate. *Structure*, **6**, 39–50.

57 Aleshin, A.E., Fromm, H.J., and Honzatko, R.B. (1998) Multiple crystal forms of hexokinase I: new insights regarding conformational dynamics, subunit interactions, and membrane association. *FEBS Lett.*, **434**, 42–46.

58 Rosano, C., Sabini, E., Rizzi, M., Deriu, D., Murshudov, G., Bianchi, M., Serafini, G. *et al.* (1999) Binding of non-catalytic ATP to human hexokinase I highlights the structural components for enzyme–membrane association control. *Structure*, **7**, 1427–1437.

59 Bosco, D., Meda, P., and Iynedjian, P.B. (2000) Glucokinase and glucokinase regulatory protein: mutual dependence for nuclear localization. *Biochem. J.*, **348**, 215–222.

60 Osbak, K.K., Colclough, K., Saint-Martin, C., Beer, N.L., Bellané-Chantelot, C., Ellard, S., and Gloyn, A.L. (2009) Update on mutations of glucokinase (GCK), which cause maturity-onset diabetes of the young, permanent neonatal diabetes, and hyperinsulinemic hypoglycemia. *Hum. Mutat.*, **30**, 1512–1526.

61 Kamata, K., Mitsuya, M., Nishimura, T., Eiki, J., and Nagata, Y. (2004) Structural basis for allosteric regulation of the monomeric allosteric enzyme human glucokinase. *Structure*, **12**, 429–438.

62 Takahashi, K., Hashimoto, N., Nakama, C., Kamata, K., Sasaki, K., Yashimoto, R., Ohyama, S. *et al.* (2009) The design and optimization of a series of 2-(pyridine-2-yl)-1H-benzimidazole compounds as allosteric glucokinase activators. *Bioorg. Med. Chem.*, **17**, 7042–7051.

63 Bebernitz, G.R., Beaulieu, V., Dale, B.A., Deacon, R., Duttaroy, A., Gao, J., Grondine, M.S. *et al.* (2009) Investigation of functionally liver selective glucokinase activators for the treatment of type 2 diabetes. *J. Med. Chem.*, **52**, 6142–6152.

64 Pfefferkorn, J.A., Guzman-Perez, A., Oates, P.J., Litchfield, J., Aspnes, G., Basak, A., Benbow, J. *et al.* (2011) Designing glucokinase activators with reduced hypoglycemia risk: discovery of *N,N*-dimethyl-5-(2-methyl-6-((5-methylpyrazin-2-yl)-carbamoyl)benzofuran-4-yloxy) pyrimidine-2-carboxamide as a clinical candidate for the treatment of type 2 diabetes mellitus. *Med. Chem. Commun.*, **2**, 828–839.

65 Xu, L.Z., Weber, I.T., Harrison, R.W., Gidh-Jain, M., and Pilkis, S.J. (1995) Sugar specificity of human beta-cell glucokinase: correlation of molecular models with kinetics measurements. *Biochemistry*, **34**, 6083–6092.

66 Cordeiro, A.T., Caceres, A.J., Vertommen, D., Concepcion, J.L., Michels, P.A.M., and Versées, W. (2007) The crystal structure of *Trypanosoma cruzi* glucokinase reveals features determining oligomerization and anomer specificity of hexose-phosphorylating enzymes. *J. Mol. Biol.*, **372**, 1215–1226.

67 Furuya, T., Kessler, P., Jardim, A., Schnaufer, A., Crudder, A., and Parsons, M. (2002) Glucose is toxic to glycosome-deficient trypanosomes. *Proc. Natl. Acad. Sci. USA*, **99**, 14177–14182.

68 Pomel, S., Luk, F.C., and Beckers, C.J. (2008) Host cell egress and invasion induce marked relocations of glycolytic enzymes in *Toxoplasma gondii* tachyzoites. *PLoS Pathog.*, **4**, e10001888.

69 Sun, A.Q., Yüksel, K.U., Jacobson, T.M., and Gracy, R.W. (1990) Isolation and characterization of human glucose-6-phosphate isomerase isoforms containing two different size subunits. *Arch. Biochem. Biophys.*, **283**, 120–129.

70 Read, J., Pearce, J., Li, X., Muirhead, H., Chirgwin, J., and Davies, C. (2001) The crystal structure of human phosphoglucose isomerase at 1.6 Å resolution: implications for catalytic mechanism, cytokine activity and haemolytic anaemia. *J. Mol. Biol.*, **309**, 447–463.

71 Cordeiro, A.T., Michels, P.A.M., Delboni, L.F., and Theimann, O.H. (2004) The crystal structure of glucose-6-phosphate isomerase from *Leishmania mexicana* reveals novel active site features. *Eur. J. Biochem.*, **271**, 2765–2772.

72 Schollen, E., Dorland, L., de Koning, T.J., Van Diggelen, O.P., Huijmans, J.G.M., Marquardt, T., Babovic-Vuksanovic, D. *et al.* (2000) Genomic organization of the human phosphomannose isomerase (MPI) gene and mutation analysis in patients with congenital disorders of glycosylation type Ib (CDG-Ib). *Hum. Mutat.*, **16**, 247–252.

73 de Lonlay, P. and Seta, N. (2009) The clinical spectrum of phosphomannose isomerase deficiency, with an evaluation of mannose treatment for CDG-1b. *Biochim. Biophys. Acta*, **1792**, 841–843.

74 Roux, C., Bhatt, F., Foret, J., de Courcy, B., Gresh, N., Piquemal, J.P., Jeffery, C.J., and Salmon, L. (2011) The reaction mechanism of type I phosphomannose isomerases: new information from inhibiton and polarizable molecular mechanics studies. *Proteins*, **79**, 203–220.

75 Dahl, R., Bravo, Y., Sharma, V., Ichikawa, M., Dhanya, R.P., Hedrick, M., Brown, B. *et al.* (2011) Potent, selective, and orally available benzoisothiazolone phosphomannose isomerase inhibitors as probe for congenital disorder of glycosylation Ia. *J. Med. Chem.*, **54**, 3661–3668.

76 Hedrick, M., Brown, B., Rascon, J., Sergienko, E., Sharma, V., Ng, B., Ichikawa, M., Freeze, H. *et al.* (2010) Therapeutic inhibitors of phosphomannose isomerase, in *Probe Reports from the NIH Molecular Libraries Program*, National Center for Biotechnology Information, Bethesda, MD.

77 Xiao, J., Guo, Z., Guo, Y., Chu, F., and Sun, P. (2006) Computational study of human phosphomannose isomerase: insights from homology modeling and molecular dynamics simulation of enzyme bound substrate. *J. Mol. Graph. Model.*, **25**, 289–295.

78 Freeze, H.H. (2009) Towards a therapy for phosphomannomutase 2 deficiency, the defect in CDG-Ia patients. *Biochim. Biophys. Acta*, **1792**, 835–840.

79 Silvaggi, N.R., Zhang, C., Lu, Z., Dai, J., Dunaway-Mariano, D., and Allen, K.N. (2006) The X-ray crystal structures of human α-phosphomannomutase 1 reveal the structural basis of congenital disorder of glycosylation type 1a. *J. Biol. Chem.*, **281**, 14918–14926.

80 Szumilo, T., Drake, R.R., York, J.L., and Elbein, A.D. (1993) GDP-mannose pyrophosphorylase: purification to homogeneity, properties and utilization to prepare photoaffinity analogs. *J. Biol. Chem.*, **268**, 17943–17950.

81 Ning, B. and Elbein, A.D. (2000) Cloning, expression and characterization of the pig liver GDP-mannose pyrophosphorylase. *Eur. J. Biochem.*, **267**, 6866–6874.

82 Perugini, M.A., Griffin, M.D.W., Smith, B. J., Webb, L.E., Davis, A.J., Handman, E. and Gerrard, J.A. (2005) Insight into the self-association of key enzymes from pathogenic species. *Eur. Biophys. J.*, **34**, 469–476.

83 Pomel, S., Rodrigo, J., Hendra, F., Cavé, C. and Loiseau, P.M. (2012) *In silico* analysis of a therapeutic target in *Leishmania infantum*: the guanosine-diphospho-D-mannose pyrophosphorylase. *Parasite*, **19**, 63–70.

84 Maeda, Y. and Kinoshita, T. (2008) Dolichol-phosphate mannose synthase: structure, function and regulation. *Biochim. Biophys. Acta*, **1780**, 861–868.

85 Imbach, T., Schenk, B., Schollen, E., Burda, P., Stutz, A., Grünewald, S., Bailie, N.M. *et al.* (2000) Deficiency of dolichol-phosphate-mannose synthase-1 causes congenital disorder of glycosylation type 1e. *J. Clin. Invest.*, **105**, 233–239.

86 Kim, S., Westphal, V., Srikrishna, G., Mehta, D.P., Peterson, S., Filiano, J., Karnes, P.S. *et al.* (2000) Dolichol phosphate mannose synthase (DPM1) mutations define congenital disorder of glycosylation Ie (CDG-Ie). *J. Clin. Invest.*, **105**, 191–198.

87 Lamani, E., Mewbourne, R.B., Fletcher, D. S., Maltsev, S.D., Danilov, L.L., Veselovsky, V.V., Lozonova, A.V. *et al.* (2006) Structural studies and mechanism of *Saccharomyces cerevisiae* dolichol-phosphate-mannose synthase: insights into the initial step of synthesis of dolichyl-phosphate-linked oligosaccharide chains in membranes of endoplasmic reticulum. *Glycobiology*, **16**, 666–678.

88 Mazhari-Tabrizi, R., Eckert, V., Blank, M., Müller, R., Mumberg, D., Funk, M., and Schwarz, R.T. (1996) Cloning and functional expression of glycosyltransferases from parasitic protozoans by heterologous complementation in yeast: the dolichol phosphate mannose synthase from *Trypanosoma brucei brucei*. *Biochem. J.*, **316**, 853–858.

89 Collier, A. and Wagner, G.K. (2008) A fast synthetic route to GDP-sugars modified at the nucleobase. *Chem. Commun.*, **14**, 178–180.

90 Kranz, C., Denecke, J., Lehle, L., Sohlbach, K., Jeske, S., Meinhardt, F., Rossi, R. *et al.* (2004) Congenital disorder of glycosylation type Ik (CDG-Ik): a defect in mannosyltransferase I. *Am. J. Hum. Genet.*, **74**, 545–551.

91 Thiel, C., Schwarz, M., Peng, J., Grzmil, M., Hasilik, M., Braulke, T., Kohlschütter, A. *et al.* (2003) A new type of congenital disorders of glycosylation (CDG-Ii) provides new insights into the early steps of dolichol-linked oligosaccharide biosynthesis. *J. Biol. Chem.*, **278**, 22498–22505.

92 Rind, N., Schmeiser, V., Thiel, C., Absmanner, B., Lübbehusen, J., Hocks, J., Apeshiotis, N. *et al.* (2010) A severe human metabolic disease caused by deficiency of the endoplasmatic mannosyltransferase hALG11 leads to congenital disorder of glycosylation-Ip. *Hum. Mol. Genet.*, **19**, 1413–1424.

93 Ilgoutz, S.C., Zawadzki, J.L., Ralton, J.E. and McConville, M.J. (1999) Evidence that free GPI glycolipids are essential for growth of *Leishmania mexicana*. *EMBO J.*, **18**, 2746–2755.

94 Ralton, J.E., Mullin, K.A., and McConville, M.J. (2002) Intracellular trafficking of glycosylphosphatidylinositol (GPI)-anchored protein and free GPIs in *Leishmania mexicana*. *Biochem. J.*, **363**, 365–375.

95 Späth, G.F., Epstein, L., Leader, B., Singer, S.M., Avila, H.A., Turco, S.J., and Beverley, S.M. (2000) Lipophosphoglycan is a virulence factor distinct from related glycoconjugates in the protozoan parasite *Leishmania major*. *Proc. Natl. Acad. Sci. USA*, **97**, 9258–9263.

96 Handford, M., Rodriguez-Furlan, C., and Orellana, A. (2006) Nucleotide-sugar transporters: structure, function and roles *in vivo*. *Braz. J. Med. Biol. Res.*, **39**, 1149–1158.

97 Capul, A.A., Hickerson, S., Barron, T., Turco, S.J., and Beverley, S.M. (2007) Comparisons of mutants lacking the Golgi UDP-galactose and GDP-mannose transporters establish that phosphoglycans are important for promastigote but not amastigote virulence in *Leishmania major*. *Infect. Immun.*, **75**, 4629–4637.

18

Transporters in Anti-Parasitic Drug Development and Resistance

Vincent Delespaux and Harry P. de Koning[*]

Abstract

In contrast to many treatments in non-infectious disease, which often act on extracellular targets such as cell surface receptors, anti-microbial chemotherapy almost invariably requires the uptake of the drug by the pathogen, in order to reach an intracellular target. The pathogen itself is often also resident within a host cell. Drug efficacy, therefore, is as much dependent on the efficient entry into the right cells as on selectivity at the target level. Entry into target cells and/or passage to target cells through host cells may be dependent on diffusion across the relevant biological membranes or on transport proteins located in these membranes. The former process is the norm for lipophilic compounds, whereas the latter is required for hydrophilic compounds, which do not appreciably diffuse across membranes. From a drug development perspective, these issues should be considered early-on and latest in the lead optimization strategy, as both options have advantages and drawbacks, which will be discussed in this chapter. Perhaps the most important issue is that transporters are highly specific in what they transport, whereas diffusion is a non-specific process, whereby a compound indiscriminately crosses any membrane dependent only on the concentration gradient. The selectivity of transport proteins can be a barrier to drug development, disallowing highly active enzyme inhibitors from entering target cells, or can allow the development of cleverly targeted drugs by engineering recognition motifs for transporters expressed only by the pathogen, allowing selective uptake and accumulation by the pathogen. In cases when this transport is energy-dependent, the drug may be concentrated against the concentration gradient. Conversely, the functional loss of such a transporter by the pathogen has often been the cause of drug resistance.

Introduction

The usual progression of drug development strategies for anti-infective agents involves the optimization of specific inhibitors of a preselected target enzyme through initial (high-throughput) screening for hit compounds, and subsequent

[*] Corresponding Author

Trypanosomatid Diseases: Molecular Routes to Drug Discovery, First edition. Edited by T. Jäger, O. Koch, and L. Flohé.
© 2013 Wiley-VCH Verlag GmbH & Co. KGaA. Published 2013 by Wiley-VCH Verlag GmbH & Co. KGaA.

optimization to increasingly potent inhibitors using medicinal chemistry and structural information of the target enzyme. Thus, the optimization to lead compound may be entirely based on assays with purified enzyme, resulting in a highly potent inhibitor – but not necessarily a good drug. Apart from absorption, distribution, metabolism, and excretion (ADME) issues and toxicological considerations that will need to be addressed for any lead compounds, the question of how the inhibitor should reach its intended intracellular target should be considered as part of the hit-to-lead strategy. An inhibitor of an essential enzyme, function, or pathway will have no anti-microbial effect if it does not reach its target, no matter how low the inhibition constant of the compound for the target may be.

This is not necessarily a matter only of uptake by the pathogen across its plasma membrane as, for eukaryotes, the target may well be located inside an organelle. Examples are the mitochondrion, the amitochondriate's hydrogenosome (e.g., *Trichomonas vaginalis*) or mitosome (*Giardia* spp.), the *Plasmodium* food vacuole, the apicomplexan apicoplast, or the kinetoplastid glycosome. Some of these have double membranes (mitochondria) or even triple membranes (apicoplasts), which the compound also needs to pass. In addition, an inhibitor may be segregated into the wrong organelle (e.g., through charge or pH), or be removed from the cytosol by ATP-binding cassette (ABC) efflux transporters or be modified by metabolic enzymes in the cytosol or through adduction with thiols such as glutathione or trypanothione, or both (an example is melarsoprol being conjugated to trypanothione and as such excreted by the trypanosome [1,2]). Such issues can undo the painstaking and expensive screening and optimization performed through enzyme inhibition assays. Some of this can be assessed through computational means (e.g., clog$P$ and polar surface area are predictors of diffusion rates across biological membranes; redox potential predicts reaction with thiols; pK_a may help predict accumulation in acidic compartments such as lysosomes and the *Plasmodium* food vacuole), but in many cases the cellular distribution is not easily predictable. This is especially the case for hydrophilic compounds that require specific, integral membrane transport proteins to cross membranes. Our knowledge of transport processes in the plasma membrane of pathogens is very incomplete and knowledge of transport processes on internal membranes is almost absent. The lead optimization strategy should therefore include one of the following options: (i) optimize for high diffusion rates by avoiding polar groups and hydrogen bonds, (ii) optimize for recognition by a known pathogen transporter, or (iii) study transport processes for the emerging class of inhibitors. This chapter aims to evaluate the various options using examples of anti-parasitic drugs.

"Rule of Five"

In 2001, Lipinski *et al.* [3] published their highly influential "Rule of Five," which described the physical properties of compounds important for "solubility and permeability in drug discovery." The authors argued that favorable physical characteristics for drug discovery would take account of the following boundaries: five or less hydrogen-bond donors, ten or less hydrogen-bond acceptors, clog $P \leq 5$ and molecular weight 500 or less. In their analysis, the authors focused mostly on permeability and oral absorption of drugs through diffusion, and stated explicitly that compound classes that are substrates for transport proteins in the relevant membranes were not bound by these rules [3]. In the following decade high-throughput screening-based drug discovery programs and library-building medicinal chemistry have to a large extent followed the Lipinski advice and concentrated on moderately lipophilic, low-mass molecules that therefore have an appreciable rate of diffusion across biological membranes. Such compounds have sufficient aqueous solubility but are also able to enter the lipophilic domain of the plasma membrane; highly lipophilic compounds (clog $P > 5$) would not be soluble and more importantly remain in the membrane environment rather than diffuse through it. The underlying assumption was that most drugs, and certainly orally active compounds, rely on diffusion through the lipid bilayer for absorption. However, this perception is at least in part a reflection of the relative lack of knowledge of transport proteins, their location, expression, and substrate selectivity in the relevant human and pathogen membranes; this is true for both cellular uptake and efflux processes [4]. Indeed, a thorough review of available evidence by Dobson and Kell [5] shows convincingly that specific transporters play a far more important role in drug uptake and excretion processes than commonly assumed. Indeed, the correlation between the octanol/water partition coefficient and uptake across the commonly used model systems (Caco-2 cell layers and parallel artificial membrane permeation assay (PAMPA)) was poor [5,6]. This reflects both the complexity of biological membranes, which consist as much of protein as of lipid (typically in a ratio of $1:1$ by mass [7]), and the profound role of many different transporters, channels, and other cell surface proteins on the distribution of pharmacologically active compounds across biological membranes.

Diffusion

Notwithstanding the above, many pharmaceutically active compounds do rely on diffusion to enter cells. From the perspective of drug development, the most obvious advantage of a compound with a high rate of diffusion is that it does not require the expression of a particular transporter in the target cell plasma membrane (and any intracellular membranes). Given that it will rarely be known whether a transporter for a potential class of new drugs is expressed by the pathogen, this advantage is considerable, especially as studies to establish the presence or absence of such transporters are costly and time-consuming. A further advantage is good oral availability, as formalized in the Rule of Five [3]. Similarly, diffusion across the blood–brain barrier (BBB) may be a requirement of the drug under development, such as in the treatment of late-stage African trypanosomiasis [8,9], where the trypanosome has entered the central nervous system (CNS) [10]. The BBB is composed of brain vascular endothelial cells sealed with tight junctions, and associated with astrocytes, microglia, and pericytes [11,12], and is believed to be all but impenetrable to most hydrophilic compounds: some 98% of all small-molecule drugs are estimated to be excluded from the CNS by this barrier [13].

Indeed, even when a drug does cross the BBB, efflux transporters such as P-glyco-protein (P-gp) and other ABC transporters often reverse the process [12,14]. This appears to be the case with the dicationic diamidine pentamidine. Its uptake must be transporter-mediated, as it cannot diffuse across membranes, but its efficacy for treatment of cerebral trypanosomiasis is fatally reduced through export by P-gp and multidrug resistance-associated proteins (MRPs) [15].

One implication of a drug with a significant diffusion rate across biological membranes is that its uptake is easily reversible and its intracellular free concentration cannot exceed the free extracellular concentration (i.e., the process is equilibrative). This means that the free plasma concentration of the active compound must not only peak at a sufficiently high concentration to drive accumulation to therapeutic levels in the target cells, but, crucially, must remain at that this level for the minimal curative time, as the drug will diffuse back out of the cell when the plasma concentration drops through the usual pharmacodynamic processes of metabolism and excretion. However, it must be stressed that this equilibrium model does allow for drug accumulation in a target cell if (i) the drug is tightly bound to an intracellular target and thus not free in the cytosol for exchange across the plasma membrane or (ii) the drug is metabolized intracellularly, particularly if modified to a form with a reduced diffusion rate (e.g., by phosphorylation). The latter mechanism also includes lyso-somotropic trapping of weak bases in an acidic compartment, which can easily be manipulated by increasing or decreasing the basicity of lead compounds.

A prominent and highly instructive example of intracellular trapping of an anti-parasitic drug through metabolism is the anti-malarial chloroquine (CQ). At neutral pH CQ is neutral and lipophilic (clog$P > 4$) allowing it to cross membranes easily. It should thus equally distribute to all cells, in equilibrium with its concentration in circulation. Yet, CQ is specifically and exclusively accumulated by erythrocytes infected by CQ-sensitive malaria parasites, to at least 20-fold the extracellular concentration [16,17], by an energy-independent process [18,19]. Homewood *et al.* [20] first proposed that CQ, a weak base, is trapped by protonation in the acidic *Plasmodium* food vacuole, rendering it charged and unable to diffuse back out of the vacuole. This model is now widely accepted [21] although it is not the whole story, as a comparative study on accumulation rates of 4-aminoquinolines found no clear correlation between either drug efficacy or drug accumulation and the log$D$ value at pH 5.0 or 7.0 [17]; instead these authors concluded that accumulation is ultimately driven by CQ binding to its (intravacuolar) target, the free heme entity ferriprotoporphyrin IX (FP) [19], the product of hemoglobin degradation by the parasite, and inhibits the formation of the hemozoin crystal [18]. A consensus model thus appears that CQ is trapped in an acidic compartment by protonation, preventing its diffusion out of the vacuole and allowing it to bind to FP or hemozoin, continually reducing the free CQ concentration in the compartment and driving ever further accumulation.

Consistent with this model, CQ resistance has been linked to a lysine-to-threonine mutation in the CQ resistance transporter (*Pf*CRT1) located in the food vacuole membrane [22,23]. This mutation, removing the charged lysine residue, is believed to allow the mutant protein to function as a carrier or channel for the protonated species of CQ, thus allowing CQ to escape from the vacuole in a transporter-mediated process [24]. *Pf*CRT is sensitive to the transport inhibitor verapamil [25], which thereby acts as a CQ-resistance reversal agent. Further complexity is given to this model by the involvement of a multidrug transporter, *Pf*MDR1 [26], demonstrating that the usual descriptor "simple diffusion" for lipophilic diffusion across membranes can be very misleading.

A good example of cellular trapping of a lipophilic drug in trypanosomatids is provided by the phosphonium salts. Despite the fact that phosphonium compounds are cations (and bisphosphonium salts are dications) such molecules can very rapidly diffuse through membranes when the positive charge is shielded and dispersed over large hydrophobic groups such as aromatic rings and long aliphatic chains [27]. Once in the cell, these compounds accumulate within the mitochondria, their accumulation driven by the strong negative-inside mitochondrial membrane potential (MMP) [28]. Indeed, the triphenylphosphonium scaffold has been extensively exploited for the delivery of covalently attached active molecules such as free radical scavengers and antioxidants to the mitochondria [28,29]. The same mechanism underlies the strong anti-leishmanial activity of a recently described series of bisphosphonium salts that exert their anti-leishmanial activity through accumulation in their mitochondria, where they inhibit Complex II [30]. A larger series, now also including monophosphonium salts, was synthesized and shown to display promising activity against *Trypanosoma brucei rhodesiense* as well, with some displaying *in vitro* EC_{50} values in the low or mid nanomolar range [31]. CoMFA (comparative molecular field analysis) modeling was employed to analyze the structure–activity relationship. As related above for the targeting of monophosphonium compounds, activity increased with better shielding and dispersal of the positive charge.

It is thus clear that the cellular trapping of diffusible compounds can be manipulated and used in rational drug design to stimulate selective accumulation even in the absence of specific transporters on the target cell. However, the use of lipophilic (pro)-drugs can equally cause inadvertent distribution to the wrong cells or tissues, where they are converted to the active, charged compounds and trapped. This may have happened with the compound DB289 (pafuramidine), the bis-*N*-methoxy prodrug of DB75 (furamidine; Immtech Pharmaceuticals), which was recently withdrawn from phase III clinical trials because of delayed nephrotoxicity [32].

Selective Uptake by Protozoan Transporters

Transporters that mediate the uptake of solutes, such as most nutrients (sugars, amino acids, nucleosides, etc.) and many drugs, fall into two main categories. They can either be energy-dependent, which makes them monodirectional and able to transport against the concentration gradient, or they can be passive, allowing the selective passage of the substrate ("permeant") in both directions. The two processes are referred to as active transport and facilitative diffusion, respectively. The differences between the two processes have important pharmacological implications.

Active transport is employed by cells for the highly efficient monodirectional uptake of specific high-value permeants, usually with high affinity. It is the combination of high transmembrane uptake rates ("catalysis") and high affinity that makes the expenditure of energy necessary. High affinity (i.e., low K_m value) means a high energy of binding and thus a low off-rate for the release of the permeant into the cell, leading to low transport rates – unless energy is expended, changing the protein conformation to a low energy state, promoting a rapid release of the permeant into the cell. Through active transport, then, permeants including drugs are quickly and efficiency concentrated in the cell.

In contrast, facilitative diffusion merely allows the bidirectional exchange of a permeant across the plasma membrane. This process is as selective as active transport, in that a permeant has to bind to a selective binding site for translocation, much as in any other protein. However, in the facilitative diffusion scenario, just as with "simple" diffusion (non-transporter-mediated), the drug transported in this way will not normally achieve higher concentrations than those in the immediate extracellular environment and exit the cell as the drug is cleared from the circulation. Exceptions are when the permeant is (i) metabolized or (de)protonated in the cell, (ii) becomes segregated in a cellular compartment or organelle, or (iii) is tightly bound to a cellular constituent, such as DNA.

A prime example of a hydrophilic anti-kinetoplastid drug is pentamidine, which has been in use against early stage West African sleeping sickness since the mid-1930s and is also used against visceral leishmaniasis [33]. Pentamidine is greatly concentrated within trypanosomes, to what would be millimolar levels if it were free in the cytosol, even when extracellular concentrations are in the low micromolar range [34]. The very rapid accumulation to intracellular levels vastly higher than the extracellular concentration is strongly suggestive of active transport and indeed pentamidine uptake was strongly reduced after a short pre-incubation with metabolic inhibitors [35]. In procyclic *T. b. brucei* [³H]pentamidine uptake correlated with the proton-motive force across the plasma membrane [36]. While our own unpublished results are absolutely consistent with active pentamidine uptake by *T. b. brucei* bloodstream forms as well, especially at low extracellular concentrations, the full picture could again be more complex than concentrative transport through a single energy-dependent transporter. First of all, we have shown that pentamidine is accumulated in trypanosomes through at least three kinetically/pharmacologically distinguishable transport activities, doubtless encoded by different genes [36,37]. These are the P2 aminopurine transporter (encoded by *TbAT1*), the high-affinity pentamidine transporter (HAPT1) and the low-affinity pentamidine transporter (LAPT1). P2 and HAPT1 have also been implicated in uptake of melaminophenyl arsenical drugs and of diminazene, and the loss of both transport activities leads to high level resistance to aromatic diamidines and melamine-linked arsenicals [37–39]. Secondly, diamidines such as pentamidine, like other cations, accumulate in the mitochondria, driven by the MMP, leading to compartmentalization and keeping free cytosolic concentrations relatively low [40,41]. A reduced MMP can therefore contribute to lower overall pentamidine accumulation, with exclusion from the cytosol mediated by an ABC-type transporter [42], leading to resistance [43,44]. The mitochondrial accumulation is further enhanced by binding of aromatic diamidines to kinetoplast DNA [45,46]. This example illustrates that active transport alone does not *necessarily* determine accumulation of active compounds to higher than extracellular levels: compartmentalization, active extrusion, and target binding still greatly influence the distribution.

Another example of a clinically essential trypanocide that relies on transporters for access to its target is difluoromethyl ornithine (DFMO; eflornithine). Recently, three groups independently identified the amino acid transporter TbAAT6 as the carrier for this drug [47–49], which is – alone or in combination with nifurtimox – the only treatment for melarsoprol-refractory late-stage sleeping sickness. Loss of this transporter was shown to lead to high levels of resistance and, conversely, the transporter had been lost independently in two DFMO-resistant strains; uptake of [^{3}H]DFMO was reduced to near-zero in resistant trypanosomes [47]. It is not currently known whether TbAAT6 is an active, accumulative transporter or not. The well-known requirement for extremely high and frequent dosages of eflornithine by intravenous infusion [50] would seem to argue against this. Indeed, before the identification of TbAAT6 as the DFMO transporter it was believed to be accumulated through passive (non-transporter-mediated) diffusion, because its uptake increased in a linear manner up to 10 mM of the compound [51]. This could now be interpreted as TbAAT6 having very low affinity for DFMO. Thus, DFMO would equilibrate across the plasma membrane and its further uptake would only be driven by its covalent binding to its target, the active site of the enzyme ornithyl decarboxylase [52]. The facilitated diffusion model would help explain why DFMO must be administered so frequently: it is rapidly cleared from the circulation [50], allowing the unbound compound to diffuse back out of the trypanosome as it is not compartmentalized or otherwise retained.

An example in *Leishmania donovani* is the transporter for miltefosine, LdMT, which was identified as an aminophospholipid translocase member of the P-type ATPases. Again, it was demonstrated that loss of LdMT activity is coupled to miltefosine resistance, as miltefosine accumulation was reduced by 97% in the resistant cells although efflux rates from preloaded cells were not affected [53,54]. Interestingly, the localization of the LdMT transporter to the plasma membrane requires a β-subunit, designated LdRos3, and thus functional loss of either protein causes miltefosine resistance [54,55]. LdMT is an example of drug accumulation by primary-active transport (i.e., directly coupled to ATP hydrolysis).

Role of Efflux Transporters

In the preceding section, it was demonstrated that loss of drug uptake into the target cell can lead to drug resistance. Equally, active extrusion of the drug from the cell will result in a reduced cellular level of the compound and hence to drug resistance. Such efflux pumps are primary active carriers of the ABC transporter family, and include the P-gp, MRPs, and breast cancer resistance protein, and play a very important role in cancer chemotherapy refractoriness [56] and many other aspects of drug distribution, such as active compound levels in the central nervous system [57].

The involvement of a *Plasmodium* efflux transporter in chloroquine resistance has been mentioned above. It has been shown that overexpression of an ABC transporter, designated *Tb*MRPA in *T. b. brucei* bloodstream forms, results in 10-fold melarsoprol resistance, as the melarsoprol–trypanothione adduct is a substrate for this transporter [58] and it was shown that this resistance level was additive with loss of the P2 uptake transporter [59]. However, *Tb*MRPA overexpression was not sufficient to give significant levels of melarsoprol resistance *in vivo* and has not been detected in melarsoprol-refractory clinical isolates [60].

Far more evidence exists for the involvement of ABC transporters in drug resistance in *Leishmania* spp. The main treatment of clinical leishmaniasis is still based on pentavalent antimony, which is reduced to the active trivalent form either in the parasite or in the host macrophages it inhabits, or both. The Sb(III) reacts with the main thiol of *Leishmania*, trypanothione [61], and it is this conjugate that is believed to be a substrate for the *Leishmania* ABC transporter, variously called PGPA, MDRA, or ABCC3 [62]. Interestingly, MDRA is an intracellular ABC transporter that appears to sequester the Sb(III)–trypanothione conjugate rather than extrude it from the cell [63]. This model was given further credibility by the finding that the *MRPA* gene was amplified in antimony-resistant field isolates, while thiol production was also upregulated in some of the isolates [64].

Miltefosine resistance in *Leishmania* can be caused by loss of uptake capacity (see above), but also by the overexpression of a different ABC transporter, called MDR1 or ABCB4 [54,65], which increases miltefosine efflux [66]. It was recently shown that drug resistance in *Leishmania* caused by overexpression of either ABC transporter (PGPA/MDRA/ABCC3 or MDR1/ABCB4) can be modulated by sublethal doses of the anti-leishmanial quinoline sitamaquine, even though this compound is not a substrate for the ABC transporters. Molecular modeling identified a sitamaquine binding site on MDR1 that overlapped with that for miltefosine [67].

Miltefosine resistance is an instructive example as it appears to always be related to impaired accumulation, but this can be mediated by (i) deletion/mutation in *Ld*MT itself, (ii) deletion/mutation of the subunit required for its correct localization, or (iii) upregulation of an ABC transporter for increased efflux.

Diagnosing Drug Resistance Through Screening of Transporter Mutations: *T. congolense* as an Example

Concept

The diagnosis of drug resistance has always been challenging, especially in protozoan parasites, which demand far more complex culture systems than bacteria. Different methods of drug resistance diagnosis in animal trypanosomes, mainly *T. congolense*, are currently available: standardized *in vivo* tests in mice or livestock, *in vitro* tests like the drug incubation *Glossina* infectivity test (DIGIT) [68] or drug incubation infectivity test (DIIT) [69], isometamidium-ELISA (enzyme-linked immunosorbent assay) [70], and more anecdotally the measure of the mitochondrial electrical potential [71]. In the last few years genotypic methods based on molecular markers have started to replace phenotypic methods. For instance, resistance to the anti-malarial drug Fansidar, a combination of pyrimethamine and sulfadoxine, can be predicted from well-characterized mutations in the respective target enzymes, dihydrofolate reductase and dihydropteroate synthetase [72]. Similarly, mutations in the food vacuole channel *PfCRT1*, particularly in codon 76, are predictive for chloroquine resistance [73,74].

Diagnosis of diminazene aceturate resistance in the livestock parasite *T. congolense* was initially performed by screening for a point mutation in the putative P2-type purine transporter *TcoAT1* by single-strand conformation polymorphism. The background to this is the discovery that in three other animal-infective trypanosomes, *T. brucei*, *T. evansi*, and *T. equiperdum*, the P2 transporter is always overwhelmingly responsible for the uptake of this key diamidine trypanocide [75–77]. Multiple mechanisms, including point mutations by which P2 functionality was lost, have been identified [78].

Further analysis by sequencing *TcoAT1* alleles in diminazene-sensitive and -resistant strains led to the identification of a single indicative $G \rightarrow A$ point mutation observed in the diminazene aceturate-resistant strains and a simple *Dpn*II-polymerase chain reaction (PCR)-restriction fragment length polymorphism (RFLP) test enabling the rapid identification of diminazene aceturate-resistant isolates from dried blood samples stored on filter papers [79,80] or from blood mixed to a 6 M guanidine hydrochloride/0.2 M EDTA buffer [81].

Evaluation

The *Dpn*II-PCR-RFLP is detecting the presence of a single point mutation in a purine transporter and a good correlation of this genotype with phenotypes *in vivo* was observed [79]. However, drug resistance can be multifactorial, as discussed in this chapter, and in practice different levels of drug resistance are observed. This, of course, cannot be measured by this method. As observed in *T. brucei* for the resistance against diamidine compounds, other transporters, particularly HAPT1, are additionally involved in the translocation of diamidines into the parasite [82]. Furthermore, it is clear that that the resistance-associated ("mutated") *TcoAT1* allele exists in *T. congolense* populations that have in all likelihood not been exposed to diminazene, having been isolated from wild animals in protected wild-life preserves, even though there is a clear trend towards homozygosity for the resistance marker in areas of increasing drug usage (Table 18.1) [83].

Sensitivity and Implementation

A trypanosome-specific 18S-PCR-RFLP is routinely used for field surveys and was described with a sensitivity of 25 trypanosomes/ml blood [84]. The *Dpn*II-PCR-RFLP will successfully diagnose around 25% of 18S-PCR-RFLP-positive samples, increasing to around 45% with an extra step of whole-genome amplification [80]. For

Table 18.1 Incidence of the *TcoAT1* resistance allele in various isolates.

Country	Area	Drug usage	Number of *TcoAT1* alleles mutated (%)			Reference
			None	One	Both	
Zambia, KwaZulu-Natal, Zimbabwe	national parks	none	3.0	61.8	35.3	[83]
Zambia	Eastern Province	moderate	10.5	26.3	63.2	[85]
Ethiopia	Ghibe Valley	high	2.7	2.7	94.6	[86]
Cameroon	Adamaoua Plateau	high	0	0	100	[87]

epidemiological surveys sensitivity can be increased by an increased sample size and mixing blood samples with a protective guanidine-EDTA buffer. The trypanosome-specific 18S-PCR-RFLP and *DpnII*-PCR-RFLP have been transferred to a network of regional reference laboratories in West, East, and Southern Africa for use in large-scale surveys to detect the presence of trypanocidal drug resistance throughout tsetse-infested Africa.

The technique is routinely used in West Africa (Burkina Faso, Benin, Côte d'Ivoire, Ghana, Mali, Nigeria, and Togo) within the framework of a recently created epidemiological network (Réseau d'épidémiosurveillance de la résistance aux trypanocides et aux acaricides en Afrique de l'Ouest/Epidemiosurveillance Network for the Resistance to Trypanocides and Acaricides in West Africa, coordinated by the Centre international de recherche-développement sur l'elevage en zone subhumide (CIRDES)).

Concluding Remarks

It is well established that the physical attributes of a drug greatly influence its distribution within the patient and thereby its activity against a target cell or organism. Yet, very often knowledge of the physical characteristics and their adherence to Lipinski's Rule of Five fails to predict cellular penetration. Our knowledge of (potential) drug transporters on human and pathogen cell surfaces is still very incomplete: not only are many transporters not yet identified, usually our knowledge of the expression pattern and the substrate specificity of known transporters is woefully incomplete. Whereas diffusion processes are easier to predict from a drug's physical characteristics than transporter-mediated uptake/efflux, this chapter has demonstrated that intracellular trapping by various devices such as sequestration, binding, protonation and metabolism of a (pro)-drug can greatly influence its total cellular accumulation. We therefore argue that drug accumulation by target and human cells should be a cost-effective part of the pre-clinical lead optimization strategy, as this would reduce failure rates later. In addition, knowledge of transport proteins involved in the drug action can give essential information and genetic markers for drug resistance and cross-resistance.

References

1 Delespaux, V. and De Koning, H.P. (2007) Drugs and drug resistance in African trypanosomiasis. *Drug Resist. Updat.*, **10**, 30–50.

2 Shahi, S.K., Krauth-Siegel, R.L., and Clayton, C. (2002) Overexpression of the putative thiol conjugate transporter TbMRPA causes melarsoprol resistance in *Trypanosoma brucei. Mol. Microbiol.*, **43**, 1129–1138.

3 Lipinski, C.A., Lombardo, F., and Dominy, B.W. (2001) Experimental and computational approaches to estimate solubility and permeability in drug discovery and development settings. *Adv. Drug Deliv. Rev.*, **46**, 3–26.

4 Sarkadi, B. and Szakács, G. (2010) Understanding transport through pharmacological barriers – are we there yet? *Nat. Rev. Drug Discov.*, **9**, 897–898.

5 Dobson, P.D. and Kell, D.B. (2008) Carrier-mediated cellular uptake of pharmaceutical drugs: an exception or the rule? *Nat. Rev. Drug. Discov.*, **7**, 205–220.

6 Balimane, P.V., Han, Y.H., and Chong, S. (2006) Current industrial practices of assessing permeability and P-glycoprotein interaction. *AAPS J.*, **8**, E1–E13.

7 Opekarová, M. and Tanner, W. (2003) Specific lipid requirements of membrane proteins – a putative bottleneck in heterologous expression. *Biochim. Biophys. Acta*, **1610**, 11–22.

8 Barrett, M.P. and Gilbert, I.H. (2002) Perspectives for new drugs against trypanosomiasis and leishmaniasis. *Curr. Top. Med. Chem.*, **2**, 471–482.

9 Enanga, B., Burchmore, R.J.S., Stewart, M. L., and Barrett, M.P. (2002) Sleeping sickness and the brain. *Cell. Mol. Life Sci.*, **59**, 845–858.

10 Barrett, M.P., Burchmore, R.J., Stich, A., Lazzari, J.O., Frasch, A.C., Cazzulo, J.J., and Krishna, S. (2003) The trypanosomiases. *Lancet*, **362**, 1469–1480.

11 Zlokovic, B.V. (2008) The blood–brain barrier in health and chronic neurodegenerative disorders. *Neuron*, **57**, 178–201.

12 Lee, G., Dallas, S., Hong, M., and Bendayan, R. (2001) Drug transporters in the central nervous system: brain barriers and brain parenchyma considerations. *Pharmacol. Rev.*, **53**, 569–596.

13 Pardridge, W.M. (2007) Blood–brain barrier delivery. *Drug Discov. Today*, **12**, 54–61.

14 De Boer, A.G., Van der Sandt, I.C.J., and Gaillard, P.J. (2003) The role of transporters at the blood–brain barrier. *Annu. Rev. Pharmacol. Toxicol.*, **43**, 629–656.

15 Sanderson, L., Dogruel, M., Rodgers, J., De Koning, H.P., and Thomas, S.A. (2009) Pentamidine movement across the murine blood–brain and blood–CSF barriers; effect of trypanosome infection, combination therapy, P-glycoprotein and MRP. *J. Pharmacol. Exp. Ther.*, **329**, 967–977.

16 Fitch, C.D. (1969) Chloroquine resistance in malaria: a deficiency of chloroquine binding. *Proc. Natl. Acad. Sci. USA*, **64**, 1181–1187.

17 Hawley, S.R., Bray, P.G., O'Neill, P.M., Park, B.K., and Ward, S.A. (1996) The role of drug accumulation in 4-aminoquinoline antimalarial potency. The influence of structural substitution and physicochemical properties. *Biochem. Pharmacol.*, **52**, 723–733.

18 Polet, H. and Barr, C.F. (1969) Uptake of chloroquine-^{3}H by *Plasmodium knowlesi in vitro. J. Pharmacol. Exp. Ther.*, **168**, 187–192.

19 Bray, P.G., Janneh, O., Raynes, K.J., Mungthin, M., Ginsburg, H., and Ward, S. A. (1999) Cellular uptake of chloroquine is dependent on binding to ferriprotoporphyrin IX and is independent

of NHE activity in *Plasmodium falciparum*. *J. Cell Biol.*, **145**, 363–376.

20 Homewood, C.A., Warhurst, D.C., Peters, W., and Baggaley, V.C. (1972) Lysosomes, pH and the anti-malarial action of chloroquine. *Nature*, **235**, 50–52.

21 Fitch, C.D. (2004) Ferriprotoporphyrin IX, phospholipids, and the antimalarial actions of quinoline drugs. *Life Sci.*, **74**, 1957–1972.

22 Sidhu, A.B., Verdier-Pinard, D., and Fidock, D.A. (2002) Chloroquine resistance in *Plasmodium falciparum* malaria parasites conferred by *pfcrt* mutations. *Science*, **298**, 210–213.

23 Lakshmanan, V., Bray, P.G., Verdier-Pinard, D., Johnson, D.J., Horrocks, P., Muhle, R.A., Alakpa, G.E. *et al.* (2005) A critical role for *Pf*CRT K76T in *Plasmodium falciparum* verapamil-reversible chloroquine resistance. *EMBO J.*, **24**, 2294–2305.

24 Bray, P.G., Mungthin, M., Hastings, I.M., Biagini, G.A., Saidu, D.K., Lakshmanan, V., Johnson, D.J. *et al.* (2006) *Pf*CRT and the trans-vacuolar proton electrochemical gradient: regulating the access of chloroquine to ferriprotoporphyrin IX. *Mol. Microbiol.*, **62**, 238–251.

25 Krogstad, D.J., Gluzman, I.Y., Kyle, D.E., Oduola, A.M., Martin, S.K., Milhous, W.K., and Schlesinger, P.H. (1987) Efflux of chloroquine from *Plasmodium falciparum*: mechanism of chloroquine resistance. *Science*, **238**, 1283–1285.

26 Duraisingh, M.T. and Cowman, A.F. (2005) Contribution of the pfmdr1 gene to antimalarial drug-resistance. *Acta Trop.*, **94**, 181–190.

27 Ross, M.F., Prime, T.A., Abakumova, I., James, A.M., Porteous, C.M., Smith, R.A., and Murphy, M.P. (2008) Rapid and extensive uptake and activation of hydrophobic triphenylphosphonium cations within cells. *Biochem. J.*, **411**, 633–645.

28 Ross, M.F., Kelso, G.F., Blaikie, F.H., James, A.M., Cochemé, H.M., Filipovska, A., Da Ros, T. *et al.* (2005) Lipophilic triphenylphosphonium cations as tools in mitochondrial bioenergetics and free radical biology. *Biochemistry (Mosc.)*, **70**, 222–230.

29 Smith, R.A., Adlam, V.J., Blaikie, F.H., Manas, A.R., Porteous, C.M., James, A.M., Ross, M.F. *et al.* (2008) Mitochondria-targeted antioxidants in the treatment of disease. *Ann. NY Acad. Sci.*, **1147**, 105–111.

30 Luque-Ortega, J.R., Reuther, P., Rivas, L., and Dardonville, C. (2010) New benzophenone-derived bisphosphonium salts as leishmanicidal leads targeting mitochondria through inhibition of respiratory complex II. *J. Med. Chem.*, **53**, 1788–1798.

31 Taladriz, A., Healy, A., Flores Pérez, E.J., Herrero García, V., Ríos Martínez, C., Alkhaldi, A.A., Eze, A.A. *et al.* (2012) Synthesis and structure–activity analysis of new phosphonium salts with potent activity against African trypanosomes. *J. Med. Chem.*, **55**, 2606–2622.

32 Paine, M., Wang, M., Boykin, D., Wilson, W.D., De Koning, H.P., Olson, C., Polig, G. *et al.* (2010) Diamidines for human African trypanosomiasis. *Curr. Opin. Investig. Drugs*, **11**, 876–883.

33 Bray, P.G., Barrett, M.P., Ward, S.A., and De Koning, H.P. (2003) Pentamidine uptake and resistance in pathogenic protozoa. *Trends Parasitol.*, **19**, 232–239.

34 Damper, D. and Patton, C.L. (1976) Pentamidine transport and sensitivity in brucei-group trypanosomes. *J. Protozool.*, **23**, 349–356.

35 Damper, D. and Patton, C.L. (1976) Pentamidine transport in *Trypanosoma brucei* – kinetics and specificity. *Biochem. Pharmacol.*, **25**, 271–276.

36 De Koning, H.P. (2001) Uptake of pentamidine in *Trypanosoma brucei brucei* is mediated by three distinct transporters. Implications for crossresistance with arsenicals. *Mol. Pharmacol.*, **59**, 586–592.

37 Bridges, D., Gould, M.K., Nerima, B., Mäser, P., Burchmore, R.J.S., and De Koning, H.P. (2007) Loss of the high affinity pentamidine transporter is responsible for high levels of cross-resistance between arsenical and diamidine drugs in African trypanosomes. *Mol. Pharmacol.*, **71**, 1098–1108.

38 Carter, N.S. and Fairlamb, A.H. (1993) Arsenical-resistant trypanosomes lack an unusual adenosine transporter. *Nature*, **361**, 173–176.

39 Teka, I.A., Kazibwe, A., El-Sabbagh, N., Al Salabi, M.I., Ward, C.P., Eze, A.A., Munday, J.C. *et al.* (2011) The diamidine diminazene aceturate is a substrate for the high affinity pentamidine transporter: implications for the development of high resistance levels. *Mol. Pharmacol.*, **80**, 110–116.

40 Lanteri, C.A., Tidwell, R.R., and Meshnick, S.R. (2008) The mitochondrion is a site of trypanocidal action of the aromatic diamidine DB75 in bloodstream forms of *Trypanosoma brucei. Antimicrob. Agents Chemother.*, **52**, 875–882.

41 Mathis, A.M., Holman, J.L., Sturk, L.M., Ismail, M.A., Boykin, D.W., Tidwell, R.R., and Hall, J.E. (2006) Accumulation and intracellular distribution of antitrypanosomal diamidine compounds DB75 and DB820 in African trypanosomes. *Antimicrob. Agents Chemother.*, **50**, 2185–2191.

42 Coelho, A.C., Beverley, S.M., and Cotrim, P.C. (2003) Functional genetic identification of PRP1, an ABC transporter superfamily member conferring pentamidine resistance in *Leishmania major. Mol. Biochem. Parasitol.*, **130**, 83–90.

43 Basselin, M., Denise, H., Coombs, G.H., and Barrett, M.P. (2002) Resistance to pentamidine in *Leishmania mexicana* involves exclusion of the drug from the mitochondrion. *Antimicrob. Agents Chemother.*, **46**, 3731–3738.

44 Mukherjee, A., Padmanabhan, P.K., Sahani, M.H., Barrett, M.P., and Madhubala, R. (2006) Roles for mitochondria in pentamidine susceptibility and resistance in *Leishmania donovani. Mol. Biochem. Parasitol.*, **145**, 1–10.

45 Wilson, W.D., Tanious, F.A., Mathis, A., Tevis, D., Hall, J.E., and Boykin, D.W. (2008) Antiparasitic compounds that target DNA. *Biochimie*, **90**, 999–1014.

46 Baraldi, P.G., Bovero, A., Fruttarolo, F., Preti, D., Tabrizi, M.A., Pavani, M.G., and Romagnoli, R. (2004) DNA minor groove binders as potential antitumor and antimicrobial agents. *Med. Res. Rev.*, **24**, 475–528.

47 Vincent, I.M., Creek, D., Watson, D.G., Kamleh, M.A., Woods, D.J., Wong, P.E., Burchmore, R.J., and Barrett, M.P. (2010) A molecular mechanism for eflornithine resistance in African trypanosomes. *PLoS Pathog.*, **6**, e1001204.

48 Baker, N., Alsford, S., and Horn, D. (2011) Genome-wide RNAi screens in African trypanosomes identify the nifurtimox activator NTR and the eflornithine transporter AAT6. *Mol Biochem Parasitol.*, **176**, 55–57.

49 Schumann Burkard, G., Jutzi, P., and Roditi, I. (2011) Genome-wide RNAi screens in bloodstream form trypanosomes identify drug transporters. *Mol. Biochem. Parasitol.*, **175**, 91–94.

50 Burri, C. and Brun, R. (2003) Eflornithine for the treatment of human African trypanosomiasis. *Parasitol. Res.*, **90**, S49–S52.

51 Bitonti, A.J., Bacchi, C.J., McCann, P.P., and Sjoerdsma, A. (1986) Uptake of α-difluoromethylornithine by *Trypanosoma brucei brucei. Biochem. Pharmacol.*, **35**, 351–354.

52 Poulin, R., Lu, L., Ackermann, B., Bey, P., and Pegg, A.E. (1992) Mechanism of the irreversible inactivation of mouse ornithine decarboxylase by alpha-difluoromethylornithine. Characterization of sequences at the inhibitor and coenzyme binding sites. *J. Biol. Chem.*, **267**, 150–158.

53 Pérez-Victoria, F.J., Gamarro, F., Ouellette, M., and Castanys, S. (2003) Functional cloning of the miltefosine transporter. A novel P-type phospholipid translocase from Leishmania involved in drug resistance. *J. Biol. Chem.*, **278**, 49965–49971.

54 Pérez-Victoria, F.J., Sánchez-Cañete, M.P., Seifert, K., Croft, S.L., Sundar, S., Castanys, S., and Gamarro, F. (2006) Mechanisms of experimental resistance of *Leishmania* to miltefosine: implications for clinical use. *Drug Resist. Updat.*, **9**, 26–39.

55 Pérez-Victoria, F.J., Sánchez-Cañete, M.P., Castanys, S., and Gamarro, F. (2006) Phospholipid translocation and miltefosine potency require both *L. donovani* miltefosine transporter and the new protein LdRos3 in *Leishmania* parasites. *J. Biol. Chem.*, **281**, 23766–23775.

56 Borst, P. and Elferink, R.O. (2002) Mammalian ABC transporters in health and disease. *Annu. Rev. Biochem.*, **71**, 537–592.

57 Begley, D.J. (2004) ABC transporters and the blood–brain barrier. *Curr. Pharm. Des.*, **10**, 1295–1312.

58 Shahi, S.K., Krauth-Siegel, R.L., and Clayton, C.E. (2002) Overexpression of the putative thiol conjugate transporter *Tb*MRPA causes melarsoprol resistance in *Trypanosoma brucei*. *Mol. Microbiol.*, **43**, 1129–1138.

59 Lüscher, A., Nerima, B., and Mäser, P. (2006) Combined contribution of *Tb*AT1 and *Tb*MRPA to drug resistance in *Trypanosoma brucei*. *Mol. Biochem. Parasitol.*, **150**, 364–366.

60 Alibu, V.P., Richter, C., Voncken, F., Marti, G., Shahi, S., Renggli, C.K., Seebeck, T. *et al.* (2006) The role of *Trypanosoma brucei* MRPA in melarsoprol susceptibility. *Mol. Biochem. Parasitol.*, **146**, 38–44.

61 Wyllie, S., Cunningham, M.L., and Fairlamb, A.H. (2004) Dual action of antimonial drugs on thiol redox metabolism in the human pathogen *Leishmania donovani*. *J. Biol. Chem.*, **279**, 39925–39932.

62 Jones, P.M. and George, A.M. (2005) Multidrug resistance in parasites: ABC transporters, P-glycoproteins and molecular modelling. *Int. J. Parasitol.*, **35**, 555–566.

63 Légaré, D., Richard, D., Mukhopadhyay, R., Stierhof, Y.D., Rosen, B.P., Haimeur, A., Papadopoulou, B., and Ouellette, M. (2001) The *Leishmania* ATP-binding cassette protein PGPA is an intracellular metal-thiol transporter ATPase. *J. Biol. Chem.*, **276**, 26301–26307.

64 Mukherjee, A., Padmanabhan, P.K., Singh, S., Roy, G., Girard, I., Chatterjee, M., Ouellette, M., and Madhubala, R. (2007) Role of ABC transporter MRPA, gamma-glutamylcysteine synthetase and ornithine decarboxylase in natural antimony-resistant isolates of *Leishmania donovani*. *J. Antimicrob. Chemother.*, **59**, 204–211.

65 Pérez-Victoria, J.M., Pérez-Victoria, F.J., Parodi-Talice, A., Jiménez, I.A., Ravelo, A. G., Castanys, S., and Gamarro, F. (2001) Alkyl-lysophospholipid resistance in multidrug-resistant *Leishmania tropica* and chemosensitization by a novel P-glycoprotein-like transporter modulator.

Antimicrob. Agents Chemother., **45**, 2468–2474.

66 Pérez-Victoria, J.M., Cortés-Selva, F., Parodi-Talice, A., Bavchvarov, B.I., Pérez-Victoria, F.J., Muñoz-Martínez, F., Maitrejean, M. *et al.* (2006) Combination of suboptimal doses of inhibitors targeting different domains of *Ltr*MDR1 efficiently overcomes resistance of *Leishmania* spp. to Miltefosine by inhibiting drug efflux. *Antimicrob. Agents Chemother.*, **50**, 3102–3110.

67 Pérez-Victoria, J.M., Bavchvarov, B.I., Torrecillas, I.R., Martínez-García, M., López-Martín, C., Campillo, M. *et al.* (2011) Sitamaquine overcomes ABC-mediated resistance to miltefosine and antimony in *Leishmania*. *Antimicrob. Agents Chemother.*, **55**, 3838–3844.

68 Clausen, P.H., Leendertz, F.H., Blankenburg, A., Tietjen, U., Mehlitz, D., Sidibe, I.A., and Bauer, B. (1999) A drug incubation *Glossina* infectivity test (DIGIT) to assess the susceptibility of *Trypanosoma congolense* bloodstream forms to trypanocidal drugs (Xenodiagnosis). *Acta. Trop.*, **72**, 111–117.

69 Kaminsky, R., Gumm, I.D., Zweygarth, E., and Chuma, F. (1990) A drug incubation infectivity test (DIIT) for assessing resistance in trypanosomes. *Vet. Parasitol.*, **34**, 335–343.

70 Eisler, M.C., Gault, E.A., Moloo, S.K., Holmes, P.H., and Peregrine, A.S. (1997) Concentrations of isometamidium in the sera of cattle challenged with drug-resistant *Trypanosoma congolense*. *Acta Trop.*, **63**, 89–100.

71 Wilkes, J.M., Mulugeta, W., Wells, C.W., and Peregrine, A.S. (1997) Modulation of mitochondrial electrical potential: A candidate mechanism for drug resistance in African trypanosomes. *Biochem. J.*, **326**, 755–761.

72 Wang, P., Lee, C.S., Bayoumi, R., Djimde, A., Doumbo, O., Swedberg, G., Dao, L.D. *et al.* (1997) Resistance to antifolates in *Plasmodium falciparum* monitored by sequence analysis of dihydropteroate synthetase and dihydrofolte reductase alleles in a large number of field samples of diverse origins. *Mol. Biochem. Parasitol.*, **89**, 161–177.

73 Fidock, D.A., Nomura, T., Talley, A.K., Cooper, R.A., Dzekunov, S.M., Ferdig, M. T., Ursos, L.M. *et al.* (2000) Mutations in the *P. falciparum* digestive vacuole transmembrane protein *Pf*CRT and evidence for their role in chloroquine resistance. *Mol. Cell*, **6**, 861–871.

74 Djimde, A., Doumbo, O.K., Cortese, J.F., Kayentao, K., Doumbo, S., Diourte, Y., Coulibaly, D. *et al.* (2001) A molecular marker for chloroquine-resistant falciparum malaria. *N. Engl. J. Med.*, **344**, 257–263.

75 Barrett, M.P., Zhang, Z.Q., Denise, H., Giroud, C., and Baltz, T. (1995) A diamidine-resistant *Trypanosoma equiperdum* clone contains a P2 purine transporter with reduced substrate affinity. *Mol. Biochem. Parasitol.*, **73**, 223–229.

76 Witola, W.H., Inoue, N., Ohashi, K., and Onuma, M. (2004) RNA-interference silencing of the adenosine transporter-1 gene in *Trypanosoma evansi* confers resistance to diminazene aceturate. *Exp. Parasitol.*, **107**, 47–57.

77 De Koning, H.P., Stewart, M., Anderson, L., Burchmore, R., Wallace, L.J.M., and Barrett, M.P. (2004) The trypanocide diminazene aceturate is accumulated predominantly through the *Tb*AT1 purine transporter; additional insights in diamidine resistance in African trypanosomes. *Antimicrob. Agents Chemother.*, **48**, 1515–1519.

78 Stewart, M.L., Burchmore, R.J., Clucas, C., Hertz-Fowler, C., Brooks, K., Tait, A., Macleod, A. *et al.* (2010) Multiple genetic mechanisms lead to loss of functional *Tb*AT1 expression in drug-resistant trypanosomes. *Eukaryot. Cell*, **9**, 336–343.

79 Delespaux, V., Chitanga, S., Geysen, D., Goethals, A., Van den Bossche, P., and Geerts, S. (2006) SSCP analysis of the P2 purine transporter *Tco*AT1 gene of Trypanosoma congolense leads to a simple PCR-RFLP test allowing the rapid identification of diminazene resistant stocks. *Acta Trop.*, **100**, 96–102.

80 Vitouley, H.S., Mungube, E.O., Allegye-Cudjoe, E., Diall, O., Bocoum, Z., Diarra, B., Randolph, T.F. *et al.* (2011) Improved PCR-RFLP for the detection of diminazene resistance in *Trypanosoma congolense* under field conditions using filter papers for sample storage. *PLoS Negl. Trop. Dis.*, **5**, e1223.

81 Avila, H., Goncalves, A.M., Nehme, N.S., Morel, C.M., and Simpson, L. (1990) Schizodeme analysis of *Trypanosoma cruzi* stocks from South and Central America by analysis of PCR-amplified minicircle variable region sequences. *Mol. Biochem. Parasitol.*, **42**, 175–187.

82 De Koning, H.P. (2008) Ever-increasing complexities of diamidine and arsenical cross-resistance in African trypanosomes. *Trends Parasitol.*, **24**, 345–349.

83 Chitanga, S., Marcotty, T., Namangala, B., Van den Bossche, P., Van den Abbeele, J., and Delespaux, V. (2011) High prevalence of drug resistance in animal trypanosomes without a history of drug exposure. *PLoS Negl. Trop. Dis.*, **5**, e1454.

84 Geysen, D., Delespaux, V., and Geerts, S. (2003) PCR-RFLP using Ssu-rDNA amplification as an easy method for species-specific diagnosis of *Trypanosoma* species in cattle. *Vet. Parasitol.*, **110**, 171–180.

85 Delespaux, V., Dinka, H., Masumu, J., Van den Bossche, P., and Geerts, S. (2008) Five-fold increase in the proportion of diminazene aceturate resistant *Trypanosoma congolense* isolates over a seven years period in Eastern Zambia. *Drug Resist. Updat.*, **11**, 205–209.

86 Moti, G.Y., Fikru, R., Van den Abbeele, J., Büscher, P., Van den Bossche, P., Duchateau, L. *et al.* (2012) Ghibe river basin in Ethiopia: present situation of trypanocidal drug resistance in *Trypanosoma congolense* using tests in mice and PCR-RFLP. *Vet. Parasitol.*, **189**, 197–203.

87 Mamoudou, A., Delespaux, V., Chepnda, V., Hachimou, Z., Andrikaye, J.P., Zoli, A., and Geerts, S. (2008) Assessment of the occurrence of trypanocidal drug resistance in trypanosomes of naturally infected cattle in the Adamaoua region of Cameroon using the standard mouse test and molecular tools. *Acta Trop.*, **106**, 115–118.

19

Peptidases in Autophagy are Therapeutic Targets for Leishmaniasis

*Roderick A.M. Williams**

Abstract

Differentiation of *Leishmania* life forms is crucial for progression and preadaptation of the parasite to the environmental conditions existing in its hosts. Autophagy is a catabolic degradation process that utilizes cytosolic ATG4s and lysosomal cathepsins to affect protein turnover and remodeling, which are crucial for parasite development, differentiation, and virulence. In this chapter, published data on the physiological roles of the cysteine peptidases involved in autophagy and virulence in *Leishmania* spp. that establishes them as therapeutic targets will be reviewed. Potential lead compounds that can modulate the activities of the cysteine peptidases for therapeutic advantage, the challenges involved, and the opportunities they provide for drug development to control leishmaniasis will be discussed.

Introduction

The two distinctive life forms of *Leishmania*, the promastigotes and amastigotes preadapt the parasite for life in the sandfly and human host, respectively [1]. Twenty *Leishmania* spp. infect humans, causing the disease collectively called leishmaniasis in approximately 12 million people in 88 countries [1,2]. The severity of leishmaniasis is a product of the metabolism of the infecting species, the host cells, and the host immune status. However, an expanding geographic frontier and the coinfections with other infecting agents such as HIV become increasingly important [3,4]. Current therapies become ineffective by their cost, toxicity, teratogenicity, drug resistance, and the absence of a sustainable national and regional control program in endemic regions [1,2,5,6]. New therapies designed on a thorough understanding of the basic biology of the parasite that could be applied to a wider group of patients are urgently required. A number of unique or functionally distinct molecular targets identified in the parasite's genome important for parasite differentiation and virulence are being characterized for essentiality and druggability in a rational drug design [7–9].

* Corresponding Author

Trypanosomatid Diseases: Molecular Routes to Drug Discovery, First edition. Edited by T. Jäger, O. Koch, and L. Flohé.
© 2013 Wiley-VCH Verlag GmbH & Co. KGaA. Published 2013 by Wiley-VCH Verlag GmbH & Co. KGaA.

A set of proteins with such potential and with an essential role in *Leishmania* spp. nutrition, differentiation, and virulence are the peptidases [10,11]. Peptidases are hydrolytic enzymes for which there are two systems for classifying them. One system of classification assigns EC numbers to peptidases based on the reactive group used to effect hydrolysis and the point on the peptide chain hydrolysis occurs [12]. In the other, peptidases with similar structure, catalytic mechanism, and substrate specificity are grouped into clans and families [13]. Peptidases with a reactive thiol group for hydrolysis, also called cysteine peptidases, are represented in *Leishmania* spp. by four clans: CA, CD, CF, and PC, which constitute approximately 1.8% of the parasite's "degradome" [10,11,14–16]. This diversity is very restrictive in comparison to humans, but the peptidases are involved in a wide range of house-keeping functions required for life [10,11,14]. In this chapter, the roles of the Clan CA cysteine peptidases involved in macroautophagy (designated here as autophagy) will be reviewed (Table 19.1).

Autophagy, first defined by Christin De Duve in the 1950s, is a catabolic process divided into four stages: induction, autophagosome biogenesis, and fusion with and degradation in the lysosome (Figure 19.1). The biogenesis and degradation of autophagosomes occur in the cytosol and lysosomes, respectively, and both require the enzymatic activities of the parasites' Clan CA cysteine peptidases at key control points (Figure 19.1a). After induction, cargoes (e.g., dysfunctional proteins) and organelles are marked and packaged into double membrane vesicles called auto-phagosomes (Figure 19.1). Digestion of the autophagosomes occurs in the lyso-some, and the metabolic substrates generated (e.g., amino acids and fatty acids) are used for protein and phospholipids synthesis during stress to maintain cellular homeostasis [17,18] (Figure 19.1). In *Trypanosoma cruzi*, *T. brucei*, *L. major*, *L. mexicana*, and *Entamoeba invadens*, autophagy is important for differentiation and virulence [19–24], but is also involved in mitochondrial integrity in *Toxoplasma gondi* and *L. major* [20,25], and in phospholipid homeostasis in *L. major* [25]. There is one instance, in *L. donovani* after treatment with anti-microbial peptides, where autophagy causes the type II programmed cell death [26]. However, it is not known if this was an attempt to avoid death and failed rather than a death process itself. Thus, more studies are required to substantiate this. The role of autophagy in differentia-tion and survival described in most studies on *Leishmania* spp. means that a downregulation of the cysteine peptidases in this pathway could potentially provide a novel target for developing chemotherapeutic agents to control leishmaniasis.

Molecular Machinery for Autophagosome Biogenesis

The autophagic pathway is an evolutionary conserved process in higher eukaryotes that requires more than 30 autophagic (ATG)-related genes or proteins [18,27,28]. Autophagosome biogenesis requires the coordinated activities of two conjugation pathways, the ATG8-lipidation and the ATG5–ATG12 conjugation pathways [18] (Figure 19.1b). In the ATG5–ATG12 conjugation pathway, the ATG5–ATG12 conjugate formed by the enzymatic activities of ATG7 and ATG10 is incorporated

Table 19.1 Potential peptidase targets in *Leishmania* spp.

Peptidases	Family	Clan	Natural substrates	Localization	Function	References
ATG4.1[a]	CA	C54	ATG8; ATG8B; ATG8C	cytosol	cleaves off the amino acids after the glycine residue at the C-terminus of ATG8; promastigote–amastigote differentiation; virulence	[24,29]
ATG4.2[a]	CA	C54	ATG8; ATG8A; ATG8–PE	cytosol	cleaves off the amino acids after the glycine residue at the C-terminus of ATG8; Cleaves PE off ATG8–PE; promastigote–amastigote differentiation; virulence; mitochondrial integrity; amastigote replication in mice	[21,24,29]
ATG12 processing	not known	not known	ATG12	not known	cleaves off the amino acids after the glycine residue at the C-terminus of ATG12	[29]
Calpain	CA	C2	not known	not known	not known	
MUP	CA	C48	SUMO	cytosol; mitochondrion	not known	[25]
MCAs[a]	CD	C14	not known	kinetoplast; cytosol; nucleus; acidocalcisome	mediate cell death; cell cycle events; amastigote replication in mice	[30–33]
CPA,[a] and CPB[a]	CA	C1	Autophagosomes; MHC molecules; host signaling components	MVT-lysosome; Host's cytosol	released to the parasitophorous vacuole to modulate host signaling and immune response; digestion of autophagosomes; digestion of sequestered MHC; mediate cell death in the cytosol; process MCAs	[10,11,23,34–38]

a) Peptidase targets in *Leishmania* spp. investigated for their role in autophagy.

(a)

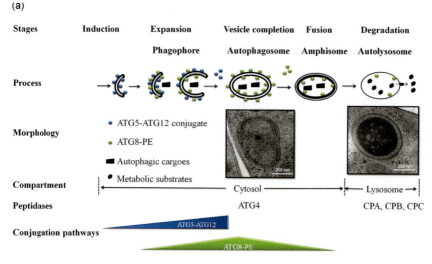

(b)

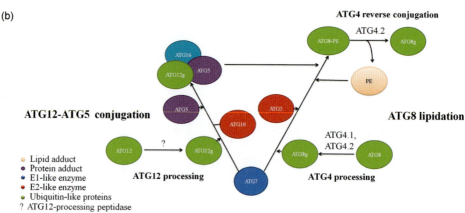

Figure 19.1 (a) Scheme of the autophagic pathway in *Leishmania* spp. The multistage autophagic process is initiated by the nucleation of the phagophore with the ATG5–ATG12 conjugate, then the ATG8–PE, which elongates, engulfs its cargo, and encloses on itself to form an autophagosome. The autophagosome fuses with the lysosomes to form the autolysosome and its contents are degraded therein. The metabolic substrates generated with the lysosome are released to the cytosol. Transmission electron microscopy images of the autophagosome and autolysosome in *Leishmania* promastigotes are shown. (b) The autophagic conjugative pathways. The ATG4–ATG8 cleavage event and interaction with the E1-like and E2-like enzymes, ATG7 and ATG3, forms the ATG8 PE, and the cleavage event between ATG4–ATG8–PE gives ATG8. ATG12 is processed by an unknown peptidase prior to interaction with the E1-like and E2-like enzymes, ATG7 and ATG10, to form the ATG5–ATG12 conjugate. This conjugate has an E3-like activity for the ATG8 lipidation reaction.

into a preautophagosomal membrane, the phagophore, to produce curvature (Figure 19.1a). The complex also has an E3-like enzymatic activity important in the second conjugation pathway (Figure 19.1b). In the ATG8-lipidation pathway, the amino acid sequences following a glycine in the C-terminal domain of ATG8 is cleaved by the Clan CA C54 family cysteine peptidase, ATG4, in a conjugation reaction. This exposed glycine is attached to phosphatidylethanolamine (PE) after the sequential catalytic actions of the ATG7, ATG3, and the ATG5–ATG12 complex, respectively, for incorporation into the phagophore [39] (Figure 19.1). ATG8–PE initiates cargo recruitment, phagophore elongation, and autophagosome completion [40–43]. The ATG5–ATG12 and ATG8–PE complexes detach from the nascent autophagosome just before closure of the autophagosome and autophagosome–lysosomal fusion (Figure 19.1) [44]. The later reaction requires the reverse conjugation reaction of ATG4 to allow the interaction of autophagosomes with the endosomal sorting complex and microtubules and recycling of ATG8 [45]. Autophagosome degradation requires the hydrolytic activities of the Clan CA C1 family of peptidases called cathepsins, which are classified as D-, B-, and L-types, each with different hydrolytic abilities [46]. This molecular autophagic machinery in *Leishmania* resembles, in part, that of their mammalian host [17,21,23,25,47,48]. The amino acid sequences of the genes of the ATG5–ATG12 conjugation pathway are distinctively different [25,29] but the ATG8-lipidation pathway has two ATG4s named ATG4.1 and ATG4.2, and four unusual ATG8 families, ATG8, ATG8A, ATG8B,, and ATG8C, for which there are 26 copies that have some similarity to the mammalian homologs [21,23,24].

ATG4 Regulates the Autophagic Pathway of *Leishmania* spp.

The specificity of the two ATG4s for the four ATG8 families are distinctively different in *L. major*; ATG4.1 has activity towards the full length proteins of ATG8, ATG8B, and ATG8C homologs, and ATG4.2 towards ATG8A (Table 19.1), but do not cleave their FRET peptides consisting of only amino acids surrounding the cleavage site following the characteristic glycine residue with such specificity [29]. Comparison of *L. major* wild-type and an individual ATG4.1-deficient line (named Δ*atg4.1*) confirmed this specificity, but showed that its contribution to the biogenesis of Green Fluorescent Protein (GFP)–ATG8-containing autophagosomes was not significant [24]. The few autophagosomes formed were sufficient for parasite function and survival (e.g., metacyclogenesis), infectivity of promastigotes to macrophages and mice, albeit less efficient than wild-type parasites [24]. Further, amastigotes of this mutant initiated lesion pathology in mice at a rate similar to wild-type [24]. These results suggest that the function of ATG4.1 is not essential but contributes to promastigote–amastigote differentiation (Table 19.1). In another *L. major* mutant line, deficient in the peptidase ATG4.2 and designated Δ*atg4.2*, ATG8A-containing autophagosomes were not formed but many ATG8-containing autophagosomes were formed that accumulated in the cytosol that should otherwise be delivered into the lysosome for degradation [21,24,29]. This block in autophagosome delivery into the lysosomes and degradation was due to the lack of the reverse conjugation activity in Δ*atg4.2* required at the late stages of autophagosome biogenesis (Figure 19.1) [21,24,29]. Δ*atg4.2* promastigotes consequently had a strong tendency to accumulate oxidized proteins within the cytosol, and displayed a fragmented mitochondrion with a prominent depolarization and production of reactive oxygen species – effects that were reversed by antioxidant, *N*-acetylcysteine, treatment [24]. This aberrant autophagic turnover substantially reduced infectivity to macrophages and lesion pathology in mice in both promastigote and amastigote infections, supporting an important role for this peptidase in promastigote and amastigote biology [24]. Some redundancy exists between the two ATG4s at the early stages of autophagosome biogenesis (Figure 19.1) [24]. However, these data show that the two ATG4s in *L. major* have distinct roles and act at two different points in the parasite's autophagic pathway (Figure 19.1). The unsuccessful attempts to generate a mutant line deficient in both peptidases argue strongly that they are essential for survival and, therefore, are drug targets (Table 19.1).

Leishmania's Cathepsins Regulates Autophagy and Virulence

In *L. mexicana* the multivesicular tubule (MVT)-lysosome has an arsenal of cysteine peptidases belonging to the Clan CA, family C1, the cathepsin L-like (CPA and CPB) and cathepsin B-like (CPC) enzymes. CPA and CPC are single-copy peptidases with limited roles in parasite virulence [10,49–51] but CPB is a polymorphic enzyme, differentially expressed in the parasite life forms and are regulated by untranslated or intracistronic sequences [52]. Many studies on *L. mexicana* have confirmed that CPB is released into the macrophages to modulate the host signaling and immune response to promote parasite survival and replication [34]. Virulence in this parasite is associated with the ability of *CPB* and to a lesser extent CPA to induce interleukin-4 to elicit a T helper 2 response [35]. This aspect of CPB has been extensively reviewed in the recent past [10,11]. Here, I will concentrate on other functions for these cysteine peptidases like autophagosome digestion, digestion of the host's major histocompatibility complex (MHC), and the ability to mediate cell death [23,36–38,53,54]. Autophagosomes are dependent on the proper functioning of the lysosomal hydrolytic enzymes for their digestion. Thus, deprivation of the activity of leishmanial lysosomal cysteine peptidases either with inhibitors or through the generation of cysteine peptidase-deficient cell lines by genetic manipulation (e.g., Δ*cpa* and Δ*cpb* deficient in the cysteine peptidases, CPA and CPB, respectively) disrupts autophagy with the autophagosomes progressing no further than the acidification stage [23]. *L. mexicana* double-cysteine peptidase mutants, named Δ*cpa/cpb*, are unable to effectively digest autophagosomes in the MVT-lysosome and accumulate damaged and non-recycled cellular constituents and GFP–ATG8-containing autophagosomes in a large structure not present in wild-type [23]. Consequently, their viability was reduced under starvation conditions presumably due to the absence of free amino acids and free fatty acids required for energy generation [23]. The absence of an effective protein turnover also compromised metacyclogenesis and differentiation to amastigotes within macrophages and in mice [23]. Like Δ*atg4.2*, amastigotes of Δ*cpa/cpb* but not the individual mutants Δ*cpa* and Δ*cpb* were less able to survive in macrophages and mice [55]. This confirms the redundancy between the two cathepsin L-like peptidases and a role for them in amastigote development and proliferation.

In the parasitophorous vacuoles of activated macrophages, intracellular amastigotes are in contact with components of the host's MHC that effectively promote their demise [36,37]. *L. donovani* endocytoses and degrades MHC molecules within the MVT-lysosomes to interrupt antigen presentation [36,37]. The mechanism by which this occurs is not known, but may require the flagellar pocket – the main site for endocytosis across the plasma membrane [14]. In higher eukaryotes autophagy and endocytosis are intrinsically linked but information for this in *Leishmania* spp. is rudimentary. In *L. major*, the vacuolar protein sorting 4 (VPS4) protein, which is localized in the endosomal compartment, is involved in sorting and autophagosome processing [21]. Mutant lines expressing a dominant-negative mutant version (VPS4^{E235Q}), defective in endosomal sorting and autophagosome processing, were susceptible to stress from nutrient deprivation and unable to differentiate from the procyclic to metacyclic life forms [21]. This result suggests that the two processes are linked and their compartments may fuse prior to the delivery of autophagosomes into the MVT-lysosome. It is not known if the MHC molecules require components of the endosomal or autophagic systems, but if they do, it may offer an additional explanation for why amastigotes of Δ*atg4.2*, defective in autophagosome processing and Δ*cpa/cpb*, which are unable to digest autophagosomes, were incapable of successfully infecting mice.

In *L. mexicana*, CBP and CPC and possibly CPA, are known to be released into the cytosol after stress- or drug-induced MVT-lysosome permeabilization to induce cell death [38,45]. In mammals the release of cysteine peptidases or caspases elicit mitochondrial outer membrane permeabilization (MOMP), release of cytochrome *c*, activation of caspase 9, and finally programmed cell death via apoptosis. In *L. mexicana* the released cysteine peptidases produce death by necrosis highlighting CPC as a death mediators [38]. *Leishmania* spp. lack caspases but have the distant homologs, the metacaspases (MCAs) from the Clan CD, family 14 in their gene content. MCAs have a distinctive substrate specificity from caspases, preference for arginine/lysine in the P1 position rather than the aspartic acid residue preferred by caspases [30], and do not bind Z-VAD-FMK like the mammalian caspases [38]. The single copy of MCA in *L. major* is localized in different cellular compartments, and is important for cell cycle progression [30] and stress-induced cell death [53]. MCA is also a death mediator in *L. donovani* [32,33], but it is not yet known if the death is caused in concert with the cathepsins. It is, however, known that *L. major* MCA cleavage, processing, and localization in the mitochondria during stress is regulated by cysteine peptidases [54], and the overexpression of MCA in *L. major* [53] and *L. donovani* [32] can impair mitochondrial function and enhance sensitivity to stress. In *T. cruzi*, the activity, function, and localization of the MCA-3 isoform is regulated by SUMOylation activities [55]. In *L. mexicana*, the function of MCA is different – it regulates parasite replication within their mammalian host [31]. *L. mexicana* MCA was not observed in the parasite's mitochondrion, which though intact has a membrane potential that was only 35% of wild-type [31]. In yeast, insoluble aggregates in the cytosol were cleared via autophagy [56] but in *L. mexicana,* MCA this was not this case [31]. Autophagic activities in the *L. mexicana* MCA-deficient line (designated Δ*mca*) were similar to wild-type [31]. It is, however, not yet known if the phenotypic differences observed between *L. major* and *L. donovani* and *L. mexicana* are due to different roles for MCA in the two species. The absence of MCA in mammals and the difference between them and caspases [57], and with a role in cell death in *L. donovani* and *L. major* though not for *L. mexicana,* may suggest that they can only be potential drug targets for therapeutic intervention to fight leishmaniasis from *L. major* and *L. donovani* [30]. Given that the diagnosis of leishmaniasis occurs long after the initial infection, targeting these cysteine peptidases with key roles in amastigote function is ideal for drug development against the life form in humans. It is also possible that inhibitors against cysteine peptidases can be synergistic with existing anti-parasitic therapy (e.g., miltefosine) in a combination therapy against leishmaniasis.

Other Possible Peptidase Targets

In contrast to other higher eukaryotes, it has been shown that *L. major* ATG12 requires processing by a peptidase prior to conjugation to ATG5 (Figure 19.1b) [25,29]. The amino acid sequences of *L. major* ATG12 show a moderate level of identity to those of ATG8 and ATG12 in other organisms, and it has amino acid sequences beyond the glycine residue required for conjugation to ATG5, typical for ATG8s [25,29]. This novel property of *L. major* ATG12 and the additional step it adds to autophagy in *Leishmania* spp., not present in any other eukaryote, is a novel regulatory point and potential target that could be investigated for its therapeutic importance (Figure 19.1b). The processing of *L. major* ATG12 does not require the hydrolytic activity of ATG4 [29], whereas the corresponding ortholog in *T. cruzi,* a related trypanosomatid, is processed by ATG4 [19,58]. Recently, it has been shown using a mutant line deficient in the protein ATG5 (named Δ*atg5*) in *L. major,* that the ATG12–ATG5 conjugation pathway is important for autophagosome biogenesis and parasite virulence [25].

Leishmania spp. contain other Clan CA peptidases with roles in ubiquitination reactions in other organisms, such as the ubiquitin C-terminus hydrolyases (C12) for which there are 19, and single copies of the ubiquitin hydrolyze (C19) and the small ubiquitin-like peptidase (C48). There are 22 peptidases with the calpain domain (C2) in *L. major* genome [14]. While the ubiquitin C-terminus hydrolyases are key determinants for protein degradation via the proteasomal system, they are also important in selective autophagy [59]; the small ubiquitin-like peptidase and calpain peptidases in mammals are important for mitochondrion activities and autophagy [60,61]. The small ubiquitin-like peptidase regulates autophagy through its SUMOylation activities on proteins involved in autophagy, such as SUMOylation of the two copies of the mammalian hypoxia-inducible factor proteins regulates autophagy in chondrocytes [60]. In *L. major,* the small ubiquitin-like peptidase, also called mitochondrion ubiquitin-like peptidase (MUP [25]) is localized to the mitochondrial membrane – the inception site for ATG5 and ATG8 during autophagosome biogenesis [25]. The contribution of this peptidase in autophagy has not yet been investigated. Calpains are important for calcium regulation functions and cell death mechanisms. In mammals, calpain activity affects autophagy in a calcium-dependent manner [62,63]. At elevated calcium levels, the activated calpain cleaves ATG5; the polypeptide fragments are translocated to the mitochondria to induce apoptotic cells death [63]. At moderate concentrations of calcium, formation of the ATG5–ATG12 conjugate and autophagy is favored [62]. Little is known about the role and regulation of ATG5 in *Leishmania* spp.

Cysteine Peptidase Inhibitors: Opportunities and Challenges

The fact that *Leishmania* cysteine peptidases can be potentially good control points in autophagy and parasite differentiation suggests that inhibitors that downregulate their activities are "good" for anti-leishmanial therapy and control. CPB has been successfully targeted with inhibitors directed against the catalytic cysteine thiolate required for hydrolysis [10,11,49,64–67]. The vinyl sulfone inhibitor, K11777 developed by McKerrow and *et al.*, that was efficacious against CPB is known to interfere with autophagosome digestion and metacyclogenesis *in vitro* [23]. *In vivo*, the efficacy of large doses of K11777 at 100 mg/kg/day for up to 28 days was modest and delayed lesion pathology in mice infected with *L. tropica* [64,68]. In *T. cruzi*, late preclinical trials for this drug candidate are ongoing by the National Institute of Allergy and Infectious Disease [68,69]. The pace for using this substance against leishmaniasis in trials is slow, presumably due to the differences between the roles of the enzymes in these two pathogens and consequently their value as drug targets. Attempts to design inhibitors with modified electrophilic Michael acceptor reactivity or different "warheads" to improve toxicity have been less successful. The inhibitory activities of the dipeptidyl α-fluorovinyl, and α-ketoheterocyclics, although active in the high nanomolar to low micromolar ranges against the recombinant *L. mexicana* cysteine peptidase CPB2.8 ΔCTE, a mutant form of the amastigote-specific CPB gene expressed without the C-terminal extension [10,70,71], were low in screens using *L. infantum* (IC_{50} 12.70 μM) [71]. The metal-based inhibitors were only effective against the promastigotes but not the amastigotes within macrophages *in vitro* due to a failure to achieve functional and molecular interspecies selectivity between humans and the parasite [72]. However, the broad range of bioactive compounds available to inhibit the hydrolytic activities of these cysteine peptidases could still inspire new compound design and synthesis with improved toxicity and selectivity profiles. Such compounds can also be active against ATG4 for which inhibitory studies are in their infancy. The reason for this is due to the lack of suitable substrates for high-throughput screening assays. FRET peptides used extensively as substrates to characterize other peptidases (e.g., CPB2.8 ΔCTE) are generally ideal substitutes for the full-length *in vivo* substrates. For ATG4s, FRET substrates comprised of the peptides surrounding the cleavage glycine residue of ATG8 are too short and cannot produce the conformational change in ATG4 [73,74] required for hydrolysis [19,29,58,75,76]. Innovative substrate designs with great screening potential are now available for the mammalian system [76,77] which, if applicable to the *Leishmania* model, could be useful for screening inhibitors and arming them with a suitable warhead (e.g., sulfone-vinyls) to confer parasite enzyme specificity.

Conclusions and Future Directions

The upregulation of autophagy during differentiation in *Leishmania* is beneficial and the interactions of the many cysteine peptidases involved are complex but present a "therapeutic window" for targeting them for leishmaniasis control (Table 19.1). As the data obtained so far show that the cysteine peptidases are important for protein turnover, autophagy, and parasite virulence, the stage is now set to analyze fully the complex interaction of the various peptidases involved in this process. However, investigations are required in our *Leishmania* model to assign functions to most of the enzymes involved in autophagy in other systems. Gaps also exist in our knowledge of potential inhibitors against these cysteine peptidases that merit clinical investigation. The development of specific and selective pharmacological agents to these cysteine peptidases is a major challenge and could be improved with the advent of structural data of these cysteine peptidases, especially ATG4 whose substrates (e.g., ATG8A–ATG8C) are unique to this parasite [29]. However, questions remain about whether the total ablation of autophagy would be adequate to totally eradicate the parasite. For example, the ATG5-null mutant ($\Delta atg5$) that is defective in autophagy was not eliminated completely by mice [25]. The reasons may be due an adaptive metabolism and robust salvage of its carbon source and energy substrates from the external milieu to circumvent the absence of autophagy. Finally, the identification of compounds with high efficacy against these parasite enzymes within increased toxicity to the pathogen but low risks to humans are continuing.

Acknowledgments

I thank Dr. L. Tetley (University of Glasgow) for help with electron microscopy analysis, and Professor G. H. Coombs and Dr. M. Weise for reading through the manuscript and their useful comments. This project was supervised by Professor G. H. Coombs and J.C. Mottram. This work was supported by Medical Research Council grants G9722968, G0000508, and G0700127.

References

1 World Health Organization (2010) Control of the leishmaniases. *World Health Organ. Tech. Rep. Ser.*, (949), xii–xiii, 1–186, back cover.

2 Croft, S.L. and Olliaro, P. (2011) Leishmaniasis chemotherapy – challenges and opportunities. *Clin. Microbiol. Infect.*, **17**, 1478–1483.

3 Reed, S.G. and Campos-Neto, A. (2003) Vaccines for parasitic and bacterial diseases. *Curr. Opin. Immunol.*, **15**, 456–460.

4 Lodge, R., Ouellet, M., Barat, C., Andreani, G., Kumar, P., and Tremblay, M.J. (2012) HIV-1 promotes intake of *Leishmania* parasites by enhancing phosphatidylserine-mediated, CD91/LRP-1-dependent phagocytosis in human macrophages. *PLoS One*, **7**, e32761.

5 Croft, S.L., Barrett, M.P., and Urbina., J.A. (2005) Chemotherapy of trypanosomiases and leishmaniasis. *Trends Parasitol.*, **21**, 508–512.

6 Alvar, J., Croft, S., and Olliaro, P. (2006) Chemotherapy in the treatment and control of leishmaniasis. *Adv. Parasitol.*, **61**, 223–274.

7 Lepesheva, G.I. and Waterman, M.R. (2011) Sterol 14alpha-demethylase (CYP51) as a therapeutic target for human trypanosomiasis and leishmaniasis. *Curr. Top. Med. Chem.*, **11**, 2060–2071.

8 Fidalgo, L.M. and Gille, L. (2011) Mitochondria and trypanosomatids: targets and drugs. *Pharm. Res.*, **28**, 2758–2770.

9 Venkatesan, S.K., Shukla, A.K., and Dubey, V.K. (2010) Molecular docking studies of selected tricyclic and quinone derivatives on trypanothione reductase of *Leishmania infantum*. *J. Comput. Chem.*, **31**, 2463–2475.

10 Mottram, J.C., Coombs, G.H., and Alexander, J. (2004) Cysteine peptidases as virulence factors of *Leishmania*. *Curr. Opin. Microbiol.*, **7**, 375–381.

11 Mottram, J.C., Helms, M.J., Coombs, G.H., and Sajid, M. (2003) Clan CD cysteine peptidases of parasitic protozoa. *Trends Parasitol.*, **19**, 182–187.

12 Schomburg, I., Chang, A., Hofmann, O., Ebeling, C., Ehrentreich, F., and Schomburg, D. (2002) BRENDA: a resource for enzyme data and metabolic information. *Trends Biochem. Sci.*, **27**, 54–56.

13 Rawlings, N.D., Barrett, A.J., and Bateman, A. (2010) MEROPS: the peptidase database. *Nucleic Acids Res.*, **38** (Database issue), D227–D233.

14 Besteiro, S., Williams, R.A., Coombs, G.H., and Mottram, J.C. (2007) Protein turnover and differentiation in *Leishmania*. *Int. J. Parasitol.*, **37**, 1063–1075.

15 Downing, T., Stark, O., Vanaerschot, M., Imamura, H., Sanders, M., Decuypere, S. *et al.* (2012) Genome-wide SNP and microsatellite variation illuminate population-level epidemiology in the *Leishmania donovani* species complex. *Infect. Genet. Evol.*, **12**, 149–159.

16 Rogers, M.B., Hilley, J.D., Dickens, N.J., Wilkes, J., Bates, P.A., Depledge, D.P. *et al.* (2011) Chromosome and gene copy number variation allow major structural change between species and strains of *Leishmania*. *Genome Res.*, **21**, 2129–2142.

17 Duszenko, M., Ginger, M.L., Brennand, A., Gualdron-Lopez, M., Colombo, M.I., Coombs, G.H. *et al.* (2011) Autophagy in protists. *Autophagy*, **7**, 127–158.

18 Klionsky, D.J., Cregg, J.M., Dunn, W.A.Jr., Emr, S.D., Sakai, Y., and Sandoval, I.V. (2003) *et al.*A unified nomenclature for yeast autophagy-related genes. *Dev. Cell*, **5**, 539–545.

19 Alvarez, V.E., Kosec, G., Sant'Anna, C., Turk, V., Cazzulo, J.J., and Turk, B. (2008) Autophagy is involved in nutritional stress response and differentiation in *Trypanosoma cruzi*. *J. Biol. Chem.*, **283**, 3454–3464.

20 Besteiro, S. (2012) Role of ATG3 in the parasite *Toxoplasma gondii*: Autophagy in an early branching eukaryote. *Autophagy*, **8**, 435–437.

21 Besteiro, S., Williams, R.A., Morrison, L.S., Coombs, G.H., and Mottram, J.C. (2006) Endosome sorting and autophagy are essential for differentiation and virulence of *Leishmania major*. *J. Biol. Chem.*, **281**, 11384–11396.

22 Picazarri, K., Nakada-Tsukui., K., and Nozaki, T. (2008) Autophagy during proliferation and encystation in the protozoan parasite *Entamoeba invadens*. *Infect. Immun.*, **76**, 278–288.

23 Williams, R.A., Tetley, L., Mottram, J.C., and Coombs, G.H. (2006) Cysteine peptidases CPA and CPB are vital for autophagy and differentiation in *Leishmania mexicana*. *Mol. Microbiol.*, **61**, 655–674.

24 Williams, R.A.M., Mottram, J.C., and Coombs, G.H. (2012) Distinct roles in autophagy and importance in autophagy of the two ATG4s of *Leishmania major*. J. Biol. Chem. Accepted.

25 Williams, R.A., Smith, T.K., Cull, B., Mottram, J.C., and Coombs, G.H. (2012) ATG5 is essential for ATG8-dependent autophagy and mitochondrial homeostasis in *Leishmania major*. *PLoS Pathog.*, **8**, e1002695.

26 Bera, A., Singh, S., Nagaraj, R., and Vaidya, T. (2003) Induction of autophagic cell death in *Leishmania donovani* by antimicrobial peptides. *Mol. Biochem. Parasitol.*, **127**, 23–35.

27 Ohsumi, Y., Ohsumi, M., and Baba, M. (1993) [Autophagy in yeast]. *Tanpakushitsu Kakusan Koso*, **38**, 46–52.

28 Tsukada, M. and Ohsumi, Y. (1993) Isolation and characterization of autophagy-defective mutants of *Saccharomyces cerevisiae*. *FEBS Lett.*, **333**, 169–174.

29 Williams, R.A., Woods, K.L., Juliano, L., Mottram, J.C., and Coombs, G.H. (2009) Characterization of unusual families of ATG8-like proteins and ATG12 in the protozoan parasite *Leishmania major*. *Autophagy*, **5**, 159–172.

30 Ambit, A., Fasel, N., Coombs, G.H., and Mottram, J.C. (2008) An essential role for the *Leishmania major* metacaspase in cell cycle progression. *Cell Death Differ.*, **15**, 113–122.

31 Castanys-Muñoz, E., Brown, E., Coombs, G.H., and Mottram, J.C. (2012) *Leishmania mexicana* metacaspase is a negative regulator of amastigote proliferation in mammalian cells. *Cell Death Dis.*, **3**, e385.

32 Lee, R.E., Brunette, S., Puente, L.G., and Megeney, L.A. (2010) Metacaspase Yca1 is required for clearance of insoluble protein aggregates. *Proc. Natl. Acad. Sci. USA*, **107**, 13348–13353.

33 Raina, P. and Kaur, S. (2012) Knockdown of LdMC1 and Hsp70 by antisense oligonucleotides causes cell-cycle defects and programmed cell death in *Leishmania donovani*. *Mol. Cell Biochem.*, **359**, 135–149.

34 Alexander, J. and Bryson, K. (2005) T helper (h)1/Th2 and *Leishmania*: paradox rather than paradigm. *Immunol. Lett.*, **99**, 17–23.

35 Alexander, J., Coombs, G.H., and Mottram, J.C. (1998) *Leishmania mexicana* cysteine proteinase-deficient mutants have attenuated virulence for mice and potentiate a T_h1 response. *J. Immunol.*, **161**, 6794–6801.

36 Antoine, J.C., Lang, T., Prina, E., Courret, N., and Hellio, R. (1999) H-2M molecules, like MHC class II molecules, are targeted to parasitophorous vacuoles of *Leishmania*-infected macrophages and internalized by amastigotes of *L. amazonensis* and *L. mexicana*. *J. Cell Sci.*, **112**, 2559–2570.

37 De Souza Leao, S., Lang, T., Prina, E., Hellio, R., and Antoine, J.C. (1995) Intracellular *Leishmania amazonensis* amastigotes internalize and degrade MHC class II molecules of their host cells. *J. Cell Sci.*, **108**, 3219–3231.

38 El-Fadili, A.K., Zangger, H., Desponds, C., Gonzalez, I.J., Zalila, H., Schaff, C. *et al.* (2010) Cathepsin B-like and cell death in the unicellular human pathogen *Leishmania*. *Cell Death Dis.*, **1**, e71.

39 Tanida, I., Mizushima, N., Kiyooka, M., Ohsumi, M., Ueno, T., Ohsumi, Y. *et al.* (1999) Apg7p/Cvt2p: A novel protein-activating enzyme essential for autophagy. *Mol. Biol. Cell*, **10**, 1367–1379.

40 Kimura, S., Noda, T., and Yoshimori, T. (2007) Dissection of the autophagosome maturation process by a novel reporter protein, tandem fluorescent-tagged LC3. *Autophagy*, **3**, 452–460.

41 Kirisako, T., Baba, M., Ishihara, N., Miyazawa, K., Ohsumi, M., Yoshimori, T. *et al.* (1999) Formation process of autophagosome is traced with Apg8/Aut7p in yeast. *J. Cell Biol.*, **147**, 435–446.

42 Kirisako, T., Ichimura, Y., Okada, H., Kabeya, Y., Mizushima, N., Yoshimori, T. *et al.* (2000) The reversible modification regulates the membrane-binding state of Apg8/Aut7 essential for autophagy and the cytoplasm to vacuole targeting pathway. *J. Cell Biol.*, **51**, 263–276.

43 Xie, Z., Nair, U., and Klionsky, D.J. (2008) Atg8 controls phagophore expansion during autophagosome formation. *Mol. Biol. Cell*, **19**, 3290–3298.

44 Kimura, S., Noda, T., and Yoshimori, T. (2008) Dynein-dependent movement of autophagosomes mediates efficient

encounters with lysosomes. *Cell Struct. Funct.*, **33**, 109–122.

45 Nowak, J., Archange, C., Tardivel-Lacombe, J., Pontarotti, P., Pebusque, M.J., Vaccaro, M.I. *et al.* (2009) The TP53INP2 protein is required for autophagy in mammalian cells. *Mol. Biol. Cell*, **20**, 870–881.

46 Zheng, X., Chu, F., Mirkin, B.L., Sudha, T., Mousa, S.A., and Rebbaa, A. (2008) Role of the proteolytic hierarchy between cathepsin L, cathepsin D and caspase-3 in regulation of cellular susceptibility to apoptosis and autophagy. *Biochim. Biophys. Acta*, **1783**, 2294–2300.

47 Rigden, D.J., Herman, M., Gillies, S., and Michels, P.A. (2005) Implications of a genomic search for autophagy-related genes in trypanosomatids. *Biochem. Soc. Trans.*, **33**, 972–974.

48 Rigden, D.J., Michels, P.A., and Ginger, M. L. (2009) Autophagy in protists: Examples of secondary loss, lineage-specific innovations, and the conundrum of remodeling a single mitochondrion. *Autophagy*, **5**, 784–794.

49 Bart, G., Frame, M.J., Carter, R., Coombs, G.H., and Mottram, J.C. (1997) Cathepsin B-like cysteine proteinase-deficient mutants of *Leishmania mexicana*. *Mol. Biochem. Parasitol.*, **88**, 53–61.

50 Denise, H., Poot, J., Jimenez, M., Ambit, A., Herrmann, D.C., Vermeulen, A.N. *et al.* (2006) Studies on the CPA cysteine peptidase in the *Leishmania infantum* genome strain JPCM5. *BMC Mol. Biol.*, **7**, 42–48.

51 Souza, A.E., Bates, P.A., Coombs, G.H., and Mottram, J.C. (1994) Null mutants for the lm*cpa* cysteine proteinase gene in *Leishmania mexicana*. *Mol. Biochem. Parasitol.*, **63**, 213–220.

52 Zangger, H., Mottram, J.C., and Fasel, N. (2002) Cell death in *Leishmania* induced by stress and differentiation: programmed cell death or necrosis? *Cell Death Differ.*, **9**, 1126–1139.

53 Zalila, H., Gonzalez, I.J., El-Fadili, A.K., Delgado, M.B., Desponds, C., Schaff, C. *et al.* (2011) Processing of metacaspase into a cytoplasmic catalytic domain mediating cell death in *Leishmania major*. *Mol. Microbiol.*, **79**, 222–239.

54 Frame, M.J., Mottram, J.C., and Coombs, G.H. (2000) Analysis of the roles of cysteine proteinases of *Leishmania mexicana* in the host–parasite interaction. *Parasitology*, **121**, 367–377.

55 Bayona, J.C., Nakayasu, E.S., Laverriere, M., Aguilar, C., Sobreira, T.J., Choi, H. *et al.* (2011) SUMOylation pathway in *Trypanosoma cruzi*: functional characterization and proteomic analysis of target proteins. *Mol. Cell Proteomics*, **10**, M110007369.

56 Lee, N., Gannavaram, S., Selvapandiyan, A., and Debrabant, A. (2007) Characterization of metacaspases with trypsin-like activity and their putative role in programmed cell death in the protozoan parasite *Leishmania*. *Eukaryot. Cell*, **6**, 1745–1757.

57 Gonzalez, I.J., Desponds, C., Schaff, C., Mottram, J.C., and Fasel, N. (2007) *Leishmania major* metacaspase can replace yeast metacaspase in programmed cell death and has arginine-specific cysteine peptidase activity. *Int. J. Parasitol.*, **7**, 161–172.

58 Alvarez, V.E., Kosec, G., Sant Anna, C., Turk, V., Cazzulo, J.J., and Turk, B. (2008) Blocking autophagy to prevent parasite differentiation: a possible new strategy for fighting parasitic infections? *Autophagy*, **4**, 361–363.

59 Shaid, S., Brandts, C.H., Serve, H., and Dikic, I. (2012) Ubiquitination and selective autophagy. *Cell Death Differ.* doi: 10.1038/cdd.2012.72

60 Yan, D., Davis, F.J., Sharrocks, A.D., and Im, H.J. (2010) Emerging roles of SUMO modification in arthritis. *Gene*, **466**, 1–15.

61 Zunino, R., Braschi, E., Xu, L., and McBride, H.M. (2009) Translocation of SenP5 from the nucleoli to the mitochondria modulates DRP1-dependent fission during mitosis. *J. Biol. Chem.*, **284**, 17783–17795.

62 Xia, H.G., Zhang, L., Chen, G., Zhang, T., Liu, J., Jin, M. *et al.* (2010) Control of basal autophagy by calpain1 mediated cleavage of ATG5. *Autophagy*, **6**, 61–66.

63 Yousefi, S., Perozzo, R., Schmid, I., Ziemiecki, A., Schaffner, T., Scapozza, L. *et al.* (2006) Calpain-mediated cleavage of Atg5 switches autophagy to apoptosis. *Nat. Cell Biol.*, **8**, 1124–1132.

64 Selzer, P.M., Pingel, S., Hsieh, I., Ugele, B., Chan, V.J., Engel, J.C. *et al.* (1999) Cysteine protease inhibitors as chemotherapy: lessons from a parasite target. *Proc. Natl. Acad. Sci. USA*, **96**, 11015–11022.

65 Mottram, J.C., Souza, A.E., Hutchison, J. E., Carter, R., Frame, M.J., and Coombs, G. H. (1996) Evidence from disruption of the *lmcpb* gene array of *Leishmania mexicana* that cysteine proteinases are virulence factors. *Proc. Natl. Acad. Sci. USA*, **3**, 6008–6013.

66 Mottram, J.C., Robertson, C.D., Coombs, G.H., and Barry, J.D. (1992) A developmentally regulated cysteine proteinase gene of *Leishmania mexicana*. *Mol. Microbiol.*, **6**, 1925–1932.

67 Mahmoudzadeh-Niknam, H. and McKerrow, J.H. (2004) *Leishmania tropica*: cysteine proteases are essential for growth and pathogenicity. *Exp. Parasitol.*, **106**, 158–163.

68 Engel, J.C., Doyle, P.S., Hsieh, I., and McKerrow, J.H. (1998) Cysteine protease inhibitors cure an experimental *Trypanosoma cruzi* infection. *J. Exp. Med.*, **188**, 725–734.

69 Doyle, P.S., Zhou, Y.M., Engel, J.C., and McKerrow, J.H. (2007) A cysteine protease inhibitor cures Chagas' disease in an immunodeficient-mouse model of infection. *Antimicrob. Agents Chemother.*, **51**, 3932–3939.

70 Steert, K., Berg, M., Mottram, J.C., Westrop, G.D., Coombs, G.H., Cos, P. *et al.* (2010) alpha-ketoheterocycles as inhibitors of *Leishmania mexicana* cysteine protease CPB. *ChemMedChem*, **5**, 1734–1748.

71 Steert, K., El-Sayed, I., Van der Veken, P., Krishtal, A., Van Alsenoy, C., Westrop, G.D. *et al.* (2007) Dipeptidyl alpha-fluorovinyl Michael acceptors: synthesis and activity against cysteine proteases. *Bioorg. Med. Chem. Lett.*, **17**, 6563–6566.

72 Vermelho, A.B., De Simone, S.G., d'Avila-Levy, C.M., Souza do Santos, A.L., Nogueira de Melo, A.C., Silva, F.P. *et al.* (2007) Trypanosomatidae peptidases: a target for drugs development. *Current Enzyme Inhibition.*, **3**, 19–48.

73 Sugawara, K., Suzuki, N.N., Fujioka, Y., Mizushima, N., Ohsumi, Y., and Inagaki, F. (2005) Structural basis for the specificity and catalysis of human Atg4B responsible for mammalian autophagy. *J. Biol. Chem.*, **280**, 40058–40065.

74 Satoo, K., Noda, N.N., Kumeta, H., Fujioka, Y., Mizushima, N., Ohsumi, Y. *et al.* (2009) The structure of Atg4B–LC3 complex reveals the mechanism of LC3 processing and delipidation during autophagy. *EMBO J.*, **28**, 1341–1350.

75 Shu, C.W., Madiraju, C., Zhai, D., Welsh, K., Diaz, P., Sergienko, E. *et al.* (2011) High-throughput fluorescence assay for small-molecule inhibitors of autophagins/Atg4. *J. Biomol. Screen*, **16**, 174–182.

76 Li, M., Hou, Y., Wang, J., Chen, X., Shao, Z.M., and Yin, X.M. (2011) Kinetics comparisons of mammalian Atg4 homologues indicate selective preferences toward diverse Atg8 substrates. *J. Biol. Chem.*, **286**, 7327–7338.

20
Proteases of *Trypanosoma brucei*

*Dietmar Steverding**

Abstract

Human African trypanosomiasis (HAT) or sleeping sickness is a parasitic infection caused by the protozoan *Trypanosoma brucei*. The disease occurs in sub-Saharan Africa where it is a major cause of morbidity and mortality in man. Combinations of toxicity and poor efficacy of current anti-sleeping sickness drugs means that new, effective, and better tolerated chemotherapies are needed for the treatment of human African trypanosomiasis. Proteases play a key role in the life cycle of *T. brucei* and in the pathogenesis of sleeping sickness. *In vitro* and *in vivo* studies over the last decades have shown that proteases are valid targets for the development of new drugs against *T. brucei*. Here, the major proteases of *T. brucei* and their cellular roles and potential as drug targets will be reviewed.

Introduction

The flagellated protozoan *Trypanosoma brucei* is the etiological agent of human African trypanosomiasis (HAT) or sleeping sickness. The parasite is transmitted by the bite of infected tsetse flies (*Glossina* spp.), and lives extracellularly in the blood and tissue fluids of humans. The occurrence of sleeping sickness is restricted to the distribution of tsetse flies, which are exclusively found in sub-Saharan Africa between 14° North and 20° South latitude [1]. In this so-called tsetse belt, millions of people living in 250 rural foci scattered over 36 African countries are at risk of contracting the disease [2,3].

Sleeping sickness occurs in two disease patterns caused by two subspecies of *T. brucei*. The chronic form of sleeping sickness is caused by *T. b. gambiense* and occurs in west and central Africa. This form of the disease accounts for about 95% of all reported cases of the infection [3]. The remaining cases are due to the acute form of sleeping sickness caused by *T. b. rhodesiense*, which is found in east and southern Africa. During the course of sleeping sickness, two disease stages can be distinguished. In the first stage, the parasites are restricted to the blood and lymph system. This hemolymphatic phase is characterized by irregular fever, headaches, joint

---

* Corresponding Author

Trypanosomatid Diseases: Molecular Routes to Drug Discovery, First edition. Edited by T. Jäger, O. Koch, and L. Flohé.
© 2013 Wiley-VCH Verlag GmbH & Co. KGaA. Published 2013 by Wiley-VCH Verlag GmbH & Co. KGaA.

pains, and itching [3]. In the second stage, parasites infect the central nervous system. Patients entering this neurological phase display the more obvious signs and symptoms of the disease, which are confusion, disturbed sleep pattern, sensory disturbances, extreme lethargy, poor condition, and coma [3]. If left untreated, sleeping sickness patients die within months when infected with *T. b. rhodesiense* or within years when infected with *T. b. gambiense* [3]. Sadly, only a few drugs (suramin, pentamidine, melarsoprol, and eflornithine (DL-α-difluoromethylornithine)) and one drug combination (eflornithine/nifurtimox) are available for chemotherapy of sleeping sickness [4]. All these drugs have major drawbacks, including poor efficacy, significant toxicity, requirement for parenteral administration, and being increasingly subject to drug resistance [5–7].

As proteases have been shown to perform important vital functions in pathogens and/or can be involved in the pathogenesis of infectious diseases, they have quickly attracted much attention as potential drug targets. Indeed, one promising line of research towards the development of new anti-sleeping sickness drugs has been the targeting of proteases. This chapter will discuss some important proteases of *T. brucei*, including their cellular role and their potential as drug targets.

Classes of Proteases

The first characterizations of proteolytic activities in *T. brucei* were carried out in the 1980s [8–14]. Subsequent research revealed that these proteolytic activities are from proteases belonging to the cysteine, serine, threonine, and metallo family of peptidases. Table 20.1 summarizes the proteases of *T. brucei* discussed in this chapter.

Cysteine Peptidases

Cysteine proteases are characterized by a common catalytic mechanism that involves a nucleophilic thiol group of a cysteine residue that is part of a catalytic cysteine–histidine dyad.

Cathepsin B- and L-Like Proteases

Cysteine cathepsins are the best-characterized cysteine peptidases and belong to the C1 family of papain-like enzymes (Table 20.1). They play a key role among lysosomal proteases and are widely distributed among living organisms, including protozoan parasites.

Perhaps the best-characterized cysteine peptidases in *T. brucei* are two proteases homologous to mammalian cathepsin B and L [15,16]. Based on the recently proposed nomenclature system for kinetoplastid C1 peptidases [15], *T. brucei* cathepsin B- and L-like proteases have been named *Tb*CATB and *Tb*CATL, respectively. In common with other C1 peptidases, both *Tb*CATB and *Tb*CATL comprise a signal peptide, a propeptide containing an I29 inhibitor domain, and a PepC1 catalytic domain, and have conserved cysteine, histidine, and asparagine

Table 20.1 Summary of *T. brucei* peptidases.

Family	Peptidase	Genetically validated	Chemically validated	Drug target
C1 (papain family)	*Tb*CATB	yes[a]	?	?
	*Tb*CATL	no[b]	yes	yes
C2 (calpain family)	*Tb*CALP1.1	no	ND[c]	?
	*Tb*CALP1.2	yes	ND	?
	*Tb*CALP1.3	no	ND	?
	*Tb*CALP1.4	no	ND	?
	*Tb*CALP4.1[d]	yes	ND	no
	*Tb*CALP8.1	yes	ND	?
C13 (legumain family)	*Tb*GPI8	yes	ND	?
C14 (caspase family)	*Tb*MCA1	ND	ND	no
	*Tb*MCA2	yes[e]	yes	?
	*Tb*MCA3	yes[e]	yes	?
	*Tb*MCA4	ND	ND	no
	*Tb*MCA5	yes[e]	ND	no
M8 (leishmanolysin family)	*Tb*MSP-B	no	?	?
S9 (prolyl oligopeptidase family)	*Tb*OPB	ND	yes	yes
	*Tb*POP	no[f]	?	?
T1 (proteasome family)	*Tb*PSB1	yes	ND	?
	*Tb*PSB2	yes	yes	yes
	*Tb*PSB5	yes	yes	yes

a) Incomplete RNAi: 60–65% of *Tb*CATB remained.
b) Incomplete RNAi: 30–35% of *Tb*CATL remained.
c) ND, not determined.
d) Procyclic forms.
e) Only simultaneous RNAi against *Tb*MCA2, *Tb*MCA3, and *Tb*MCA5 showed a phenotype.
f) Incomplete RNAi: 20% of *Tb*POP remained.

residues in the active site that are embedded in highly conserved peptide motifs [15,17]. In addition, other amino acids and peptide sequences are also conserved in both *Tb*CATB and *Tb*CATL, including several cysteine residues that form disulfide bonds [15].

The length of the prepro-*Tb*CATB is 340 amino acids and thus similar to the length of human cathepsin B (339 amino acids) [15]. The enzyme is encoded by a single-copy gene for which expression is regulated at the level of mRNA stability and is greatest in bloodstream forms [18].

At 450 amino acids, the length of the prepro-*Tb*CATL is significantly longer than that of human cathepsin L (333 amino acids) [14]. This is due to a 108-amino-acid C-terminal extension on the parasite enzyme [19] for which a definitive biological function is not yet known. *Tb*CATL is encoded by more than 20 genes arranged in long tandem array [19,20]. The expression of *Tb*CATL is developmentally regulated with the highest activity levels found in bloodstream forms [21,22].

Calpain-Like Proteins

Calpains are a large family of calcium-dependent cysteine proteases (C2 family of calpain-like enzymes) that are involved in a wide range of differentiation and cell regulatory processes. They are heterodimeric proteins consisting of an 80-kDa subunit and a 28-kDa subunit [23]. The large subunit is typically divided into an N-terminal domain of unknown function, a protease domain containing the catalytic triad of cysteine, histidine, and asparagine, a linker domain, and a calcium-binding domain [23].

Systematic analysis of the genome of *T. brucei* revealed a large and diverse family of calpain-like proteins in this parasite (*Tb*CALPs; Table 20.1) [24]. Based on their structural features, *Tb*CALPs were categorized into five groups [24]. Only *Tb*CALPs of group 1 and 2 are four-domain proteins resembling the general structure of mammalian calpains, while *Tb*CALPs of group 3 consist only of the N-terminal domain, and *Tb*CALPs of group 4 and 5 are highly divergent proteins [24,25]. Interestingly, the catalytic triad is only conserved in one member of the *Tb*CALPs, suggesting that most of these proteins probably do not act as cysteine proteases [24]. In addition, the C-terminal domain of all *Tb*CALPs does not show any similarity to the calcium-binding domain of conventional calpains [24]. Several *Tb*CALPs contain N-terminal dual myristoylation/palmitoylation signals, indicating that they might be membrane-associated, and some *Tb*CALPs are differentially expressed in bloodstream and procyclic forms [25].

Metacaspases

Metacaspases are a new family of cysteine proteases (C14 family of caspase-like enzymes) that are homologous to mammalian caspases, and are found in plants, fungi, and protozoa [26]. Metacaspases are predicted to have a similar structure to caspases with conserved histidine and cysteine residues in the active site [26]. However, they have a strict arginine or lysine substrate specificity and lack asparagine specificity, which is a characteristic of caspases [27,28].

To date, five metacaspases (*Tb*MCA1–*Tb*MCA5; Table 20.1) have been identified in *T. brucei* [29]. Interestingly, *Tb*MCA1 and *Tb*MCA4 have a serine residue in place of a cysteine residue in their catalytic site [30], suggesting that these metacaspases might be inactive. In addition, *Tb*MCA4 is both myristoylated and palmitoylated, and primarily expressed in bloodstream forms [31]. For *Tb*MCA2 it has been shown that cysteine peptidase activity is calcium dependent [28]. *Tb*MCA2 and *Tb*MCA3, which are located in a tandem repeat on chromosome 6, are only expressed in bloodstream forms, while *Tb*MCA5 is also expressed in procyclic forms [32].

GPI : Protein Transamidase

GPI : protein transamidases are enzyme complexes that catalyze the attachment of GPI (glycosylphosphatidylinositol) anchors to proteins. The subunit responsible for the protein–GPI anchoring reaction is GPI8, a cysteine peptidase containing cysteine and histidine residues in its active site. GPI8 belongs to the C13 family of legumain-like enzymes.

The homolog of GPI8 in *T. brucei*, *Tb*GPI8 (Table 20.1), has been identified, and the corresponding gene cloned and expressed [33,34]. *Tb*GPI8 is encoded by a single-copy gene, and is expressed by both procyclic and bloodstream forms [34]. The enzymatic activity of recombinant *Tb*GPI8 was shown to be strongly affected by the sulfhydryl alkylating agent *p*-chloro-mercuriphenyl-sulfonic acid, indicating that the enzyme is a cysteine protease [33].

Serine Peptidases

In serine proteases, the hydroxyl group of a serine residue in the active site acts as a nucleophile that attacks the carbonyl carbon of the scissile peptide bond of the substrate protein. So far, two serine proteases, oligopeptidase B (*Tb*OPB) and prolyl-oligopeptidase (*Tb*POP) have been characterized in *T. brucei*, both belonging to the S9 family of prolyl oligopeptidase-like enzymes (Table 20.1). Oligopeptidases are endopeptidases that cleave peptides but not proteins. That oligopeptidases cannot cleave proteins is due to their structure: their active site is located at the end of a narrow cavity, which is only accessible for peptides.

*Tb*OPB is a soluble serine oligopeptidase that is released into the bloodstream during infection [35,36]. *Tb*OPB is optimally active at alkaline pH and does not hydrolyze proteins larger than 4 kDa [35]. The protease exhibits activity towards trypsin-like enzyme substrates but not towards prolyl oligopeptidase substrates [36]. Unlike most serine peptidases, the activity of *Tb*OPB is inhibited by thiol-blocking reagents and enhanced by reducing agents and polyamines [36]. The reactive cysteine residues for thiol-inhibiting and -activating *Tb*OPB activity have been identified as C256, and as C559 and C597, respectively [37].

*Tb*POP is also a soluble serine oligopeptidase that is discharged into the bloodstream of *T. brucei*-infected mice [38]. *Tb*POP hydrolyzes peptide bonds at the C-terminal side of proline and alanine residues at slightly alkaline pH [38]. Unlike most other prolyl oligopeptidases, *Tb*POP can also cleave collagen [38].

Metalloproteases

The catalytic mechanism of metalloproteases involves a metal, which in most cases is zinc. The metal ion is coordinated by three ligands, which can be histidine, glutamate, aspartate, lysine or arginine. The fourth coordination position is taken up by a labile water molecule.

The genome of *T. brucei* contains three gene families encoding major surface proteases, *Tb*MSP-A, *Tb*MSP-B, and *Tb*MSP-C, which belong to the M8 family of leishmanolysin-like enzymes (Table 20.1) [39]. Each of these proteases displays about 33% sequence identity with the major surface protease of *Leishmania* species, GP63 [39]. In all three sequences the positions of 20 cysteine residues, 10 proline residues, and the zinc-binding motif HEXXH are conserved [39]. *Tb*MSP-A and *Tb*MSP-B families comprise five and four genes, respectively, whereas the *Tb*MSP-C family contains only one gene [39]. *Tb*MSP-B is transcribed in both bloodstream forms and procyclic forms [39] but its mRNA accumulates to a 50-fold higher steady level in bloodstream trypanosomes [40].

In contrast to *TBMSP-B, TbMSP-A* and *TbMSP-C* are transcribed only in bloodstream forms [39].

Threonine Proteases

Like serine proteases, threonine proteases also have a hydroxyl group in their active site that acts as a nucleophile to cleave a peptide bond. However, the hydroxyl group comes from a threonine residue and not from a serine residue. The archetype members of this class of proteases are the catalytic subunits of the proteasome, which belong to the T1 family of proteasome β subunit-like enzymes.

The proteasome is a multifunctional enzyme complex that plays an important role in the degradation of intracellular proteins [41]. The proteasome of *T. brucei* resembles structurally and functionally those of other eukaryotic cells [42]. The 20S core particle of the trypanosomal proteasome has a barrel-shape structure and is made up of four rings [43]. By using mass spectrometric techniques and bioinformatics, all essential seven α-subunits and seven β-subunits have been identified as part of the trypanosomal 20S proteasome [44]. This suggests that the two outer and the two inner rings of the trypanosomal 20S proteasome are each made up of the seven α-subunits and seven β-subunits, respectively, like any other eukaryotic 20S proteasome. Affinity-labeling experiments confirmed that also for the trypanosomal 20S proteasome the trypsin-like activity is associated with the β2 subunit (*Tb*PSB2; Table 20.1) and the chymotrypsin-like activity with the β5 subunit (*Tb*PSB5; Table 20.1) [45]. With respect to substrate specificity and inhibitor sensitivity, the trypanosomal proteasome differs from the mammalian proteasome. Whereas the proteasome of *T. brucei* exhibits a high trypsin-like activity but a low chymotrypsin-like activity, the reverse is true for the proteasome of mammalian cells [43]. Likewise, the trypanosomal and mammalian proteasome are particularly sensitive to inhibition of the trypsin-like activity and the chymotrypsin-like activity, respectively [46,47].

Cellular Functions

*Tb*CATB and *Tb*CATL

Both *Tb*CATB and *Tb*CATL are found in the lysosome of bloodstream forms [22,48], whereas their subcellular localization in procyclic forms is unknown. In bloodstream forms of *T. brucei*, both enzymes are involved in the degradation of phagocytosed host proteins and are essential for survival [18,48]. In addition, *Tb*CATL seems to facilitate trans-endothelial entry of bloodstream forms into the brain. The ability of bloodstream forms of *T. brucei* to cross an *in vitro* model of a human blood–brain barrier (BBB) was reduced by RNA interference (RNAi) against *Tb*CATL and blocked by the cysteine protease inhibitor *N*-methylpiperazine-urea-phenylalanyl-homophenylalanine-vinylsulfone-benzene (K11777; Figure 20.1) [49,50].

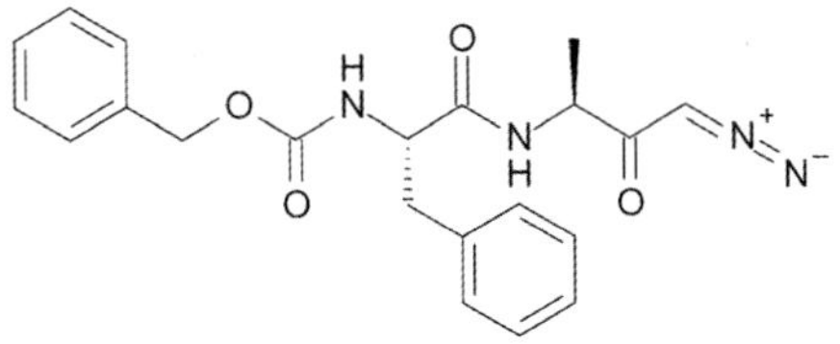

Cbz-Phe-Ala-CHN₂

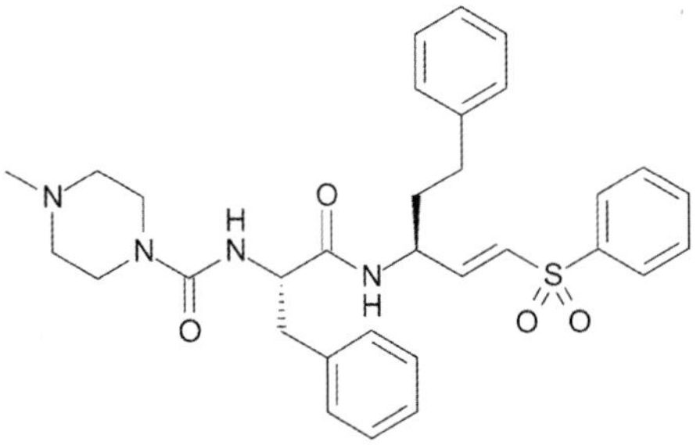

K11777

Figure 20.1 Structures of peptidyl cysteine protease inhibitors with *in vitro* and *in vivo* activity against bloodstream forms of *T. brucei* [48,58].

*Tb*CALPs

Three principle types of subcellular localization for *Tb*CALPs were identified: the flagellum, the cell body and the subpellicular cytoskeleton [25]. *Tb*CALP1.3 is localized to the tip of the flagellum, which suggests a possible involvement in sensory functions [25]. *Tb*CALP1.4, *Tb*CALP4.2, and *Tb*CALP6.1 occur throughout the cell body, but their functions remain to be determined [25]. *Tb*CALP4.1 and *Tb*CALP8.1 are associated to the cytoskeleton, and are essential and required for correct cell morphogenesis and organelle positioning in the parasite [51]. *Tb*CALP4.1 fulfils this function in procyclic forms, whereas *Tb*CALP8.1 is responsible for this role in bloodstream forms [51].

*Tb*MCAs

*Tb*MCA2, *Tb*MCA3, and *Tb*MCA5 are found to colocalize with RAB11, a marker for recycling endosomes, whereas *Tb*MCA4 is associated with the flagellum [32]. The subcellular localization of *Tb*MCA2, *Tb*MCA3, and *Tb*MCA5 rules out any involvement of these metacaspases in programmed cell death [32]. Simultaneous RNAi against *Tb*MCA2, *Tb*MCA3, and *Tb*MCA5 led to an immediate growth arrest in bloodstream forms, indicating that they play an essential role for the parasite [32]. Recently, it has been shown that *Tb*MCA3 is involved in the processing of *Tb*MCA4 during which the latter metacaspase is released from the parasite [31]. Reverse genetics revealed that TbMCA4 has roles in both cell cycle progression and parasite virulence during murine infection [31]. In addition, overexpression of TbMCA4 in yeast led to growth inhibition, mitochondrial dysfunction, and cell death, supporting the role of this metacaspase in controlling cellular proliferation in connection with mitochondrial biogenesis [29].

TbGPI8

TbGPI8 localizes within the tubular structures of the endoplasmic reticulum [33], where the addition of GPI anchors usually occurs. TbGPI8 plays an essential role in both procyclic and bloodstream forms [34]. Procyclic mutants deficient in TbGPI8 lack the major GPI-anchored surface protein, procyclin, but accumulate a pool of unlinked GPI molecules [34]. Although viable in culture, these mutants are unable to establish an infection in the midgut of tsetse flies, confirming the important role of GPI-anchored proteins for the insect–parasite interaction [34]. Inducible RNAi against TbGPI8 in bloodstream forms results in a severe growth deficiency of the parasites followed by cell death [34]. The development of multinuclear, multi-kinetoplast and multiflagellar phenotypes in these cells suggests a block in cytokinesis [34]. These data indicate that TbGPI8 is important for correct cell cycle progression in T. brucei.

TbOPB and TbPOP

Both TbOPB and TbPOP are released into the host bloodstream and contribute to the pathogenesis of African trypanosomiasis [35,36,38].

TbOPB is not secreted by live trypanosomes but released from dead or dying parasites into the circulation where it retains full activity [36]. This serine peptidase has been implicated in the hydrolysis of the atrial natriuretic factor [36], a peptide hormone involved in the homeostatic control of body water, sodium, potassium, and fat. The cleavage of the atrial natriuretic factor by TbOPB has been suggested from the observations that the peptide hormone is a substrate for the enzyme *in vitro* [35] and that its level is reduced in the plasma of T. brucei-infected dogs [52]. A reduction of the atrial natriuretic factor would explain the observed hypervolemia and, thus, the cardiomyopathy known to occur in African trypanosomiasis [53].

Like TbOPB, released TbPOP retains its activity in the plasma of infected rodents. In the bloodstream the enzyme mediates the degradation of several hormones and neuropeptides, including bradykinin, β-endorphin, gonadotropin-releasing hormone, neurotensin, and thyrotropin-releasing hormone [38]. The collagenolytic activity of TbPOP could help the parasite to cross the BBB and thus to establish an infection of the central nervous system [38]. These features may indicate that TbPOP plays an important role in the development and maintenance of a T. brucei infection within a mammalian host [38].

TbMSP-B

The metalloprotease *Tb*MSP-B is an integral membrane protein that is involved in the release of the variant surface glycoprotein (VSG) during differentiation of bloodstream forms to procyclic forms [54]. Using RNAi, it was shown that *Tb*MSP-B can release a recombinant VSG from transgenic procyclic trypanosomes [39]. In bloodstream-form mutants deficient in *Tb*MSP-B, the VSG was removed more slowly and in a non-truncated form during differentiation [54]. This latter result, however, indicated that *Tb*MSP is not solely responsible for the release of VSG during the differentiation process. In fact, it has been shown that *Tb*MSP-B and a phospholipase C (GPI-PLC) act synergistically in removal of VSG molecules from the cell surface during the differentiation of bloodstream trypanosomes to procyclic forms [54].

Proteasome

The main function of the proteasome is the degradation of regulatory proteins targeted for breakdown by ubiquitin conjunction. In *T. brucei*, the proteasome fulfils a similar role. For example, inhibition of the activity of the proteasome by lactacystin blocks the turnover of ubiquitinated proteins in intact cells of *T. brucei* [55]. In addition, inhibition of the proteasome activity arrests procyclic forms in G_2 and bloodstream forms in both G_1 and G_2 phases of the cell cycle, indicating that the proteasome is essential for driving cell cycle progression in *T. brucei* [56].

Proteases as Drug Targets

TbCATB and TbCATL

The lysosomal cysteine protease activity of *T. brucei* has been chemically validated as a drug target (Table 20.1). Studies with peptidyl diazomethylketones, peptidyl chloromethylketones, peptidyl fluoromethylketones, and peptidyl vinyl sulfones have shown that these irreversible cysteine protease inhibitors kill cultured bloodstream forms at low micromolar concentrations [48,57]. Furthermore, treatment of *T. brucei*-infected mice with carbobenzyloxyphenylalanyl-alanine diazomethylketone (Cbz-Phe-Ala-CHN$_2$; Figure 20.1) and N-methylpiperazine-urea-phenylalanyl-homophenylalanine-vinylsulfone-benzene (K11777; Figure 20.1) leads to a reduction in parasitemia and a prolongation of survival [48,58]. The killing of the parasites *in vivo* was found to be correlated with the inactivation of lysosomal cysteine protease activity [48]. However, genetic validation of *Tb*CATB and *Tb*CATL requirement for survival has been confounded by a lack of complete RNAi silencing of the target transcript (Table 20.1). Although RNAi against *TbCATB* was shown to be toxic *in vitro* [18] and to rescue mice from an otherwise lethal *T. brucei* infection [49], the observed modest reduction of 32% of *Tb*CATB protein [18] raises the question as to whether the RNAi-induced lethality had anything to do with the cysteine protease. RNAi against *TbCATL* was shown not to produce any phenotype *in vitro* [18] and not to rescue mice from a lethal *T. brucei* infection [49]. This is probably not surprising as RNAi of *TbCATL* never resulted in a complete ablation of the enzyme *in vitro* and *in vivo* (only 60–65% reduction of the protein) [18,49]. On the other hand, recent chemical validation using specific peptidyl inhibitors revealed that *TbCATL*, rather than *TbCATB*, is essential to the survival of bloodstream forms of *T. brucei* and, therefore, the appropriate drug target [59]. However, considering that non-specific cysteine protease inhibitors are therapeutic *in vivo* and show excellent selectivity indices *in vitro* [48,58], it may not be necessary to design compounds that act selectively against either *TbCATB* or *TbCATL*.

TbCALPs

A systematic RNAi study of chromosome 1 genes revealed growth phenotypes for *TbCALP1.2* but not for *TbCALP1.1*, *TbCALP1.3*, and *TbCALP1.4* in bloodstream forms of *T. brucei* (Table 20.1) [25,60]. Depletion of *TbCALP4.1* and *TbCALP8.1* using RNAi (Table 20.1) was shown to interfere with cytokinesis, organelle positioning and cell growth in procyclic and bloodstream forms, respectively [51], demonstrating the requirement of these calpain-related proteins in distinct life-cycle stages of *T. brucei*. However, because of the lack of chemical validation, it remains to be shown whether *TbCALPs* are good drug targets for the treatment of sleeping sickness.

TbMCAs

Their absence in humans and their marked difference from the orthologous human caspases make *TbMCAs* attractive new drug targets for anti-trypanosomal chemotherapeutics. This suggestion is corroborated by the observation that *TbMCA2*, *TbMCA3*, and *TbMCA5* are essential for bloodstream forms of *T. brucei* (Table 20.1) [32]. The apparent essentiality of metacaspases in *T. brucei* has led to the development of a series of inhibitors for *TbMCA2* and *TbMCA3* on the basis of known substrate specificity and the predicted catalytic mechanism of these enzymes. Some of the newly developed compounds (derived from α-amino-protected arginine with an α-ketoheterocyclic P1' warhead; Figure 20.2) inhibit the enzymatic activity of *TbMCA2* and *TbMCA3* with IC_{50} values in the low micromolar range and display modest trypanocidal activities *in vitro* with low cytotoxicity [61]. Further optimization and *in vivo* testing of the compounds are necessary before *TbMCAs* can be regarded as validated drug targets for HAT.

TbGPI8

Although *TbGPI8* has been shown to be essential for bloodstream forms of *T. brucei* (Table 20.1) [34], it remains to be demonstrated whether the differences between

α-amino protected arginine derivative compound 18

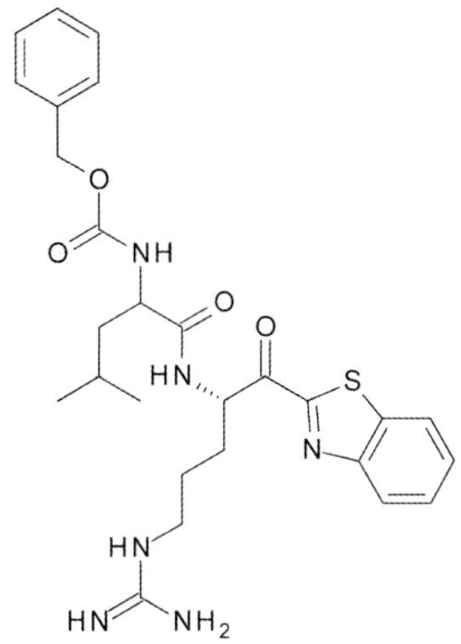

Figure 20.2 Structure of an α-amino-protected arginine with an α-ketobenzothiazole P1′ warhead and a leucine residue at the level of the P2 position with inhibitory activity against *Tb*MCA2 and *in vitro* trypanocidal activity against bloodstream forms of *T. brucei*. The designation "compound 18" refers to notation used in [61].

substrate specificities and functions of mammalian and parasite enzymes are sufficient for the development of selective inhibitors.

*Tb*OPB and *Tb*POP

As yet, *Tb*OPB has not been genetically validated to be essential for the survival of *T. brucei* (Table 20.1). Studies with peptidyl chloromethylketones and peptidyl phosphonate diphenyl esters, two groups of irreversible serine peptidase inhibitors, have been shown to inhibit trypsin-like protease activity of bloodstream forms of *T. brucei* and to display modest trypanocidal activities *in vitro* [62]. Active-site labeling studies revealed that both groups of inhibitors primarily target an 80-kDa protein, indicative of *Tb*OPB [62]. One of these inhibitors, carbobenzyloxyglycyl-4-amidino-phenylglycine phosphonate diphenyl ester (Cbz-Gly-(4-AmPhGly)^P(OPh)$_2$; Figure 20.3), was able to cure a *T. brucei* infection in mice at a dosage of 5 mg/kg/day [62]. These findings indicate that *Tb*OPB may represent a potential chemotherapeutic target in *T. brucei*.

Prolylisoxazoles (Figure 20.4), prolylisoxazolines (Figure 20.4), and JTP-4819, specific inhibitors of prolyloligopeptidases were shown to inhibit the growth of bloodstream forms of *T. brucei in vitro* with 50% growth inhibition values in the low micromolar range [38,63]. As the inhibitors are not toxic to mammalian cells

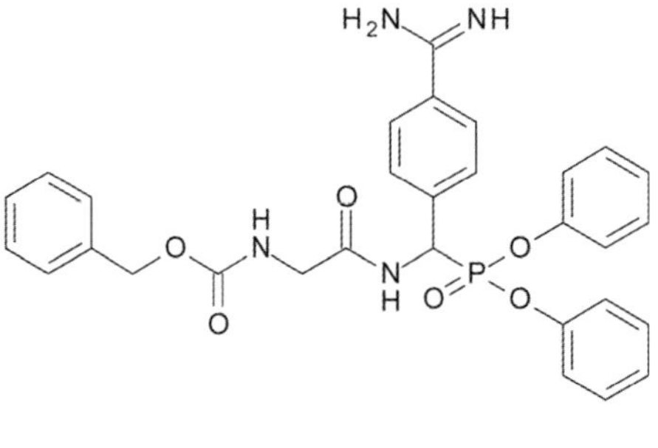

Cbz-Gly-(4-AmPhGly)^P(OPh)$_2$

Figure 20.3 Structure of a peptidyl serine peptidase inhibitor with inhibitory activity against *Tb*OPB, and *in vitro* and *in vivo* activity against bloodstream forms of *T. brucei* [62].

at the concentrations used in the tests [38], it is likely that the observed trypanocidal activities of the compounds are due to the inhibition of *Tb*POP. On the other hand, RNAi against *Tb*POP did not produce any phenotype in bloodstream and procyclic forms (Table 20.1) [38], raising questions about the requirement of *Tb*POP for *T. brucei*. However, as the ablation of *Tb*POP was incomplete, the remaining activity of about 20% of the protein could explain the survival of the parasites [38]. Further research on the action of mechanism of *Tb*POP inhibitors is necessary to establish structure–activity relationships of these compounds.

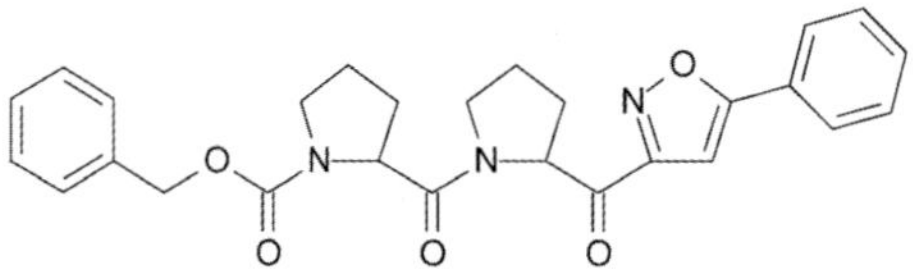

Prolylisoxazole derivative compound 3d

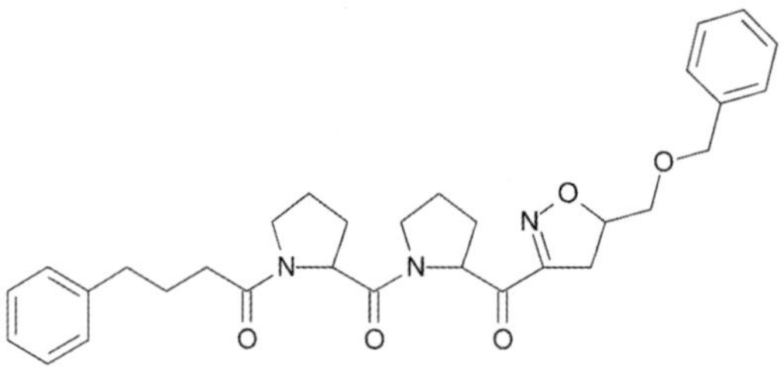

Prolylisoxazoline derivative compound 3f

Figure 20.4 Structure of prolylisoxazole and prolylisoxazoline compounds with *in vitro* trypanocidal activity against bloodstream forms of *T. b. rhodesiense*. The designations "compound 3d" and "compound 3f" refer to denotations used in [63].

*Tb*MSP-B

Bloodstream form Δ*msp-b* mutants, in which all four tandem *TbMSP-B* genes from both chromosomal alleles were deleted, show no significant difference in growth *in vitro* compared to wild-type bloodstream forms (Table 20.1) [54]. This finding indicates that *Tb*MSP-B is not essential for normal growth of *T. brucei* bloodstream forms. Nevertheless, some peptidomimetic inhibitors of mammalian zinc metalloproteases (SmithKline Beecham Pharmaceuticals compounds BRL29808, BRL49244, BRL57240, and SB201140; Figure 20.5) were found to be trypanocidal *in vitro* with growth inhibitory activities in the low micromolar range [64]. Although three of these compounds (BRL29808, BRL57240, and SB201140) were able to inactivate GP63, the *Tb*MSP-B homolog of *Leishmania major* [64], this observation does not prove that the *Tb*MSP-B is the inhibition target in bloodstream-form trypanosomes. It is also possible that these peptidomimetic inhibitors exert their trypanocidal activities against bloodstream forms of *T. brucei* by targeting other enzymes than metalloproteases.

Proteasome

The necessity of the proteasome for survival of *T. brucei* has been genetically and chemically validated (Table 20.1). By using RNAi against all β-subunits genes of the

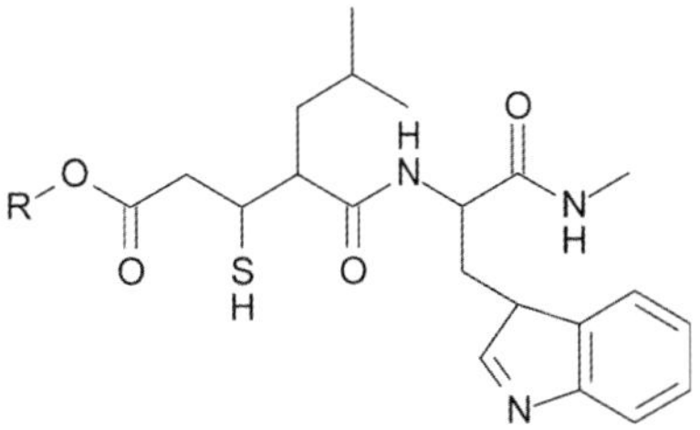

BRL49244: $R = CH_3$
BRL57240: $R = CH(CH_3)_2$
SB201140: $R = 4\text{-}CH_2C_6H_4OCH_3$

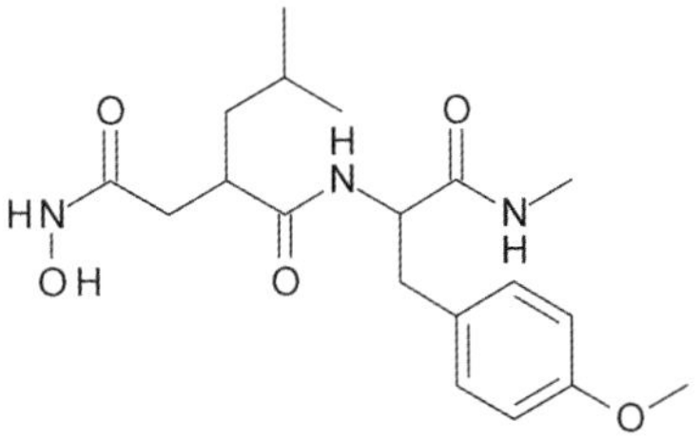

BRL29808

Figure 20.5 Structures of peptidomimetic zinc metalloproteases inhibitors with *in vitro* trypanocidal activity against bloodstream forms of *T. brucei* [64].

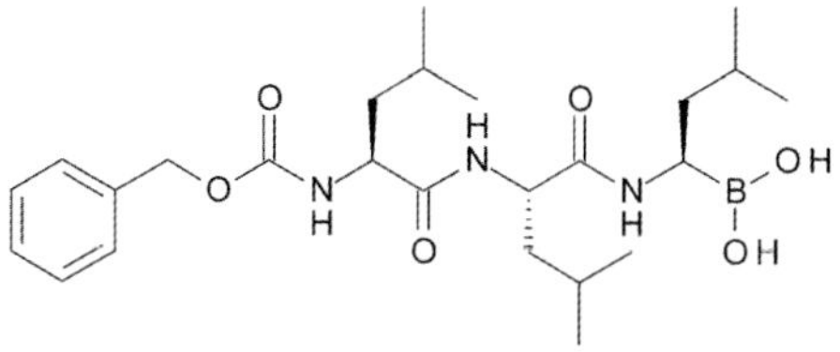

MG-262

Figure 20.6 Structure of the proteasome inhibitor MG-262 with promising *in vitro* and *in vivo* activity against bloodstream forms of *T. brucei* [42].

proteasome, it was shown that the three catalytic active β1-, β2-, and β5-subunits (*Tb*PSB1, *Tb*PSB2, and *Tb*PSB5) are vital for *T. brucei* [55]. All proteasome inhibitors tested so far displayed substantial trypanocidal activities with 50% growth inhibition values in the nanomolar range [46,47,65–68]. In addition, the peptide boronate inhibitor MG-262 (Figure 20.6) was shown to slow the growth of *T. brucei* in the blood of infected mice [42] indicating that proteasome inhibitors display trypanocidal activity *in vivo*. The observed differences in peptidase activity, substrate specificity, and inhibitor sensitivity between the trypanosomal and the mammalian proteasome [42] makes this enzyme complex an interesting drug target for sleeping sickness. As the trypanosomal proteasome is particularly sensitive to inhibitors of the trypsin-like activity [46,47,66], agents targeting this activity would be the rational choice for future anti-trypanosomal drug development.

Conclusion

Proteases have been validated as targets for the development of new drugs against HAT. Importantly, proteases are druggable targets as verified by the development of anti-protease drugs as effective therapies for many human diseases. The most promising targets for anti-trypanosomal drugs are the lysosomal cysteine protease *Tb*CATL and the proteasome. The research to target *Tb*CATL and the proteasome should benefit from the intense interest by pharmaceutical companies to design protease inhibitors as therapeutics for arthritis, osteoporosis, and various cancers. In addition, the development of new inhibitors to target proteases for the treatment of other protozoan infections will provide new avenues for novel trypanocidal agents.

References

1 Molyneux, D.H., Pentreath, V., and Doua, F. (1996) African trypanosomiasis in man, in *Manson's Tropical Diseases* (ed. G.C. Cook), Saunders, London, pp. 1171–1196.

2 World Health Organization (2005) *Control of human African trypanosomiasis: a strategy for the African region. AFRO (AFR/RC55/11)*, WHO, Geneva.

3 World Health Organization (2010) *African trypanosomiasis (sleeping sickness). Fact Sheet 259*, WHO, Geneva.

4 Steverding, D. (2010) The development of drugs for treatment of sleeping sickness: a historical review. *Parasit. Vectors*, **3**, 15.

5 Fairlamb, A.H. (2003) Chemotherapy of human African trypanosomiasis: current and future prospects. *Trends Parasitol.*, **19**, 488–494.

6 Matovu, E., Seebeck, T., Enyaru, J.C., and Kaminsky, R. (2001) Drug resistance in *Trypanosoma brucei* ssp., the causative agents of sleeping sickness in man and nagana in cattle. *Microbes Infect.*, **3**, 763–770.

7 Delespaux, V. and de Koning, H.P. (2007) Drugs and drug resistance in African trypanosomiasis. *Drug Resist. Updat.*, **10**, 30–50.

8 Steiger, R.F., Van Hoof, F., Bontemps, J., Nyssens-Jadin, M., and Druetz, J.E. (1979) Acid hydrolases of trypanosomatid flagellates. *Acta Trop.*, **36**, 335–341.

9 North, M.J., Coombs, G.H., and Barry, J.D. (1983) A comparative study of the proteolytic enzymes of *Trypanosoma brucei, T. equiperdum, T. evansi, T. vivax, Leishmania tarentolae* and *Crithidia fasciculate. Mol. Biochem. Parasitol.*, **9**, 161–180.

10 Lonsdale-Eccles, J.D. and Mpimbaza, G.W. (1986) Thiol-dependent proteases of African trypanosomes. Analysis by electrophoresis in sodium dodecyl sulphate/polyacrylamide gels co-polymerized with fibrinogen. *Eur. J. Biochem.*, **155**, 469–473.

11 Lonsdale-Eccles, J.D. and Grab, D.J. (1987) Lysosomal and non-lysosomal peptidyl hydrolases of the bloodstream forms of *Trypanosoma brucei brucei. Eur. J. Biochem.*, **169**, 467–475.

12 Boutignon, F., Huet-Duvillier, G., Demeyer, D., Richet, C., and Degand, P. (1990) Study of proteolyitc activities released by incubation of trypanosomes (*Trypanosoma brucei brucei*) in pH 5.5 and 7.0 phosphate/glucose buffers. *Biochim. Biophys. Acta*, **1035**, 369–377.

13 Robertson, C.D., North, M.J., Lockwood, B. C., and Coombs, G.H. (1990) Analysis of the proteinases of *Trypanosoma brucei. J. Gen. Microbiol.*, **136**, 921–925.

14 Mbawa, Z.R., Gumm, I.D., Fish, W.R., and Lonsdale-Eccles, J.D. (1991) Endopeptidase variations among different life-cycle stages of African trypanosomes. *Eur. J. Biochem.*, **195**, 183–190.

15 Caffrey, C.R. and Steverding, D. (2009) Kinetoplastid papain-like cysteine peptidases. *Mol. Biochem. Parasitol.*, **167**, 12–19.

16 Caffrey, C.R., Lima, A.P., and Steverding, D. (2011) Cysteine peptidases of kinetoplastid parasites. *Adv. Exp. Med. Biol.*, **712**, 84–99.

17 Lecaille, F., Kaleta, J., and Brömme, D. (2002) Human and parasitic papain-like cysteine proteases: their role in physiology and pathology and recent developments in inhibitor design. *Chem. Rev.*, **102**, 4459–4488.

18 Mackey, Z.B., O'Brien, T.C., Greenbaum, D.C., Blank, R.B., and McKerrow, J.H. (2004) A cathepsin B-like protease is required for host protein degradation in *Trypanosoma brucei. J. Biol. Chem.*, **279**, 48426–48433.

19 Mottram, J.C., North, M.J., Barry, J.D., and Coombs, G.H. (1989) A cysteine proteinase cDNA from *Trypanosoma brucei* predicts an enzyme with an unusual C-terminal extension. *FEBS Lett.*, **258**, 211–215.

20 Berriman, M., Ghedin, E., Hertz-Fowler, C., Blandin, G., Renauld, H., Bartholomeu, D.C., Lennard, N.J. *et al.* (2005) The genome of the African trypanosome *Trypanosoma brucei. Science*, **309**, 416–422.

21 Pamer, E.G., So, M., and Davis, C.E. (1989) Identification of a developmentally regulated cysteine protease of *Trypanosoma brucei. Mol. Biochem. Parasitol.*, **33**, 27–32.

22 Caffrey, C.R., Hansell, E., Lucas, K.D., Brinen, L.S., Alvarez Hernandez, A., Cheng, J., Gwaltney, S.L.2nd *et al.* (2001) Active site mapping, biochemical properties and subcellular localization of rhodesain, the major cysteine protease of *Trypanosoma brucei rhodesiense. Mol. Biochem. Parasitol.*, **118**, 61–73.

23 Goll, D.E., Thompson, V.F., Li, H., Wei, W., and Cong, J. (2003) The calpain system. *Physiol. Rev.*, **83**, 731–801.

24 Ersfeld, K., Barraclough, H., and Gull, K. (2005) Evolutionary relationships and protein domain architecture in an expanded calpain superfamily in kinetoplastid parasites. *J. Mol. Evol.*, **61**, 742–757.

25 Liu, W., Apagyi, K., McLeavy, L., and Ersfeld, K. (2010) Expression and cellular localisation of calpain-like proteins in *Trypanosoma brucei*. *Mol. Biochem. Parasitol.*, **169**, 20–26.

26 Uren, A.G., O'Rourke, K., Aravind, L.A., Pisabarro, M.T., Seshagiri, S., Koonin, E.V., and Dixit, V.M. (2000) Identification of paracaspases and metacaspases: two ancient families of caspase-like proteins, one of which plays a key role in MALT lymphoma. *Mol. Cell*, **6**, 961–967.

27 Vercammen, D., van de Cotte, B., De Jaeger, G., Eeckhout, D., Casteels, P., Vandepoele, K., Vandenberghe, I. *et al.* (2004) Type II metacaspases Atmc4 and Atmc9 of Arabidopsis thaliana cleave substrate after arginine and lysine. *J. Biol. Chem.*, **279**, 45329–45336.

28 Moss, C.X., Westrop, G.D., Juliano, L., Coombs, G.H., and Mottram, J.C. (2007) Metacaspase 2 of *Trypanosoma brucei* is a calcium-dependent cysteine peptidase active without processing. *FEBS Lett.*, **581**, 5635–5639.

29 Szallies, A., Kubata, B.K., and Duszenko, M. (2002) A metacaspase of *Trypanosoma brucei* causes loss of respiration competence and clonal death in the yeast *Saccharomyces cerevisiae*. *FEBS Lett.*, **517**, 144–150.

30 Mottram, J.C., Helms, M.J., Coombs, G.H., and Sajid, M. (2003) Clan CD cysteine peptidases of parasitic protozoa. *Trends Parasitol.*, **19**, 182–187.

31 Proto, W.R., Castanys-Munoz, E., Black, A., Tetley, L., Moss, C.X., Juliano, L., Coombs, G.H., and Mottram, J.C. (2011) *Trypanosoma brucei* metacaspase 4 is a pseudopeptidase and a virulence factor. *J. Biol. Chem.*, **286**, 39914–39925.

32 Helms, M.J., Ambit, A., Appleton, P., Tetley, L., Coombs, G.H., and Mottram, J.C. (2006) Bloodstream form *Trypanosoma brucei* depend upon multiple metacaspases associated with RAB11-positive endosomes. *J. Cell Sci.*, **119**, 1105–1117.

33 Kang, X., Szallies, A., Rawer, M., Echner, H., and Duszenko, M. (2002) GPI anchor transamidase of *Trypanosoma brucei*:

in vitro assay of the recombinant protein and VSG anchor exchange. *J. Cell Sci.*, **115**, 2529–2539.

34 Lillico, S., Field, M.C., Blundell, P., Coombs, G.H., and Mottram, J.C. (2003) Essential roles for GPI-anchored proteins in African trypanosomes revealed using mutants deficient in GPI8. *Mol. Biol. Cell*, **14**, 1182–1194.

35 Troeberg, L., Pike, R.N., Morty, R.E., Berry, R.K., Coetzer, T.H., and Lonsdale-Eccles, J.D. (1996) Proteases from *Trypanosoma brucei brucei*. Purification, characterisation and interactions with host regulatory molecules. *Eur. J. Biochem.*, **238**, 728–736.

36 Morty, R.E., Lonsdale-Eccles, J.D., Mentele, R., Auerswald, E.A., and Coetzer, T.H. (2001) Trypanosome-derived oligopeptidase B is released into the plasma of infected rodents, where it persists and retains full catalytic activity. *Infect. Immun.*, **69**, 2757–2761.

37 Morty, R.E., Shih, A.Y., Fülöp, A., and Andrews, N.W. (2005) Identification of the reactive cysteine residues in oligopeptidase B from *Trypanosoma brucei*. *FEBS Lett.*, **579**, 2191–2196.

38 Bastos, I.M., Motta, F.N., Charneau, S., Santana, J.M., Dubost, L., Augustyns, K., and Grellier, P. (2010) Prolyl oligopeptidase of *Trypanosoma brucei* hydrolyzes native collagen, peptide hormones and is active in the plasma of infected mice. *Microbes Infect.*, **12**, 457–466.

39 LaCount, D.J., Gruszynski, A.E., Grandgenett, P.M., Bangs, J.D., and Donelson, J.E. (2003) Expression and function of the *Trypanosoma brucei* major surface protease (GP63) genes. *J. Biol. Chem.*, **278**, 24658–24664.

40 El-Sayed, N.M. and Donelson, J.E. (1997) African trypanosomes have differentially expressed genes encoding homologues of the *Leishmania* GP63 surface protease. *J. Biol. Chem.*, **272**, 26742–26748.

41 Coux, O., Tanaka, K., and Goldberg, A.L. (1996) Structure and function of the 20S and 26S proteasome. *Annu. Rev. Biochem.*, **65**, 801–847.

42 Steverding, D. (2007) The proteasome as a potential target for chemotherapy of African trypanosomiasis. *Drug Dev. Res.*, **68**, 205–212.

43 Hua, S., To, W.Y., Nguyen, T.T., Wong, M.L., and Wang, C.C. (1996) Purification and characterization of proteasomes from *Trypanosoma brucei*. *Mol. Biochem. Parasitol.*, **78**, 33–46.

44 Huang, L., Jacob, R.J., Pegg, S.C., Baldwin, M.A., Wang, C.C., Burlingname, A.L., and Babbitt, P.C. (2001) Functional assignment of the 20 S proteasome from *Trypanosoma brucei* using mass spectrometry and new bioinformatics approaches. *J. Biol. Chem.*, **276**, 28327–28339.

45 Wang, C.C., Bozdech, Z., Liu, C.L., Shipway, A., Backes, B.J., Harris, J.L., and Bogyo, M. (2003) Biochemical analysis of the 20 S proteasome of *Trypanosoma brucei*. *J. Biol. Chem.*, **278**, 15800–15808.

46 Glenn, R.J., Pemberton, A.J., Royle, H.J., Spackmann, R.W., Smith, E., Rivett, A.J., and Steverding, D. (2004) Trypanocidal effect of α′,β′-epoxyketones indicates that trypanosomes are particularly sensitive to inhibitors of proteasome trypsin-like activity. *Int. J. Antimicrob. Agents*, **24**, 286–289.

47 Steverding, D., Pemberton, A.J., Royle, H., Spackman, R.W., and Rivett, A.J. (2006) Evaluation of the anti-trypanosomal activity of tyropeptin A. *Planta Med.*, **72**, 761–763.

48 Scory, S., Caffrey, C.R., Stierhof, Y.-D., Ruppel, A., and Steverding, D. (1999) *Trypanosoma brucei*: killing of bloodstream forms *in vitro* and *in vivo* by the cysteine proteinase inhibitor Z-Phe-Ala-CHN$_2$. *Exp. Parasitol.*, **91**, 327–333.

49 Abdulla, M.H., O'Brien, T., Mackey, Z.B., Sajid, M., Grab, D.J., and McKerrow, J.H. (2008) RNA interference of *Trypanosoma brucei* cathepsin B and L affects disease progression in a mouse model. *PLoS Negl. Trop. Dis.*, **2**, e298.

50 Nikolskaia, O.V., Lima de A., A.P., Kim, Y.V., Lonsdale-Eccles, J.D., Fukuma, T., Scharfstein, J., and Grab, D.J. (2006) Blood–brain barrier traversal by African trypanosomes requires calcium signalling induced by parasite cysteine protease. *J. Clin. Invest.*, **116**, 2739–2747.

51 Olego-Fernandez, S., Vaughan, S., Shaw, M.K., Gull, K., and Ginger, M.L. (2009) Cell morphogenesis of *Trypanosoma brucei* requires the paralogous, differentially expressed calpain-related proteins CAP5.5 and CAP5.5V. *Protist*, **160**, 576–590.

52 Ndung'u, J.M., Wright, N.G., Jennings, F.W., and Murray, M. (1992) Changes in atrial natriuretic factor and plasma rennin activity in dogs infected with *Trypanosoma brucei*. *Parasitol. Res.*, **78**, 553–556.

53 Antoine-Moussiaux, N., Büscher, P., and Desmecht, D. (2009) Host-parasite interactions in trypanosomiasis: on the way to an antidisease strategy. *Infect. Immun.*, **77**, 1276–1284.

54 Grandgenett, P.M., Otsu, K., Wilson, H.R., Wilson, M.E., and Donelson, J.E. (2007) A function for a specific zinz metalloprotease of African trypanosomes. *PLoS Pathog.*, **3**, 1432–1445.

55 Li, Z., Zou, C.B., Yao, Y., Hoyt, M.A., McDonough, S., Mackey, Z.B., Coffino, P., and Wang, C.C. (2002) An easily dissociated 26 S proteasome catalyzes an essential ubiquitin-mediated protein degradation pathway in *Trypanosoma brucei*. *J. Biol. Chem.*, **277**, 15486–15498.

56 Mutomba, M.C., To, W.Y., Hyun, W.C., and Wang, C.C. (1997) Inhibition of proteasome activity blocks cell cycle progression at specific phase boundaries in African trypanosomes. *Mol. Biochem. Parasitol.*, **90**, 491–504.

57 Troeberg, L., Morty, R.E., Pike, R.N., Lonsdale-Eccles, J.D., Palmer, J.T., McKerrow, J.H., and Coetzer, T.H. (1999) Cysteine proteinase inhibitors kill cultured bloodstream forms of *Trypanosoma brucei brucei*. *Exp. Parasitol.*, **91**, 349–355.

58 Caffrey, C.R., Scory, S., and Steverding, D. (2000) Cysteine proteinases of trypanosome parasites: novel targets for chemotherapy. *Curr. Drug Target*, **1**, 155–162.

59 Steverding, D., Sexton, D.W., Wang, X., Gehrke, S.S., Wagner, G.K., and Caffrey, C.R. (2012) *Trypanosoma brucei*: chemical evidence that cathepsin L is essential for survival and a relevant drug target. *Int. J. Parasitol.*, **42**, 481–488.

60 Subramaniam, C., Veazey, P., Redmond, S., Hayes-Sinclair, J., Chambers, E., Carrington, M., Gull, K. *et al.* (2006) Chromosome-wide analysis of gene function by RNA interference in the African trypanosome. *Eukaryot. Cell*, **5**, 1539–1549.

61 Berg, M., Van der Veken, P., Joossens, J., Muthusamy, V., Breugelmans, M., Moss,

C.X., Rudplf, J. *et al.* (2010) Design and evaluation of *Trypanosoma brucei* metacaspase inhibitors. *Bioorg. Med. Chem. Lett.*, **20**, 2001–2006.

62 Morty, R.E., Trcobcrg, L., Powers, J.C., Ono, S., Lonsdale-Eccles, J.D., and Coetzer, T.H. (2000) Characterisation of the antitrypanosomal activity of peptidyl α-aminoalkyl phosphonate diphenyl esters. *Biochem. Pharmacol.*, **60**, 1497–1504.

63 Bal, G., Van der Veken, P., Antonov, D., Lambier, A.M., Grellier, P., Croft, S.L., Augustyns, K., and Haemers, A. (2003) Prolylisoxazoles: potent inhibitors of prolyloligopeptidase with antitrypanosomal activity. *Bioorg. Med. Chem. Lett.*, **13**, 2875–2878.

64 Bangs, J.D., Ransom, D.A., Nimick, M., Christie, G., and Hooper, N.M. (2001) *In vitro* cytocidal effects on *Trypanosoma brucei* and inhibition of *Leishmania* major GP63 by peptidomimetic metalloprotease inhibitors. *Mol. Biochem. Parasitol.*, **114**, 111–117.

65 Nkemgu-Njinkeng, J., Rosenkranz, V., Wink, M., and Steverding, D. (2002) Antitrypanosomal activities of proteasome inhibitors. *Antimicrob. Agents Chemother.*, **46**, 2038–2040.

66 Steverding, D., Spackman, R.W., Royle, H.J., and Glenn, R.J. (2005) Trypanocidal activities of trileucin methyl vinyl sulfone proteasome inhibitors. *Parasitol. Res.*, **95**, 73–76.

67 Steverding, D., Baldisserotto, A., Wang, X., and Marastoni, M. (2011) Trypanocidal activity of peptidyl vinyl ester derivatives selective for inhibition of mammalian proteasoem trypsin-like activity. *Exp. Parasitol.*, **128**, 444–447.

68 Steverding, D., Wang, X., Potts, B.C., and Palladino, M.A. (2012) Trypanocidal activity of β-lactone-γ-lactam proteasome inhibitors. *Planta Med.*, **78**, 131–134.

Part Four
Examples of Target-Based Approaches and Compounds Under Consideration

Trypanosomatid Diseases: Molecular Routes to Drug Discovery, First edition. Edited by T. Jäger, O. Koch, and L. Flohé.
© 2013 Wiley-VCH Verlag GmbH & Co. KGaA. Published 2013 by Wiley-VCH Verlag GmbH & Co. KGaA.

21
Screening Approaches Towards Trypanothione Reductase

Mathias Beig, Frank Oellien, R. Luise Krauth-Siegel, and Paul M. Selzer[*]

Abstract

Trypanosomes and *Leishmania*, the causative agents of African sleeping sickness, Chagas disease, and Leishmaniasis, are responsible for over half a million human deaths per year in subtropical and tropical regions around the world. Only a handful of chemotherapeutics are available, and their efficacy suffers from drug resistance and serious side-effects. Therefore, new inhibiting compounds of essential targets are urgently needed. Trypanosomes lack both glutathione reductase and thioredoxin reductase, but possess the phylogenetically related trypanothione reductase (TR), a validated drug target and key enzyme of the unique trypanothione-based thiol metabolism. By inhibiting this essential flavoenzyme the parasite becomes vulnerable against oxidative stress induced by the host defense system and drug treatment. Here, we provide an overview of published TR screenings, and present an alternative approach combining *in silico* and *in vitro* experiments. Starting from an *in vitro* screen of 2816 highly diverse compounds, 21 novel TR actives could be identified. These inhibitors were used as the starting point to identify similar substances within a compound library of 200 000 available chemicals by a ligand-based *in silico* screening. *In vitro* screening of the resulted *in silico*-enriched dataset led to the identification of 61 additional TR actives. All 82 TR inhibitors showed IC_{50} values down to the nanomolar range. Subsequently, the dataset of known actives was used to implement a novel structure-based *in silico* screening approach that might identify further potential novel TR inhibitors.

Introduction

Parasitic Diseases Caused by Trypanosomatids

The most relevant Kinetoplastida for human and animal health belong to the genera *Trypanosoma* and *Leishmania*. African sleeping sickness occurs in 36 sub-Saharan countries coinciding with the presence of tsetse flies that transmit the disease. *T. brucei gambiense* is found in west and central Africa and causes the chronic form of

[*] Corresponding Author

Trypanosomatid Diseases: Molecular Routes to Drug Discovery, First edition. Edited by T. Jäger, O. Koch, and L. Flohé.
© 2013 Wiley-VCH Verlag GmbH & Co. KGaA. Published 2013 by Wiley-VCH Verlag GmbH & Co. KGaA.

sleeping sickness accounting for more than 95% of reported cases. *T. b. rhodesiense* occurs in east and southern Africa, and infects domestic livestock and wildlife. In humans, this zoonotic parasite results in an acute form of sleeping sickness, which represents less than 5% of reported cases. Any untreated sleeping sickness is fatal. *T. b. brucei, T. vivax* and *T. congolense* cause Nagana (Surra) cattle disease. Although not infective for humans, the parasites have an enormous economic impact on the agricultural development in Africa [1].

In the New World, *T. cruzi* is responsible for Chagas disease, a zoonosis, also called human American trypanosomiasis. The acute stage after infection with high parasitemia lasts for about 2 months. A majority of those infected during childhood remain asymptomatic for decades or even life-long. However, in about one-third of cases chronic Chagas disease develops with heart failure as the most frequent and severe clinical manifestation [2].

Leishmania spp. occur worldwide and are the causative agents for a broad spectrum of diseases. Clinical syndromes are cutaneous leishmaniasis (oriental sore) caused by *L. major* and *L. tropica* infections. *L. brasiliensis* is responsible for muco-cutaneous leishmaniasis (espundia). Visceral leishmaniasis, also known as kala-azar or black fever, is caused by *L. donovani* and *L. infantum.* It is the most severe form and fatal if left untreated. Trypanosomatids affect about 30 million people and account for half a million of fatalities per year [3]. The different manifestations of trypanosomiasis and leishmaniasis represent neglected tropical diseases (NTDs). Currently, the World Health Organization (WHO) counts 17 NTDs. All of them are diseases that thrive in impoverished settings, especially in the heat and humidity of tropical climates. NTDs are preventable infectious diseases that have been largely neglected by major stakeholders including media, governments, and organizations working in the health sector [4]. Despite their medical importance, commercial drug development approaches were/are negligible.

Present Chemotherapy of Trypanosomiasis and Leishmaniasis

Less than a dozen drugs are currently available for the chemotherapy of trypanoso-matid-related diseases. Many of them were introduced more than 50 years ago and suffer from severe adverse effects and/or increasing resistance development. Early-stage sleeping sickness caused by *T. b. gambiense* is treated by pentamidine. The aromatic diamidine accumulates in the parasite to millimolar concentrations [5] and tightly interacts with DNA, but numerous other targets have been proposed as well [6]. *T. b. rhodesiense* infections are treated with suramin. At physiological pH, suramin bears six negative charges and inhibits many enzymes by electrostatic interactions [6]. As soon as the parasites have crossed the blood–brain barrier (BBB), pentamidine and suramin are no longer effective. In this second/late stage of sleeping sickness chemotherapy is based on melarsoprol, a trivalent arsenical responsible for drug-related death in about 5% of treatments. The arsenical forms a stable adduct with trypanothione, $T(SH)_2$, named MelT [7]. A recent genome-scale RNA interference (RNAi) target sequencing screen identified a link between melarsoprol resistance and trypanothione synthetase (TryS) and trypanothione reductase (TR), suggesting that MelT is toxic for the parasite [8]. On the other hand, depletion of the cellular $T(SH)_2$ levels results in an increased sensitivity of *T. brucei* to melarsen oxide, the antimonial triostam, as well as nifurtimox [9], indicating that the dithiol plays a central role in the mode of action of different anti-trypanosomal drugs.

In the case of a *T. b. gambiense* infection, difluoromethylornithine (DFMO, eflornithin) is an alternative drug. The specificity of this suicide inhibitor of ornithine decarboxylase (ODC) is due to the fact that the *T. b. gambiense* enzyme has an *in vivo* half-live of about 18 h in contrast to the rapidly turned-over mammalian ODC [10]. A novel approach towards safer treatment of late-stage *T. b. gambiense* infections is a nifurtimox–eflornithine combination therapy (NECT) [11].

Treatment of Chagas disease is based on nifurtimox and benznidazol (Radanil$^®$), nitroheterocyclic prodrugs [12]. *T. cruzi* and *T. brucei* possess a type I nitroreductase (NTR) that catalyzes the two-electron reduction of nifurtimox [13], the final product being a toxic unsaturated open-chain nitrile [14]. Since type I NTRs are missing in mammalian cells, this mechanism could explain the selectivity of the drug towards the parasites. The anti-parasitic mechanism of benznidazole may be similar to that of nifurtimox.

For the past seven decades, pentavalent antimonials such as sodium stibogluconate and meglumine antimoniate have been the standard first-line treatment for visceral leishmaniasis. These chelates of Sb(V) require reductive activation to the Sb(III) state [15,16]. Several modes of actions have been proposed [17], one being the direct interference with the parasite thiol metabolism [18]. Other drugs against visceral leishmaniasis are the antibiotics amphotericin B and paromomycin, and the alkylphosphocholine miltefosine. Improved lipid formulations of the compounds have been obtained [19]. Unfortunately, these new drugs are very expensive and thus unavailable for the majority of patients. Taken together, several of the current drugs against trypanosomatids, such as DFMO, melarsoprol, and the antimonials, directly or indirectly interfere with the parasite thiol redox metabolism, underlining the essential role of the trypanothione system.

Unique Thiol Redox Metabolism of Trypanosomatids as a Target Area for Future Drug Development

Trypanosomatids show a large number of biochemical, morphological, and genetic peculiarities, one being their thiol redox metabolism. Trypanosomatids lack glutathione reductase (GR) and thioredoxin reductase (TrxR) as well as catalase and selenocysteine-containing glutathione peroxidases (GPXs). While in most organisms the glutathione (GSH)/GR and thioredoxin (Trx)/TrxR systems maintain the cellular thiol homeostasis, trypanosomatids possess a redox metabolism that is based on trypanothione (bis(glutathionyl)spermidine; $T(SH)_2$) [20] and the flavoenzyme TR [21–24].

$T(SH)_2$ is synthesized from glutathione and spermidine. Glutathione itself is generated by two reactions catalyzed by γ-glutamylcysteine synthetase (GSH1) and glutathione synthetase (GSH2), enzymes common to those in mammalian cells. In *T. brucei*, spermidine is also obtained by *de novo* synthesis while *T. cruzi* and *Leishmania* mainly take up polyamines from their host cell [23]. The final conjugation of two GSH molecules with spermidine is catalyzed by TryS [3] (Figure 21.1).

$T(SH)_2$ is an excellent spontaneous reductant of dehydroascorbate, GSSG, and ovothiol disulfide, and acts as cofactor in the parasite glyoxalase system. Many of the $T(SH)_2$-dependent reactions are mediated by tryparedoxin (Tpx), a distant relative of thioredoxins and glutaredoxins. Tpx transfers the reducing equivalents from $T(SH)_2$ to ribonucleotide reductase, methionine sulfoxide reductase as well as 2-Cys-peroxiredoxins (2-Cys-Prxs) and non-selenium GPX-type enzymes (nsGPXs) [23].

The absence of the trypanothione system from mammals and the lack of a functional redundancy within the parasite render the components of this metabolism attractive drug target molecules [3,25,26]. All proteins of the trypanothione system studied so far such as GSH1 [27,28], ODC [29], spermidine synthase [29], TryS [9,30], TR [31–33], Tpx [34,35] as well as the cytosolic 2-Cys-Prx and nsGPX-type enzymes [34,36,37] have been shown to be essential, and several of them are currently investigated as putative drug targets [3].

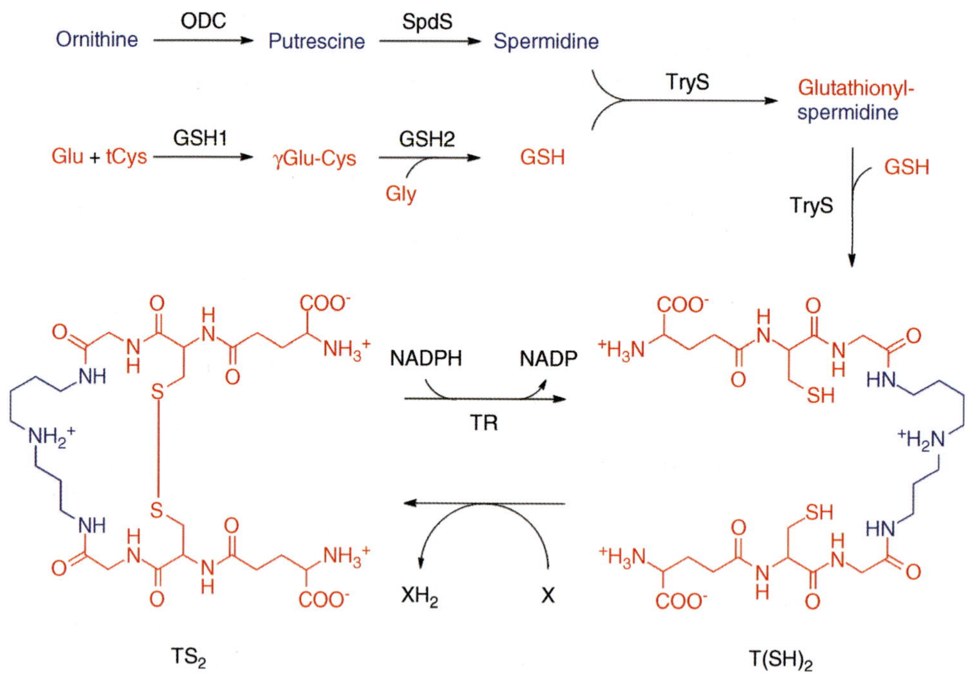

Figure 21.1 Synthesis and reduction of trypanothione in African trypanosomes. ODC, ornithine decarboxylase; SpdS, spermidine synthase; GSH1, γ-glutamylcysteine synthetase; GSH2, glutathione synthetase; TryS, trypanothione synthetase; TR, trypanothione reductase; $T(SH)_2$, trypanothione; TS_2, trypanothione disulfide; X, oxidized substrate, XH_2, reduced substrate.

TR is a Validated Drug Target

Since trypanosomatids lack GR and TrxR, TR is the only enzyme that connects the NADPH- and thiol-redox systems [22–24]. The enzyme is essential for all trypanosomatids studied so far. Viable *L. donovani* devoid of TR activity could not be obtained and gene replacement was only possible upon episomal coexpression of the TR-coding sequence [32]. *Leishmania* with 15% remaining TR activity did not show a growth defect under axenic culture conditions but their survival inside activated macrophages was significantly impaired [31]. In conditional knockout cell lines of bloodstream *T. brucei*, the TR activity could be lowered to less than 10% of wild-type activity. These parasites became highly sensitive to exogenous hydrogen peroxide and were avirulent in an animal infection model [33].

Essentiality is a prerequisite for a drug target molecule but a number of other criteria have to be achieved as well [38,39]. Most of them are perfectly fulfilled by TR. The recombinant protein is available in large quantities and highly stable. The same is true for trypanothione disulfide (TS$_2$), its unique substrate [40]. The active sites of TR and human GR, the closest related host enzyme, are sufficiently different. A drawback may be that the activity of TR has to be lowered by 90% or more to affect parasite survival [33]. This implies that a competitive inhibitor must have a very high affinity, a conclusion corroborated by a recent metabolic control analysis [38]. Thus, non-competitive or irreversible inhibitors may be attractive alternatives. Drugs that covalently attach to their target are traditionally considered as unfavorable. However, covalent inhibitors have proved to be successful therapies for various indications and about one third of all approved covalent drugs are anti-infectives [41].

Structural Comparison of TR and Human GR

TR and GR are both members of the large protein family of FAD-dependent disulfide oxidoreductase comprising also TrxR and lipoamide dehydrogenase. The enzymes are homodimers whose subunits fold into four domains: FAD-binding, NAD(P)H-binding, central, and interface domains. The three-dimensional (3-D) structures of free human GR and of several ligand complexes are known [25]. Crystal structures of TR have been solved for the free enzyme [42–45], with bound trypanothione [46] and NADPH [43], with a covalently bound mepacrine mustard [47] as well as in complex with mepacrine [48], the first tricyclic ligand shown to inhibit TR [49]. Most recently, the 3-D structure of TR in complex with a dihydroquinazoline has been obtained [50].

Despite an overall sequence identity of about 40% and closely related three-dimensional structures, TR and GR show a mutually exclusive specificity with respect to their disulfide substrates. TS$_2$ differs from glutathione disulfide (GSSG) by the presence of the spermidine bridge and thus may require more space in the active site. Indeed, TR has a rather extended active site with dimensions of about $15 \times 15 \times 20\,\text{Å}^3$ (Figure 21.2) [42]. The most important difference between both substrates is that GSSG carries a net charge of -2, whereas TS$_2$ has an overall charge of $+1$. This is mirrored by the opposite charge distribution in the active sites of the

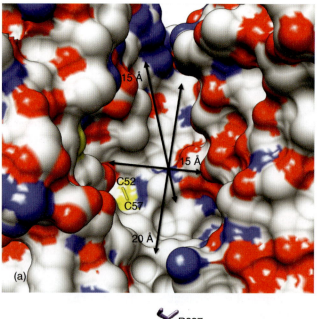

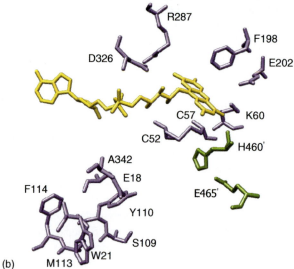

Figure 21.2 Schematic presentation of the active site of *T. cruzi* TR. (a) Top view into the large trypanothione disulfide binding site having dimensions of about $15 \times 15 \times 20\,\text{Å}^3$ (arrows). The disulfide bridge between C52 and C57 in the oxidized form of the enzyme is indicated. The cofactor FAD is not visible because it is buried in the protein structure. On the solvent-accessible surface nitrogen atoms are depicted in blue, oxygens in red, and sulfur atoms in yellow. (b) The isoalloxazine ring of the cofactor FAD (yellow) forms the center of the active site.

NADPH binds at the re-site, while TS$_2$ binds at the si-site of the flavin ring where also the redox active dithiol/disulfide couple of C52–C57 is located. E18 (A34 in human GR), W21 (R37), S109 (I113), M113 (N117), and A342 (R347) are the five residues in the active site that are not conserved when comparing TR with human GR. Primed residues (green) are provided by the second subunit of the homodimeric protein. The substitution of A34 and R37 by Glu and Trp, respectively, converts human GR in an enzyme with TR activity and vice versa.

enzymes. GR has a hydrophilic, positively charged region that interacts with the glycine carboxylates of GSSG, while the active site of TR is lined by hydrophobic and negatively charged residues to accommodate the spermidine moiety of TS_2 (Figure 21.2b). Mutation of two or three residues (most important: A34 → E18 and R37 → W21, additionally R347 → A343) in the active sites of both proteins is sufficient to convert GR into an enzyme with TR activity and vice versa [51–53]. Charge has been shown to be also a major discriminating factor for GR versus TR inhibitors [54]. Since the discovery of trypanothione in 1985 [20], a large number of compounds have been detected that inhibit TR but not the host GR [25,55–59]. In summary, the development of compounds that inhibit TR but do not interfere with human GR is clearly feasible.

Screening Approaches Towards TR

Current State of the Art

TR has been subjected to a number of virtual and chemical screening campaigns. The first virtual screening approach [60] employed a rigid-body docking algorithm to predict binding affinities of ligands to TR. In total, 500 molecular sketches were analyzed, resulting in a variety of compounds that proved to have some inhibitory potency. Most of the compounds possessed typical features of TR inhibitors, namely the presence of aromatic groups and (poly) amino chains [60]. Virtual screening of about 1 million commercially available chemicals towards the TS_2-binding site of TR revealed 25 *in silico* hits. In the subsequent kinetic analysis two structurally new types of ligands emerged, the anti-microbial chlorhexidine (competitive, $K_i = 2\,\mu M$) and a piperidine derivative (mixed type, $K_i = 6.2\,\mu M$ and $K_i' = 8.5\,\mu M$) [61]. A computational approach combining ligand similarity and protein docking methods identified several novel chemotypes that inhibit *T. cruzi* and *T. brucei* TR. The best inhibitor was a dibenzooxathiepine which in the 5,5'-dithiobis(2-nitrobenzoic acid) (DTNB; Ellman's reagent)-coupled assay (see Section Combined *In Vitro/In Silica Screening Campaign*) showed an IC_{50} value of $11\,\mu M$ [62]. Ligand- and structure-based methodologies were recently combined to develop a fast virtual screening protocol. Nineteen known competitive inhibitors of TR with different scaffolds and physicochemical properties were selected, and for each of the ligands up to 500 conformations were docked into the active site of the enzyme. Subsequently the ASINEX database (www.asinex.com) was screened for molecules with a shape similar to that of the reference inhibitors. The resulting compounds were evaluated for a correct alignment of electrostatic fields between reference and database ligands. The best inhibitor showed a K_i value of $5.7\,\mu M$ against recombinant *T. cruzi* TR. Docking approaches suggest that the extended phenyl-imidazol substituent of the compound is partially inserted in the tunnel that connects the TS_2-binding site with the cavity at the 2-fold axis of the homodimer [63].

For real high-throughput screening approaches, an automated protocol was developed that is based on a TR assay in which a low TS_2 concentration, usually

$6\,\mu M$ or less, is kept constant by the presence of excess DTNB. The apparent K_m value of *T. cruzi* TR for TS$_2$ has been reported to be 9.1 [64], 1.5 [65] or 10.4 μM [45] in comparison to values of 18 [66] or 29.6 μM [45] measured in the direct assay. The main rational for the development of this coupled assay system was to reduce the high costs for TS$_2$ [64]. However, the system also has some problems. Compounds may react with DTNB [67] or weak competitive inhibitors may be selected and indicate artificially low K_i values. We have recently established an enzymatic method for the production of TS$_2$ in large quantities at costs that are less than 1% of the commercial product [40]. This should allow future high-throughput screenings using the direct assay.

Based on the coupled assay system, various screenings have been reported. Analysis of a library of 62 000 diverse compounds identified five series of putative hit compounds. For two series based on a quinoline and pyrimidopyridazine, respectively, a large number of analogs was synthesized. Most of the derivatives inhibited TR with IC$_{50}$ or K_i values in the low micromolar range and did not affect human GR. Unfortunately, none of the compounds had a potency that was likely to be of therapeutic significance [55]. The analysis of a chemical library of 100 000 "lead-like" structures identified 120 compounds with IC$_{50}$ values ranging from 1 to 67 μM, which belonged to 12 distinct structural classes. Based on their activities in whole-cell assays, five classes were selected for further investigations. However, no correlation between the anti-parasitic effect and inhibition of TR was observed [65]. Screening of 1266 pharmacologically active compounds from the Sigma-Aldrich LOPAC 1280 library against TR, followed by evaluation of the 22 most potent molecules against human GR as well as cultured *T. brucei*, revealed three new classes of TR inhibitors. One of the compounds was a piperazine with a diphenylmethane substituent. Cyclization of this moiety resulted in a potent competitive inhibitor of TR ($K_i = 331$ nM) that affected the growth of *T. brucei* with an EC$_{50}$ value of 775 nM [57] and kept inactivity towards the host GR. The second hit compound was indatraline, also acting as a linear competitive inhibitor of TR. Indatraline is a monoamine reuptake inhibitor and thus active in the central nervous system. This rendered the molecule suitable as a starting point for the development of compounds against late-stage African sleeping sickness. Novel analogs of indatraline were synthesized but none of them showed improved potency as TR inhibitor when compared to the original lead [68]. The third hit was BTCP, a dopamine uptake inhibitor. BTCP was considered to be a promising starting molecule for further development due to its low molecular mass and its ability to cross the BBB. Newly synthesized analogs retained the potency to act as competitive inhibitors of TR but were only marginally more active against *T. brucei* compared to mammalian cells [69]. A modeling-based *de novo* synthesis of compounds linking BTCP with diaryl sulfide-based inhibitors resulted in conjugates with improved inhibitory potency that probably occupy two different binding sites within the wide active center of TR [70]. The compounds displayed activity towards different trypanosomatids but also the malarial parasite *Plasmodium falciparum*, and thus no correlation between TR inhibition and *in vitro* activity. In summary, for most of the TR inhibitors identified so far a low correlation between enzyme inhibition and anti-parasitic activity has been observed, indicating that the reductase may not be the main cellular target. However, this could also, at least partially, be due to the uptake profiles of the individual compounds in the parasite and/or the screening system employed.

Combined *In Vitro/In Silico* Screening Campaign

In target-based drug discovery projects, virtual screening or *in silico* screenings are alternative or complementary approaches to *in vitro* screening campaigns. They provide several advantages compared to their assay-based counterparts: (i) there is almost no limitation on the number of compounds that can be analyzed (several millions of compounds can be screened with common high-performance computing clusters), (ii) virtual screenings are cheap, because testing is done without purchasing any compounds, and (iii) virtual screening can be performed on enumerated combinatorial libraries without the requirements of a physically available compound. If the 3-D structure of the target to be addressed is known like in the case of TR, *in silico* screening campaigns usually try to identify novel inhibitors by high-throughput docking approaches or structure-based pharmacophore searches [71–73]. Although several crystal structures of TR are available in the Protein Data Bank [74], their applicability for common straight structure-based *in silico* screenings is very limited or even inappropriate. In comparison to other druggable protein targets like kinases or proteases, the active site of TR is an extremely wide building a cleft of $15 \times 15 \times 20 \, \text{Å}^3$, which allows many different binding modes and the simultaneous binding of more than one ligand (Figure 21.2a). In addition, the large hydrophobic cavity does not provide many directed interactions like hydrogen bonds between the protein and the ligand, and the hydrophobic moieties are not well defined. Therefore, the binding mode of even very similar compounds is unpredictable and docking approaches often result in numerous different ligand conformations spread all over the active site without showing a favored binding mode. As a result, docking applications are not able to discriminate between active and non-active structures. On the other hand, common ligand-based pharmacophore searches are also not applicable, because known TR inhibitors are structurally diverse and do not share the same pharmacophore. As a consequence, many computational screening approaches showed modest results in the past. More successful virtual screening approaches as described above faced the limitations by implementing hybrid methods that combine ligand- and structure-based screening methods or to incorporate other ligand information retrieved from known TR inhibitors. In all these approaches the ligand-based filters result in a small focused dataset of potential TR inhibitors that are subsequently docked into the active site of TR while often using some kinds of additional constraints.

Here, we describe an alternative strategy that combines *in vitro* and *in silico* methods (Figure 21.3) [75]. In a first step, an *in vitro* screening campaign of a structurally highly diverse compound set was performed to identify novel *in vitro* hits that are able to inhibit TR. The identified chemical entities were then used as a starting point for further ligand-based *in silico* screening campaigns that led to an

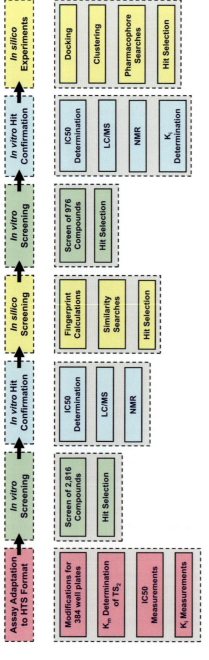

Figure 21.3 Workflow combining *in vitro* and *in silico* approaches to identify novel TR inhibitors.

enriched focused dataset containing *in silico* hits with an increased potential towards TR. The focused dataset was again tested in a following *in vitro* screening. The result was a dataset with numerous novel and validated TR inhibitors. Finally, the knowledge of these structurally diverse inhibitors was used in a novel *in silico* approach that established a new access towards structure-based virtual screening of TR like high-throughput docking and pharmacophore searches.

TR Assay Adaptation

The *in vitro* screening was based on a photometric assay composed of TS_2, NADPH, and TR following NADPH consumption at 340 nm [66]. This assay is known to produce highly reliable data and avoids putative site reactions that may occur in coupled setups. As the conventional assay in a 1-ml cuvette format was not suited for the screening of a large compound library, it was adapted to a 50-µl format in 384-well plates. Bovine serum albumin (0.1 mg/ml) and 0.01% detergent were added to stabilize the enzyme and to prevent adhesion, reduce surface tensions in the wells, and the formation of droplets at the pipetting steps. In addition, high concentrations of the substrate TS_2 were used to mimic high oxidative stress conditions, to enlarge the measurement window, and to discriminate against weak competitive inhibitors. To evaluate the successful adaptation of the assay, the measured kinetic data were compared with those obtained in a cuvette-based format [66]. Our measurements were carried out as end-point determinations using the total Δ of absorption decrease at 340 nm after 30 min for calculating the kinetic constants. The obtained K_m value for TS_2 and K_i values for three known inhibitors (chlorhexidine, mepacrine, and BG237 (compound 8 in [76])) were in excellent agreement with the published values [49,61,76].

In Vitro Screening

After the adaption of the assay for high-throughput purposes, an initial *in vitro* screen with 2816 compounds was conducted. The substances represented a structurally highly diverse subset of a screening library containing 200 000 chemicals. The three known TR inhibitors mepacrine, BG237, and chlorhexidine were included as controls. All compounds were studied at a concentration of 20 µM in the presence of 150 µM TS_2. The final concentration of dimethylsulfoxide in the assay was 2%. Statistical assay data analysis revealed $Z' \geq 0.87$ that proved the robustness of the assay. By using an inhibition threshold of 30% we obtained 64 *in vitro* hits, which resulted in a reasonable hit rate of 1.8% [75].

To confirm the identified hits, IC_{50} determinations and structure verification experiments were performed. For the IC_{50} values, 11 substance concentrations ranging from 100 µM to 10 nM were studied. In total, 29 *in vitro* hits were validated by IC_{50} measurements and 21 compounds passed the structural validation by liquid chromatography-mass spectrometry (LC-MS) and nuclear magnetic resonance (NMR). The 21 actives showed IC_{50} values down to 1.15 µM and thus were more

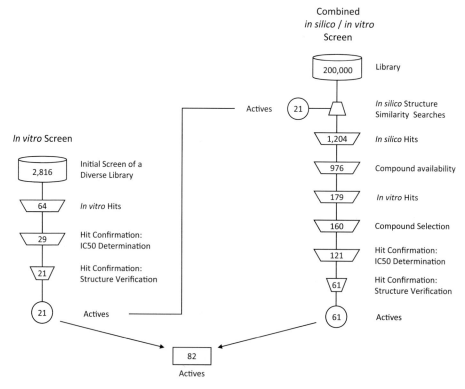

Figure 21.4 Results of the *in vitro/in silico* screening workflow. After screening the highly diverse compound set of 2816 compounds, 21 active compounds could be identified, and their structure and purity confirmed by LC-MS and NMR. The actives were then used as the query base for an *in silico* structure similarity search with the aim to create an activity-enriched compound set. The set of 1204 compounds resulted in additional 61 actives, leading to a total of 82 novel TR inhibitors.

potent than the known competitive inhibitor chlorhexidine with a K_i of 2 μM [61] and an IC_{50} of 45 μM. Taken together, this initial *in vitro* setup resulted in a set of 21 novel, highly active TR inhibitors that were then used as basis for the following *in silico* screening campaign [75] (Figure 21.4).

In Silico Screening

Similarity searches were performed for the 21 confirmed hits on a database of 200 000 compounds. As the molecular properties responsible for the on-target activity of these compounds were not known, six fingerprints were used instead of only one molecular descriptor. The fingerprints were selected to cover different structural aspects of the hits such as similar topology, similar structural fragments, and pharmacophoric features. The similarity search workflow itself was implemented within the software Pipeline Pilot (www.accelrys.com). Only the 13 best *in silico* hits per query compound and fingerprint were selected, and duplicates retrieved by different similarity searches were removed. Finally, a focused compound dataset was generated containing 1204 novel potential structures that could be tested in the next *in vitro* screen [75] (Figure 21.4).

Second *In Vitro* Screen

Only 976 of the 1204 compounds identified in the *in silico*-enriched dataset were available in reasonable amounts and thus could be studied in the second *in vitro* screening campaign. While the first *in vitro* screening resulted in 64 hits, the second screening was capable of identifying additional 179 hits showing an inhibition of 30% or more, although the first dataset was almost 3 times as large (2816 versus 976 compounds) (Figure 21.4). This corresponds to a hit rate of 17%, which was nearly 10 times higher than that in the initial screen and clearly demonstrates the success of the *in silico* virtual screening cycle to deliver an activity-enriched dataset (Figure 21.5). In total, 160 hits were selected manually for hit confirmation. After determining the IC_{50} values with 11 concentrations ranging from 200 μM to 3 nM, and after structural confirmation, 61 additional, newly confirmed actives were identified. In summary, our combined *in vitro/in silico* approach led to the

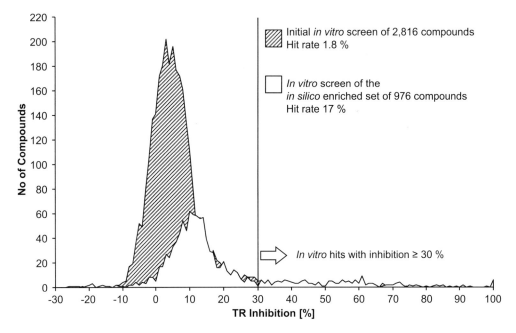

Figure 21.5 Activity distribution of the performed *in vitro* screenings. Histogram showing the percentage of TR inhibition plotted against the number of compounds. The overall activity of the *in silico*-enriched dataset is shifted to the right when compared with the initial *in vitro* screen dataset. Importantly, the second screen delivered more *in vitro* hits that showed an inhibition of 30% or more.

identification of 82 novel TR inhibitors with IC_{50} values down to the nanomolar range. Currently, the 10 most active and structurally diverse TR inhibitors are being tested in parasite cell culture assays.

Consensus Pharmacophore Building

The detailed kinetic analysis of the most potent inhibitors revealed an uncompetitive type of inhibition [75]. This together with the pronounced structural similarity of all actives suggested that most compounds bind in the active site and probably share similar binding modes. To validate this hypothesis, a set of 120 compounds (the 82 actives plus 38 additional related compounds) was prepared for docking using the Gold docking-software [77]. The X-ray structure of *T. cruzi* TR [46] was prepared for the docking using the software MOE (www.chemcomp.com) by removing the substrate and water molecules, and assigning hydrogens and ionizations states. Each ligand structure was docked into a grid around the active site with a radius of 1.5 nm leading to a maximum of 50 poses per compound. All resulting 6000 poses were inspected and showed no accumulation into specific parts of the pocket. Moreover, several highly similar compounds showed high-scored poses in different areas of the pocket with different orientations (Figure 21.6a). Nevertheless, we were confident to find an inherent higher degree of order within the poses that was not obvious by this first visual overview. To detect the hidden presence of predominant binding modes, all poses were analyzed regarding existing pose clusters using the Drugscore^{Maps} approach [78]. Here, the docking poses are clustered by means of a protein–ligand fingerprint [79] and emergent self-organizing maps [80]. Using this approach, the high-dimensional protein–ligand interaction space is projected into a two-dimensional (2-D) landscape representation that visualizes binding mode clusters in an intuitive way. In a preliminary step, the fconv application [81] was used to create a decreased dataset of 600 poses. The poses for each molecule were clustered regarding the root mean square deviation between the poses. For each cluster, a representative was chosen for each cluster and the five best-scored representative poses were chosen for the Drugscore^{Maps} clustering. In the final 2-D landscape visualization (Figure 21.6b), clusters of poses with similar binding modes can easily be identified as green valleys that are separated by brown hills from other pose clusters with different binding modes. Indeed several major clusters could be identified by manual inspection proving the success of our search for the "needle" in the former "haystack." Additional investigations showed that the most active *in vitro* compound is represented in two different major pose clusters with high-scored docking poses sharing interactions with other active compounds of the corresponding cluster. These two binding poses might be considered as potential binding modes [75].

These initial and promising results led to a more detailed analysis of all clusters and their corresponding protein–ligand binding modes, which is still ongoing. As a preliminary result, the protein–ligand interaction fingerprints tool of the MOE package was used to aggregate the ligand–protein interactions observed in manually selected binding mode clusters. Hereby, interactions like hydrogen bonds, ionic

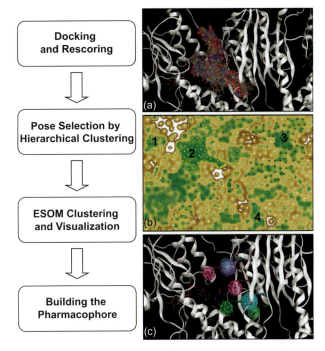

Docking and Rescoring

Pose Selection by Hierarchical Clustering

ESOM Clustering and Visualization

Building the Pharmacophore

Figure 21.6 Building of a consensus pharmacophore by docking and clustering experiments. (a) Active compounds were docked in the active site of TR using the docking program Gold. (b) After a pose selection by a hierarchical clustering, the protein–ligand interaction fingerprints of the selected poses were calculated and clustered using Drugscore^Maps. The data was analyzed by the map in which each dot represents a docking pose. The poses can either be located in green valleys or are separated by brownish hills. If docking poses fall together in one valley, they share the same space and interactions within the binding site. Finally, four separate pose clusters (1–4) were identified including the most frequent interactions with the target. (c) The resulting clusters were analyzed using the Protein Ligand Interaction Fingerprints of MOE and a consensus pharmacophore derived from the observed interaction was built. Green spheres represent a hydrophobic feature, magenta spheres represent hydrogen-bond donor heavy atom and cyan spheres represent hydrogen-bond acceptor heavy atom. The purple spheres represent either a hydrogen-bond donor or acceptor atom.

interactions, and surface contacts of protein–ligand complexes were classified according to the protein residue of origin and translated into a corresponding pharmacophore feature. Finally, this led to a consensus pharmacophore representing probably potential interaction features and excluded volumes (Figure 21.6c). In a structure-based virtual screening campaign this pharmacophore query was used to search a database containing 4 million compounds available from various suppliers. Finally, the pharmacophore approach resulted in 1189 *in silico* hits that were subsequently docked into the active site of TR using the Gold docking software [77]. The 100 top-ranked docking hits were selected and are currently in the process of *in vitro* testing.

Conclusion

TR is a validated target protein and was addressed in various target-based screening approaches in the past leading to the identification of novel inhibitors. The active site of TR is an extremely wide cleft with only few directed interaction features. Unfortunately, this fact prevents a successful and rational application of structure-based *in silico* screening approaches. We could overcome this situation by combining *in vitro* and ligand-based *in silico* methods, and were able to identify 82 novel TR inhibitors by this combined approach. Future experiments will show the potential of these compounds on the parasite itself.

References

1 Ilemobade, A.A. (2009) Tsetse and trypanosomosis in Africa: the challenges, the opportunities. *Onderstepoort J. Vet. Res.*, **76**, 35–40.

2 Rassi, A. and Marin-Neto, J.A. (2010) Chagas disease. *Lancet*, **375**, 1388–1402.

3 Flohé, L. (2011) The trypanothione system and the opportunities it offers to create drugs for the neglected kinetoplast diseases. *Biotechnol. Adv.*, **30**, 294–301.

4 Pokhrel, S., Reidpath, D., and Allotey, P. (2011) Social sciences research in neglected tropical diseases 3: investment in social science research in neglected diseases of poverty: a case study of Bill and Melinda Gates Foundation. *Health Res. Policy Syst.*, **9**, 2.

5 Carter, N.S., Berger, B.J., and Fairlamb, A.H. (1995) Uptake of diamidine drugs by the P2 nucleoside transporter in melarsen-sensitive and -resistant *Trypanosoma brucei brucei*. *J. Biol. Chem.*, **270**, 28153–28157.

6 Denise, H. and Barrett, M.P. (2001) Uptake and mode of action of drugs used against sleeping sickness. *Biochem. Pharmacol.*, **61**, 1–5.

7 Fairlamb, A.H., Henderson, G.B., and Cerami, A. (1989) Trypanothione is the primary target for arsenical drugs against African trypanosomes. *Proc. Natl. Acad. Sci. USA*, **86**, 2607–2611.

8 Alsford, S., Eckert, S., Baker, N., Glover, L., Sanchez-Flores, A., Leung, K.F., Turner, D. J. *et al.* (2012) High-throughput decoding of antitrypanosomal drug efficacy and resistance. *Nature*, **482**, 232–236.

9 Ariyanayagam, M.R., Oza, S.L., Guther, M. L., and Fairlamb, A.H. (2005) Phenotypic analysis of trypanothione synthetase knockdown in the African trypanosome. *Biochem. J.*, **391**, 425–432.

10 Iten, M., Mett, H., Evans, A., Enyaru, J.C., Brun, R., and Kaminsky, R. (1997) Alterations in ornithine decarboxylase characteristics account for tolerance of *Trypanosoma brucei rhodesiense* to D,L-alpha-difluoromethylornithine. *Antimicrob. Agents Chemother.*, **41**, 1922–1925.

11 Priotto, G., Kasparian, S., Mutombo, W., Ngouama, D., Ghorashian, S., Arnold, U., Ghabri, S. *et al.* (2009) Nifurtimox–eflornithine combination therapy for second-stage African *Trypanosoma brucei gambiense* trypanosomiasis: a multicentre, randomised, phase III, non-inferiority trial. *Lancet*, **374**, 56–64.

12 Wilkinson, S.R., Bot, C., Kelly, J.M., and Hall, B.S. (2011) Trypanocidal activity of nitroaromatic prodrugs: current treatments and future perspectives. *Curr. Top. Med. Chem.*, **11**, 2072–2084.

13 Wilkinson, S.R., Taylor, M.C., Horn, D., Kelly, J.M., and Cheeseman, I. (2008) A mechanism for cross-resistance to nifurtimox and benznidazole in trypanosomes. *Proc. Natl. Acad. Sci. USA*, **105**, 5022–5027.

14 Hall, B.S., Bot, C., and Wilkinson, S.R. (2011) Nifurtimox activation by trypanosomal type I nitroreductases generates cytotoxic nitrile metabolites. *J. Biol. Chem.*, **286**, 13088–13095.

15 Zhou, Y., Messier, N., Ouellette, M., Rosen, B.P., and Mukhopadhyay, R. (2004) *Leishmania major* LmACR2 is a pentavalent antimony reductase that confers sensitivity to the drug pentostam. *J. Biol. Chem.*, **279**, 37445–37451.

16 Denton, H., McGregor, J.C., and Coombs, G.H. (2004) Reduction of anti-leishmanial pentavalent antimonial drugs by a parasite-specific thiol-dependent reductase, TDR1. *Biochem. J.*, **381**, 405–412.

17 Castillo, E., Dea-Ayuela, M.A., Bolas-Fernandez, F., Rangel, M., Gonzalez-Rosende, M.E., Bolás-Fernández, F., and González-Rosende, M.E. (2010) The kinetoplastid chemotherapy revisited: current drugs, recent advances and future perspectives. *Curr. Med. Chem.*, **17**, 4027–4051.

18 Wyllie, S., Cunningham, M.L., and Fairlamb, A.H. (2004) Dual action of antimonial drugs on thiol redox metabolism in the human pathogen *Leishmania donovani*. *J. Biol. Chem.*, **279**, 39925–39932.

19 World Health Organization (2010) Control of the leishmaniases. *World Health Organ. Tech. Rep. Ser.*, (949), xii–xiii, 1–186, back cover.

20 Fairlamb, A.H., Blackburn, P., Ulrich, P., Chait, B.T., and Cerami, A. (1985) Trypanothione: a novel bis(glutathionyl) spermidine cofactor for glutathione reductase in trypanosomatids. *Science*, **227**, 1485–1487.

21 Fairlamb, A.H., Smith, K., and Hunter, K.J. (1992) The interaction of arsenical drugs with dihydrolipoamide and dihydrolipoamide dehydrogenase from arsenical resistant and sensitive strains of *Trypanosoma brucei brucei*. *Mol. Biochem. Parasitol.*, **53**, 223–231.

22 Krauth-Siegel, R.L. and Comini, M.A. (2008) Redox control in trypanosomatids, parasitic protozoa with trypanothione-based thiol metabolism. *Biochim. Biophys. Acta*, **1780**, 1236–1248.

23 Krauth-Siegel, L. and Leroux, A.E. (2012) Low molecular mass antioxidants in parasites. *Antioxid. Redox Signal*, **17**, 583–607.

24 Fairlamb, A.H. and Cerami, A. (1992) Metabolism and functions of trypanothione in the Kinetoplastida. *Ann. Rev. Microbiol.*, **46**, 695–729.

25 Krauth-Siegel, R.L., Bauer, H., and Schirmer, R.H. (2005) Dithiol proteins as guardians of the intracellular redox milieu in parasites: old and new drug targets in trypanosomes and malaria-causing plasmodia. *Angew. Chem. Int. Ed. Engl.*, **44**, 690–715.

26 Jaeger, T. and Flohé, L. (2006) The thiol-based redox networks of pathogens: unexploited targets in the search for new drugs. *BioFactors*, **27**, 109–120.

27 Huynh, T.T., Huynh, V.T., Harmon, M.A., and Phillips, M.A. (2003) Gene knockdown of gamma-glutamylcysteine synthetase by RNAi in the parasitic protozoa *Trypanosoma brucei* demonstrates that it is an essential enzyme. *J. Biol. Chem.*, **278**, 39794–39800.

28 Mukherjee, A., Roy, G., Guimond, C., and Ouellette, M. (2009) The gamma-glutamylcysteine synthetase gene of *Leishmania* is essential and involved in response to oxidants. *Mol. Microbiol.*, **74**, 914–927.

29 Xiao, Y., McCloskey, D.E., and Phillips, M. A. (2009) RNA interference-mediated silencing of ornithine decarboxylase and spermidine synthase genes in *Trypanosoma brucei* provides insight into regulation of polyamine biosynthesis. *Eukaryot. Cell*, **8**, 747–755.

30 Comini, M.A., Guerrero, S.A., Haile, S., Menge, U., Lunsdorf, H., and Flohe, L. (2004) Validation of *Trypanosoma brucei* trypanothione synthetase as drug target. *Free Radic. Biol. Med.*, **36**, 1289–1302.

31 Dumas, C., Ouellette, M., Tovar, J., Cunningham, M.L., Fairlamb, A.H., Tamar, S., Olivier, M. *et al.* (1997) Disruption of the trypanothione reductase gene of *Leishmania* decreases its ability to survive oxidative stress in macrophages. *EMBO J.*, **16**, 2590–2598.

32 Tovar, J., Wilkinson, S., Mottram, J.C., and Fairlamb, A.H. (1998) Evidence that trypanothione reductase is an essential enzyme in *Leishmania* by targeted replacement of the *tryA* gene locus. *Mol. Microbiol.*, **29**, 653–660.

33 Krieger, S., Schwarz, W., Ariyanayagam, M. R., Fairlamb, A.H., Krauth-Siegel, R.L., and

Clayton, C. (2000) Trypanosomes lacking trypanothione reductase are avirulent and show increased sensitivity to oxidative stress. *Mol. Microbiol.*, **35**, 542–552.

34 Wilkinson, S.R., Horn, D., Prathalingam, S.R., and Kelly, J.M. (2003) RNA interference identifies two hydroperoxide metabolizing enzymes that are essential to the bloodstream form of the African trypanosome. *J. Biol. Chem.*, **278**, 31640–31646.

35 Comini, M.A., Krauth-Siegel, R.L., and Flohe, L. (2007) Depletion of the thioredoxin homologue tryparedoxin impairs antioxidative defence in African trypanosomes. *Biochem. J.*, **402**, 43–49.

36 Schlecker, T., Schmidt, A., Dirdjaja, N., Voncken, F., Clayton, C., and Krauth-Siegel, R.L. (2005) Substrate specificity, localization, and essential role of the glutathione peroxidase-type tryparedoxin peroxidases in *Trypanosoma brucei*. *J. Biol. Chem.*, **280**, 14385–14394.

37 Diechtierow, M. and Krauth-Siegel, R.L. (2011) A tryparedoxin-dependent peroxidase protects African trypanosomes from membrane damage. *Free Rad. Biol. Med.*, **51**, 856–868.

38 Olin-Sandoval, V., Moreno-Sanchez, R., and Saavedra, E. (2010) Targeting trypanothione metabolism in trypanosomatid human parasites. *Curr. Drug Targets*, **11**, 1614–1630.

39 Wyatt, P.G., Gilbert, I.H., Read, K.D., and Fairlamb, A.H. (2011) Target validation: linking target and chemical properties to desired product profile. *Curr. Top. Med. Chem.*, **11**, 1275–1283.

40 Comini, M.A., Dirdjaja, N., Kaschel, M., and Krauth-Siegel, R.L. (2009) Preparative enzymatic synthesis of trypanothione and trypanothione analogues. *Int. J. Parasitol.*, **39**, 1059–1062.

41 Singh, J., Petter, R.C., Baillie, T.A., and Whitty, A. (2011) The resurgence of covalent drugs. *Nat. Rev. Drug Discov.*, **10**, 307–317.

42 Kuriyan, J., Kong, X.P., Krishna, T.S., Sweet, R.M., Murgolo, N.J., Field, H., Cerami, A. *et al.* (1991) X-ray structure of trypanothione reductase from *Crithidia fasciculata* at 2.4-A resolution. *Proc. Natl. Acad. Sci. USA*, **88**, 8764–8768.

43 Lantwin, C.B., Schlichting, I., Kabsch, W., Pai, E.F., and Krauth-Siegel, R.L. (1994) The structure of *Trypanosoma cruzi* trypanothione reductase in the oxidized and NADPH reduced state. *Proteins*, **18**, 161–173.

44 Zhang, Y., Bond, C.S., Bailey, S., Cunningham, M.L., Fairlamb, A.H., and Hunter, W.N. (1996) The crystal structure of trypanothione reductase from the human pathogen *Trypanosoma cruzi* at 2.3 A resolution. *Protein Sci.*, **5**, 52–61.

45 Jones, D.C., Ariza, A., Chow, W.H., Oza, S.L., and Fairlamb, A.H. (2010) Comparative structural, kinetic and inhibitor studies of *Trypanosoma brucei* trypanothione reductase with *T. cruzi*. *Mol. Biochem. Parasitol.*, **169**, 12–19.

46 Bond, C.S., Zhang, Y., Berriman, M., Cunningham, M.L., Fairlamb, A.H., and Hunter, W.N. (1999) Crystal structure of *Trypanosoma cruzi* trypanothione reductase in complex with trypanothione, and the structure-based discovery of new natural product inhibitors. *Structure*, **7**, 81–89.

47 Saravanamuthu, A., Vickers, T.J., Bond, C.S., Peterson, M.R., Hunter, W.N., and Fairlamb, A.H. (2004) Two interacting binding sites for quinacrine derivatives in the active site of trypanothione reductase: a template for drug design. *J. Biol. Chem.*, **279**, 29493–29500.

48 Jacoby, E.M., Schlichting, I., Lantwin, C.B., Kabsch, W., and Krauth-Siegel, R.L. (1996) Crystal structure of the *Trypanosoma cruzi* trypanothione reductase.mepacrine complex. *Proteins*, **24**, 73–80.

49 Krauth-Siegel, R.L., Lohrer, H., Bücheler, U.S., and Schirmer, R.H. (1991) The antioxidant enzymes glutathione reductase and trypanothione reductase as drug targets, in *Biochemical Protozoology* (eds G. Coombs and M. North), Taylor & Francis, London, pp 493–505.

50 Patterson, S., Alphey, M.S., Jones, D.C., Shanks, E.J., Street, I.P., Frearson, J.A., Wyatt, P.G. *et al.* (2011) Dihydroquinazolines as a novel class of *Trypanosoma brucei* trypanothione reductase inhibitors: discovery, synthesis, and characterization of their binding mode by protein crystallography. *J. Med. Chem.*, **54**, 6514–6530.

51 Sullivan, F.X., Sobolov, S.B., Bradley, M., and Walsh, C.T. (1991) Mutational analysis of parasite trypanothione reductase: acquisition of glutathione reductase activity in a triple mutant. *Biochemistry*, **30**, 2761–2767.

52 Bradley, M., Bücheler, U.S., and Walsh, C.T. (1991) Redox enzyme engineering: conversion of human glutathione reductase into a trypanothione reductase. *Biochemistry*, **30**, 6124–6127.

53 Stoll, V.S., Simpson, S.J., Krauth-Siegel, R.L., Walsh, C.T., and Pai, E.F. (1997) Glutathione reductase turned into trypanothione reductase: structural analysis of an engineered change in substrate specificity. *Biochemistry*, **36**, 6437–6447.

54 Faerman, C.H., Savvides, S.N., Strickland, C., Breidenbach, M.A., Ponasik, J.A., Ganem, B., Ripoll, D. *et al.* (1996) Charge is the major discriminating factor for glutathione reductase versus trypanothione reductase inhibitors. *Bioorg. Med. Chem.*, **4**, 1247–1253.

55 Spinks, D., Shanks, E.J., Cleghorn, L.A., McElroy, S., Jones, D., James, D., Fairlamb, A.H. *et al.* (2009) Investigation of trypanothione reductase as a drug target in *Trypanosoma brucei*. *Chem. Med. Chem.*, **4**, 2060–2069.

56 Eberle, C., Burkhard, J.A., Stump, B., Kaiser, M., Brun, R., Krauth-Siegel, R.L., and Diederich, F. (2009) Synthesis, inhibition potency, binding mode, and antiprotozoal activities of fluorescent inhibitors of trypanothione reductase based on mepacrine-conjugated diaryl sulfide scaffolds. *Chem. Med. Chem.*, **4**, 2034–2044.

57 Richardson, J.L., Nett, I.R., Jones, D.C., Abdille, M.H., Gilbert, I.H., and Fairlamb, A.H. (2009) Improved tricyclic inhibitors of trypanothione reductase by screening and chemical synthesis. *Chem. Med. Chem.*, **4**, 1333–1340.

58 Schmidt, A. and Krauth-Siegel, R.L. (2002) Enzymes of the trypanothione metabolism as targets for antitrypanosomal drug development. *Curr. Top. Med. Chem.*, **2**, 1239–1259.

59 Moreira, D.R.M., Leite, A.C.L., Santos, R.R., and dos and Soares, M.B.P. (2009) Approaches for the development of new anti-*Trypanosoma cruzi* agents. *Curr. Drug Targets*, **10**, 212–231.

60 Horvath, D. (1997) A virtual screening approach applied to the search for trypanothione reductase inhibitors. *J. Med. Chem.*, **40**, 2412–2423.

61 Meiering, S., Inhoff, O., Mies, J., Vincek, A., Garcia, G., Kramer, B., Dormeyer, M. *et al.* (2005) Inhibitors of *Trypanosoma cruzi* trypanothione reductase revealed by virtual screening and parallel synthesis. *J. Med. Chem.*, **48**, 4793–4802.

62 Perez-Pineiro, R., Burgos, A., Jones, D.C., Andrew, L.C., Rodriguez, H., Suarez, M., Fairlamb, A.H. *et al.* (2009) Development of a novel virtual screening cascade protocol to identify potential trypanothione reductase inhibitors. *J. Med. Chem.*, **52**, 1670–1680.

63 Maccari, G., Jaeger, T., Moraca, F., Biava, M., Flohe, L., and Botta, M. (2011) A fast virtual screening approach to identify structurally diverse inhibitors of trypanothione reductase. *Bioorg. Med. Chem. Lett.*, **21**, 5255–5258.

64 Hamilton, C.J., Saravanamuthu, A., Eggleston, I.M., and Fairlamb, A.H. (2003) Ellman's-reagent-mediated regeneration of trypanothione *in situ*: substrate-economical microplate and time-dependent inhibition assays for trypanothione reductase. *Biochem. J.*, **369**, 529–537.

65 Holloway, G.A., Charman, W.N., Fairlamb, A.H., Brun, R., Kaiser, M., Kostewicz, E., Novello, P.M. *et al.* (2009) Trypanothione reductase high-throughput screening campaign identifies novel classes of inhibitors with antiparasitic activity. *Antimicrob. Agents Chemother.*, **53**, 2824–2833.

66 Jockers-Scherübl, M.C., Schirmer, R.H., and Krauth-Siegel, R.L. (1989) Trypanothione reductase from *Trypanosoma cruzi*. Catalytic properties of the enzyme and inhibition studies with trypanocidal compounds. *Eur. J. Biochem.*, **180**, 267–272.

67 Martyn, D.C., Jones, D.C., Fairlamb, A.H., and Clardy, J. (2007) High-throughput screening affords novel and selective trypanothione reductase inhibitors with anti-trypanosomal activity. *Bioorg. Med. Chem. Lett.*, **17**, 1280–1283.

68 Walton, J.G., Jones, D.C., Kiuru, P., Durie, A.J., Westwood, N.J., and Fairlamb, A.H. (2011) Synthesis and evaluation of indatraline-based inhibitors for trypanothione reductase. *Chem. Med. Chem.*, **6**, 321–328.

69 Patterson, S., Jones, D.C., Shanks, E.J., Frearson, J.A., Gilbert, I.H., Wyatt, P.G., and Fairlamb, A.H. (2009) Synthesis and evaluation of 1-(1-(benzo[*b*]thiophen-2-yl)cyclohexyl)piperidine (BTCP) analogues as inhibitors of trypanothione reductase. *Chem. Med. Chem.*, **4**, 1341–1353.

70 Eberle, C., Lauber, B.S., Fankhauser, D., Kaiser, M., Brun, R., Krauth-Siegel, R.L., and Diederich, F. (2011) Improved inhibitors of trypanothione reductase by combination of motifs: synthesis, inhibitory potency, binding mode, and antiprotozoal activities. *Chem. Med. Chem.*, **6**, 292–301.

71 Selzer, P.M. (2006) Structure-based rational drug design: Neue Wege der modernen Wirkstoffentwicklung, in *Allgemeine Parasitologie* (eds T. Hiepe, R. Lucius, and B. Gottstein), Parey, Stuttgart, pp 422–427.

72 Selzer, P.M., Brutsche, S., Wiesner, P., Schmid, P., and Mullner, H. (2000) Target-based drug discovery for the development of novel antiinfectives. *Int. J. Med. Microbiol.*, **290**, 191–201.

73 Marhöfer, R.J., Oellien, F., and Selzer, P.M. (2011) Drug discovery and the use of computational approaches for infectious diseases. *Future Med. Chem.*, **3**, 1011–1025.

74 Berman, H.M., Westbrook, J., Feng, Z., Gilliland, G., Bhat, T.N., Weissig, H., Shindyalov, I.N. *et al.* (2000) The protein data bank. *Nucleic Acids Res.*, **28**, 235–242.

75 Beig, M., Bender, F., Gassel, M., Krauth-Siegel, R.L., and Selzer, P.M. (2012) *Trypanothione reductase: a target protein for a combined* in silico *and* in vitro *screening approach.* Submitted.

76 Bonse, S., Santelli-Rouvier, C., Barbe, J., and Krauth-Siegel, R.L. (1999) Inhibition of *Trypanosoma cruzi* trypanothione reductase by acridines: kinetic studies and structure–activity relationships. *J. Med. Chem.*, **42**, 5448–5454.

77 Verdonk, M.L., Cole, J.C., Hartshorn, M.J., Murray, C.W., and Taylor, R.D. (2003) Improved protein–ligand docking using GOLD. *Proteins*, **52**, 609–623.

78 Koch, O., Neudert, G., and Klebe, G. (2009) Drugscore[Maps]: visualizing similarities in protein–ligand interactions. *Chem. Central J.*, **3** (Suppl. 1), P61.

79 Neudert, G. and Klebe, G. (2011) DSX: a knowledge-based scoring function for the assessment of protein–ligand complexes. *J. Chem. Inf. Model.*, **51**, 2731–2745.

80 Ultsch, A. and Moerchen, F. (2006) *ESOM-Maps: tools for clustering, visualization, and classification with Emergent SOM. Technical Report 46*, Marburg, Department of Mathematics and Computer Science, Philipps-University of Marburg.

81 Neudert, G. and Klebe, G. (2011) fconv: format conversion, manipulation and feature computation of molecular data. *Bioinformatics*, **27**, 1021–1022.

22
Redox-Active Agents in Reactions Involving the Trypanothione/Trypanothione Reductase-based System to Fight Kinetoplastidal Parasites

Thibault Gendron, Don Antoine Lanfranchi, and Elisabeth Davioud-Charvet[*]

Abstract

African trypanosomiasis, Chagas disease, and leishmaniasis are human infectious diseases caused by various kinetoplastid parasites. Trypanothione reductase (TR) is a flavoenzyme unique to these parasites that is responsible for maintaining trypanothione (bis(glutathionyl)spermidine) in its reduced dithiol form. This enzyme plays a crucial role in the thiol redox metabolism and is essential *in vivo* for all trypanosomatids living in the human host studied so far. These findings make the flavoenzyme a promising target for anti-kinetoplastidal drug development. In this chapter, we examine the work published in the field of redox-active agents acting as substrates of the NADPH-dependent TR-based system. We also highlight our own work on trypanothione-reactive agents and discuss how these compounds might be developed as potential specific lead compounds to fight kinetoplastidal parasites.

Introduction

Flavin-disulfide oxidoreductases are responsible for maintaining the reducing intracellular milieu and thus protect the cell from oxidative injuries. Interference with these antioxidant enzymes is a promising approach for the development of new anti-parasitic drugs [1,2]. The glutathione and the thioredoxin systems represent the two major antioxidant and redox-regulatory principles in mammal cells. Nearly all organisms, including mammals and *Plasmodium falciparum*, the causative agent of tropical malaria, have both, glutathione/glutathione reductase (GR) and thioredoxin/thioredoxin reductase (TrxR) systems (Figure 22.1) [3,4].

By contrast, an alternative central player of these systems is the NADPH-dependent flavoenzyme trypanothione reductase (TR), exclusively found in all kinetoplastideae parasites and *Euglena* algae cells [5–8]. Trypanosomatids include the causative agents of African sleeping sickness (*Trypanosoma brucei gambiense, T. b. rhodesiense*), South American Chagas disease (*T. cruzi*), and Nagana cattle disease (*T. congolense, T. b. brucei, T. vivax*), and the different *Leishmania* species causing the various forms of leishmaniasis, such as Oriental sore (*L. tropica*) or kala-azar (*L. donovani*). These

---

[*] Corresponding Author

Trypanosomatid Diseases: Molecular Routes to Drug Discovery, First edition. Edited by T. Jäger, O. Koch, and L. Flohé.
© 2013 Wiley-VCH Verlag GmbH & Co. KGaA. Published 2013 by Wiley-VCH Verlag GmbH & Co. KGaA.

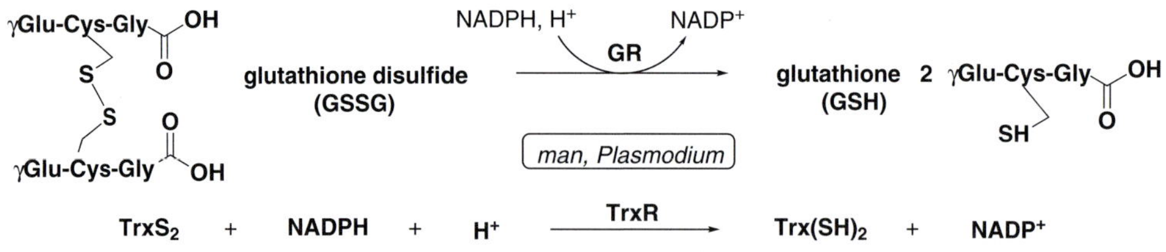

γGlu-Cys-Gly OH
S O
S O
γGlu-Cys-Gly OH
glutathione disulfide
(GSSG)
NADPH, H+
NADP+
GR
man, Plasmodium
glutathione
(GSH)
2 γGlu-Cys-Gly OH
SH O
TrxS2 + NADPH + H+
TrxR
Trx(SH)2 + NADP+

Figure 22.1 NADPH-dependent glutathione/GR and thioredoxin/TrxR systems in the human host.

flagellated protozoa have a unique trypanothione/TR system instead of the GR and TrxR systems (Figure 22.2).

In addition, there are major differences in structure and reactivity of the reductant species governing the flux of the thiols in the antioxidant network of these parasites: the parasitic enzyme system is dependent on trypanothione and other glutathionylspermidines [5,6] as substrates, whereas the corresponding host enzyme system is based on glutathione [9]. Most probably, the trypanothione system not only replaces the glutathione system but also a full thioredoxin system in these protozoa. *T. brucei* has a thioredoxin [10] but the nearly completed genome projects did not reveal a TrxR gene in any trypanosomatid organism.

Both GR and TR proteins belong to the family of homodimeric pyridine nucleotide-disulfide oxidoreductases, which also includes flavoenzymes such as lipoamide dehydrogenase, TrxR, and mercuric ion reductase (Figure 22.3). Based on their central function in redox homeostasis, NADPH-dependent disulfide reductases are most promising candidates for structure-based drug development [11–15]. Whereas the mechanism and the structure of TR and GR are very similar, with about 40% identities in the primary sequences, they are mutually exclusive toward their respective substrates, trypanothione versus glutathione [16]. Unlike the GR active site, which is mainly cationic, the TR active site exhibits a negatively charged anchor residue (Glu18). Thus, it appears that a basic or positively charged substituent, combined with a flexible aliphatic chain, can efficiently potentiate the binding of the inhibitor inside the active site, as exemplified by mepacrine [17]. In addition, TR possesses a large hydrophobic pocket (Trp21–Leu17–Met113) that is the subject of intensive recent efforts in molecular modeling [18,19].

γGlu-Cys-Gly
H
N
O
HN
S
S
O
γGlu-Cys-Gly
N
H
trypanothione disulfide
(T(S)2)
NADPH, H+
NADP+
TR
kinetoplastids
trypanothione
(T(SH)2)
γGlu-Cys-Gly
HS
HS
γGlu-Cys-Gly

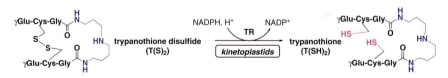

Figure 22.2 NADPH-dependent flavoenzyme TR in kinetoplastid parasites.

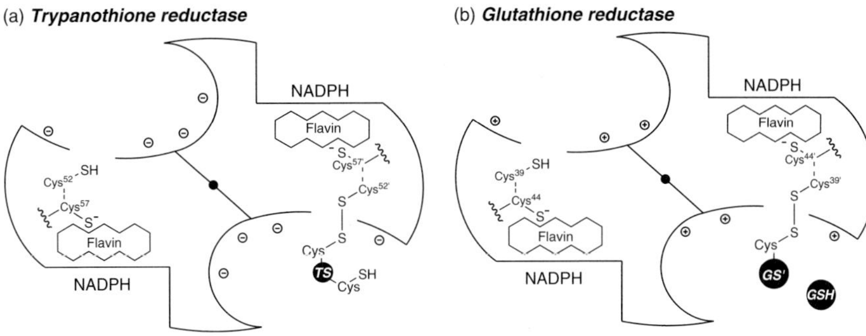

(a) *Trypanothione reductase*   (b) *Glutathione reductase*

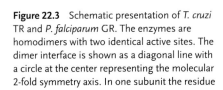

Figure 22.3 Schematic presentation of *T. cruzi* TR and *P. falciparum* GR. The enzymes are homodimers with two identical active sites. The dimer interface is shown as a diagonal line with a circle at the center representing the molecular 2-fold symmetry axis. In one subunit the residue numbers are primed. The schemes depict the reaction intermediate in which a mixed disulfide is formed between the enzyme and the respective disulfide substrate: (a) TR with bound trypanothione (TS) and (b) GR with bound glutathione (GS II) [2].

TR as a Drug Target Molecule

TR is the key enzyme of trypanothione metabolism. The known sensitivity of trypanosomatids towards oxidative stress and the absence of the enzyme from the mammalian host render TR an attractive target molecule for the development of new anti-trypanosomal drugs. As shown previously, trypanothione metabolism is not only involved in resistance mechanisms but also in the mode of action of antimonial drugs used for the treatment of leishmaniasis for more than a decade [20].

One of the prerequisite for an enzyme to be employed as a drug target molecule is that it is essential for the developmental stage of the respective microorganism causing the disease. This condition is not the absolute one that identifies the protein as a drug target. Different genetic (RNA interference, knockout) [21,22], chemical (inhibitors) and metabolomics (analysis of the trypanothione and polyamine pathways) approaches have unequivocally shown that TR is essential. Bloodstream African trypanosomes with less than 10% of wild-type TR activity were unable to grow although the levels of reduced trypanothione and total thiols remained constant. The parasites were highly sensitive towards hydrogen peroxide and were unable to initiate parasitemia in mice [22]. The *de novo* synthesis of trypanothione and residual levels of TR are sufficient to maintain resting thiol levels, but insufficient to cope with oxidative stress situations. It is not the absolute thiol concentration but the regeneration of trypanothione by the reductase that becomes rate limiting when the enzyme activity drops below 10% [22]. To facilitate drug screening programs on TRs, analogs of 5,5′-dithiobis(2-nitrobenzoic acid) (DTNB; Ellman's reagent) have been developed and tested as artificial disulfide substrates [23]. The most effective alternative substrate, 5,5′-dithiobis(2-nitrobenzamide) (DTNBA), has k_{cat}/K_m values in the same range as the values found for trypanothione disulfide, TS_2, and gives an accurate measure of TR activities and inhibitor sensitivity. Finally, the cost of this assay is very low compared with the assays utilizing TS_2 as physiological substrate. Another assay based on Ellman's-reagent-mediated regeneration of trypanothione *in situ* has been set up as an economical microplate and time-dependent inhibition assay for TR [24].

Turncoat Inhibitors (Subversive Substrates or Redox Cyclers) of TR as Anti-Trypanosomal Drugs

Subversive substrates or turncoat inhibitors are compounds that are reduced by the flavoenzymes in a single-electron step (Equation 22.1) to the respective radical, which then spontaneously reacts with molecular oxygen to yield superoxide anion radicals:

$$NADPH + 2X \rightarrow NADP^+ + 2X^{\bullet-} + H^+ \tag{22.1}$$

$$2X^{\bullet-} + 2O_2 \rightarrow 2X + 2O_2^{\bullet-}. \tag{22.2}$$

In the case of TR, the physiological reduction of TS_2 is concomitantly inhibited, NADPH and O_2 are wasted, and the thiol/disulfide ratio is lowered. Since the reaction of the radical intermediate with molecular oxygen regenerates the subversive substrate, the compounds act as catalysts producing oxidative stress and are thus expected to have a strong impact on the redox equilibrium of the parasites. In addition, reduced subversive substrates can transfer the electrons to a physiological oxidant or an electron acceptor in a reaction that can continuously shift the redox equilibrium at the expense of NADPH. Such continuous redox cycling has been recently exemplified with anti-malarial subversive substrates of both human and parasitic GR from *Plasmodium*-infected red blood cells [25–28]. See Figure 22.4.

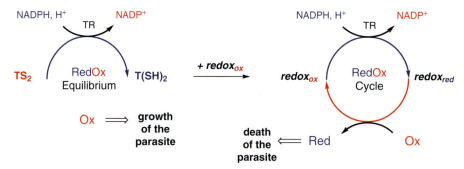

Figure 22.4 Schematic NADPH-dependent redox cycling of a subversive substrate of TR (or redox-active compound) affecting redox homeostasis leading to the death of the parasite. RedOx means redox-active compound with Ox and Red in subscript to indicate if the compound acts in its oxidized or its reduced state. Ox stands for oxidant or electron acceptor and Red for reductant. In the absence of the redox cycler, the redox equilibrium is maintained by the trypanothione/TR system and Ox should be a selected combined target essential for the growth of the parasite. In the presence of the redox-active agent under its reduced state, the redox homeostasis would be destroyed if the reduced species Red is lethal to the parasite.

Well-known subversive substrates are nitrofuran and naphthoquinone (NQ) derivatives. Many NQ drugs display notable anti-parasitic activities. TR, TrxR, lipoamide dehydrogenase (LipDH) as well as GR interact with NQs by catalyzing their reduction in the presence of oxygen in a futile redox cycle. In the case of TR, menadione, plumbagin, and other 1,4-NQs act as inhibitors and subversive substrates [12,29–31]. Towards GR, 1,4-NQ derivatives were mainly observed as reversible non/uncompetitive inhibitors [32] and weak subversive substrates of human GR. The pronounced ability of LipDII to reduce quinones is well known since the yeast enzyme was first described as menadione reductase [33]. The potency of turncoat inhibitors can be evaluated by the catalytic efficiency k_{cat}/K_m in the absence of the disulfide substrate and the K_i (and IC_{50} values) in the presence of the disulfide substrate. In both assays, oxidation of NADPH is measured continuously. Inhibition of the disulfide substrate reduction can be merely seen as a reporter activity of the NQ reduction but quantitative correlation should be avoided because these assays are done in open air and NQ binding might occur at various sites of the flavoenzyme simultaneously.

1,4-NQs as Trypanocidal Agents

Quinones can be activated by one or two-electron reduction steps (Figure 22.5). Reduction of 1,4-NQs was studied by cyclic voltammetry [34–36] and in enzymatic assays by measuring the oxidation of NAD(P)H, which yields the sum of one- and two-electron reduction rates of the compounds (Figure 22.5) [12,32,34–36]. When R^1 is a methyl group, the presence of halogen atoms at the methyl side-chain of menadione derivatives shifts both one- and two-electron reduction waves to more positive potentials, rendering the halogenomethyl menadione derivatives more reducible than the non-halogeno analogs [34,36].

Crystallographic studies revealed a substantial structural similarity between TR and human erythrocyte GR [37]. These enzymes possess two distinct binding sites for pyridine nucleotide and disulfide substrate, separated by the isoalloxazine core of FAD (Figure 22.6). The crystallographic analysis of human GR has revealed that certain non/uncompetitive inhibitors bind in a cavity at the dimer interface, distinct from the disulfide and NADPH binding sites. This "third site" is situated at the

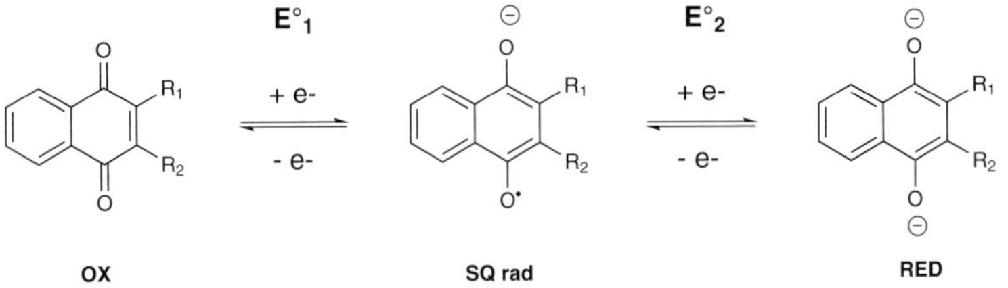

Figure 22.5 Oxidoreduction of 1,4-NQs. OX, oxidized form; RED, reduced form; SQ rad, semiquinone radical.

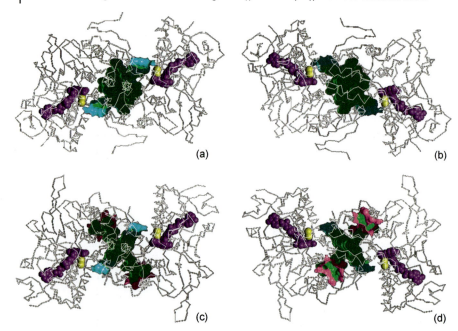

Figure 22.6 Front (a and c, respectively) and back (b and d, respectively) views of the protein backbone depicted for *T. cruzi* TR (TcTR) and human GR(hGR), showing the cavity at the dimer interface (green area). The cavity, also called the "third site," is connected to the two disulfide substrate (TS₂ and GSSG, respectively)-binding sites through two short channels (blue area). These channels emerge at the bottom of the V-shaped catalytic crevices in close proximity to the redox-active disulfide bridges. The redox-active disulfide bridges (Cys53 and Cys58 in TcTR; Cys58 and Cys63 in hGR) and the FAD molecules are shown as yellow and purple hard spheres, respectively. As indicated by the CAST calculation [12], two additional channels that connect the cavity with the protein surface in a region distinct from the two catalytic sites are detectable in the GR structure (pink area).

2-fold symmetry axis of the homodimeric protein [38] and is the locus of binding of menadione [39]. Three mechanisms accounting for NQ reduction were envisioned: (i) dithiol reduction, (ii) hydride ion reduction from the N^5 position of FADH⁻, and (iii) one-electron reduction from reduced forms of FAD. The most probable mechanism seems to be the third one since alkylation of the dithiol in TR by iodoacetamide [40], or in human GR by fluoromethyl NQ, increased the rate of menadione reduction [34].

Interestingly, it should be noted that TR is 10-fold more efficient in the one-electron reduction of quinones than is GR. The mechanism of reduction of several (naphtho) quinones has been investigated with *T. congolense* TR [40] and the putative site of reduction has been discussed by several groups (see Fairlamb, Krauth-Siegel, and Davioud-Charvet's works). A comparison of both TR and GR "third-site" structures has been discussed [12]. TR possesses at least two binding sites: one for the disulfide substrate and another for pyridine nucleotide, each of them separated by the isoalloxazine core of FAD. Taken together, experimental findings and crystal structures suggest that quinone reduction might occur at the NADPH-reduced flavin even if NQs were observed to bind to the "third site" in human GR as well [39].

The obtained steady-state kinetic parameters for reduction of quinones by TR enlighten several facts [40]: (i) there is an observed hyperbolic dependence of the log V/K_m values of quinones on their single-electron reduction potentials (E^1), which is characteristic of an outer-sphere single-electron transfer reaction; (ii) anaerobic reductive alkylation of Cys52 of reduced TR nearly abolish the TS_2 reducing activity but the alkylated TR is still able to reduce quinone substrates; and (iii) an excess of $NADP^+$ inhibits the reduction of TS_2 whereas it increases the V/K_m values of quinones. At $[NADP^+]/[NADPH]$ ratio greater than 10 reduction of benzoquinone by one-electron transfer occurs with 80% of the electrons introduced into TR by NADPH. Moreover, the reduced TR (EH_2) is oxidized by benzoquinone compounds 100 times faster in the presence of $NADP^+$ than in its absence. Thus, these data show that occupancy of the nicotinamide-binding pocket by $NADP^+$ is mandatory to increase the rate of quinone reduction.

Knowing that several NQs were substrates of GR, Henderson *et al.* postulated, by analogy, that TR might reduce functional groups other than disulfides [29]. As TR and GR share the same catalytic mechanism to reduce their respective physiological disulfide substrates, albeit with a difference in the charge of the active site, three NQs were prepared, possessing two side-chain carboxylic acid residues, one side-chain guanidine residue, and two side-chain guanidine residues, respectively (Figure 22.7). The guanidine NQs **2** and **3** were revealed to act as substrates of *Crithidia fasciculata* TR and their reduced forms were readily reoxidized by molecular oxygen, and thus the redox-active compounds undergo classical enzyme-catalyzed redox cycling. This was confirmed in aerobic condition by monitoring oxygen consumption directly, cytochrome c reduction by superoxide, and the concomitant NADPH consumption (which was approximately stoichiometric with oxygen consumption). The authors identified such compounds as "subversive" substrates. When these redox-active NQs interact with the TR enzyme they do not inactivate the enzyme but cause an important consumption of NADPH, inhibiting TS_2 reduction and generating the production of free radicals. *In vitro* experiments evidenced that pretreatment of cultured *T. cruzi* trypomastigotes with the bisguanidine NQ prevented infection of human saphenous vein smooth muscle cells by the parasite: 14% infected cells at 0.5 µM and 0% infection at 1 µM of the drug.

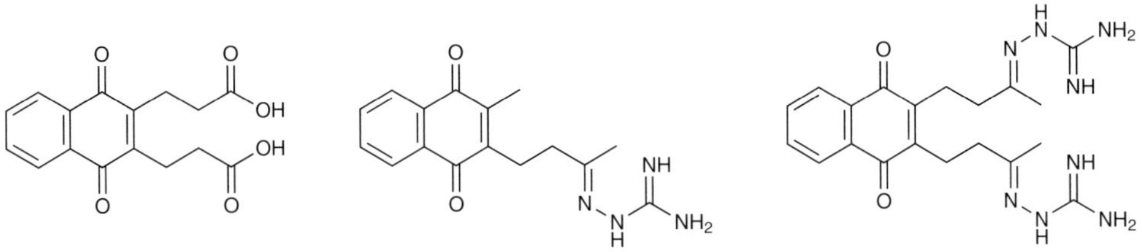

Figure 22.7 Structures of trypanocidal 1,4-NQs acting as subversive substrates of TR.

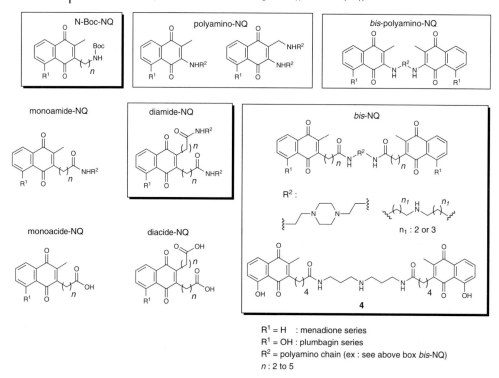

Figure 22.8 Structures of 1,4-NQs derived from menadione, plumbagin, and juglone designed as subversive substrates of TR.

A large set of NQ derivatives were further synthesized to study their trypanocidal activities against the intracellular amastigote stages of both *T. cruzi* and *L. donovani*, and upon the bloodstream-form trypomastigotes from *T. brucei* (Figure 22.8) [12,31]. The goal of this work was aimed at the design of efficient turncoat TR inhibitors having a high selectivity for TcTR versus hGR, and the identification of a correlation between redox cycling activities and *in vitro* anti-trypanosomal activities. When tested as potential inhibitors of the TR-catalyzed TS$_2$ reduction most of them (mono- or diacid-NQ, diamide-NQ, (bis)polyamino-NQ, N-Boc-NQ, etc.) were ineffective, with no or very little *T. cruzi* TR inhibition at concentration of up to 50 μM. However, most of the bis-1,4-NQs that are linked by a polyamino(biscarbonylbutyl or pentyl) spacer (bis-NQ) behaved as very potent inhibitors in the low micromolar range (IC$_{50}$ < 5 μM in the presence of 57 μM TS$_2$) [12]. The most powerful TR inhibitor was the bis-NQ **4** with a K_i of 0.45 μM, exhibiting an uncompetitive inhibition type toward both TS$_2$ and NADPH. An uncompetitive inhibitor of TR is expected to have a strong effect on the thiol redox balance and thus on the viability of the parasites since the resulting accumulation of the substrate even enhances inhibition of the enzyme *in vivo* [41].

Moreover, the bis-NQ **4** behaved as a very efficient subversive substrate for *T. cruzi* TR with a k_{cat}/K_m value of $11.4 \times 10^4 \, M^{-1} s^{-1}$. The strongest trypanocidal activity was observed with compounds that combined high redox cycling activity with efficient inhibition of TS$_2$ reduction. Interestingly, the plumbagin derivative **4** showed ED$_{50}$ values of 4.3 and 1.1 µM in parasitic assays using *T. cruzi* and *T. brucei* in cultures, respectively [12].

Nitrofurans

Nitroaromatic compounds have long been known to possess several biological activities. Regarding the treatment of parasitic diseases, their use is well documented; more particularly, the use of nitroheterocycles such as nitrofurans or nitroimidazoles (Figure 22.9).

The development of new anti-trypanosomal drugs based on these series started in the 1950s and 1960s. Nitrofurazone was one of the first nitrofurans to be assessed in clinical trials [42]. Despite a high anti-parasitic activity, the use of this compound was stopped due to its toxicity. However, new nitroheterocycles were developed and nifurtimox (Figure 22.10) was licensed for use against *T. cruzi*, the causative agent of Chagas disease. Also active on *T. brucei*, this molecule was also identified in 2003 to be used in combination with eflornithine in treating melarsoprol-refractory trypanosomiasis [43]. However, even for the marketed drug nifurtimox, host toxicity remains. This toxicity is one of the first causes of premature arrest of the treatment, sometimes by the medical team but, most often, by patients that are reluctant to endure the side-effects. These premature treatment arrests are also responsible for the appearance of parasitic resistance to nifurtimox [44]. These issues have driven researchers to gain a better understanding of the mechanism of action of nitrofurans, with the aim to develop new molecules with better therapeutic index. Here, we summarize key facts and recent advances on this topic.

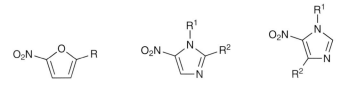

Figure 22.9 General structures of anti-parasitic nitrofurans (left) and nitroimidazoles.

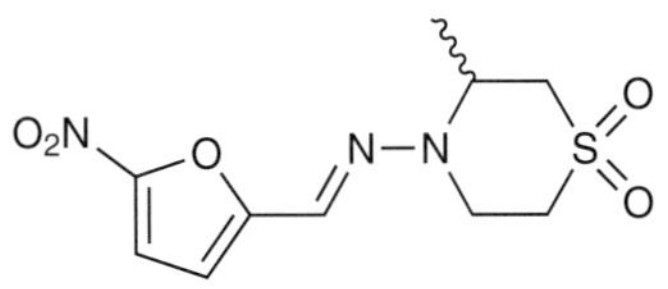

Figure 22.10 Structure of nifurtimox.

Parasitic Targets and Mechanism of Action of Nitrofurans

Nitrofurans are known to interact with TR [29,45]. Interestingly, two modes of inhibition have been described depending on oxygen supply [29]. In aerobic conditions, the inhibition was uncompetitive versus NADPH and either non-competitive or uncompetitive versus TS_2 when a saturated solution of NADPH was used [45]. In addition, the inhibition was fully reversible as the complete activity of the enzyme was recovered after dialysis of the nitrofuran from the medium [29]. In anaerobic conditions, the enzyme activity was reduced to 7% of the original TR activity, even after nitrofuran dialysis. Thus, in the absence of O_2, nitrofurans irreversibly inhibit the enzyme [29]. With the improvements of the physicochemical tools, and especially in electrochemistry, a better understanding of the redox properties and behavior of the nitro group was reached. The one-electron reduction of the nitro group leads to the formation of a radical anion (Equation 22.1, where $X = RNO_2$) [46]. Subsequent quenching of this nitro-anion radical can follow two different pathways. The radical anion can react with molecular oxygen, leading to the formation of the initial nitrofuran and superoxide anion (Equation 22.2, where $X = RNO_2$) [47], or it can dismutate into the derived nitroso compound, the initial nitrofuran and water (Equation 22.3) [46]:

$$2\,R\text{-}NO_2^{\bullet -} + 2\,H^+ \rightarrow R\text{-}NO_2 + RNO + H_2O. \tag{22.3}$$

Electrochemical studies have demonstrated that the kinetics of the reaction with molecular oxygen is very fast, thus privileging the first pathway (Equation 22.2, where $X = RNO_2$) versus the second one (Equation 22.3) [47]. On the other hand, under anaerobic conditions the first pathway is blocked; the radical anion decays by dismutation, leading to the formation of a highly electrophilic nitroso species [46]. This nitroso intermediate immediately reacts with any surrounding nucleophilic entities and particularly with thiols. This could be an explanation for the enzyme inactivation in anaerobic conditions as the nitroso might alkylate nucleophilic residues, such as cysteine, that are essential for the enzyme activity.

Trypanothione inhibition is only one part of the mechanism of action of nitrofurans. According to Equation 22.2 (where $X = RNO_2$), the decay of the radical anion leads to the formation of superoxide and the initial nitrofuran. As the parasite is particularly sensitive to reactive oxygen species (ROS), the production of superoxide might participate in the anti-parasitic effect of nitrofurans. In addition, is noteworthy that the nitrofuran is regenerated in the course of this reaction with molecular oxygen and thus available for a new redox cycle. This roughly constant concentration of oxidized nitrofuran clearly enhances oxygen uptake and NADPH consumption [46]. To summarize, nitrofurans have three main deleterious effects on parasite metabolism [29]: as observed with NQs (i) they inhibit the reduction of thiols such as trypanothione, (ii) they trigger the production of ROS and free radicals, and (iii) they cause futile consumption of NADPH. Thus, nitrofurans perfectly meet the criteria of subversive substrates of TR and their redox cycle activity can be summarized as shown in Figure 22.11. As discussed in relation to NQs,

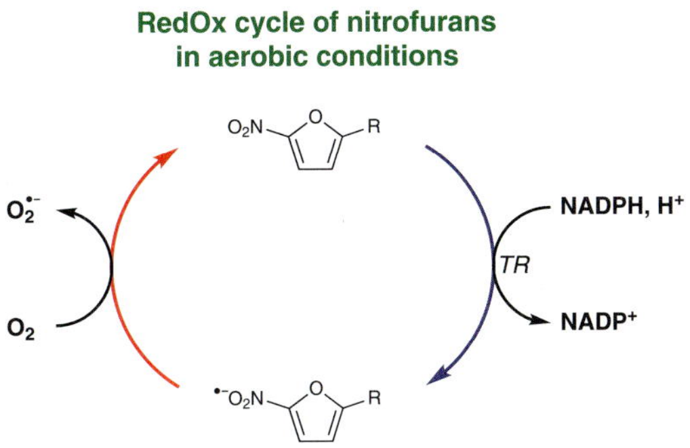

**RedOx cycle of nitrofurans
in aerobic conditions**

Figure 22.11 Redox cycle of nitrofurans in presence of molecular oxygen.

nitrofurans were also proposed to bind to TR enzyme in the "third site" at the dimer interface, but the site where reduction occurs is still a matter of debate [13,14,45].

Most of the authors agree to consider this redox cycle activity as the main mechanism of action of the anti-parasitic activity of nitrofurans. However, direct thiol depletion was recently evidenced as an alternative mechanism of action; it would result in direct thiol alkylation by electrophilic species and nitroso species upon bioactivation of the reduced nitrofuran. Recently, a new cytotoxic metabolite of nifurtimox was isolated and characterized, as the result of two-electron reduction of the nitrofuran moiety by a trypanosomal type I nitroreductase [48]. The exact target and mechanism of action of this unsaturated nitrile metabolite remain to be determined. The nitrofuran reductase activity is absolutely mandatory for the redox cycle and a prerequisite for further metabolic bioactivation.

Recent Lead Nitrofuran Prodrugs

The nitrofuran chemistry has been extensively developed in the last three decades, and numerous derivatives have been evaluated and selected, albeit with low therapeutic index. In order to increase selectivity toward the trypanosomes versus the host cells, the targeting of specific parasitic transporters was investigated. It is well known that trypanosomes have a specific transporter for diamidine and particularly the P2 transporter, which has a great affinity for melamine-based residue [49]. With the aim to target these transporters, melamine-based nitrofurans have been synthesized (Figure 22.12) [50,51].

Results from the STIB 795 *T. b. brucei*-infected murine model *in vivo* with the melamine-derived nitrofuran **5a** showed that all mice were cured at a dose of 20 mg/kg for 4 days. Interestingly, the P2-deficient trypanosome mutants were as sensitive to the drug as the wild-type parasites, suggesting that other transporters could be responsible for the uptake of this melamine-based nitrofuran. Additional structure–activity relationships were studied from derivatives with one alkylated amine residue of the melamine moiety (compounds **5b** and **5c**). These compounds

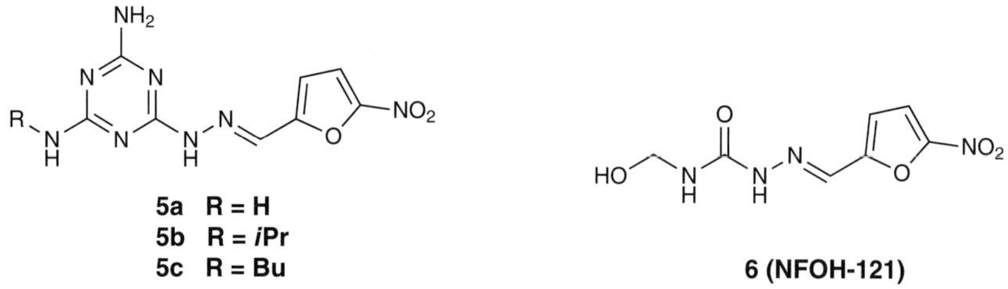

5a R = H
5b R = iPr
5c R = Bu

6 (NFOH-121)

Figure 22.12 Example of recently developed nitrofurans with anti-parasitic activity.

resulted in similar activity on *T. b. rhodesiense in vitro* while the *in vitro* activity on *T. cruzi* was up to 10-fold higher. Although the dosage was higher (50 mg/kg intraperitoneally for 4 days), STIB 900 *T. b. rhodesiense*-infected mice were cured with an appreciable survival time (greater than 30 days) in the STIB 795 model whereas in the STIB 900 model 25% of mice were cured, resulting in an average survival time of 27 and 41 days for compounds **5b** and **5c**, respectively. In spite of an increase in the toxicity over L6 cells, no overt sign of toxicity was found in mice [51]. In conclusion, melamine-based nitrofurans are promising lead compounds with general anti-parasitic activity over the different strains of *Trypanosoma*.

Nitrofurazone was one the first nitrofurans used in the treatment of African trypanosomiasis. However, this molecule is highly toxic and the overall mortality due to the drug was unacceptable. Thus, the drug was withdrawn from the market. Recently, a prodrug of nitrofurazone was synthesized by *N*-hydroxymethylation of the terminal amine of the semicarbazone fragment of nitrofurazone (Figure 22.13) and evaluated for its anti-parasitic activity.

Nitrofurazone is reduced by *T. cruzi* LipDH and to a much less extent by TR [30]. Interestingly, the activity of the prodrug NFOH-121 was similar to nifurtimox or benznidazole against *T. cruzi* trypomastigotes, but higher against amastigote forms [52]. The activity of NFOH-121 was next evaluated *in vivo* in a murine model of Chagas disease [53]. Four groups of Swiss mice were infected by *T. cruzi*, and were, respectively, treated with placebo, benznidazole, NFOH-121, and nitrofurazone. The group treated with the prodrug displayed the lowest mortality (16%), followed by benznidazole (33%), placebo (66%), and finally nitrofurazole (75%). NFOH-121 was effective in reducing the parasite load as polymerase chain reaction analyses of blood samples were negative after 180 days post-treatment. In these studies, the prodrug NFOH-121 led to a comparable survival and cure level as with treatment with benznidazole or nifurtimox. Therefore, this molecule emerges as a promising candidate for anti-trypanosomal treatments.

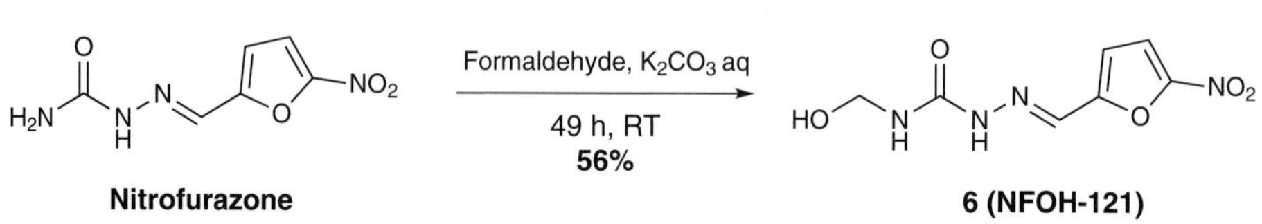

Nitrofurazone

Formaldehyde, K$_2$CO$_3$ aq

49 h, RT
56%

6 (NFOH-121)

Figure 22.13 Synthesis of hydroxymethylnitrofurazone from nitrofurazone.

Other Subversive Substrates

2,2,4-Trimethyl-1,2-dihydroquinolines

A screening program supported by WHO/TDR identified a series of 2,2,4-trimethyl-1,2-dihydroquinolines (THQs) with promising anti-trypanosomal activity [54]. One of these 1,2-dihydroquinolines **7** (Figure 22.14) displayed potent and selective anti-trypanosomal activity *in vitro* against the *T. b. rhodesiense* strain STIB 900 ($IC_{50} = 0.054\ \mu M$, SI = 300), but unfortunately **7** was inactive in a murine *T. b. brucei* model. With a view to obtain *in vivo* active compounds against *T. b. rhodesiense* bloodstream trypomastigotes, the authors undertook the preparation of more than 50 analogs at the N1 and C6 position of the 1,2-dihydroquinoline core (Figure 22.14). Several N^1-substituted derivatives displayed nanomolar IC_{50} values *in vitro*, with selectivity indexes, relative to L6 rat myoblasts, up to 18 000. The most potent compound was **8** with an IC_{50} of 7 nM. The results of *in vivo* evaluation revealed that THQ **9** was the most active compound (murine model: *T. b. brucei* STIB 795, intraperitoneal injection at a daily dose of 50 mg/kg for 4 days). By day 14, each of the mice receiving compound **9** was still alive. However, from day 10, they relapsed and were positive for parasites.

The *in vitro* anti-trypanosomal structure–activity relationship (SAR) study highlighted the importance of a 6-oxygen atom for anti-trypanosomal activity in this series of THQs. Indeed, compounds lacking the 6-oxygen atom or bearing an oxygen atom at the 7-position were far less potent than their 6-oxygen counterpart. Based on these SAR studies and the fact that 6-hydroxy-1,2-dihydroquinolines are prone to auto-oxidize into quinone imine compounds, the authors expected ROS to be involved in the mechanism of action of these agents. *In vitro* fluorescence experiments in *T. b. brucei* confirmed that 6-oxygen-THQs were able to generate ROS. Thus, they proposed that compounds esterified at the 6-oxygen atom were hydrolyzed rapidly by trypanosomal esterases, followed by two-electron oxidation to a quinone imine species (Figure 22.15). As quinones, quinone imines are known to undergo a single-electron reduction to form semiquinones, suggesting that they

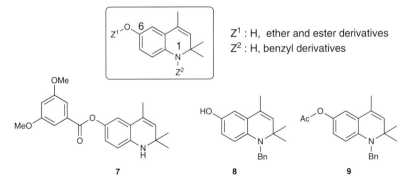

Z¹ : H, ether and ester derivatives
Z² : H, benzyl derivatives

7   **8**   **9**

Figure 22.14 THQs with anti-trypanosomal activities.

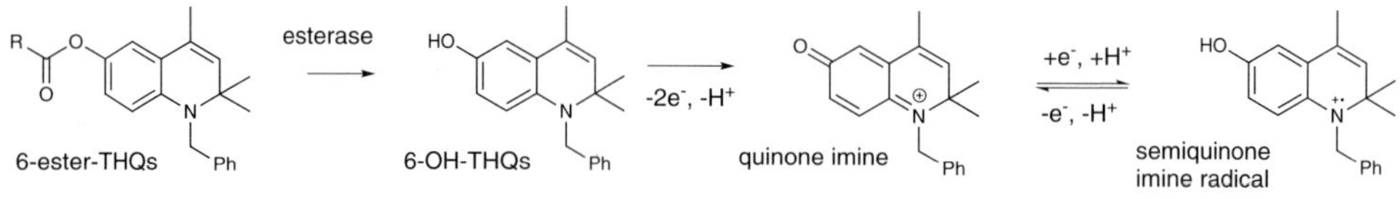

Figure 22.15 Proposed anti-trypanosomal mechanism of THQs.

might act as subversive substrates of TR, or other flavoenzymes, with redox cycling activity (Figure 22.15). It should be noted that this TR substrate hypothesis was not further investigated but was just speculated. The ability of quinone imine species to act as subversive substrates of TR is still an open question.

Methylene Blue

Methylene blue (MB, Figure 22.16) is an old, well-known molecule that belongs to the phenothiazine family. It has been extensively researched for medicinal applications, such as in cancer therapy, for the treatment of methemoglobinemia, as an inhibitor of Tau protein aggregation, and as an anti-malarial drug [55]. MB was also found to be active against African trypanosomes *in vitro* [56]. This was an incentive to investigate the mechanism of action of MB. Thus, it was demonstrated that MB is a non-competitive inhibitor of *T. cruzi* TR with a K_i of $1.9\,\mu M$ in TS_2 reduction assays [57]. Furthermore, MB can be effectively reduced by TR in its colorless leuco-methylene blue reduced form. In the presence of oxygen leucomethylene blue is highly unstable and instantaneously auto-oxidizes into MB, which is able to be reduced once again by TR, closing the redox cycle (Figure 22.17, path A).

In the same study, the authors demonstrated that MB readily oxidized reduced forms of thiols like trypanothione, glutathione, or glutathionylspermidine. This oxidation is non-enzymatic and is a two-step chemical process as described in Figure 22.17 (path B) [57]. This alternative redox activity of MB can also be considered as a deleterious redox cycle as it generates ROS and a considerable amount of oxidized thiols. It is reasonable to assume that both pathways might contribute to the anti-trypanosomal activity of MB. Regarding the fact that MB is cheap, available, and a well-tolerated molecule – its use has been approved for the treatment of methemoglobinemia – its application as anti-trypanosomal drug has to be carefully considered.

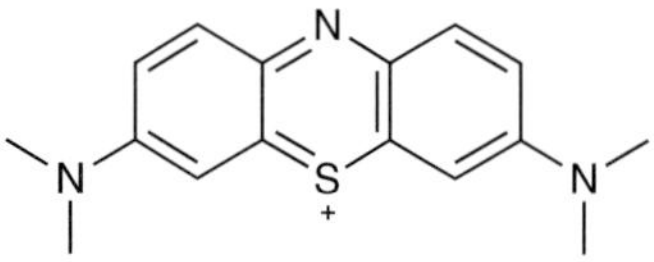

Figure 22.16 Structure of MB.

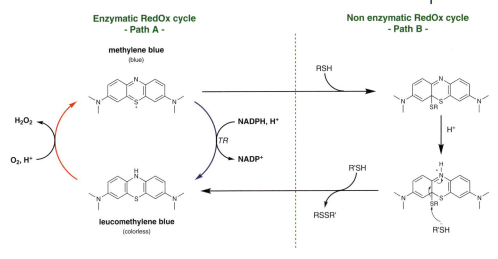

Figure 22.17   Two redox cycles of MB.

Chinifur

The first reported synthesis of chinifur, namely (*E*)-*N*-(5-(diethylamino)pentan-2-yl)-3-(2-(5-nitrofuran-2-yl)vinyl)isoquinoline-4-carboxamide (Figure 22.18), dates from the beginning of the 1980s. It was patented as part of a series of molecules with anti-blastic activity [58]. As it also possesses a nitrofuran, chinifur was screened for anti-parasitic activity. Enzymatic studies revealed that chinifur acts in the same way as the classical substituted nitrofurans. *T. congelense* TR was proven to have a great affinity for this substrate, which acts as a non-competitive inhibitor towards TS$_2$ [45]. As a result, chinifur exhibits the most potent inhibition of TS$_2$ reduction, with a degree of inhibition as high as 97% on *T. cruzi* TR, whereas nifurtimox only lowered by 37% the reduction in the same experimental conditions [30]. The binding site of chinifur in the enzyme remains unclear, and it is usually assumed that the molecule binds both at the trypanothione binding site and at the interface site [45]. In addition to its inhibitory activity, chinifur also induced a high oxidase activity. In the same way as the other nitrofurans, it enters a redox cycle through the nitro group, generating ROS while consuming the NADPH [30]. To our knowledge, and despite these promising results, no *in vivo* studies have been performed for this molecule.

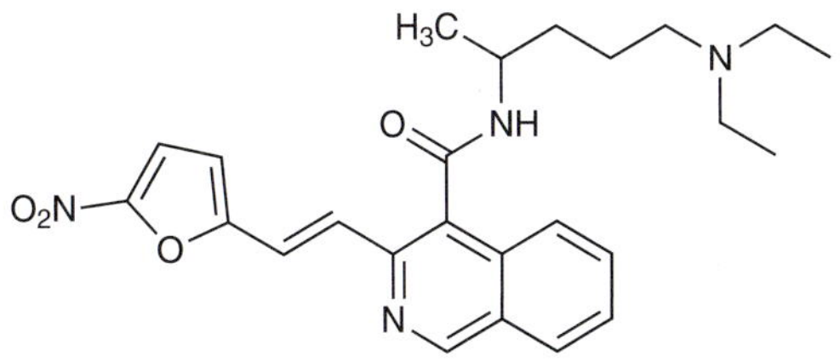

Figure 22.18   Structure of chinifur.

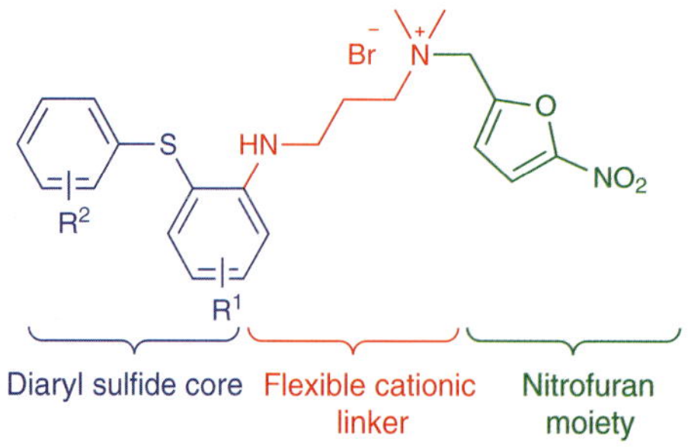

Figure 22.19 Structure of diaryl sulfide-based subversive substrates.

Diaryl Sulfides

Diaryl sulfides were described as inhibitors of TR in 1995 [59]. Starting from this core, a new class of dual drug has been developed by introducing a 5-nitrofurfuryl unit as substituent (Figure 22.19) [15]. Conceptually, the design of these molecules fulfills three structural features: a diaryl sulfide core to enhance the affinity for TR, a flexible cationic linker to meet the criteria for helping the binding in the anionic pocket of TR, and finally a nitrofuran to give a redox cycling effect. Four products were synthesized and evaluated both in biochemical and *in vitro* cell assays. In enzymatic studies, compounds displayed a mixed competitive and uncompetitive mode of inhibition toward TS_2. In addition, the introduction of the nitrofuran moiety was successful, as an important increase in NADPH oxidase activity was observed (up to 14 times). Anti-parasitic assays against *T. b. rhodesiense* STIB 900 strain revealed a high potency with IC_{50}s ranging from 0.6 to 1 μM and cytotoxicity (evaluated over L6 myoblast cells) starting at 27 and rising above 170 μM. This ongoing series should be soon evaluated in *in vivo* growth inhibition studies.

Trypanothione-Reactive Agents (Susceptible to Enter Redox Cycling Following Double Michael Addition) as Anti-Trypanosomal Drugs

Unsaturated Mannich Bases as Dithiol-Alkylating Agents

From a screening of 350 000 compounds of the Pfizer library, unsaturated Mannich bases were identified to be efficient time-dependent inhibitors of *P. falciparum* TrxR [60,61]. Recently, we showed that unsaturated Mannich bases such as compound **10** (Figure 22.20) are also potent irreversible inhibitors of *T. cruzi* TR [33,62]. Although TrxR and TR are structurally and mechanistically related enzymes, the mode of inactivation is strikingly different depending on the presence of two vicinal cysteines and their solvent exposure. The same discrepancy occurs when comparing the dithiol trypanothione and the monothiol glutathione. In the case of the *Plasmodium* TrxR enzyme [61] or of trypanothione [62,63], one of thiols (of the cysteines at the C-terminus of TrxR) attacks the double bond of **10** to generate the first reversible adduct

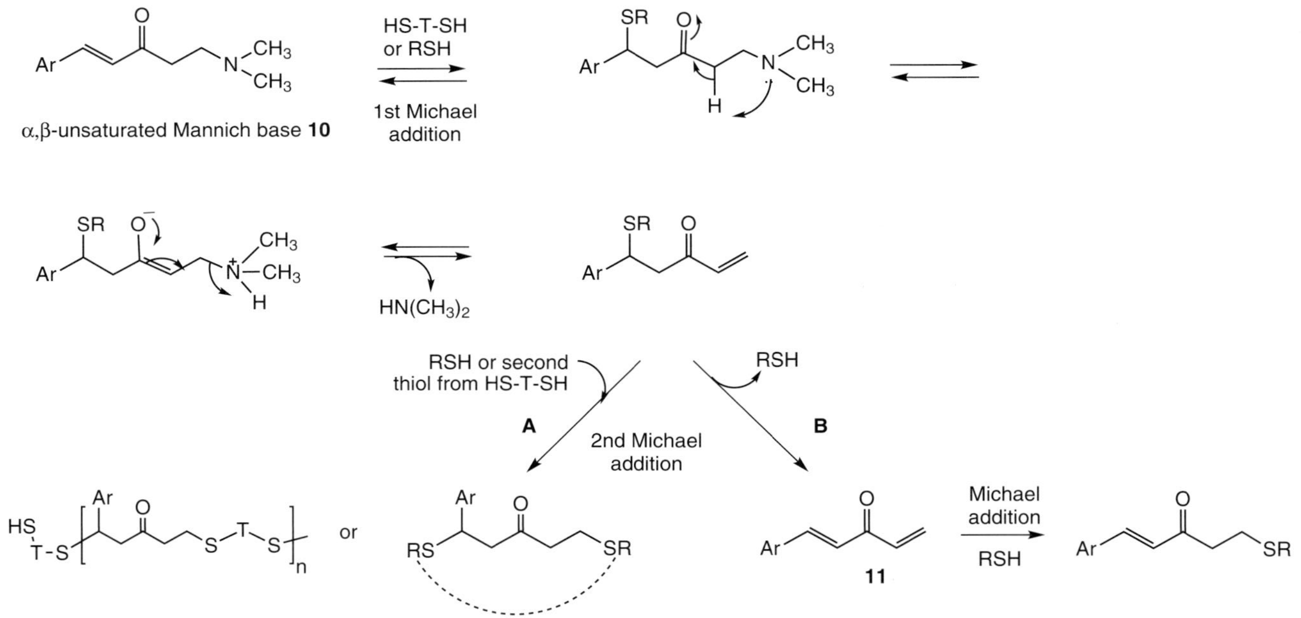

Figure 22.20 Proposed reaction mechanisms for the modification of protein thiols (RSH) by an unsaturated Mannich base such as **8** (Ar, 2-chlorophenyl). Mechanism A: in the case of two vicinal reactive protein thiols, such as, Cys535 and Cys540 in *P. falciparum* TrxR or with trypanothione. Mechanism B: in the case of a single reactive protein thiol, such as Cys52 in *T. cruzi* TR.

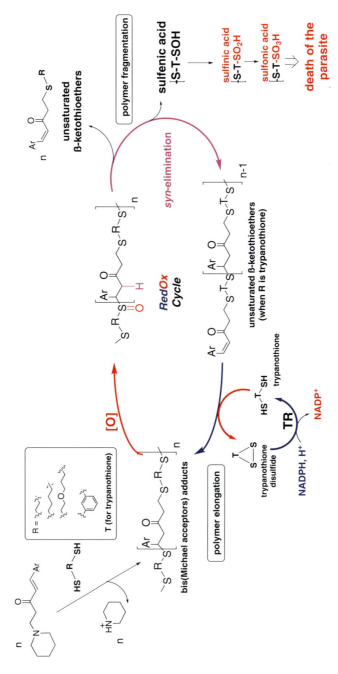

Figure 22.21 Postulated mechanism for polymer formation and fragmentation from an unsaturated Mannich base and a dithiol In the case of a physiological dithiol like trypanothione, polymer elongation is proposed to be maintained at the expense of trypanothione regeneration catalyzed by the NADPH-dependent TR. Continuous redox cycling under oxidative conditions and polymer fragmentation, upon *syn*-elimination of the regenerated reactive unsaturated ketone, is expected to contribute to polymer elongation. Overoxidation of the released sulfenic acid might lead to sulfinic and sulfonic acids of trypanothione and other thiol species responsible for the death of the parasite.

(Figure 22.20, upper line). Following base-catalyzed elimination of the *N*,*N*-dialkyla-mino moiety and formation of a new highly reactive Michael acceptor, addition of a second enzyme thiol (or a vicinal thiol) to the double bond of the enone enables the inhibitor to bind irreversibly (mechanism A). The postulated reaction product is a macrocyclic adduct composed of the inhibitor and the thiol redox pair Cys535 and Cys540, or an oligomer of (trypanothione/unsaturated β-ketothioether)adducts following intermolecular Michael additions. In TR, the situation varies a little bit. The enzyme has the redox active dithiol/disulfide (Cys52–Cys57 in *T. cruzi* TR) adjacent to the flavin cofactor but lacks an additional C-terminal cystine redox pair. In the presence of NADPH, *T. cruzi* TR is irreversibly inactivated by unsaturated Mannich bases. Interestingly, when a stock solution of **10** that was stored for 2 days at 4 °C was used, inhibition of *T. cruzi* was faster and much more complete. Within 5 min, 5 μM of **10** inhibited TR to 80%, in comparison to a fresh sample of **10** that caused only 37% inactivation. The active principle for TR inactivation by the unsaturated Mannich bases proved to be the divinylketone **11** (Figure 22.20). Electrospray ionization mass spectrometry and matrix-assisted laser desorption/ionization-time of flight mass spectrometry analyses of TR modified by **10** and **11**, respectively, revealed a single identical 5-(2′-chlorophenyl)-oxo-4-pentenyl group bound to Cys52 in accordance with reaction mechanism B in Figure 22.20. The visible absorption spectra of TR modified by **10** or **11** showed charge transfer absorption around 530 nm, and thus confirmed that Cys57 has not been modified [62].

Sulfoxides or sulfones are known metabolites of sulfides *in vivo* [44,64,65]; they can undergo β-elimination, which in the case of unsaturated Mannich base dithiols adducts S-oxides, regenerates the unsaturated β-ketothioethers following polymer fragmentation and the release of sulfenic acids (Figure 22.21). The latter might be overoxidized in sulfinic and sulfonic acids [64].

Quinols

Recently, quinols were also developed as double Michael acceptors, forming two covalent bonds with their protein target(s) (Figure 22.22 and 22.23). They were shown to be very potent against *T. brucei*, although the counter-screen against human cell line MRC5 revealed insufficient selectivity to be of therapeutic value against these parasites [66]. However, the strategy for preparing melamine- and

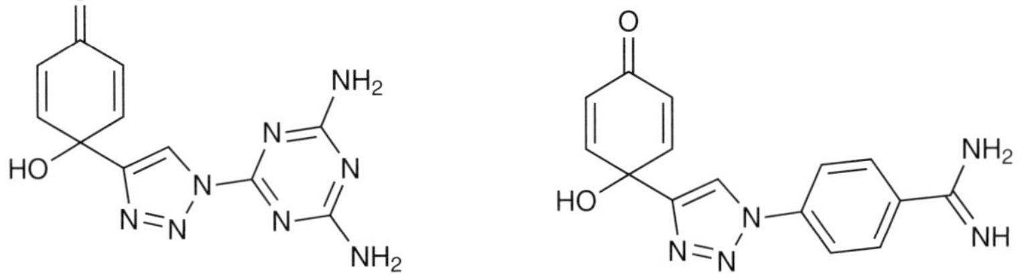

Figure 22.22 Structure of melamine- and benzamidine-derived quinols.

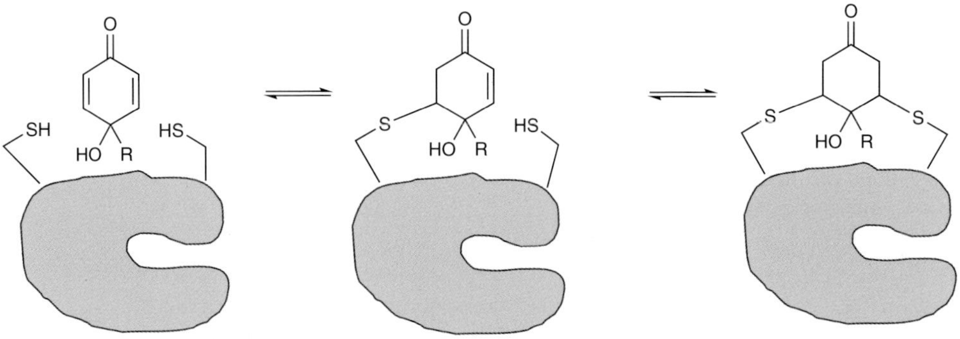

Figure 22.23 Proposed mode of action of the quinols. Cysteine residues are abbreviated to —SH.

benzamidine-derived compounds incorporating the purine P2 transporter-targeting motif demonstrated that it was possible to improve their selectivity, but this proved to be at the expense of anti-trypanosomal potency.

Conclusions

TR is one of the most attractive targets for the comprehensive concept of redox cyclers to fight trypanosomatid parasites. Uncompetitive inhibitors *vis-à-vis* NADPH or TS_2 or subversive substrates are most promising drug candidates because physiological compensation like an increase in substrate flux or in the expression of the enzyme does not overcome TR inhibition [41]. A novel approach will be the development of a lead drug that interferes with the trypanothione/TR system and is selectively uptaken by transporters in all pathogenic kinetoplastids. The simultaneous interaction with the NADPH-dependent TR-catalyzed reactions and another electron acceptor essential for the parasite should have synergistic effects on the redox metabolism of the parasite and may prevent or at least slow down drug resistance development.

Acknowledgments

Our work is supported in part by the Centre National de la Recherche Scientifique, Strasbourg University and the International Center for Frontier Research in Chemistry icFRC in Strasbourg (www.icfrc.fr). The chapter is an updated version of a previous review written by Krauth-Siegel and Davioud-Charvet, 2005. The authors are grateful to Didier Belorgey for careful scientific reading of the manuscript.

References

1 Schirmer, R.H., Müller, J.G., and Krauth-Siegel, R.L. (1995) Disulfide-reductase inhibitors as chemotherapeutic agents: the design of drugs for Trypanosomiasis and Malaria. *Angew. Chem. Int. Ed. Engl.*, **34**, 141–154.

2 Krauth-Siegel, R.L., Bauer, H., and Schirmer, R.H. (2005) Dithiol proteins as guardians of the intracellular redox milieu in parasites: old and new drug targets in trypanosomes and malaria-causing plasmodia. *Angew. Chem. Int. Ed.*, **44**, 690–715.

3 Williams, C.H.J. (1991) Lipoamide dehydrogenase, glutathione reductase, thioredoxin reductase, and mercuric ion reductase – a family of flavoenzyme transhydrogenases, in *Chemistry and Biochemistry of Flavoenzymes* (ed. F. Müller), CRC Press, Boca Raton, FL, vol. **III**, pp. 121–211.

4 Argyrou, A. and Blanchard, J. (2004) Flavoprotein disulfide reductases: advances in chemistry and function. *Prog. Nucleic Acid Res. Mol. Biol.*, **78**, 89–142.

5 Fairlamb, A., Blackburn, P., Ulrich, P., Chait, B., and Cerami, A. (1985) Trypanothione: a novel bis(glutathionyl) spermidine cofactor for glutathione reductase in trypanosomatids. *Science*, **227**, 1485–1487.

6 Fairlamb, A., Henderson, G., and Cerami, A. (1986) The biosynthesis of trypanothione and N^1-glutathionylspermidine in *Crithidia fasciculata*. *Mol. Biochem. Parasitol.*, **21**, 247–257.

7 Shames, S.L., Fairlamb, A.H., Cerami, A., and Walsh, C.T. (1986) Purification and characterization of trypanothione reductase from *Crithidia fasciculata*, a new member of the family of disulfide-containing flavoprotein reductases. *Biochemistry*, **25**, 3519–3526.

8 Montrichard, F., Le Guen, F., Laval-Martin, D.L., and Davioud-Charvet, E. (1999) Evidence for the co-existence of glutathione reductase and trypanothione reductase in the non-trypanosomatid Euglenozoa: *Euglena gracilis* Z. *FEBS Lett.*, **442**, 29–33.

9 Schirmer, R.H., Schöllhammer, T., Eisenbrand, G., and Krauth-Siegel, R.L. (1987) Oxidative stress as a defense mechanism against parasitic infections. *Free Radic. Res.*, **3**, 3–12.

10 Schmidt, H. and Krauth-Siegel, R.L. (2003) Functional and physicochemical characterization of the thioredoxin system in *Trypanosoma brucei*. *J. Biol. Chem.*, **278**, 46329–46336.

11 Bond, C.S., Zhang, Y., Berriman, M., Cunningham, M.L., Fairlamb, A.H., and Hunter, W.N. (1999) Crystal structure of *Trypanosoma cruzi* trypanothione reductase in complex with trypanothione, and the structure-based discovery of new natural product inhibitors. *Structure*, **7**, 81–89.

12 Salmon-Chemin, L., Buisine, E., Yardley, V., Kohler, S., Debreu, M.-A., Landry, V., Sergheraert, C. *et al.* (2001) 2- and 3-Substituted 1,4-naphthoquinone derivatives as subversive substrates of trypanothione reductase and lipoamide dehydrogenase from *Trypanosoma cruzi*: synthesis and correlation between redox cycling activities and *in vitro* cytotoxicity. *J. Med. Chem.*, **44**, 548–565.

13 Vega-Teijido, M., Caracelli, I., and Zukerman-Schpector, J. (2006) Conformational analyses and docking studies of a series of 5-nitrofuran- and 5-nitrothiophen-semicarbazone derivatives in three possible binding sites of trypanothione and glutathione reductases. *J. Mol. Graph. Model.*, **24**, 349–355.

14 Iribarne, F., González, M., Cerecetto, H., Aguilera, S., Tapia, O., and Paulino, M. (2007) Interaction energies of nitrofurans with trypanothione reductase and glutathione reductase studied by molecular docking. *J. Mol. Struct.*, **818**, 7–22.

15 Stump, B., Kaiser, M., Brun, R., Krauth-Siegel, R.L., and Diederich, F. (2007) Betraying the parasite's redox system: diaryl sulfide-based inhibitors of trypanothione reductase: subversive substrates and antitrypanosomal properties. *ChemMedChem*, **2**, 1708–1712.

16 Faerman, C.H., Savvides, S.N., Strickland, C., Breidenbach, M.A., Ponasik, J.A., Ganem, B., Ripoll, D. *et al.* (1996) Charge is the major discriminating factor for glutathione reductase versus trypanothione reductase inhibitors. *Bioorg. Med. Chem.*, **4**, 1247–1253.

17 Jacoby, E.M., Schlichting, I., Lantwin, C.B., Kabsch, W., and Krauth-Siegel, R.L. (1996) Crystal structure of the *Trypanosoma cruzi* trypanothione reductase-mepacrine complex. *Proteins*, **24**, 73–80.

18 Khan, M.O.F., Austin, S.E., Chan, C., Yin, H., Marks, D., Vaghjiani, S.N., Kendrick, H. *et al.* (2000) Use of an additional

hydrophobic binding site, the Z site, in the rational drug design of a new class of stronger trypanothione reductase inhibitor, quaternary alkylammonium phenothiazines. *J. Med. Chem.*, **43**, 3148–3156.

19 Aguirre, G., Cabrera, E., Cerecetto, H., Di Maio, R., González, M., Seoane, G., Duffaut, A. *et al.* (2004) Design, synthesis and biological evaluation of new potent 5-nitrofuryl derivatives as anti-*Trypanosoma cruzi* agents. Studies of trypanothione binding site of trypanothione reductase as target for rational design. *Eur. J. Med. Chem.*, **39**, 421–431.

20 Wyllie, S., Cunningham, M.L., and Fairlamb, A.H. (2004) Dual action of antimonial drugs on thiol redox metabolism in the human pathogen leishmania donovani. *J. Biol. Chem.*, **279**, 39925–39932.

21 Dumas, C., Ouellette, M., Tovar, J., Cunningham, M.L., Fairlamb, A.H., Tamar, S., Olivier, M. *et al.* (1997) Disruption of the trypanothione reductase gene of Leishmania decreases its ability to survive oxidative stress in macrophages. *EMBO J.*, **16**, 2590–2598.

22 Krieger, S., Schwarz, W., Ariyanayagam, M.R., Fairlamb, A.H., Krauth-Siegel, R.L., and Clayton, C. (2000) Trypanosomes lacking trypanothione reductase are avirulent and show increased sensitivity to oxidative stress. *Mol. Microbiol.*, **35**, 542–552.

23 Davioud-Charvet, E., Becker, K., Landry, V., Gromer, S., Logé, C., and Sergheraert, C. (1999) Synthesis of 5,5′-dithiobis(2-nitrobenzamides)as alternative substrates for trypanothione reductase and thioredoxin reductase: a microtiter colorimetric assay for inhibitor screening. *Anal. Biochem.*, **268**, 1–8.

24 Hamilton, C.J., Saravanamuthu, A., Eggleston, I.M., and Fairlamb, A.H. (2003) Ellman's-reagent-mediated regeneration of trypanothione *in situ*: substrate-economical microplate and time-dependent inhibition assays for trypanothione reductase. *Biochem. J.*, **369**, 529–537.

25 Müller, T., Johann, L., Jannack, B., Brückner, M., Lanfranchi, D.A., Bauer, H., Sanchez, C. *et al.* (2011) Glutathione reductase-catalyzed cascade of redox

reactions to bioactivate potent antimalarial 1,4-naphthoquinones – a new strategy to combat malarial parasites. *J. Am. Chem. Soc.*, **133**, 11557–11571.

26 Davioud-Charvet, E. and Lanfranchi, D.A. (2011) Subversive substrates of glutathione reductases from *Plasmodium falciparum*-infected red blood cells as antimalarial agents, in *Apicomplexan Parasites* (ed. K. Becker), Wiley-VCH Verlag GmbH, Weinheim, pp 373–396.

27 Johann, L., Lanfranchi, D.A., Davioud-Charvet, E., and Elhabiri, M. (2012) A physico-biochemical study with redox-cyclers as antimalarial and anti-schistosomal drugs. *Curr. Pharm. Des.*, **18**, 3539–3566.

28 Blank, O., Davioud-Charvet, E., and Elhabiri, M. (2012) Interactions of the antimalarial drug methylene blue with methemoglobin and heme targets in plasmodium falciparum: a physico-biochemical study. *Antioxid. Redox Signal.*, **17**, 544–554.

29 Henderson, G.B., Ulrich, P., Fairlamb, A.H., Rosenberg, I., Pereira, M., Sela, M., and Cerami, A. (1988) 'Subversive' substrates for the enzyme trypanothione disulfide reductase: alternative approach to chemotherapy of Chagas disease. *Proc. Natl. Acad. Sci. USA*, **85**, 5374–5378.

30 Blumenstiel, K., Schöneck, R., Yardley, V., Croft, S.L., and Krauth-Siegel, R.L. (1999) Nitrofuran drugs as common subversive substrates of *Trypanosoma cruzi* lipoamide dehydrogenase and trypanothione reductase. *Biochem. Pharmacol.*, **58**, 1791–1799.

31 Salmon-Chemin, L., Lemaire, A., De Freitas, S., Deprez, B., Sergheraert, C., and Davioud-Charvet, E. (2000) Parallel synthesis of a library of 1,4-naphthoquinones and automated screening of potential inhibitors of trypanothione reductase from *Trypanosoma cruzi*. *Bioorg. Med. Chem. Lett.*, **10**, 631–635.

32 Biot, C., Bauer, H., Schirmer, R.H., and Davioud-Charvet, E. (2004) 5-substituted tetrazoles as bioisosteres of carboxylic acids. Bioisosterism and mechanistic studies on glutathione reductase inhibitors as antimalarials. *J. Med. Chem.*, **47**, 5972–5983.

33 Krauth-Siegel, R.L. and Davioud-Charvet, E. (2005) Trypanothione reductase and other flavoenzymes as targets of antiparasitic drugs, in *Flavins and Flavoproteins 2005* (eds T. Nishino, R. Miura, M. Tanokura, and K. Fukui), ARchiTect, Tokyo, pp 867–876.

34 Bauer, H., Fritz-Wolf, K., Winzer, A., Kühner, S., Little, S., Yardley, V., Vezin, H. *et al.* (2006) A fluoro analogue of the menadione derivative 6-[2′-(3′-methyl)-1′4′-naphthoquinolyl]hexanoic acid is a suicide substrate of glutathione reductase. Crystal structure of the alkylated human enzyme. *J. Am. Chem. Soc.*, **128**, 10784–10794.

35 Morin, C., Besset, T., Moutet, J.-C., Fayolle, M., Brückner, M., Limosin, D., Becker, K. *et al.* (2008) The aza-analogues of 1,4-naphthoquinones are potent substrates and inhibitors of plasmodial thioredoxin and glutathione reductases and of human erythrocyte glutathione reductase. *Org. Biomol. Chem.*, **6**, 2731–2742.

36 Lanfranchi, D.A., Belorgey, D., Müller, T., Vezin, H., Lanzer, M., and Davioud-Charvet, E. (2012) Exploring the trifluoromenadione core as a template to design antimalarial redox-active agents interacting with glutathione reductase. *Org. Biomol. Chem.*, **10**, 4795–4806.

37 Pai, E.F., Karplus, P.A., and Schulz, G.E. (1988) Crystallographic analysis of the binding of NADPH, NADPH fragments, and NADPH analogues to glutathione reductase. *Biochemistry*, **27**, 4465–4474.

38 Karplus, P.A. and Schulz, G.E. (1987) Refined structure of glutathione reductase at 1.54 Å resolution. *J. Mol. Biol.*, **195**, 701–729.

39 Karplus, P.A., Pai, E.F., and Schulz, G.E. (1989) A crystallographic study of the glutathione binding site of glutathione reductase at 0.3-nm resolution. *Eur. J. Biochem.*, **178**, 693–703.

40 Cenas, N.K., Arscott, D., Williams, C.H., and Blanchard, J.S. (1994) Mechanism of reduction of quinones by *Trypanosoma congolense* trypanothione reductase. *Biochemistry*, **33**, 2509–2515.

41 Cornish-Bowden, A. (1986) Why is uncompetitive inhibition so rare? *FEBS Lett.*, **203**, 3–6.

42 Apted, F.I.C. (1960) Nitrofurazone in the treatment of sleeping sickness due to *Trypanosoma rhodesiense. Trans. R. Soc. Trop. Med. Hyg.*, **54**, 225–228.

43 Simarro, P.P., Diarra, A., Ruiz Postigo, J.A., Franco, J.R., and Jannin, J.G. (2011) The Human African Trypanosomiasis Control and Surveillance Programme of the World Health Organization 2000–2009: The Way Forward. *PLoS Negl. Trop. Dis.*, **5**, e1007.

44 Sokolova, A.Y., Wyllie, S., Patterson, S., Oza, S.L., Read, K.D., and Fairlamb, A.H. (2010) Cross-resistance to nitro drugs and implications for treatment of human African trypanosomiasis. *Antimicrob. Agents Chemother.*, **54**, 2893–2900.

45 Cenas, N., Bironaite, D., Dickancaite, E., Anusevicius, Z., Sarlauskas, J., and Blanchard, J.S. (1994) Chinifur, a selective inhibitor and 'subversive substrate' for *Trypanosoma congolense* trypanothione reductase. *Biochem. Biophys. Res. Commun.*, **204**, 224–229.

46 Maya, J.D., Bollo, S., Nuñez-Vergara, L.J., Squella, J.A., Repetto, Y., Morello, A., Périé, J. *et al.* (2003) *Trypanosoma cruzi*: effect and mode of action of nitroimidazole and nitrofuran derivatives. *Biochem. Pharmacol.*, **65**, 999–1006.

47 Julião, M.S., da, S., Ferreira, E.I., Ferreira, N.G., and Serrano, S.H.P. (2006) Voltammetric detection of the interactions between RNO_2^- and electron acceptors in aqueous medium at highly boron doped diamond electrode (HBDDE). *Electrochim. Acta*, **51**, 5080–5086.

48 Hall, B.S., Bot, C., and Wilkinson, S.R. (2011) Nifurtimox activation by trypanosomal type I nitroreductases generates cytotoxic nitrile metabolites. *J. Biol. Chem.*, **286**, 13088–13095.

49 Carter, N.S. and Fairlamb, A.H. (1993) Arsenical-resistant trypanosomes lack an unusual adenosine transporter. *Nature*, **361**, 173–176.

50 Stewart, M.L., Bueno, G.J., Baliani, A., Klenke, B., Brun, R., Brock, J.M., Gilbert, I.H. *et al.* (2004) Trypanocidal activity of melamine-based nitroheterocycles. *Antimicrob. Agents Chemother.*, **48**, 1733–1738.

51 Baliani, A., Peal, V., Gros, L., Brun, R., Kaiser, M., Barrett, M.P., and Gilbert, I.H. (2009) Novel functionalized melamine-based nitroheterocycles: synthesis and activity against trypanosomatid parasites. *Org. Biomol. Chem.*, **7**, 1154.

52 Chung, M.-C., Güido, R.V.C., Martinelli, T.F., Gonçalves, M.F., Polli, M.C., Botelho, K.C.A., Varanda, E.A. *et al.* (2003) Synthesis and *in vitro* evaluation of potential antichagasic hydroxymethylnitrofurazone (NFOH-121): a new nitrofurazone prodrug. *Bioorg. Med. Chem.*, **11**, 4779–4783.

53 Davies, C., Cardozo, R.M., Negrette, O.S., Mora, M.C., Chung, M.C., and Basombrio, M.A. (2010) Hydroxymethylnitrofurazone is active in a murine model of Chagas disease. *Antimicrob. Agents Chemother.*, **54**, 3584–3589.

54 Fotie, J., Kaiser, M., Delfín, D.A., Manley, J., Reid, C.S., Paris, J.-M., Wenzler, T. *et al.* (2010) Antitrypanosomal activity of 1,2-dihydroquinolin-6-ols and their ester derivatives. *J. Med. Chem.*, **53**, 966–982.

55 Schirmer, R.H., Adler, H., Pickhardt, M., and Mandelkow, E. (2011) 'Lest we forget you — methylene blue . . . '. *Neurobiol. Aging*, **32**, 2325.e7–2325.e16.

56 Boda, C., Enanga, B., Courtioux, B., Breton, J.-C., and Bouteille, B. (2006) Trypanocidal activity of methylene blue. *Chemotherapy*, **52**, 16–19.

57 Buchholz, K., Comini, M.A., Wissenbach, D., Schirmer, R.H., Krauth-Siegel, R.L., and Gromer, S. (2008) Cytotoxic interactions of methylene blue with trypanosomatid-specific disulfide reductases and their dithiol products. *Mol. Biochem. Parasitol.*, **160**, 65–69.

58 Sukhova, N.M., Lidaka, M.J., Voronova, V.A., Zidermane, A.A., Kravchenko, I.M., Dauvarte, A.Z., Preisa, I.E. *et al.* (1979) amides substitués d'acides 2'-(2'-(5''nitrofuranyl-2'')vinyl et 4-(5''-nitrofuranyl-2'')-1,3-butadienyl)quinoléine-4-carboxyliques, leur procédé de préparation et leur application thérapeutique. French Patent FR19780026058.

59 Fernandez-Gomez, R., Moutiez, M., Aumercier, M., Bethegnies, G., Luyckx, M., Ouaissi, A., Tartar, A. *et al.* (1995) 2-Amino diphenylsulfides as new inhibitors of trypanothione reductase. *Int. J. Antimicrob. Agents*, **6**, 111–118.

60 Davioud-Charvet, E., McLeish, M.J., Veine, D., Giegel, D., Andricopulo, A.D., Becker, K., and Müller, S. (2002) Mechanism-based inactivation of thioredoxin reductase from Plasmodium falciparum by Mannich bases. Implications for drug design, in *Flavins and Flavoproteins 2002* (eds S. Chapman, R. Perham, and N. Scrutton), Weber, Berlin, pp 845–851.

61 Davioud-Charvet, E., McLeish, M.J., Veine, D.M., Giegel, D., Arscott, L.D., Andricopulo, A.D., Becker, K. *et al.* (2003) Mechanism-based inactivation of thioredoxin reductase from *Plasmodium falciparum* by Mannich bases. Implication for cytotoxicity. *Biochemistry*, **42**, 13319–13330.

62 Lee, B., Bauer, H., Melchers, J., Ruppert, T., Rattray, L., Yardley, V., Davioud-Charvet, E. *et al.* (2005) Irreversible inactivation of trypanothione reductase by unsaturated Mannich bases: a divinyl ketone as key intermediate. *J. Med. Chem.*, **48**, 7400–7410.

63 Wenzel, I.N., Wong, P.E., Maes, L., Müller, T.J.J., Krauth-Siegel, R.L., Barrett, M.P., and Davioud-Charvet, E. (2009) Unsaturated Mannich bases active against multidrug-resistant *Trypanosoma brucei brucei* strains. *ChemMedChem*, **4**, 339–351.

64 Angiolini, L., Ghedini, N., and Tramontini, M. (1985) The Mannich bases in polymer synthesis. 10. Synthesis of poly (β-ketothioethers) and their behaviour towards hydroperoxide reagents. *Polymer Commun.*, **26**, 218–221.

65 Wyllie, S., Patterson, S., Stojanovski, L., Simeons, F.R.C., Norval, S., Kime, R., Read, K.D. *et al.* (2012) The anti-trypanosome drug fexinidazole shows potential for treating visceral leishmaniasis. *Sci. Transl. Med.*, **4**, 119re1–119re1.

66 Capes, A., Patterson, S., Wyllie, S., Hallyburton, I., Collie, I.T., McCarroll, A.J., Stevens, M.F.G. *et al.* (2012) Quinol derivatives as potential trypanocidal agents. *Bioorg. Med. Chem.*, **20**, 1607–1615.

23
Inhibition of Trypanothione Synthetase as a Therapeutic Concept

Oliver Koch, Timo Jäger, Leopold Flohé, and Paul M. Selzer*

Abstract

Trypanothione synthetase (TryS) has been shown to synthesize both steps of trypanothione biosynthesis in all trypanosomatids so far investigated, to be essential for sustaining the entire trypanothione system and for survival of *Trypanosoma brucei* and likely of other trypanosomatids, proved to be druggable, and is therefore considered a most attractive target for the design of trypanocidal drugs. More recent insights into structure, catalytic mechanism, and substrate binding of TryS are briefly reviewed in respect of drug design options, and related achievements are compiled. Lead compounds corroborating the therapeutic concept of trypanothione synthesis inhibition have been identified. The growing knowledge on the enzyme's mechanism of action and structure offers ample further chances to design trypanocidal drugs that, due to the target's peculiarities, can be expected to be as efficacious as safe.

Introduction

As has been amply reviewed ([1–5] and Chapter 9 of this volume) the protozoan parasites of the genus *Trypanosoma* and *Leishmania*, the causative agents of Chagas' disease, African sleeping sickness, and the various forms of leishmaniasis, respectively, are *inter alia* unique in having an unusual redox metabolism. In these parasites, glutathione (GSH) is transformed into trypanothione (T(SH)$_2$, N^1, N^8-bis(glutathionyl)spermidine) and the latter, either by itself or with the aid of the thioredoxin homolog "tryparedoxin" (TXN), plays a key role in all metabolic pathways that depend on GSH and/or thioredoxin in their mammalian hosts. Many of the T(SH)$_2$-dependent enzymes could be demonstrated to be essential for parasite survival by genetic techniques (for latest review, see Chapter 9 of this volume). Out of the T(SH)$_2$-dependent pathways the metabolism of hydroperoxides ([6] and Chapter 10 of this volume) and the reduction of ribonucleotides, a pivotal step of DNA biosynthesis [7], are of vital importance. Inhibition of T(SH)$_2$ biosynthesis should affect the entire trypanothione system and, accordingly, is

---

* Corresponding Author

Trypanosomatid Diseases: Molecular Routes to Drug Discovery, First edition. Edited by T. Jäger, O. Koch, and L. Flohé.
© 2013 Wiley-VCH Verlag GmbH & Co. KGaA. Published 2013 by Wiley-VCH Verlag GmbH & Co. KGaA.

considered an attractive strategy to create trypanocidal drugs. The validity of this concept was indeed corroborated by knocking down trypanothione synthetase (TryS) expression [8,9], and related inhibitor studies in *T. brucei* [10] and *L. infantum* [11].

For *T. brucei*, and likely for *L. infantum*, TryS is thus considered a genetically and chemically validated drug target. Whether this quality holds true for TryS in all trypanosomatids remains to be verified, since the biosynthesis of $T(SH)_2$ may differ between species. In fact, the conjugation of two GSH molecules with spermidine to yield $T(SH)_2$ has for long been believed to be catalyzed by two distinct enzymes, a glutathionyl spermidine synthetase (GspS) and a TryS acting on glutathionylsper-midine (Gsp) [12]. More recently, however, TryS of *T. cruzi* [13], *T. brucei* [14], *Crithidia fasciculata* [15], *L. major* [16], *L. donovani* [17], and *L. infantum* [11] were recognized to catalyze both conjugation steps, leaving the role of GspS, which coexists in some trypanosomatids, undefined (see Chapter 9 of this volume). Another corollary is the bifunctionality of GspS [18] and TryS [19]: these enzymes also catalyze the breakdown of Gsp and $T(SH)_2$ into spermidine and GSH. The ligase activity, though, predominates [8,14,15], while the amidase activity appears to be dispensable [20].

Despite the still fragmentary knowledge on $T(SH)_2$ biosynthesis, considerable efforts were undertaken to detect or synthesize TryS inhibitors. After a first X-ray structure of TryS had been solved [19], the synthetic efforts have increasingly made use of structure-based rational design. This chapter focuses on the functional and structural characteristics of TryS with respect to inhibitor design, and compiles the approaches and achievements in the search for TryS inhibitors.

Functional and Structural Characteristics of TryS

The biosynthesis of $T(SH)_2$ (Figure 23.1) is catalyzed by the bifunctional trypano-thione synthetase amidase. The X-ray structure of *Lm*TryS [19] revealed that the two enzymatic functions reside in two distinct domains – a C-terminal synthetase domain and an N-terminal amidase domain (Figure 23.2), the latter one being less important in the present context. The synthetase moiety of TryS catalyzes the ligation of two GSH molecules to spermidine with the consumption of two ATP. As in other C–N ligases, the carboxylic function, here of the glycine of GSH, has to be phosphorylated by Mg^{2+}/ATP, before carboxamide formation with one of the terminal amino groups of spermidine can proceed, Gsp is formed as an intermedi-ate. However, since spermidine is asymmetric, two different intermediates may be formed: N^1- or N^8-Gsp, both yielding $T(SH)_2$ by a second analogous glutathiony-lation step [21]. N^8-Gsp, though, appeared to be the better interim substrate for *Cf* TryS, as evident from a lower K_m [22].

The substrate specificity of TryS, however, is not particularly strict. Apart from spermidine, TryS also accepts other polyamines and spermidine analogs (Table 23.1). *Tc*TryS can also convert aminopropylcadaverine into homotrypanothione [23] and shows a 5-fold higher activity with spermine (yielding N^1,N^{12}-bis(glutathionyl)

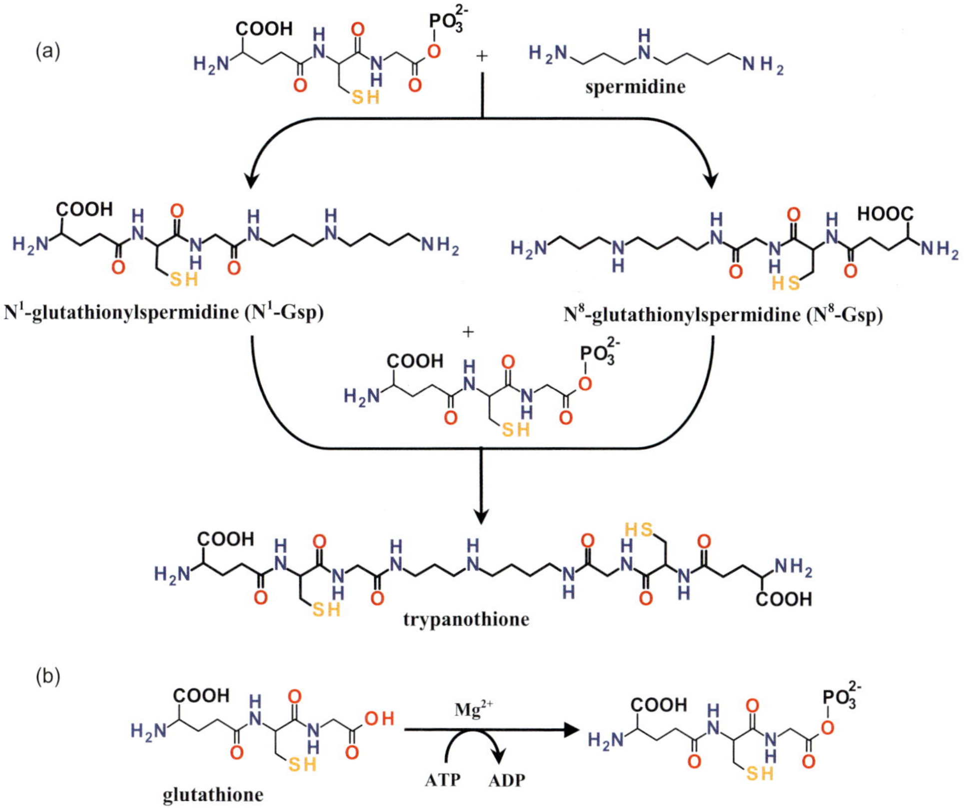

Figure 23.1 (a) Alternative routes of T(SH)$_2$ biosynthesis. Owing to the asymmetry of spermidine, the first step of trypanothione biosynthesis can lead to two different glutathionylspermidines, N^1-Gsp or N^8-Gsp. (b) Activation of glutathione by phosphorylation.

cadaverine) than with spermidine [24]. Spermine is also a substrate for *Tb*TryS [25] and *Cf*TryS [26]. Both conjugates are also physiological substrates of trypanothione reductase [23,24] and therefore can replace trypanothione in the case of spermidine shortage. Distinct polyamine specificities have been discussed to result from selective pressure exerted by the host environment [16]. The specificity of TryS for thiols has not been investigated. However, a certain tolerance in GSH specificity can be expected from specificity studies with GspS, which is homologous and quite similar to TryS. GspS is capable of processing glutathione analogs and derivatives (see Table 23.1) [27,28]. S-substitution of cysteine with methyl or ethyl or a replacement of cysteine by valine or isoleucine is well tolerated, indicating that a hydrophobic subpocket can be filled, whereas larger groups such as a butyl substituent at the cysteine lead to decrease of affinity and result in inhibition (see Section "Turncoat Inhibitors (Subversive Substrates or Redox Cyclers) of TR as Anti-Trypanosomal Drugs" of Chapter 22). While corresponding physiological substrates are missing, this data may be instrumental for TryS inhibitor design.

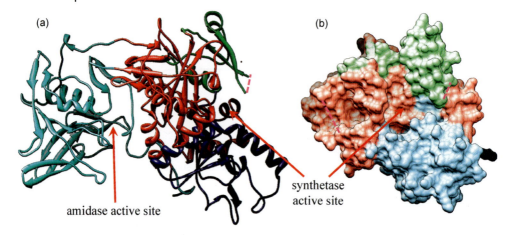

(a) amidase active site

(b) synthetase active site

Figure 23.2 TryS-amidase X-ray structure. The magenta dashed lines indicate unsolved loop regions (residues 253–261 and 552–578). The coloring indicates domains (N-terminal amidase domain of residues 1–215 and 634–652: turquoise; C-terminal synthetase domain of residues 216–393 and 595–633 (subdomain A: red), residues 394–511 (subdomain B: blue), and residues 512–594 (subdomain C: green)). Reproduced from the dataset (Protein Data Bank (PDB) ID: 2vpm) from Fyfe *et al.* [19].

Unfortunately, the molecular explanation of TryS catalysis and specificity must still rely on two X-ray structures only: the one of *Lm*TryS [19] and that of *Ec*GspS [18], a homolog of TryS from *Escherichia coli* that can only synthesize Gsp and not $T(SH)_2$ [29]. The later enzyme is, however, of interest, since its structure might disclose the difference in reaction specificity of GspS and TryS. The former structure provided important insights into the mechanism of TryS, but left some questions unanswered, because a few critical parts of the sequence (residues 251–261 and 552–578) proved to be disordered and, thus could not be solved. Starting from these two X-ray structures, an exhaustive molecular dynamics simulation has recently been performed, which corroborated mechanistic assumptions derived from previous studies, and provided further insights into substrate binding and catalysis [30].

Both enzymes, GspS and TryS, consist of two domains, a C-terminal amidase domain and an N-terminal ligase (or synthetase) domain (Figure 23.1). *Ec*GspS structures with substrate analogs bound were also obtained, from which reliable substrate binding modes for GSH, Mg^{2+}/ATP, and spermidine could be deduced [31]. Unfortunately, cocrystallization of *Lm*TryS with substrates or analogs has so far failed, but based on the pronounced similarity to *Ec*GspS homologous substrate binding could be proposed: a triangular arrangement of GSH, ATP, and spermidine in a way that activation of GSH and glutathionyl transfer to spermidine, as outlined above, appears feasible [19]. In both cases, well-structured binding sites for GSH were identified, while the binding region for spermidine seemed less characteristic in line with the broad polyamine specificity of these enzymes. The ATP is caught in

Table 23.1 Spermidine and glutathione analogs as substrates in $T(SH)_2$ biosynthesis: relative k_{cat} values in comparison to spermidine as substrate are given; "substrate" means that conversion to Gsp or a trypanothione analog was observed without kinetic analysis.

	Relative K_{cat} for TryS	Relative K_{cat} for GspS	Relative K_{cat} for GspS/TryS complex
Spermidine analog			
Spermine	substrate[d] 5.1[e]	0.8[a]	0.2[b]
N-acetyl spermine	2.3[e]	0.7[a]	
N^1-Acetylspermidine	0.07[e]	0[a]	
N^8-Acetylspermidine	0.86[e]		
Aminopropylcadaverine	substrate[c]		
N-Propyl-1,3-propanediamine		0.7[a]	
3,3-Iminobispropylamine		0.5[a]	0.176[b]
N-Methylpropanediamine		0.25[a]	
N-Cycloheyl-1,3-propanediamine		0.25[a]	
1-Propyl-1,4-diaminobutane			0.30[b]
1,7-Diaminoheptane		0[a]	0.075[b]
1,3-Diaminopropane	0.17[e]	0[a]	0.06[b]
Putrescine	0.02[e]	0[a]	0.04[b]
GSH analogs			
H-Glu-Abu-Gly-OH	0.8[a]	0.6[a]	
H-Abu-Gly-OH	0[a]	0.2[a]	
Cys-Gly	0.041[a]	0.041[a]	
Glu-Cys(S-methyl)-Gly		4.1[f]	
Glu-Cys(S-ethyl)-Gly		3.8[f]	
Glu-Cys(S-propyl)-Gly		1.0[f]	
Glu-Cys(S-butyl)-Gly		0.04[f]	
Glu-Gly-Gly		0.04[f]	
Glu-Val-Gly		1.1[f]	
Glu-Ile-Gly		1.5[f]	

a) Tested on *Cf*GspS [12].
b) Tested on co-purified *Cf*GspS and TryS [22].
c) Tested on *Tc*TryS [13].
d) Tested on *Tb*TryS [25].
e) Tested on *Tc*TryS [24].
f) Tested on *Cf*GspS [27].

an ATP-grasp fold, as is found in several C–N ligases [32]. The typical feature of the ATP-grasp proteins is a loop region that is assumed to serve as a lid after ATP binding. In TryS, this lid shields the reaction center from the solvent and is thought to minimize futile hydrolysis of ATP and/or glutathionylphosphate, before all substrates required for Gsp synthesis have been bound [15,31,33]. Almost logically, this flexible loop (residues 552–578) remained unordered, and is missing in the X-ray structure of substrate-free *Lm*TryS [19] (Figure 23.3a) and *Ec*GspS [31], while it

(a)

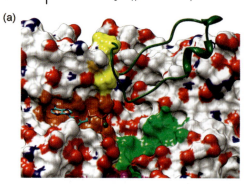

(b)

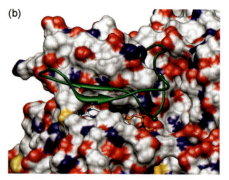

Figure 23.3 ATP-grasp fold loop. (a) Modeled loop region (green) of *Lm*TryS that is missing in the X-ray structure of *Lm*TryS [19] (surface color similar to Figure 23.4; brown: ATP binding region; light green: GSH binding region; yellow: solved residues outside loop region). (b) Loop (green) that serves as a lid in the *Ec*GspS X-ray structure (PDB ID: 2io7) [31].

was clearly resolved in the *Ec*GspS structure, when analyzed in the presence of the (inhibiting) product Mg^{2+}/ADP [31] (Figure 23.3b). It can therefore safely be assumed that the ATP binding mode in *Ec*GspS and TryS is essentially identical. In respect of inhibitor design, the ATP binding mode of ATP-grasp proteins has an important consequence: ATP mimics that bind similarly are not competed out by the abundant cellular ATP.

The molecular dynamics approach, thus, fully confirmed the substrate binding modes for the first step of the TryS reaction, as deduced from the X-ray structure. The second step had left questions open. In fact, it was hard to understand how a single enzyme could ligate two GSH molecules to the remote ends of spermidine and Comini *et al.* [15] had discussed that this might in principle be achieved by three distinct mechanisms: either (i) the enzyme has two reaction centers, (ii) a single reaction center is flexible enough to move the activated GSH to either site of the spermidine molecule, or (iii) the interim product Gsp has to change its position to offer its still free amino terminus to the reaction center. The X-ray structure, though, did not provide any evidence for two reaction centers, ruling out the first possibility; the identified sites for substrate binding appeared rigid enough to shed doubt on the second possibility and, therefore, re-binding of interim product was proposed as the only realistic option [19]. Yet docking of an inverted Gsp into a productive position for the second glutathionylation proved to be difficult, if not impossible, when the unmodified X-ray structure of *Lm*TryS was used. Extensive molecular dynamics, however, disclosed a second GSH binding pocket, which was separated from the reaction center by the spermidine binding site, and further a discrete flexibility of spermidine binding site residues. This second GSH binding site together with the prerecognized spermidine site builds an ideal binding area for N^8-Gsp. N^1-Gsp can also be bound, although its possible poses appear less productive [30]. Interestingly, the site for binding of the glutathionyl part of Gsp is made up from the second unresolved loop of the *Lm*TryS X-ray structure (residues 253–261), pointing to its substantial flexibility in the absence of substrates. It is therefore tempting to speculate that the Gsp binding area does not adopt its ideal conformation until after Gsp formation. Moreover, the loop that critically contributes to the Gsp pocket is completely different and, in fact, partially deleted in *Ec*GspS, thus explaining why this enzyme does not catalyze the second step of $T(SH)_2$ synthesis.

Figure 23.4 shows the *Lm*TryS model containing Mg^{2+}/ATP, GSH, and N^8-GSP, as obtained by molecular modeling and molecular dynamics simulation. As proposed for the first step of the catalysis, the substrates are bound in a triangular manner bringing their functional groups in sufficient contact for smooth interaction. In conclusion, the X-ray studies on *Ec*GspS [31] and *Lm*TryS [19] expanded by molecular dynamics simulations [30] and, complemented by kinetic analyses of TryS [15,25,33], suggest the following reaction mechanism (Figure 23.4). In a first step, Mg^{2+}/ATP, GSH, and spermidine bind to the S1, S2, and S3 pockets, respectively. GSH is phosphorylated and ligates to spermidine, preferentially to its N^8, yielding N^8-Gsp. ATP thereby hydrolyzed can leave the ATP-grasp cage as ADP to allow renewed ATP binding. For the second step, the glutathionyl part of N^8-Gsp moves from the S2 to the S4 site. Thereby the S2 site is cleared for renewed GSH binding

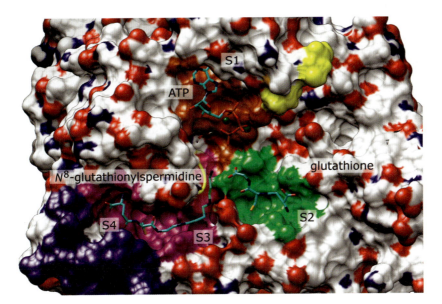

Figure 23.4 *Lm*TryS model structure containing ATP, 2 Mg^{2+}, glutathione, and N^8-Gsp according to [30]. The purple region indicates the flexible loop region that represents an important part of the Gsp binding pocket. The flexible ATP-grasp fold loop region was removed for clarity (yellow surface). The surface of residues 619/620 was set to transparent for the sake of clarity (yellow ribbon).

and the spermidine part of N^8-Gsp now occupies the S3 pocket in an inverse orientation to get its N^1 glutathionylated. Evidently the reaction sequence is accompanied by major remodeling of binding pockets, which is likely triggered by partial reactions in a still unclear manner.

TryS Inhibitor Design

Without any structural knowledge on TryS, early attempts to design inhibitors started off with derivatives or analogs of substrates, in particular of GSH. This starting point was *inter alia* chosen because GSH itself had been recognized to inhibit TryS [13,15–17,25] – a phenomenon that in retrospect is likely explained by competition for the Gsp-binding pocket (S4 in Figure 23.4). Early studies were also compromised by the misconception that TryS only catalyzes the second step of T(SH)$_2$ synthesis [12]. Inhibition of the initial step of T(SH)$_2$ synthesis appeared more attractive and, accordingly, GspS was considered a drug target of choice. However, since TryS, in its first reaction step, acts as a GspS, studies on GspS inhibition might also be relevant to TryS inhibitor design and will be considered in this chapter.

One of the first detailed analyses was presented by Verbruggen *et al.* [28] who tested phosphinic and phosphonic acid analogs of glutathione on *Cf*GspS (Table 23.2; compounds **1–6**). Later, de Creacker *et al.* [27] recognized that modifications of the cysteine or glycine moiety of GSH cannot only lead to substrates with high affinity (Table 23.1) but also to inhibitors of *Cf*GspS (Table 23.2; compounds **7–11**). A replacement of Cys against bulky hydrophobic residues (Leu/Phe) or polar ones leads to TryS inhibitors. It can be assumed that the inhibitory effect is based on a change of binding mode so that this analog can no longer be phosporylated, since smaller hydrophobic modifications yield substrates (Table 23.1). Later, Amisson *et al.* described further GSH-Gly modifications with inhibitory activity on *Cf*GspS (see Table 23.2, compounds **12–19**) [34,35]. Other glutathione derivatives were also reported to be active against *T. brucei*, *T. cruzi*, or *L. donovani* [36,37], but their precise effect on T(SH)$_2$ biosynthesis remains to be established.

Special efforts were devoted to the design of compounds to mimic the tetrahedral transition state presumed to occur during Gsp synthesis [37–39]. As compiled in Table 23.3, some of these compounds showed reasonable or even good inhibitory activity against *Ec*GspS (compounds **20–24**), *Cf*GspS (compound **21**), or TryS of different trypanosomatid species (compound **20**). The phosphina-analog of Gsp (compound **20**) also proved to be instrumental to clarify the binding pockets for GSH and spermidine in *Ec*GspS, and, as a transition state mimic, became indeed further phosphorylated at the GspS active site [31].

The ATP-grasp nature of TryS appeared to justify a search for ATP mimics that might inhibit the enzyme [40]. Screening protein kinase inhibitors, which bind ATP similarly, led to a series of paullones that inhibited *Cf*TryS. Paullones are a group of compounds preferentially targeting the ATP binding pocket of cyclin-dependent kinases [41]. In particular, N^5-substituted paullones seemed to be attractive leads

Table 23.2 GSH analogs with inhibitory activity on GspS or TryS.

	Compound	Inhibition: percentage, IC_{50} or K_i
1	γ-L-Glu-L-Val—N(H)—...P(=O)(OH)(H)	50%[a)]
2	γ-L-Glu-L-Val—N(H)—...P(=O)(OH)(OH)	78%[a)]
3	γ-L-Glu-L-Val—N(H)—...P(=O)(OH)—O—...—OCH$_3$	71%[a)]
4	γ-L-Glu-L-Leu—N(H)—...P(=O)(OH)(OH)	86%[a)], $K_i = 60\,\mu M^{c)}$
5	γ-L-Glu-L-Leu—N(H)—...(C=O)...P(=O)(OH)(OH)	62%[a)]
6	γ-L-Glu-L-Leu—N(H)—...P(=O)(O—Phenyl)(O—Phenyl)	76%[a)]
7	γ-L-Glu-L-Ser-Gly	50%[b)]
8	γ-L-Glu-L-Leu-Gly	58%[b)]
9	γ-L-Glu-L-Phe-Gly	73%[b)]
10	γ-L-Glu-L-Val-Ala	58%[b)]
11	γ-L-Glu-L-Leu-Ala	95%[b)]
12	γ-L-Glu-L-Leu-L-Dap	$K_i = 7.2\,\mu M$, $K_i' = 21\,\mu M^{c)}$
13	γ-L-Glu-L-Leu-L-Dab	$K_i = 10.4\,\mu M$, $K_i' = 24\,\mu M^{c)}$
14	γ-L-Glu-L-Leu-L-Orn	$K_i = 10\,\mu M$, $K_i' = 39\,\mu M^{c)}$
15	γ-L-Glu-L-Leu-L-Lys	$K_i = 27\,\mu M$, $K_i' = 48\,\mu M^{c)}$
16	γ-L-Glu-L-Leu-L-Arg	$K_i = 6,4\,\mu M$, $K_i' = 17\,\mu M^{c)}$
17	γ-L-Glu-L-Leu-L-Ser	$K_i = 14\,\mu M$, $K_i' = 25\,\mu M^{c)}$
18	γ-L-Glu-L-Leu-NHCH$_2$-5-tetrazole	$IC_{50} = 138\,\mu M^{d)}$
19	γ-L-Glu-L-Leu-NHCH$_2$-B(OH)$_2$ HCl	$K_i = 81\,\mu M$, $K_i' = 18\,\mu M^{d)}$

a) Tested on *Cf*GspS with 5 mM compound [28].
b) Tested on *Cf*GspS with 5 mM compound [27].
c) Tested on *Cf*GspS [34].
d) Tested on *Cf*GspS [38].

inhibiting *Cf* TryS at low nanomolar concentration (Figure 23.5). As expected for a ATP-grasp pocket binder, the inhibition was not competed out by ATP at all, thus demonstrating that such ATP mimics might indeed be useful TryS inhibitors. Unfortunately, it turned out that the most active compounds with more bulky substituents at N^5 preferentially inhibited *Cf* TryS, but hardly the TryS of pathogenic trypanosomatids. Docking of these inhibitors to various TryS structures obtained by homology modeling revealed that their high affinity to *Cf* TryS was due to binding of the substituent to a cleft near the active site of *Cf* TryS that was substantially smaller

Table 23.3 Gsp analogs presumed to mimic the transition state during Gsp formation. Inhibitory activity was tested on GspS and TryS, as indicated.

Compound	K_i
20	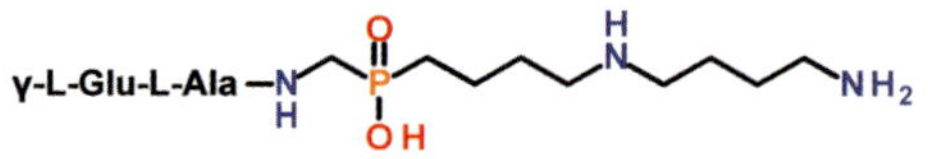 *Ec*GspS: $K_i = 3.2\,\mu M$, $K_i^* = 7.8\,nM$[b] *Cf*GspS: $K_i = 29\,nM$[c] *C*TrySS: $K_i = 1330\,nM$[c] *Lm*TryS: $K_i = 580\,nM$[c] *Tc*TryS: $K_i = 490\,nM$[c] *Tb*TryS: $K_i = 1200\,nM$[c]
21	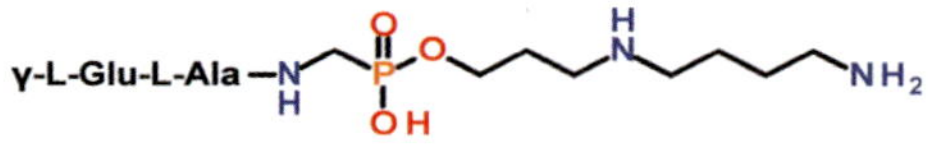 *Ec*GspS: $K_i = 6.0\,\mu M$, $K_i' = 14\,\mu M$[a] *Cf*GspS: $K_i = 156\,\mu M$[c]
22	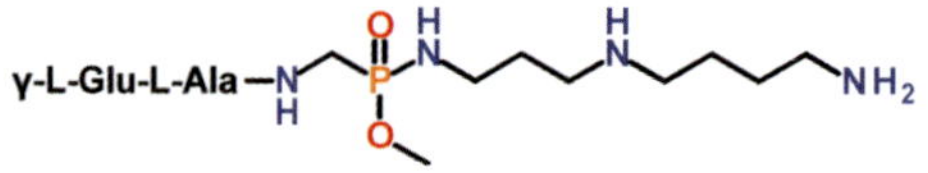 $K_i = 24.0\,\mu M$, $K_i^* = 0.88\,\mu M$[a]
23	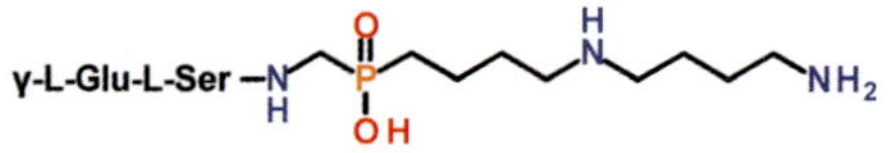 $K_i = 4.8\,\mu M$, $K_i^* = 9.2\,nM$[b]
24	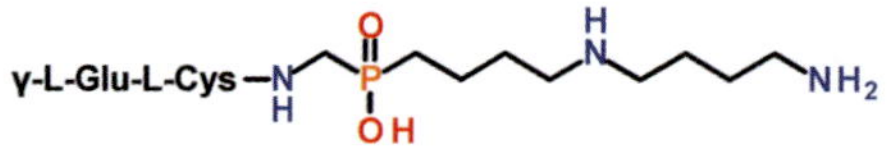 $K_i = 2.1\,\mu M$, $K_i^* = 3.1\,nM$[b]

a) *Ec*GspS [39].
b) *Ec*GspS [38].
c) *Cf*GspS and TryS from different species [33]. K_i', calculated as K for enzyme/substrate/inhibitor complex according to Chen *et al.* [39]; K_i^*, recalculated for "slow-binding inhibitors" according to Chen *et al.* [39].

in the TryS of all other species [42]. Trimming down the substituent led to compounds that also inhibit the TryS of *T. brucei, T. cruzi* (unpublished data), and *L. infantum* [11], although with so far disappointing potency.

A variety of TryS inhibitors were obtained by random screening of a library with 63 362 compounds (Table 23.4). Overall 725 confirmed hits were identified that showed greater than 33% inhibition of *Tb*TryS at a concentration of 30 μM. In total, 174 compounds were selected for further investigation leading to three series of lead

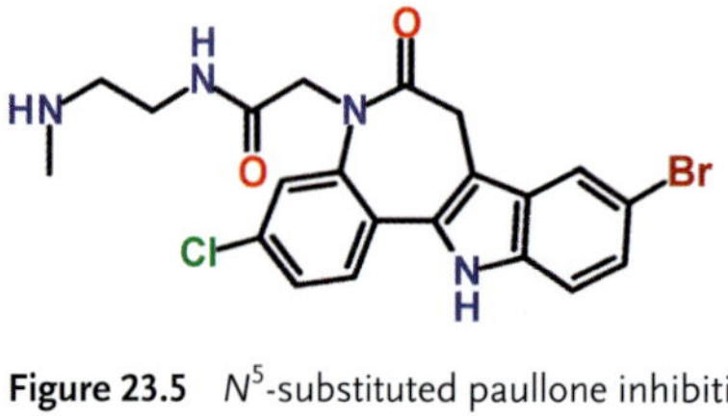

Figure 23.5 N^5-substituted paullone inhibiting *Cf* TryS with an IC$_{50}$ of 30 nM.

Table 23.4 TryS inhibitors derived from random screening.

	Compound	IC$_{50}$	EC$_{50}$
25	DDD66604	19 μM[a)]	
26	DDD60632	0.273 μM[a)]	27.1 μM
27	DDD73385	0.317 μM[a)]	21.2 μM
28	DDD85811	0.095 μM[a)]	8.8 μM
29	DDD86243	0.140 μM[a)]	5.1 μM
30	DDD86439	0.045 μM[b)]	

a) From [10].
b) From [43].
IC$_{50}$ = concentration yielding 50% inhibition of *Tb*TryS; EC$_{50}$ = concentration yielding 50% growth inhibition of bloodstream *T. brucei* after 72 h.

Table 23.5 Natural product with inhibitory activity on *Ld*TryS (IC_{50}) and activity on *L. donovani* (EC_{50}) [17].

Compound	TryS K_i	EC_{50}
Tomatione	12.54 µM	18.02 µM
	3.12 µM	13.42 µM

Conessine	3.55 µM	11.23 µM

Uvaol	6.33 µM	11.71 µM

Betulin

structures (see Table 23.4, compounds **26–29**) that were also active in a proliferation test with bloodstream *T. brucei* [10,43]. The most potent lead compound DD86243 was selected for first chemical validation of *Tb*TryS by Torrie *et al.* [10]. Expectedly, exposure of bloodstream *T. brucei* to this compound resulted in a decrease of intracellular level of $T(SH)_2$ and an increase of GSH, as had previously been observed in *T. brucei* with the TryS gene knocked down [8,9]. Moreover, the efficacy of the compound varied in a predicted manner when the TryS activity of the parasites was manipulated by genetic techniques [10].

So far, the natural product collections have only contributed few compounds that could be considered encouraging enough for further development. Some examples of *Ld*TryS inhibitors with anti-leishmanial activity are compiled in Table 23.5.

Conclusions

TryS inhibition must be rated as an attractive strategy to create novel trypanocidal drugs. The target enzyme is unique in sequence and structure, is a low-abundance protein, and has been validated genetically and chemically. Related rational inhibitor design, however, is just in its infancy, which is explained by a long-lasting confusion about the enzyme's biological role and the lack of any structural information. Only in recent years has related drug design gotten into its swing due to the first elucidation of a TryS structure and "proof of principle" by means of inhibitors that precisely fulfill theory-based predictions. Many options the target molecule offers have not yet been exploited: neither targeting its unique Gsp binding site has systematically been tried nor has the search for ATP mimics that keep the lid of its ATP-grasp pocket closed been successful. It is hoped that the chances offered by recent insights will be used to speed up the drug discovery process.

References

1 Fairlamb, A.H. (2003) Chemotherapy of human African trypanosomiasis: current and future prospects. *Trends Parasitol.*, **19**, 488–494.

2 Fairlamb, A.H. and Cerami, A. (1992) Metabolism and functions of trypanothione in the Kinetoplastida. *Annu. Rev. Microbiol.*, **46**, 695–729.

3 Flohé, L. (2012) The trypanothione system and the opportunities it offers to create drugs for the neglected kinetoplast diseases. *Biotechnol. Adv.*, **30**, 294–301.

4 Krauth-Siegel, L.R., Comini, M.A., and Schlecker, T. (2007) The trypanothione system. *Subcell. Biochem.*, **44**, 231–251.

5 Irigoin, F., Cibils, L., Comini, M.A., Wilkinson, S.R., Flohé, L., and Radi, R. (2008) Insights into the redox biology of *Trypanosoma cruzi*: trypanothione metabolism and oxidant detoxification. *Free Radic. Biol. Med.*, **45**, 733–742.

6 Castro, H. and Tomas, A.M. (2008) Peroxidases of trypanosomatids. *Antioxid. Redox. Signal.*, **10**, 1593–1606.

7 Dormeyer, M., Reckenfelderbäumer, N., Lüdemann, H., and Krauth-Siegel, R.L. (2001) Trypanothione-dependent synthesis of deoxyribonucleotides by *Trypanosoma brucei* ribonucleotide reductase. *J. Biol. Chem.*, **276**, 10602–10606.

8 Comini, M.A., Guerrero, S.A., Haile, S., Menge, U., Lünsdorf, H., and Flohé, L. (2004) Validation of *Trypanosoma brucei* trypanothione synthetase as drug target. *Free Radic. Biol. Med.*, **36**, 1289–1302.

9 Ariyanayagam, M.R., Oza, S.L., Guther, M. L., and Fairlamb, A.H. (2005) Phenotypic analysis of trypanothione synthetase knockdown in the African trypanosome. *Biochem. J.*, **391**, 425–432.

10 Torrie, L.S., Wyllie, S., Spinks, D., Oza, S. L., Thompson, S., Harrison, J.R., Gilbert, I. H., Wyatt, P.G., Fairlamb, A.H., and Frearson, J.A. (2009) Chemical validation of trypanothione synthetase: a potential drug target for human trypanosomiasis. *J. Biol. Chem.*, **284**, 36137–36145.

11 Sousa, A., Jaeger, T., Flohé, L., Tomas, A. M., and Castro, H. (2011) Functional characterization of the trypanothione biosynthetic pathway of *Leishmania infantum*. Paper presented at the *New drugs for neglected diseases. COST CM0801 Annual Meeting*, Modena.

12 Smith, K., Nadeau, K., Bradley, M., Walsh, C., and Fairlamb, A.H. (1992) Purification of glutathionylspermidine and trypanothione synthetases from *Crithidia fasciculata*. *Protein Sci.*, **1**, 874–883.

13 Oza, S.L., Tetaud, E., Ariyanayagam, M.R., Warnon, S.S., and Fairlamb, A.H. (2002) A single enzyme catalyses formation of Trypanothione from glutathione and spermidine in *Trypanosoma cruzi*. *J. Biol. Chem.*, **277**, 35853–35861.

14 Comini, M., Menge, U., and Flohé, L. (2003) Biosynthesis of trypanothione in *Trypanosoma brucei brucei*. *Biol. Chem. Hoppe Seyler.*, **384**, 653–656.

15 Comini, M., Menge, U., Wissing, J., and Flohé, L. (2005) Trypanothione synthesis in *Crithidia* revisited. *J. Biol. Chem.*, **280**, 6850–6860.

16 Oza, S.L., Shaw, M.P., Wyllie, S., and Fairlamb, A.H. (2005) Trypanothione biosynthesis in *Leishmania major*. *Mol. Biochem. Parasitol.*, **139**, 107–116.

17 Saudagar, P. and Dubey, V.K. (2011) Cloning, expression, characterization and inhibition studies on trypanothione synthetase, a drug target enzyme, from *Leishmania donovani*. *Biol. Chem.*, **392**, 1113–1122.

18 Bollinger, J.M. Jr., Kwon, D.S., Huisman, G.W., Kolter, R., and Walsh, C.T. (1995) Glutathionylspermidine metabolism in *Escherichia coli*. Purification, cloning, overproduction, and characterization of a bifunctional glutathionylspermidine synthetase/amidase. *J. Biol. Chem.*, **270**, 14031–14041.

19 Fyfe, P.K., Oza, S.L., Fairlamb, A.H., and Hunter, W.N. (2008) *Leishmania* trypanothione synthetase-amidase structure reveals a basis for regulation of conflicting synthetic and hydrolytic activities. *J. Biol. Chem.*, **283**, 17672–17680.

20 Wyllie, S., Oza, S.L., Patterson, S., Spinks, D., Thompson, S., and Fairlamb, A.H. (2009) Dissecting the essentiality of the bifunctional trypanothione synthetase-amidase in *Trypanosoma brucei* using chemical and genetic methods. *Mol. Microbiol.*, **74**, 529–540.

21 Fairlamb, A.H., Henderson, G.B., and Cerami, A. (1986) The biosynthesis of trypanothione and N^1-glutathionylspermidine in *Crithidia fasciculata*. *Mol. Biochem. Parasitol.*, **21**, 247–257.

22 Henderson, G.B., Yamaguchi, M., Novoa, L., Fairlamb, A.H., and Cerami, A. (1990) Biosynthesis of the trypanosomatid metabolite trypanothione: purification and characterization of trypanothione synthetase from *Crithidia fasciculata*. *Biochemistry*, **29**, 3924–3929.

23 Hunter, K.J., Le Quesne, S.A., and Fairlamb, A.H. (1994) Identification and biosynthesis of N^1,N^9-bis(glutathionyl) aminopropylcadaverine (homotrypanothione) in *Trypanosoma cruzi*. *Eur. J. Biochem.*, **226**, 1019–1027.

24 Ariyanayagam, M.R., Oza, S.L., Mehlert, A., and Fairlamb, A.H. (2003) Bis (glutathionyl)spermine and other novel trypanothione analogues in *Trypanosoma cruzi*. *J. Biol. Chem.*, **278**, 27612–27619.

25 Oza, S.L., Ariyanayagam, M.R., Aitcheson, N., and Fairlamb, A.H. (2003) Properties of trypanothione synthetase from *Trypanosoma brucei*. *Mol. Biochem. Parasitol.*, **131**, 25–33.

26 Comini, M.A., Dirdjaja, N., Kaschel, M., and Krauth-Siegel, R.L. (2009) Preparative enzymatic synthesis of trypanothione and trypanothione analogues. *Int. J. Parasitol.*, **39**, 1059–1062.

27 De Craecker, S., Verbruggen, C., Rajan, P.K., Smith, K., Haemers, A., and Fairlamb, A.H. (1997) Characterization of the peptide substrate specificity of glutathionylspermidine synthetase from *Crithidia fasciculata*. *Mol. Biochem. Parasitol.*, **84**, 25–32.

28 Verbruggen, C., De Craecker, S., Rajan, P., Jiao, X.-Y., Borloo, M., Smith, K., Fairlamb, A.H., and Haemers, A. (1996) Phosphonic acid and phosphinic acid tripeptides as inhibitors of glutathionylspermidine synthetase. *Bioorg. Med. Chem. Lett.*, **6**, 253–258.

29 Tabor, H. and Tabor, C.W. (1975) Isolation, characterization, and turnover of glutathionylspermidine from *Escherichia coli*. *J. Biol. Chem.*, **250**, 2648–2654.

30 Koch, O., Cappel, D., Nocker, M., Jäger, T., Flohé, L., Sotriffer, C.A., and Selzer, P.M., Molecular dynamics reveal binding mode of glutathionylspermidine by trypanothione synthetase, PLOS One, Accepted.

31 Pai, C.H., Chiang, B.Y., Ko, T.P., Chou, C.C., Chong, C.M., Yen, F.J., Chen, S., Coward, J.K., Wang, A.H., and Lin, C.H. (2006) Dual binding sites for translocation catalysis by *Escherichia coli* glutathionylspermidine synthetase. *EMBO J.*, **25**, 5970–5982.

32 Fawaz, M.V., Topper, M.E., and Firestine, S.M. (2011) The ATP-grasp enzymes. *Bioorg. Chem.*, **39**, 185–191.

33 Oza, S.L., Chen, S., Wyllie, S., Coward, J.K., and Fairlamb, A.H. (2008) ATP-dependent ligases in trypanothione biosynthesis – kinetics of catalysis and inhibition by phosphinic acid pseudopeptides. *FEBS J.*, **275**, 5408–5421.

34 Amssoms, K., Oza, S.L., Augustyns, K., Yamani, A., Lambeir, A.M., Bal, G., Van der Veken, P., Fairlamb, A.H., and Haemers, A. (2002) Glutathione-like tripeptides as inhibitors of glutathionylspermidine

synthetase. Part 2: substitution of the glycine part. *Bioorg. Med. Chem. Lett.*, **12**, 2703–2705.

35 Amssoms, K., Oza, S.L., Ravaschino, E., Yamani, A., Lambeir, A., Rajan, P., Bal, G., Rodriguez, J., Fairlamb, A.H., Augustyns, K., and Haemers, A. (2002) Glutathione-like tripeptides as inhibitors of glutathionylspermidine synthetase. Part 1: Substitution of the glycine carboxylic acid group. *Bioorg. Med. Chem. Lett.*, **12**, 2553–2556.

36 Daunes, S., D'Silva, C., Kendrick, H., Yardley, V., and Croft, S.L. (2001) QSAR study on the contribution of log$P$ and E_s to the *in vitro* antiprotozoal activity of glutathione derivatives. *J. Med. Chem.*, **44**, 2976–2983.

37 Ravaschino, E.L., Docampo, R., and Rodriguez, J.B. (2006) Design, synthesis, and biological evaluation of phosphinopeptides against *Trypanosoma cruzi* targeting trypanothione biosynthesis. *J. Med. Chem.*, **49**, 426–435.

38 Lin, C.H., Chen, S., Kwon, D.S., Coward, J. K., and Walsh, C.T. (1997) Aldehyde and phosphinate analogs of glutathione and glutathionylspermidine: potent, selective binding inhibitors of the *E. coli* bifunctional glutathionylspermidine synthetase/amidase. *Chem. Biol.*, **4**, 859–866.

39 Chen, S., Lin, C.H., Kwon, D.S., Walsh, C. T., and Coward, J.K. (1997) Design, synthesis, and biochemical evaluation of phosphonate and phosphonamidate analogs of glutathionylspermidine as inhibitors of glutathionylspermidine synthetase/amidase from *Escherichia coli*. *J. Med. Chem.*, **40**, 3842–3850.

40 Flohé, L. (2009) In search of trypanocidal drugs, in *Antiparasitic and Antibacterial Drug Discovery: From Molecular Targets to Drug Candidates* (ed. P.M. Selzer), Wiley-VCH GmbH Verlag, Weinhein, pp. 211–226.

41 Schultz, C., Link, A., Leost, M., Zaharevitz, D.W., Gussio, R., Sausville, E.A., Meijer, L., and Kunick, C. (1999) Paullones, a series of cyclin-dependent kinase inhibitors: synthesis, evaluation of CDK1/cyclin B inhibition, and *in vitro* antitumor activity. *J. Med. Chem.*, **42**, 2909–2919.

42 Koch, O., Jaeger, T., Heller, K., Stuhlmann, F., Flohé, L., and Selzer, P.M. (2009) What makes the difference? A computational approach to explain varying paullone activity on trypanothione synthetase from different species. Paper presented at the *10th Drug Design and Development Seminar and COST Action CM0801 Workshop "New Drugs for Neglected Diseases"*, Rauischholzhausen Castle.

43 Spinks, D., Torrie, L.S., Thompson, S., Harrison, J.R., Frearson, J.A., Read, K.D., Fairlamb, A.H., Wyatt, P.G., and Gilbert, I. H. (2012) Design, synthesis and biological evaluation of *Trypanosoma brucei* trypanothione synthetase inhibitors. *ChemMedChem*, **7**, 95–106.

24

Targeting the Trypanosomatidic Enzymes Pteridine Reductase and Dihydrofolate Reductase

Stefania Ferrari, Valeria Losasso, Puneet Saxena, and Maria Paola Costi*

Abstract

Drugs currently in use against *Leishmania* and *Trypanosoma* infections have limitations in terms of efficacy, safety, duration of treatment, toxicity, and resistance. It is therefore mandatory to identify molecular targets to be specifically inhibited. Folate is an essential cofactor in the biosynthesis of DNA and amino acids. The inhibition of its metabolism leads to alterations of cell replication and function. Only a few trypanosomatid enzymes of the folate pathway are presently discussed as potential targets, among them the bifunctional enzyme dihydrofolate reductase-thymidylate synthase (DHFR-TS) and pteridine reductase (PTR1). The identification of a specific enzyme such as PTR1, able to reduce folates other than biopterins, allowed the understanding of the resistance of trypanosomatids against known anti-folate drugs. In most cases only the inhibition of both enzymes, DHFR-TS and PTR1, would fully arrest the pathway's metabolic function. The proposed combination therapy opens up a novel approach: repositioning of the well-established anti-folate strategy for the treatment of trypanosomatid diseases by the discovery of novel anti-folates that complement the efficacy profile of known drugs. The present chapter compiles the existing medicinal chemistry approaches specifically targeting the folate pathway in trypanosomatids, in particular PTR1 and the DHFR activity of DHFR-TS. It covers the structural biology of the targets, related computational studies, core structure synthesis, and biological inhibitor characterization.

Introduction

Enzymes belonging to the folate pathway are among the most-studied biological targets not only in the field of anti-parasitic, but also for anti-microbial and anti-tumoral drugs. They are among the best-ranking targets within the TDR Targets database (www.dndi.org and www.who.int) [1]. Some of the enzymes belonging to this pathway, such as thymidylate synthase (TS), dihydrofolate reductase (DHFR), and pteridine reductase (PTR1), are of interest as targets for the design of new inhibitors, because they are involved in the biosynthesis of reduced folate, which is

---

* Corresponding Author

Trypanosomatid Diseases: Molecular Routes to Drug Discovery, First edition. Edited by T. Jäger, O. Koch, and L. Flohé.
© 2013 Wiley-VCH Verlag GmbH & Co. KGaA. Published 2013 by Wiley-VCH Verlag GmbH & Co. KGaA.

an essential cofactor for the synthesis of the 2′-deoxythymidine-5′-monophosphate (dTMP) necessary for DNA synthesis (Figure 24.1). TS catalyzes the reductive methylation of 2′-deoxyuridine-5′-monophosphate (dUMP) to dTMP, using the cofactor N^5,N^{10}-methylenetetrahydrofolate (mTHF) as a carbon donor and reducing agent. DHFR restores the 5,6,7,8-tetrahydrofolate (THF) pool through the NADPH-dependent reduction of the 7,8-dihydrofolate previously produced. In trypanosomatids the DHFR and TS activities are achieved by a single bifunctional enzyme, DHFR-TS. Folate analogs acting as DHFR inhibitors were ineffective in the control of infections caused by the *Leishmania* and *Trypanosoma* parasites, due to different resistance mechanisms, including reduced uptake mediated by folate transporters, modulation of the level of polyglutamylated folates, and the presence of PTR1 [2]. PTR1 belongs to the family of short-chain dehydrogenases/reductases (SDRs), and reduces both folate and unconjugated pterin (biopterin) [3]. Reduced biopterins are essential for several cellular metabolic cycles, whereas the ability of PTR1 to reduce folates acts as a metabolic bypass when DHFR is inhibited. Under physiological conditions PTR1 is responsible for the reduction of 10% of the folic acid required by the cell, but when classic anti-folate drugs inhibit DHFR-TS, PTR1 is upregulated, thus providing the amount of reduced folates necessary for parasite survival. In *T. brucei*, PTR1 was demonstrated to be a promising drug target by itself or when DHFR is simultaneously inhibited [4]. However, a *L. major* PTR1-null mutant was shown to be viable; consequently in *L. major*, PTR1 is not a drug target on its own, if DHFR-TS is not inhibited [5,6], whereas a combination strategy has been demonstrated to work [7,8] *in vitro*. Therefore, identifying a specific inhibitor of PTR1 and using that inhibitor in combination with known anti-folates to optimize anti-parasitic efficacy appears to be a valid concept [7]. Many anti-folates are available as approved or investigational drugs or lead compounds from previous discovery programs. Many pteridine and pyrimidine derivatives have also been tested against the *Trypanosoma* and *Leishmania* parasites, and often exhibited anti-parasitic activities. However, the usually poor selectivity for the parasitic enzyme(s) and related toxicity has remained a matter of concern. In this chapter, medicinal chemistry approaches to generate anti-folates targeting PTR1 and DHFR proteins will be compiled.

X-Ray Crystal Structures of DHFR and PTR1

Structural Studies of PTR1

The primary sequences of PTR1 show identity percentages in the range of 72–95% among *Leishmania* species, and 41–46% between the *Leishmania* and *Trypanosoma* parasites. The PTR1 sequences from *Trypanosoma* species share a 53% identity, whereas the sequences of PTR1 and PTR2 in *T. cruzi* are almost identical (95% identity), with only nine residues differing (Table 24.1 and Figure 24.2). The first three-dimensional (3-D) structure of a PTR, the ternary complex of *Lm*PTR1, NADPH, and methotrexate (MTX), was deposited in the Protein Data Bank

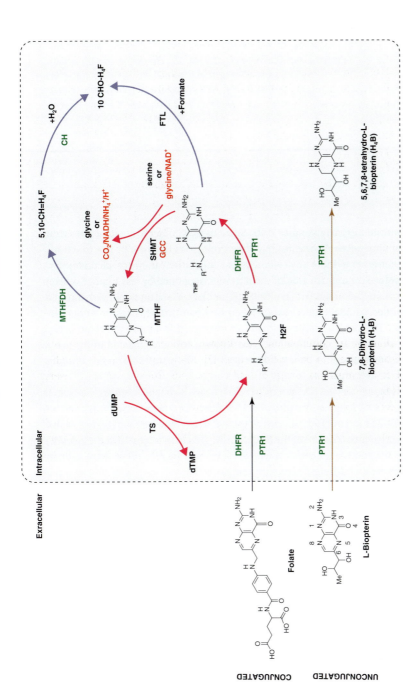

Figure 24.1 Schematic representation of several pathways involving PTR1 and DHFR. The cosubstrates folic acid and biopterin are salvaged and activated by *Leishmania* using both PTR1 and DHFR. The biopterin reduction pathway is shown with brown arrows, whereas the initial involvement of folic acid is depicted in black. The DHFR/PTR1 pathway is shown in pink arrows while the MTHFDH (methylene-H_4F dehydrogenase/methenyl-H_4F cyclohydrolase) is represented in purple color. SHMT: serine hydroxymethyltransferase; GCC: glycine cleavage complex; FTL: formyltetrahydrofolate ligase; MTHFDH: methylene tetrahydrofolate dehydrogenase; CH: cyclohydrolase.

Table 24.1 Percentage of identity (and similarity) among the PTR1 sequences from 10 trypanosomatidic parasites.

	Lb	Ld	Li	Lm	Lme	Lt	Ltr	Tb	Tc (1)	Tc (2)
L. amazonensis	72 (83)	91 (94)	91 (94)	91 (94)	88 (91)	79 (86)	95 (96)	41 (58)	45 (60)	45 (60)
L. braziliensis		74 (84)	74 (84)	72 (83)	74 (83)	73 (83)	75 (85)	45 (58)	46 (60)	46 (60)
L. donovani			99 (99)	90 (94)	90 (94)	82 (87)	95 (97)	42 (58)	45 (60)	46 (60)
L. infantum				90 (94)	90 (94)	82 (87)	95 (97)	42 (58)	45 (60)	46 (60)
L. major					87 (91)	80 (87)	93 (96)	43 (59)	45 (60)	45 (60)
L. mexicana						82 (87)	92 (93)	43 (58)	45 (60)	45 (59)
L. tarentolae							82 (88)	44 (60)	45 (60)	46 (60)
L. tropica								42 (59)	45 (60)	45 (60)
T. brucei									53 (69)	54 (69)
T. cruzi (PTR1)										95 (97)

(PDB) (www.rcsb.org) in September 2001. Since then, 38 other X-ray structures from five different kinetoplastid parasites have been released (Table 24.2). The functional enzyme is a tetramer without any evidence for cooperativity in the mechanism. Two active sites colocalize on each side of the tetramer, separated by less than 25 Å. Each monomer has a α/β-domain with typical SDR topology based on the Rossmann fold: a seven-stranded parallel β-sheet sandwiched between three helices on either side (Figure 24.3). The catalytic center is mainly constructed from a single chain except for the side-chain of Arg 287 (*Lm*PTR1 numbering), which is located in the active site of the partner subunit, where it interacts with the substrates through a bridging water molecule (Figure 24.4).

The catalytic center lies in a curved cleft – an L-shaped depression that is approximately 30 Å long, 22 Å wide, and 15 Å deep. The loop between β6 and α6 (residues 225–233 in *Lm*PTR1), known as the substrate-binding loop (Figure 24.3b), is a common structural feature of the SDR family. This loop is located at the entrance of the active site and makes contacts with substrates or ligands present at the active site. A comparison of different structures suggests that this loop is flexible and that its conformation depends on its interactions with the substrate or inhibitors, respectively [5,11]. However, the comparison of different crystallographic 3-D structures shows that there is a high level of structural conservation of the protein, irrespective of whether PTR1 is in a binary or a ternary complex or whether a substrate, product or inhibitor is bound. The PTR1 catalytic center appears to be relatively rigid, with the correct alignment of functional groups to support catalysis. Seven residues (Arg17, Ser111, Phe113, Asp181, Tyr194, Lys198, and Arg287′; *Lm*PTR1 numbering) are important for creating the active site or substrate binding or have been implicated in catalysis [5] (Figure 24.2 and Figure 24.4a). A network of hydrogen bonds organizes the active site and serves to position the cosubstrate NADPH [10]. The interaction between PTR1 and NADPH differs from that of other SDRs in two respects: (i) in the consensus coenzyme-binding motif, GxxxGxG (where x is any amino acid), which is involved in cofactor recognition, and (ii) in the cofactor binding motif   NADPH specificity

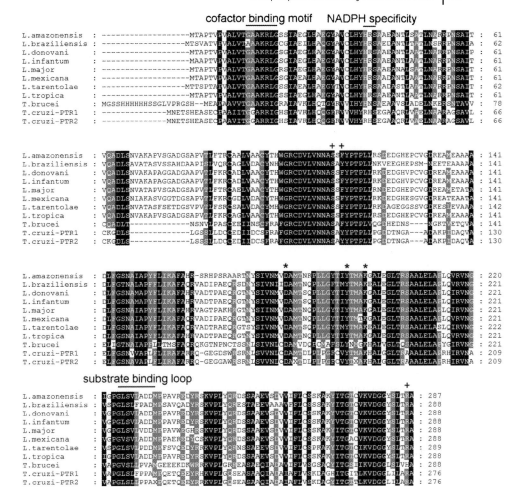

Figure 24.2 Alignment of 11 PTR1 sequences from 10 different trypanosomatid species. Residues conserved (identity or strong similarity) among all the 11 sequences are represented with black background; residues conserved among at least nine out of 11 sequences are represented with gray background. Important motifs and regions cited in the text are labeled: *residues form the catalytic triad; +other residues important for creating the active site, substrate binding, or implicated in catalysis. Source: NCBI-Protein database (http://www.ncbi.nlm.nih.gov/protein); accession codes: 2196544, 134062149, 317455034, 134069808, 16975355, 322491891, 34810072, 83701129, 270346627, 2842819, and 38492443.

pattern determining the nucleotide (NADH versus NADPH) specificity. PTR1 has an Arg residue (Arg17 in LmPTR1) instead of the second Gly residue (Figure 24.2), and it confers specificity using three residues of the main-chain (His38, Arg39, and Ser40 in *Lm*PTR1) to generate a 2′-phosphate-binding pocket instead of having two basic side-chains interacting with NADPH [4] (Figure 24.2). In substrates binding,

Table 24.2 List of crystallographic structures of PTR1 available in the PDB.

Source	Cofactor/substrate/ligand present in the structure	PDB ID
L. donovani	–	2XOX [9]
L. major	NADPH, MTX	1E7W [4]
	NADP⁺, DHB	1E92 [4]
	NADP⁺, TAQ	1WOC [10]
	NADP⁺, DHB	2BF7 [5]
	NADPH, CB3717	2BFA [5]
	NADPH, trimethoprim	2BFM [5]
	NADPH	2BFO [5]
	NADP⁺, tetrahydrobiopterin	2BFP [5]
	NADP⁺, methyl 1-(4-{[(2,4-diaminopteridin-6-yl)methyl](methyl)amino}benzoyl)piperidine-4-carboxylate	2QHX [7]
	NADP⁺, methyl 1-(4-{[(2,4-diaminopteridin-6-yl)methyl]amino}benzoyl)piperidine-4-carboxylate	3H4V [7]
L. tarentolae	NADPH, MTX	1P33 [11]
T. brucei	NADP⁺, 6,7-bis(1-methylethyl)pteridine-2,4-diamine	3JQ6 [8]
	NADP⁺, 6-phenylpteridine-2,4,7-triamine	3JQ7 [8]
	NADP⁺, 6,7,7-trimethyl-7,8-dihydropteridine-2,4-diamine	3JQ8 [8]
	NADP⁺, 2-amino-6-(1,3-benzodioxol-5-yl)-4-oxo-4,7-dihydro-H-pyrrolo[2,3-*d*]pyrimidine-5-carbonitrile	3JQ9 [8]
	NADP⁺, 2-amino-1,9-dihydro-6H-purine-6-thione	3JQA [8]
	NADP⁺, 2-amino-5-(2-phenylethyl)-3,7-dihydro-4H-pyrrolo[2,3-*d*]pyrimidin-4-one	3JQB [8]
	NADP⁺, 2-amino-6-bromo-4-oxo-4,7-dihydro-3H-pyrrolo[2,3-*d*]pyrimidine-5-carbonitrile	3JQC [8]
	NADP⁺, 2-amino-4-oxo-6-phenyl-4,7-dihydro-3H-pyrrolo[2,3-*d*]pyrimidine-5-carbonitrile	3JQD [8]
	NADP⁺, 2-amino-6-(4-methoxyphenyl)-4-oxo-4,7-dihydro-3H-pyrrolo[2,3-*d*]pyrimidine-5-carbonitrile	3JQE [8]
	NADP⁺, 1,3,5-triazine-2,4,6-triamine	3JQF [8]
	NADP⁺, 6-[(4-methoxybenzyl)sulfanyl]pyrimidine-2,4-diamine	3JQG [8]
	NADP⁺, MTX	2C7V [12]
	NADP⁺, folic acid	3BMC [8]
	NADP⁺, N^2-cyclopropyl-1,3,5-triazine-2,4,6-triamine	3BMN [8]
	NADP⁺, 6-[(4-methylphenyl)sulfanyl]pyrimidine-2,4-diamine	3BMO [8]
	NADP⁺, 6-(benzylsulfanyl)pyrimidine-2,4-diamine	3BMQ [8]
	NADP⁺, 6-chloro-1H-benzimidazol-2-amine	2WD7 [13]
	NADP⁺, 1-(3,4-dichlorobenzyl)-7-phenyl-1H-benzimidazol-2-amine	2WD8 [13]
	NADP⁺, 6-(4-methylphenyl)quinazoline-2,4-diamine	2VZ0 [14]
	NADP⁺, 1H-benzimidazol-2-amine	3GN1 [13]
	NADP⁺, 1-(3,4-dichlorobenzyl)-1H-benzimidazol-2-amine	3GN2 [13]
	NADP⁺, 5-[2-(2,5-dimethoxyphenyl)ethyl]thieno[2,3-d]pyrimidine-2,4-diamine	3MCV [15]
	NADP⁺, 2-{4-[2-(2-amino-4-oxo-4,7-dihydro-3H-pyrrolo[2,3-d]pyrimidin-5-yl)-ethyl]-benzoylamino}-pentanedioic acid	2X9G [15]
	NADP⁺, TMQ	2X9V [15]
	NADP⁺, N^2-cyclopropyl-1,3,5-triazine-2,4,6-triamine	2X9N [15]
T. cruzi	NADPH, MTX	1MXF [16]
	NADP⁺, dihydrofolic acid	1MXH [16]

(a)

(b)

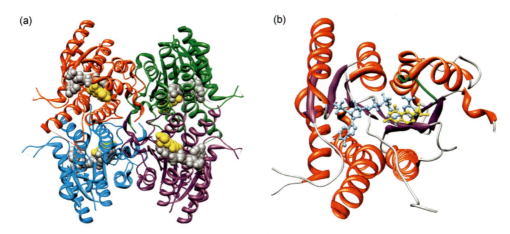

Figure 24.3 *Lm*PTR1 structure (PDB ID: 1E92). (a) Tetrameric structure of *Lm*PTR1. Each subunit is colored with a different color. The cofactor (in gray) and the substrate (in yellow) are represented in spheres. (b) Monomer of *Lm*PTR1 in ribbon representation (Rossmann fold). The substrate-binding loop is highlighted in green. The cosubstrate (in cyan) and the substrate (in yellow) are represented in ball and stick.

the pterin is sandwiched between Phe113 (*Lm*PTR1 numbering) and nicotinamide and all eight functional groups are involved in hydrogen -bond interactions, five of which directly with the cosubstrate. Such extensive interaction between the substrate and cosubstrate is unique to PTR1 among the SDR family members [4]. In the binary complex (LmPTR1) and (NADPH), the pterin-binding site is occupied by water molecules, and ethylene glycol binds to Asp181 and Arg287′ [5]. As much of

(a)

(b)

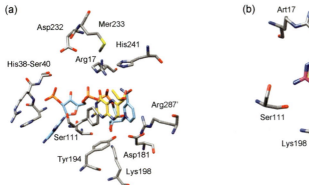
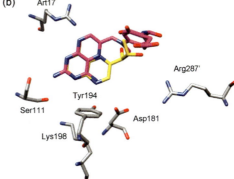

Figure 24.4 Residues forming the *Lm*PTR1 active site (PDB ID: 1E92). Each protein residue and molecule is colored by atom: N, blue; O, red; S, yellow; C, gray. (a) *Lm*PTR1 active site with bound NADP^{+} (C atom in cyan) and DHB (C atom in yellow). (b) Comparison of substrate (DHB, C atom in yellow) and MTX (C atom in magenta, from PDB ID: 1E7W) binding orientation.

the pterin-binding site is formed by nicotinamide, the substrate can only bind effectively after the formation of the protein–cofactor complex. Such an ordered, sequential mechanism is common in SDRs [4].

In PTR, both reductions (to the dihydro derivative and tetrahydro derivative) have been shown to utilize the same substrate orientation. PTR1 accomplishes two modes of reduction in a single active site. The first reduction, similar to that of other SDR family members, utilizes a catalytic triad formed by a Tyr, a Lys, and an Asp (Tyr194, Lys198, and Asp181 in *Lm*PTR1) (Figure 24.2 and Figure 24.4a) to (i) position the nicotinamide of NADPH for hydride transfer (Lys), (ii) acquire a proton from the solvent (Asp), and (iii) pass the proton over onto the substrate (Tyr). The Lys residue with its basic side-chain may also reduce the pK_a of Tyr and thereby assist catalysis. The second reduction presents similarities with DHFR: the proton source is a suitably positioned water molecule and the pK_a has been proposed to be decreased by an interaction with the acidic 4-hydroxy group of the enolized substrate. The enolization is favored by the interaction between the NADPH diphosphate and an Arg residue (Arg17 in *Lm*PTR1, Figure 24.2 and Figure 24.4a) [4].

PTR1s from different species display different activities: *Lm*PTR1 is known to be able to catalyze all four reductions (folates and biopterins), whereas *Tb*PTR1 is equally active with biopterin and dihydrobiopterin (DHB) as substrates but relatively inefficient with folate and dihydrofolate (DHF). The slower catalysis of folates and weaker inhibition displayed by MTX against *Tb*PTR1 may be due to the presence of a less flexible and more restricted binding pocket in that enzyme compared with that of *Lm*PTR1. *Tb*PTR1 and *Lm*PTR1 show 51% identity and a closely related topology; however, few structural differences are responsible for the different enzymatic activities and inhibition profiles of these enzymes [5,8,12]. In 2003, Senkovich *et al.* expressed a recombinant PTR from *T. cruzi* (*Tc*PTR2) that can reduce only dihydropteridines but not oxidized pteridine [17]. This protein differs from the previously reported *Tc*PTR1 [3] at only nine amino acid positions in the primary sequence and the comparison of the two crystallographic structures could not explain the inability of *Tc*PTR2 to catalyze the first reduction step [16].

A number of structures of PTR1 complexed with different ligands have been obtained, (Table 24.2). The binding of MTX to PTR1/NADPH is dominated by interactions with the cosubstrate through five hydrogen bonds. The pteridine ring of MTX binds in a different orientation, rotated about the N^2–N^5 axis by 180° relative to the binding orientation observed for DHB (Figure 24.4b). CB3717 is an N^{10}-substituted, conjugated, pterin-like molecule similar to MTX but with two significant differences: it is a 2-amino-4-oxoquinazoline and it has a prop-2-inyl (propargyl) group as the N^{10} substituent. The 2-amino-4-oxoquinazoline adopts a pterin-like binding mode [5], and is sandwiched between the cosubstrate's nicotinamide and Phe113 (*Lm*PTR1 numbering), a position at which all of its functional groups participate in hydrogen bonding. In both crystallographic structures, an ethylene glycol molecule is present, which replaces several of the highly conserved and ordered water molecules observed in the other structures [5]. The *p*-aminobenzoate (pABA)-glutamate tail of these inhibitors is poorly ordered, as reflected by their thermal parameters and the less well-defined electron density associated with this group [4]. This feature is likely a consequence of the shape of the PTR1 ligand-binding cavity, which is relatively wide just above the catalytic center with a concomitant lack of specific interactions formed between the ligand and the enzyme. A biological consequence of this wide entry into the active site is that PTR1 is a broad-spectrum enzyme that can process a range of pteridine compounds, including conjugated pteridines such as DHF. However, the shape of the cavity also explains why ligands such as MTX and CB3717 are more potent inhibitors of DHFR and TS, respectively [5]. The lack of affinity of PTR1 for the pABA-Glu tail of MTX is demonstrated indirectly by the inhibitor 2,4,6-triaminoquinazoline (TAQ), which simply is the pterin component of MTX. Notably, TAQ, despite being a much smaller molecule than MTX, displays a comparable level of inhibition (IC_{50} values of 2.0 and 1.1 µM, respectively, towards *Lm*PTR1). The overlay of the crystal structures of these molecules in complex with *Lm*PTR1 indicates that their pterin-like head groups bind to the active site of the enzyme in a very similar fashion [10]. The interaction of trimethoprim (IC_{50} of 12 µM) with PTR1 is very different. The diaminopyrimidine is displaced by approximately 2.5 Å from the pterin-equivalent binding position, which can be explained by steric restrictions imposed on the trimethoxyphenyl tail of the inhibitor [5]. Few aminobenzimidazole derivatives, crystallized in complex with *Tc*PTR1, showed distinct binding modes in the PTR1 active site depending on their substituents [13]. Only one of these resembles the previously observed binding modes, suggesting a further synthetic elaboration of known ligands to exploit the alternative observed binding modes.

Structural Studies of DHFR

In the bifunctional enzyme DHFR-TS of trypanosomatids the N-terminal DHFR domain (residues 1–232 in *Tc*DHFR-TS) is joined by a linker to the TS domain (residues 235–521 in *Tc*DHFR-TS). The *Tc*DHFR domain possesses only 36% identity with its human counterpart and has an additional 20 amino acid residues at the N-terminus. Moreover, several key residues involved in binding anti-folates in human DHFR (*Hs*DHFR) are replaced by other amino acids in equivalent positions in the *T. cruzi* protein [18]. The active site in the *Tc*DHFR domain appears to be more hydrophobic than the site in *Hs*DHFR, suggesting that the former should favor the binding of lipophilic inhibitors. The overall structure of *Tc*DHFR-TS is very similar to that of *L. major* DHFR-TS (*Lm*DHFR-TS), with a 68.8% sequence identity [18].

Ten structures of trypanosomatid DHFRs have been deposited in the PDB since 2008 (Table 24.3). Other crystallographic structures of *Tc*DHFR and *Lm*DHFR are known from the literature, but are not publically available [19,20].

The overall structure of *Tc*DHFR-TS is very flexible. There is evidence of functional interactions between the domains, via conformational changes of the two domains, as revealed in the rotation angles between different subunits [18]. Owing to the short linker connecting the two domains, the orientation of the DHFR domains relative to the TS domains is restricted and the two active sites are on the same side of the structure [18] (Figure 24.5). The fold of the DHFR domain is characterized by a mixed

Table 24.3 List of crystallographic structures of DHFR available from the PDB (the structures of *T. cruzi* are the complete bifunctional DHFR-TS enzyme).

Source	Cofactor/substrate/ligand present in the structure	PDB ID:
T. brucei	NADPH, 5-(4-chloro-phenyl)-6-ethyl-pyrimidine-2,4-diamine	3QFX [21]
	NADPH, 6,6-dimethyl-1-[3-(2,4,5-trichlorophenoxy)propoxy]-1,6-dihydro-1,3,5-triazine-2,4-diamine	3RG9 [21]
T. cruzi	NADP$^+$, dUMP	2H2Q [18,19]
	NADP$^+$, MTX + dUMP	3CL9 [18,19]
	NADP$^+$, TMQ	3CLB/3HBB[a] [18,19]
	NADP$^+$, ethyl 4-(5-{[(2,4-diaminoquinazolin-6-yl)methyl]amino}-2-methoxyphenoxy)butanoate	3KJS [22]
	NADPH, 1-[3-(2,3-dichlorophenoxy)propoxy]-6,6-dimethyl-1,6-dihydro-1,3,5-triazine-2,4-diamine + dUMP	3INV [23]
	1-(4-chlorophenyl)-6,6-dimethyl-1,6-dihydro-1,3,5-triazine-2,4-diamine	3IRM [23]
	NADPH, 1-(4-chlorophenyl)-6,6-dimethyl-1,6-dihydro-1,3,5-triazine-2,4-diamine	3IRN [23]
	NADPH, 5-[3-(3-fluorophenoxy)propoxy]quinazoline-2,4-diamine	3IRO [23]

a) These refer to two different refinements of the same structure.

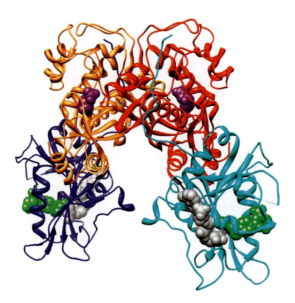

Figure 24.5 Crystallographic structure of TcDHFR-TS (PDB ID: 3CL9) in complex with dUMP (purple), NADP$^+$ (gray), and MTX (green). The two TS domains are colored in orange and red; the two DHFR domains are colored in cyan and blue; the short linking region between the two domains is shown in black.

β-sheet of eight strands (order 43251687), with strand 8 being antiparallel to the rest [18]. The cosubstrate specificity is determined by several contacts between the adenine phosphate O atoms and particular protein residues (Thr102, Ser100, Ser101, and Arg78). Other hydrogen bonds between the cosubstrate and the protein involve the following residues: Ala28, Thr80, Ser158, and Gly157. Hydrophobic interactions are formed between the adenine ring and the protein [18].

The N-terminal extension (residues 1–20) of the *Tc*DHFR domain folds back on the TS domain; its modulation of the catalytic activity of the two domains has been shown in *L. major* and *Plasmodium falciparum* enzymes [18,24] (Figure 24.5). Senkowich *et al.* [18] suggested a possible role of the C-terminal end of this loop in transmitting the information due to its contact with two helices of the DHFR domain (residues 132–145 and 156–171 in *Tc*DHFR), the conformation of which may be sensitive to the presence of the bound cosubstrate. A comparison of the *Tc*DHFR domain in the binary and ternary complexes demonstrates a closure of the binding pocket upon inhibitor binding; there are movements in Met49, Asp48, Phe52, Ile84, Phe88, Leu91, and the nicotinamide moiety of the cosubstrate [18,19].

A study by Vanichtanankul *et al.* [21] highlighted the similarity of *Tb*DHFR to a mutant of the *P. falciparum* enzyme (*Pf*DHFR) that is associated with pyrimethamine (PYR) resistance. This similarity has been suggested to explain the substantially higher inhibition constants of *Tb*DHFR for rigid anti-folates, including PYR. The crystal structure of *Tb*DHFR complexed with PYR has shown that Thr86 (in *Tb*DHFR corresponding to Ser108 in PYR-sensitive *Pf*DHFR) is responsible for a displacement of the rigid PYR ligand, which then causes movements in the Leu90 and the Pro91–Phe94 loop. The same study showed that this displacement does not happen with more flexible inhibitors [21]. The search for effective trypanosomal DHFR inhibitors should benefit from the development of new *Pf*DHFR inhibitors that are being developed to overcome PYR-resistance.

Discovery and Development of PTR1 Inhibitors

Pteridine-Like Compounds

The pteridine-like compounds resemble the substrate structure. Modulation of the folate core can significantly change the activity profile. Beverley *et al.* [25] described the inhibition profile and anti-leishmanial activity of three series of compounds: diaminopteridines, quinazolines, and 5-deazapteridines. Some of the compounds very effectively inhibited PTR1 (Table 24.4 , compounds **1** and **2**) but showed limited efficacy against the *L. major* strain LT252 clone CC1. They were also tested against mutants of *Leishmania* lacking DHFR-TS (*dhfr-ts⁻*) or PTR1 (*ptr1⁻*) to gain information regarding their mechanism of action.

Compounds with similar structures (diaminopteridines and quinoxalines) have also been studied by Cavazzuti *et al.* [7]. A medium-throughput screening approach was performed against *Lm*PTR1 and *Tc*PTR1. The trypanosomatid studies were enlarged to a panel of microbial enzymes and the corresponding human enzymes

Table 24.4 Chemical structures and activity values for PTR1 inhibitors.

ID	Structure		Activities
1		$W = NH_2$, $NH\text{-}CH_3$, $NH\text{-}Ac$, OH, H, CH_3 $X = NH_2$, $NH\text{-}Ac$, OH, H $Y = N$, CH, CH_2 $Z = N$, $N\text{-}CH_3$, CH, CH_2	best compounds of this series showed IC_{50} versus LmPTR1 $= 0.4\,\mu M$
2			best compounds of this series showed IC_{50} versus LmPTR1 $= 0.4\,\mu M$
3			K_i versus LmPTR1: $0.1\,\mu M$ K_i versus TcPTR1: $7\,\mu M$ K_i versus HsTS: no inhibition at $190\,\mu M$ K_i versus HsDHFR: $10\,\mu M$
4			K_i versus LmPTR1: $0.037\,\mu M$ K_i versus HsDHFR: $0.8\,\mu M$
5			[a] IC_{50} versus *L. donovani* promastigote: $0.101\,M$ [a] IC_{50} versus *L. donovani* amastigote: $0.0231\,M$
6			[a] IC_{50} versus *L. donovani* promastigote: $0.0908\,M$ [a] IC_{50} versus *L. donovani* amastigote: $0.018\,M$

7

K_i versus *Ld*PTR1: 0.428 μM
IC$_{50}$ versus *L. donovani*
amastigote: 10 μM

8

best compounds of this series
showed:
IC$_{50}$ versus *L. donovani*
promastigote: 0.22 μg/ml
IC$_{50}$ versus *L. donovani*
amastigote: 0.75 μg/ml

9

best compounds of this series
showed:
IC$_{50}$ versus *L. donovani*
promastigote: 4.17 μg/ml
IC$_{50}$ versus *L. donovani*
amastigote: 14.35 μg/ml

10

best compounds of this series
showed:
IC$_{50}$ versus *L. donovani*
promastigote: 121 μM

11

best compounds of this series
showed:
IC$_{50}$ versus *L. donovani*
promastigote: 29 μM
IC$_{50}$ versus *L. donovani*
amastigote: 3 μM

12

IC$_{50}$ versus *Lm*PTR1 = 1.1 μM
IC$_{50}$ versus
*Tc*DHFR = 0.0038 nM
EC$_{50}$ versus *L. major*
promastigote: 0.3 μM
EC$_{50}$ versus *T. cruzi* amastigote:
9.2 μM

(continued)

Table 24.4 (*Continued*)

ID	Structure	Activities
13		IC_{50} versus *Lm*PTR1 = 2.0 µM
14		IC_{50} versus *Lm*PTR1 = 5.6 mM
15		IC_{50} versus *Lm*PTR1 = 50 µM
16		K_i^{app} versus *Tb*PTR1: 10.6 µM
17		K_i^{app} versus *Tb*PTR1: 288 µM
18		K_i^{app} versus *Tb*PTR1: 0.4 µM
19		K_i^{app} versus *Tb*PTR1: 0.007 µM K_i^{app} versus *Tb*DHFR: >50 µM K_i^{app} versus *Hs*DHFR: >50 µM EC_{50} versus *T. brucei* = 9.9 µM EC_{50} versus MRC5 ≥ 30 µM
20		K_i^{app} versus *Tb*PTR1: 0.047 µM K_i^{app} versus *Tb*DHFR: >30 µM K_i^{app} versus *Hs*DHFR: >50 µM EC_{50} versus *T. brucei* = 9.6 µM EC_{50} versus MRC5 = 21 µM

a) These data are reported in [26]. The numbers are obtained through flow cytometry test.

Table 24.5 Chemical structures and reported activity values for DHFR inhibitors.

ID	Structure	Activities
21		K_i versus *Lm*DHFR: 0.12 μM K_i versus *Tc*DHFR: 1 μM K_i versus *Tb*DHFR: 0.01 μM EC_{50} versus *L. major* promastigote: 175 μM EC_{50} versus *L. donovani* amastigote: 160 μM
22		K_i versus *Lm*DHFR: 5.8 μM EC_{50} versus *L. major* promastigote: >500 μM EC_{50} versus *L. donovani* amastigote: >100 μM
23		K_i versus *Lm*DHFR: 0.25 μM K_i versus *Tc*DHFR: 0.1 μM K_i versus *Tb*DHFR: 0.01 μM EC_{50} versus *L. major* promastigote: 32 μM EC_{50} versus *L. donovani* amastigote: 34 μM
24		IC_{50} versus *L. mexicana* DHFR: 0.2–2 μM EC_{50} versus *L. mexicana* promastigote: 12–24 μM
25	 R = nonyl, dodecyl, CH_2O-1-naphthyl	EC_{50} versus *L. major* promastigote: 1–500 μM

(continued)

Table 24.5 (Continued)

ID	Structure	Activities
26		EC_{50} versus *L. major* promastigote: 5.6 μM EC_{50} versus *L. donovani* amastigote: 4.6 μM
27	R_1 = Me, Et R_2 = in 3′: C_nH_{2n+1} n = 0–10, $CH(CH_3)_2$, CH_2-Ph, THP, in 4′: Et, Pr	K_i versus *Lm*DHFR: 48–750 nM K_i versus *Tc*DHFR: 23–3110 nM K_i versus *Tb*DHFR: 3.6–131 nM K_i versus *Hs*DHFR: 400–6000 nM best compounds of this series showed: 99% inhibition of *L. infantum* amastigote at 12.5 μM 100% inhibition of *T. cruzi* amastigote at 3.13 μM IC_{50} versus *T. b. rhodesiense*: 1 μM
28	R_1 = Me, Et R_2 = Ph, p-Cl-Ph, 1-naphthyl	41–47% inhibition of *L. mexicana* DHFR at 0.22–0.27 μM EC_{50} versus *L. major* amastigote: 0.04–25 nM toxicity (TD_{50}) = 3.6–17.9 μM
29	R_1 = C_6H_{13}; R_2 = C_3H_7, C_8H_{17} R_1 = R_2 = C_3H_7, C_6H_{13}, C_8H_{17}, $C_{10}H_{21}$ R_1 = H; R_2 = H, CH_3, CH_2Ph, C_nH_{2n+1} n = 5–10, THP	in enzymatic assay, best compounds of this series showed: K_i versus *Lm*DHFR: 7 nM K_i versus *Tc*DHFR: 30 nM K_i versus *Hs*DHFR: 2400–2500 nM *in vitro*, best compounds of this series showed: IC_{50} versus *L. donovani* amastigote: 3.7 μM IC_{50} versus *T. cruzi* amastigote: 1.2 μM

(continued)

30

IC$_{50}$ versus *T. b. rhodesiense*: 0.73 μM
cytotoxicity: 5.5–14 μM
K$_i$ versus *Tc*DHFR: 20.2 ± 6.6 nM
K$_i$ versus *Hs*DHFR: 80.9 ± 12.5 nM
LD$_{90}$ versus *T. cruzi* trypomastigote: 36 nM
LD$_{50}$ versus *T. cruzi* amastigote: 26 nM

31

$n = 3$–5; R = H, Et

K$_i$ versus *Tc*DHFR: 0.107–55.7 nM
K$_i$ versus *Hs*DHFR: 1.45–485 nM
IC$_{50}$ versus *T. cruzi* amastigote: from 11.5 to >171 μM

32

K$_i$ versus *Tc*DHFR: 3.3 ± 0.6 nM
K$_i$ versus *Hs*DHFR: 24.5 ± 4.3 nM

33

R = H, Et, Bu, Hex, octyl, decyl, CH$_2$-Ph

K$_i$ versus *Lm*DHFR: 1.4–170 nM
K$_i$ versus *Hs*DHFR: 34–1288 nM
selectivity index: 7.3–50.7
IC$_{50}$ versus *L. donovani* amastigote: 1.7–79.9 μM
IC$_{50}$ versus *T. cruzi* amastigote: 0.041–0.22 μM
IC$_{50}$ versus *T. b. rhodesiense*: 0.054–0.67 μM

Table 24.5 (Continued)

ID	Structure	Activities
34		cytotoxicity: 0.82–3.8 μM K_i versus *Lm*DHFR: 212 nM K_i versus *Hs*DHFR: 908 nM selectivity index: 4.28 IC_{50} versus *L. donovani* amastigote: 0.53 μM IC_{50} versus *T. cruzi* amastigote: 0.18 μM IC_{50} versus *T. b. rhodesiense*: 0.17 μM
35		cytotoxicity: 1.6 μM IC_{50} versus *L. donovani* amastigote: 1.6 μM IC_{50} versus *T. cruzi* amastigote: 0.50 μM IC_{50} versus *T. b. rhodesiense*: 0.42 μM cytotoxicity: 4.9 μM
36		40% of inhibition of *Tc*DHFR at 15 μM 25% of inhibition of *Hs*DHFR at 15 μM MIC versus *T. cruzi* amastigote: 54 μM IC_{50} versus *T. b. rhodesiense*: 3.6 μM cytotoxicity: > 163 μM

(continued)

37

IC$_{50}$ versus *TcDHFR* at 95 μM
MIC versus *T. cruzi* amastigote: 55 μM
IC$_{50}$ versus *T. b. rhodesiense*: 1.0 μM
cytotoxicity: > 166 μM

38

R = Me, Et

32–50% of inhibition of *TcDHFR* at 100 μM
21–43% of inhibition of *HsDHFR* at 15–100 μM
IC$_{50}$ versus *L. donovani*: 47–56 μM
IC$_{50}$ versus *T. cruzi*: 8.6–30 μM
IC$_{50}$ versus *T. brucei*: 15–16 μM
cytotoxicity: >296 μM

39

24% of inhibition of *TcDHFR* at 100 μM
16% of inhibition of *HsDHFR* at 100 μM
IC$_{50}$ versus *L. donovani*: <21 μM
IC$_{50}$ versus *T. cruzi*: 53 μM
IC$_{50}$ versus *T. brucei*: 108 μM
cytotoxicity: 181 μM

Table 24.5 (*Continued*)

ID	Structure	Activities
40		28% of inhibition of *Tc*DHFR at 100 μM 10% of inhibition of *Hs*DHFR at 100 μM IC_{50} versus *L. donovani*: 54 μM IC_{50} versus *T. cruzi*: 60 μM IC_{50} versus *T. brucei*: 35 μM cytotoxicity: >265 μM
41		50% of inhibition of *Tc*DHFR at 100 μM 37% of inhibition of *Hs*DHFR at 50 μM IC_{50} versus *L. donovani*: 69 μM IC_{50} versus *T. cruzi*: 35 μM IC_{50} versus *T. brucei*: 11 μM cytotoxicity: 208 μM

MIC, minimum inhibitory concentration.

(*Hs*TS, *Hs*DHFR) to gain information on compound selectivity. The most active compounds bear a glutamic acid chain embedded in a rigid piperidine nucleus (Table 24.4, compounds **3** and **4**). Compounds **3** and **4** were also active against *T. cruzi* amastigote form. When tested in combination with PYR, a known DHFR inhibitor, the compounds showed additive activity, suggesting a potential use in combination therapy. The pteridine and quinoxaline scaffolds, therefore, deserve further interest for the development of PTR1 inhibitors.

From DHFR to PTR1 Inhibitors

In 2008, Kumar *et al.* [26] tried to understand the role of pteridine metabolism in the chemotherapy of *L. donovani* infections by integrating experimental studies with computational techniques. The unavailability of the X-ray crystallographic structure of *L. donovani* PTR1 (*Ld*PTR1) led these researchers to build a homology model based on *Lm*PTR1 (PDB ID: 1E7W), which has a sequence identity of 91%. They synthesized 20 pyrimidine thiones, a kind of scaffold already known to generate inhibitors of DHFR. Two compounds: ((4-flour-phenyl)-6-methyl-2-thioxo-1,2,3,4-tetrahedron-pyrimidine-5-carboxylic acid ethyl ester) (Tables 24.4, compound **5**) and (4-(3-*O*-benzyl-1,2-*O*-isopropylidene-β-ʟ-threo-furano-4-yl)-2,6-dimethyl-1,4-dihy-dro-pyridine-3,5-dicarboxylic acid ethyl ester) (Table 24.4, compound **6**) showed good activity. Docking studies on compounds **5** and **6** indicated that their carboxylic acid ethyl ester group of the pyridine moiety plays an important role in binding to PTR1. None of these inhibitors directly interacted with NADPH. However, docking studies without NADPH in the PTR1 active site were not successful. The results suggest that NADPH affects the conformation of the enzyme in a way that facilitates binding of these inhibitors.

In 2010, Kaur *et al.* [27,28] reported on analogous docking studies with monastrol (4-[3-hydroxyphenyl]-6-methyl-2-thioxo-1,2,3,4-tetrahedron-4H-pyramidine-5-carboxylic acid ethyl ester; Table 24.4, compound **7**), a compound inhibiting recombinant *Ld*PTR1 and growth of amastigotes with no host cytotoxicity and now considered a drug candidate in pre-clinical development. When it was docked into the active site of the homology model of *Ld*PTR1, docking poses compatible with similar affinities for both enantiomeric forms of monastrol were obtained. As in the earlier study, the carboxylic acid ethyl ester group of the pyridine moiety showed an important role in binding to PTR1: the carbonyl oxygen atom acts as hydrogen bond acceptor interacting with Arg17 and Ala230. The hydroxyl group of the phenyl ring interacts with PTR1 via hydrogen bonding with Tyr194. The binding of monastrol to the *Ld*PTR1 is further stabilized by a π-stacking between its phenyl ring and the nicotinamide moiety of NADPH [27,28].

Also in 2010, Pandey *et al.* [29], starting from compound **6** (Table 24.4), synthesized a series of 1-phenyl-4-glycosyl-dihydropyridines of which *inter alia* compounds **8** and **9** (Table 24.4) were active against *L. donovani in vitro* and *in vivo*. Docking studies revealed that all highly active dihydropyrimidine derivatives occupy similar spatial arrange-ments. Modeling studies on two classes of compounds, the dihydropyridines **8** and **9**

(Table 24.4) and 12 compounds from Baylis–Hillman chemistry (Table 24.4, compounds **10** and **11**) [29,30], showed that the phenyl ring from the former as well as the hexahydro pyrimido pyrimidinone ring of **11** fit well in the hydrophobic pocket formed by residues Ala230, Tyr191, Tyr194, Phe113, Pro224 and Leu18. Further, Phe113 possibly acts as a π-donor site involved in edge to face π–π-stacking interaction.

Non-Pteridine-Like PTR1 Inhibitors

In 2004, McLuskey *et al.* solved the crystal structure of TAQ (Table 24.4, compound **13**) in complex with PTR1 [10]. TAQ shows an inhibition constant very similar to that of MTX (Table 24.4, compound **12**) and occupies the pteridine binding pocket, sandwiched between the cosubstrate's nicotinamide and Phe113, with five functional groups participating in hydrogen-bond interactions. The 6-amino group interacts with highly conserved water molecules. The binding modes thus obtained suggested that the main anchor of both inhibitors is the pteridine ring. Therefore, fragment-based drug design approaches were undertaken to generate new PTR1 inhibitors.

Accordingly, a virtual screening approach has been performed to identify a new scaffold for the inhibition of *Lm*PTR1 [31]. Fifty-six compounds were selected for testing, and 2-ammino-thiadiazole (Table 24.4, compound **14**) was chosen for chemical development because of its chemical tractability, low molecular weight, and suitability to incremental fragment-based approach. Twenty-six thiazole derivatives were further studied together with a few more compounds selected to extend the hydrophobic interaction. Riluzole (Table 24.4, compound **15**) emerged as a potential new lead. It inhibits the enzyme with a K_i of 7 μM [31].

In 2009, Brenk *et al.* [13] started a new program aiming at inhibitors of *Tb*PTR1. Most of the known PTR1 inhibitors were derived from DHFR inhibitors; it is therefore not surprising that many of them also inhibit human and parasitic DHFR with inhibition constants in the low micromolar to nanomolar range. This broad spectrum activity is, of course, undesirable with respect to safe therapy. Until recently, though, conventional assays did not discriminate between inhibition of PTR1 and DHFR. Therefore a sequential assay has been set up to meet this goal (Guerrieri, personal communication). Also, known core structures mostly have a relatively high polar surface area (PSA), which prevents permeation of the blood–brain barrier, as is required to treat the second stage of African sleeping sickness. The virtual screening campaign for fragments inhibiting PTR1 that considered the possible complications yielded two novel chemical series: aminobenzothiazole and aminobenzimidazole derivatives. One of the hits (2-amino-6-chloro-benzimidazole; Table 24.4, compound **16**) was subjected to crystal structure analysis in complex with PTR1, confirming the predicted binding mode. However, the crystal structures of two analogs (2-aminobenzimidazole and 1-(3,4-dichloro-benzyl)-2-amino-benzimidazole; Table 24.4, compounds **17** and **18**) in complex with PTR1 revealed two alternative binding modes due to previously unobserved protein movements and the occurrence of water-mediated protein-ligand contacts. On the basis of the alternative binding mode of 1-(3,4-dichloro-benzyl)-2-amino-benzimidazole, further derivatives were designed, and selective PTR1 inhibitors with efficacies in the low nanomolar range and favorable physicochemical properties were obtained [32]. The most potent compounds of this series have appropriate drug-like properties and are highly selective (above 7000-fold) for PTR1 over human or trypanosomal DHFR. Two compounds (Table 24.4, compounds **19** and **20**) are the most potent and selective *Tb*PTR1 inhibitors so far disclosed in the literature.

Inhibition of DHFR

Anti-folates are roughly grouped into two classes: (i) classical anti-folates, i.e. structural analogs of folic acid with a polar glutamate side-chain, which require a carrier-mediated active transport system for entering the cell, and (ii) non-classical anti-folates that lack the glutamate side-chain, called lipophilic anti-folates. They are known to enter the cell via passive diffusion.

Most clinically used DHFR inhibitors (such as MTX, trimethoprim, cycloguanil, and PYR; Tables 24.4 and 24.5 , compounds **12** and **21–23**) are either not selective or not active at all against the parasitic DHFR [33]. Only few inhibitors that selectively inhibit the parasitic bifunctional DHFR-TS (Table 24.5, compounds **24–28**) have been reported in the literature [25,34–37]. Sirawaraporn *et al.* reported a milestone work on some 2,4-diaminopyrimidines as selective inhibitors of *Lm*DHFR. These compounds also showed some *in vitro* activity against *L. donovani* amastigotes. The most active compound that inhibited the parasite enzyme with a selectivity factor of 130 was the 3-octyloxy derivative (Table 24.5, compound **26**) [36].

Gilbert *et al.* obtained and tested 5-benzyl-2,4-diaminopyrimidines (Table 24.5, compound **27**) against recombinant DHFR from *L. major*, *T. cruzi*, *T. brucei*, and humans [38]. An interaction between the 2,4-diaminopyrimidine moiety and an aspartic acid residue in the enzyme's active site could be identified to be of critical importance. Along the same line, a new series of 2,4-diaminopyrimidines (Table 24.5, compound **29**) were synthesized by Gilbert to optimize potency, selectivity, and the PSA [39]. These series showed broad potency against *L. major* and *T. cruzi* DHFR. Having two substituents on the aromatic ring generally did not yield selective compounds.

In 2005, Senkovich *et al.* expressed and purified the *Tc*DHFR-TS protein, thus providing an essential tool for any related drug design strategy. Then they chose trimetrexate (TMQ, Table 24.5, compound **30**) as a template for the design of derivatives with improved selectivity. TMQ is a lipophilic anti-folate, which is a US Food and Drug Administration-approved drug for the treatment of *Pneumocystis carinii* infection in AIDS patients, but also a potent inhibitor of *T. cruzi* DHFR activity and highly effective against *T. cruzi* [40]. In fact, the activity of TMQ against *T. cruzi* is about 100- to 200-fold higher than that of the currently used drugs, benznidazole ($LD_{50} = 6\,\mu M$ against trypomastigotes) and nifurtimox ($LD_{50} = 3.4\,\mu M$ against amastigotes) [41,42]. However, TMQ has not yet been tested in an animal model of Chagas disease. TMQ is also a good inhibitor of human DHFR; further improvement of the selectivity of this drug would therefore be necessary [40]. Based on the differences in the active site of *T. cruzi* and human enzymes and the binding mode of MTX, six new compounds (Table 24.5, compound **31**) have been designed and synthesized by Zuccotto *et al.* as inhibitors of *Tc*DHFR. However, none of the compounds proved to be reasonably selective for the parasite enzyme or sufficiently active against *T. cruzi* amastigotes [37].

In 2009, finally, 3-D structures of the entire *Tc*DHFR-TS were reported: (i) the folate-free state of the enzyme, (ii) the complex with the lipophilic anti-folate TMQ, and (iii) the complex with the classical anti-folate MTX. They show subtle differences compared with the human counterpart. The differences between the DHFR domain of the *Tc*DHFR-TS and *Hs*DHFR (see above) could now be systematically exploited for the development of more specific anti-folates [18,19]. Schormann *et al.* used the structural information to generate 3-D quantitative structure–activity relationship models of *Tc*DHFR-TS (30 inhibitors in the learning set) and *Hs*DHFR (36 inhibitors in the learning set) which showed good agreement between experimental and predicted enzyme inhibition data. Following the medicinal chemistry work started in 2005, they designed and synthesized six novel TMQ derivatives [22]. One of these compounds, ethyl 4-(5-[(2,4-diamino-6-quinazolinyl)methyl]amino-2-methoxyphenoxy)butanoate (Table 24.5, compound **32**), was co-crystallized with the bifunctional *Tc*DHFR-TS and the crystal structure of the ternary enzyme–cosubstrate–inhibitor complex was determined. Molecular docking was used to analyze the potential interactions of all inhibitors with *Tc*DHFR-TS and *Hs*DHFR. Binding affinities of each inhibitor for the respective enzymes were calculated, based on the experimental or docked binding mode. An estimated 60–70% of the total binding energy turned out to be contributed by the 2,4-diaminoquinazoline scaffold. In consequence, these compounds showed low nanomolar affinity (K_i in the low nanomolar range) for the parasitic enzyme, but unfortunately low specificity with respect to the human enzyme (selectivity index = 1–3), thus revealing the need to improve the selectivity and also the difficulties in transforming a human DHFR inhibitor used as an anti-cancer drug into a useful anti-parasitic drug.

Another series of 2,4-diaminoquinazolines (Table 24.5, compounds **33–35**) evaluated as inhibitors of leishmanial DHFR [43] was, however, more promising. All compounds showed potent activity against recombinant *Lm*DHFR. Those compounds that have a benzylidene group instead of a benzyl group at the terminal position (e.g. **34** in Table 24.5) were less effective than the benzyl analog **33** (Table 24.5), since the rigid alkene group in **34** likely prevents the compound from adopting an optimal conformation. The compounds were all quite selective for the parasite enzyme.

Also non-folate-related DHFR inhibitors have been designed and tested against *T. cruzi*. They bear a heterocyclic pyrimidine or triazine [44]. Virtual screening methods were applied to discover novel parasite DHFR inhibitors not based on the 2,4-diamminopyrimidine motif. Zuccotto *et al.* [45] identified in particular two compounds (Table 24.5, compounds **36** and **37**) active against *T. cruzi* enzyme and also *T. brucei* trypomastigote. Chowdhury *et al.* [46] used the *L. major* active site for docking and identified compounds with weak activity (Table 24.5, compounds **38–41**).

Conclusions and Perspectives

The unusual primary resistance of trypanosomatids against anti-folates can be explained by overlapping activities of PTR1 and DHFR-TS, which guarantee a sufficient supply of THF as long as only one of the enzymes is inhibited. Experimentally, a combined inhibition of PTR1 and of the DHFR activity of DHFR-TS leads to efficient eradication of the parasites and is therefore considered to be a promising approach to treat trypanosomatid diseases. In view of the broad experience in the design of anti-folates developed as anti-cancer drugs or anti-bacterial agents and the substantial structural knowledge on the pivotal trypanosomatid enzymes, the development of a combination therapy appear to be a realistic concept. The structural differences between trypanosomatid PTR1 and DHFR-TS and their mammalian congeners are pronounced enough to enable selective inhibition and, thus, render the proposed combination therapy a perspective towards an efficacious and safe therapy.

References

1 Agüero, F., Al-Lazikani, B., Aslett, M., Berriman, M., Buckner, F.S., Campbell, R.K., Carmona, S., Carruthers, I.M., Chan, A.W., Chen, F., Crowther, G.J., Doyle, M. A., Hertz-Fowler, C., Hopkins, A.L., McAllister, G., Nwaka, S., Overington, J.P., Pain, A., Paolini, G.V., Pieper, U., Ralph, S.A., Riechers, A., Roos, D.S., Sali, A., Shanmugam, D., Suzuki, T., Van Voorhis, W.C., and Verlinde, C.L. (2008) Genomic-scale prioritization of drug targets: the TDR Targets database. *Nat. Rev. Drug Discov.*, **7**, 900–907.

2 Vickers, T.J. and Beverley, S.M. (2011) Folate metabolic pathways in *Leishmania*. *Essays Biochem.*, **51**, 63–80.

3 Robello, C., Navarro, P., Castanys, S., and Gamarro, F. (1997) A pteridine reductase gene *ptr1* contiguous to a P-glycoprotein confers resistance to antifolates in *Trypanosoma cruzi*. *Mol. Biochem. Parasitol.*, **90**, 525–535.

4 Gourley, D.G., Schuettelkopf, A.W., Leonard, G.A., Luba, J., Hardy, L.W., Beverley, B.M., and Hunter, W.N. (2001) Pteridine reductase mechanism correlates pterin metabolism with drug resistance in trypanosomatid parasites. *Nat. Struct. Biol.*, **8**, 521–525.

5 Schuettelkopf, A.W., Hardy, L.W., Beverley, S.M., and Hunter, W.N. (2005) Structures

of *Leishmania major* pteridine reductase complexes reveal the active site features important for ligand binding and to guide inhibitor design. *J. Mol. Biol.*, **352**, 105–116.

6 Ong, H.B., Sienkiewicz, N., Wyllie, S., and Fairlamb, A.H. (2011) Dissecting the metabolic roles of pteridine reductase 1 in *Trypanosoma brucei* and *Leishmania major*. *J. Biol. Chem.*, **286**, 10429–10438.

7 Cavazzuti, A., Paglietti, G., Hunter, W.N., Gamarro, F., Piras, S., Loriga, M., Alleca, S., Corona, P., McLuskey, K., Tulloch, L., Gibellini, F., Ferrari, S., and Costi, M.P. (2008) Discovery of potent pteridine reductase inhibitors to guide antiparasite drug development. *Proc. Natl. Acad. Sci. USA*, **105**, 1448–1453.

8 Tulloch, L.B., Martini, V.P., Iulek, J., Huggan, J.K., Hwan Lee, J., Gibson, C.L., Smith, T.K., Suckling, C.J., and Hunter, W.N. (2010) Structure-based design of pteridine reductase inhibitors targeting African sleeping sickness and the leishmaniases. *J. Med. Chem.*, **53**, 221–229.

9 Barrack, K.L., Tulloch, L.B., Burke, L.-A., Fyfe, P.K., and Hunter, W.N. (2011) Structure of recombinant *Leishmania donovani* pteridine reductase reveals a disordered active site. *Acta Crystalogr. F*, **67**, 33–37.

10 McLuskey, K., Gibellini, F., Carvalho, P., Avery, M.A., and Hunter, W.N. (2004) Inhibition of *Leishmania major* pteridine reductase by 2,4,6-triaminoquinazoline: structure of the NADPH ternary complex. *Acta Crystalogr. D*, **60**, 1780–1785.

11 Zhao, H., Bray, T., Ouellette, M., Zhao, M., Ferre, R.A., Matthews, D., Whiteley, J.M., and Varughese, K.I. (2003) Structure of pteridine reductase (PTR1) from *Leishmania tarentolae. Acta Crystalogr. D*, **59**, 1539–1544.

12 Dawson, A., Gibellini, F., Sienkiewicz, N., Tulloch, L.B., Fyfe, P.K., McLusley, K., Fairlamb, A.H., and Hunter, W.N. (2006) Structure and reactivity of *Trypanosoma brucei* pteridine reductase: inhibition by the archetypal antifolate methotrexate. *Mol. Microbiol.*, **61**, 1457–1468.

13 Mpanhanga, C.P., Spinks, D., Tulloch, L.B., Shanks, E.J., Robinson, D.A., Collie, I.T., Fairlamb, A.H., Wyatt, P.G., Frearson, J.A., Hunter, W.N., Gilbert, I.H., and Brenk, R. (2009) One scaffold, three binding modes: novel and selective pteridine reductase 1 inhibitors derived from fragment hits discovered by virtual screening. *J. Med. Chem.*, **52**, 4454–4465.

14 Shanks, E.J., Ong, H.B., Robinson, D.A., Thompson, S., Sienkiewicz, N., Fairlamb, A.H., and Frearson, J.A. (2010) Development and validation of a cytochrome *c*-coupled assay for pteridine reductase 1 and dihydrofolate reductase. *Anal. Biochem.*, **396**, 194–203.

15 Dawson, A., Tulloch, L.B., Barrack, K.L., and Hunter, W.N. (2010) High-resolution structures of *Trypanosoma brucei* pteridine reductase ligand complexes inform on the placement of new molecular entities in the active site of a potential drug target. *Acta Crystalogr. D*, **66**, 1334–1340.

16 Schormann, N.S., Biswajit, P., Senkovich, O., Carson, M., Howard, A., Smith, C., DeLucas, L., and Chattopadhyay, D. (2005) Crystal structure of *Trypanosoma cruzi* pteridine reductase 2 in complex with a substrate and an inhibitor. *J. Struct. Biol.*, **152**, 64–75.

17 Senkovich, O., Pal, B., Schormann, N., and Chattopadhyay, D. (2003) *Trypanosoma cruzi* genome encodes a pteridine

reductase 2 protein. *Mol. Biochem. Parasitol.*, **127**, 89–92.

18 Senkovich, O., Schormann, N., and Chattopadhyay, D. (2009) Structures of dihydrofolate reductase-thymidylate synthase of *Trypanosoma cruzi* in the folate-free stata and in complex with two antifolate drugs, trimetrexate and methotrexate. *Acta Crystalogr. D.*, **65**, 704–716.

19 Schormann, N., Senkovich, O., Walker, K., Wright, D.L., Anderson, A.C., Rosowsky, A., Ananthan, S., Shinkre, B., Velu, S., and Chattopadhyay, D. (2008) Structure-based approach to pharmacophore identification, *in silico* screening, and three-dimensional quantitative structure–activity relationship studies for inhibitors of *Trypanosoma cruzi* dihydrofolate reductase function. *Proteins*, **73**, 889–901.

20 Knighton, D.R., Kan, C.C., Howland, E., Janson, C.A., Hostomska, Z., Welsh, K.M., and Matthews, D.A. (1994) Structure of and kinetic channelling in bifunctional dihydrofolate reductase-thymidylate synthase. *Nat. Struct. Biol.*, **1**, 186–194.

21 Vanichtanankul, J., Taweechai, S., Yuvaniyama, J., Vilaivan, T., Chitnumsub, P., Kamchonwongpaisan, S., and Yuthavong, Y. (2011) Trypanosoma dihydrofolate reductase reveals natural antifolate resistance. *ACS Chem. Biol.*, **6**, 905–911.

22 Schorman, N., Velu, S.E., Murugesan, S., Senkovich, O., Walker, K., Chenna, B.C., Shinkre, B., Desai, A., and Chattopadhyay, D. (2010) Synthesis and characterization of potent inhibitors of *Trypanosoma cruzi* dihydrofolate reductase. *Bioorg. Med. Chem.*, **18**, 4056–4066.

23 Chitnumsub, P., Yuvaniyama, J., Chahomchuen, T., Vilaivan, T., and Yuthavong, Y. (2009) Crystallization and preliminary crystallographic studies of dihydrofolate reductase-thymidylate synthase from *Trypanosoma cruzi*, the Chagas disease pathogen. *Acta Crystalogr. F*, **65**, 1175–1178.

24 Dasgupta, T. and Anderson, K.S. (2008) Probing the role of parasite-specific, distant structural regions on communication and catalysis in the bifunctional thymidylate synthase-dihydrofolate reductase from

Plasmodium falciparum. Biochemistry, **47**, 1336–1345.

25 Hardy, L.W., Matthews, W., Nare, B., and Beverley, S.M. (1997) Biochemical and genetic tests for inhibitors of *Leishmania* pteridine pathways. *Exp. Parasitol.*, **87**, 158–170.

26 Kumar, P., Kumar, A., Verma, S.S., Dwivedi, N., Singh, N., Siddiqi, M.I., Tripathi, R.P., Dube, A., and Singh, N. (2008) *Leishmania donovani* pteridine reductase 1: biochemical properties and structure-modeling studies. *Exp. Parasitol.*, **120**, 73–79.

27 Singh, N., Kaur, J., Kumar, P., Gupta, S., Singh, N., Ghosal, A., Dutta, A., Kumar, A., Tripathi, R., Siddiqi, M.I., Mandal, C., and Dube, A. (2009) An orally effective dihydropyrimidone (DHPM) analogue induces apoptosis-like cell death in clinical isolates of *Leishmania donovani* overexpressing pteridine reductase 1. *Parasitol. Res.*, **105**, 1317–1325.

28 Kaur, J., Sundar, S., and Singh, N. (2010) Molecular docking, structure–activity relationship and biological evaluation of the anticancer drug monastrol as a pteridine reductase inhibitor in a clinical isolate of *Leishmania donovani. J. Antimicrob. Chemother.*, **65**, 1742–1748.

29 Pandey, V.P., Bisht, S.S., Mishra, M., Kumar, A., Siddiqi, M.I., Verma, A., Mittal, M., Sane, S.A., Gupta, S., and Tripathi, R.P. (2010) Synthesis and molecular docking studies of 1-phenyl-4-glycosyl-dihydropyridines as potent antileishmanial agents. *Eur. J. Med. Chem.*, **45**, 2381–2388.

30 Kaur, J., Kumar, P., Tyagi, S., Pathak, R., Batra, S., Singh, P., and Singh, N. (2011) *In silico* screening, structure–activity relationship, and biologic evaluation of selective pteridine reductase inhibitors targeting visceral leishmaniasis. *Antimicrob. Agents Chemother.*, **55**, 659–666.

31 Ferrari, S., Morandi, F., Motiejunas, D., Nerini, E., Henrich, S., Luciani, R., Venturelli, A., Lazzari, S., Calò, S., Gupta, S., Hannaert, V., Michels, P.A., Wade, R.C., and Costi, M.P. (2011) Virtual screening identification of nonfolate compounds, including a CNS drug, as antiparasitic agents inhibiting pteridine reductase. *J. Med. Chem.*, **54**, 211–221.

32 Spinks, D., Ong, H.B., Mpamhanga, C.P., Shanks, E.J., Robinson, D.A., Collie, I.T., Read, K.D., Frearson, J.A., Wyatt, P.G., Brenk, R., Fairlamb, A.H., and Gilbert, I.H. (2011) Design, synthesis and biological evaluation of novel inhibitors of *Trypanosoma brucei* pteridine reductase 1. *ChemMedChem*, **6**, 302–308.

33 Nare, B., Luba, J., Hardy, L.W., and Beverley, S. (1997) New approaches to *Leishmania* chemotherapy: pteridine reductase 1 (PTR1) as a target and modulator of antifolate sensitivity. *Parasitology*, **114** (Suppl.), S101–S110.

34 Gilbert, I.H. (2002) Inhibitors of dihydrofolate reductase in leishmania and trypanosomes. *Biochim. Biophys. Acta*, **1587**, 249–257.

35 Daubersies, P., Thomas, A.W., Millet, P., Brahimi, K., Langermans, J.A., and Ollomo, B. (2000) Inhibition of sporozoite invasion and inhibition of intra-hepatic development. *Nat. Med.*, **6**, 1258–1263.

36 Sirawaraporn, W., Sertsrivanich, R., Booth, R.G., Hansch, C., Neal, R.A., and Santi, D.V. (1988) Selective inhibition of *Leishmania* dihydrofolate reductase and *Leishmania* growth by 5-benzyl-2,4-diaminopyrimidines. *Mol. Biochem. Parasitol.*, **31**, 79–85.

37 Zuccotto, F., Brun, R., Gonzalez Pacanowska, D., Ruiz Perez, L.M., and Gilbert, I.H. (1999) The structure-based design and synthesis of selective inhibitors of *Trypanosoma cruzi* dihydrofolate reductase. *Bioorg. Med. Chem. Lett.*, **9**, 1463–1468.

38 Chowdhury, S.F., Villamor, V.B., Guerrero, R.H., Leal, I., Brun, R., Croft, S.L., Goodman, J.M., Maes, L., Ruiz- Perez, L.M., Pacanowska, D.G., and Gilbert, I.H. (1999) Design, synthesis, and evaluation of inhibitors of trypanosomal and leishmanial dihydrofolate reductase. *J. Med. Chem.*, **42**, 4300–4312.

39 Pez, D., Leal, I., Zuccotto, F., Boussard, C., Brun, R., Croft, S.L., Yardley, V., Ruiz-Perez, L.M., Gonzalez Pacanowska, D., and Gilbert, I.H. (2003) 2,4-Diaminopyrimidines as inhibitors of leishmanial and trypanosomal dihydrofolate reductase. *Bioorg. Med. Chem.*, **11**, 4693–4711.

40 Senkovich, O., Bhatia, V., Garg, N., and Chattopadhyay, D. (2005) Lipophilic antifolate trimetrexate is a potent inhibitor of *Trypanosoma cruzi*: prospect for chemotherapy of Chagas' disease. *Antimicrob. Agents Chemother.*, **49**, 234–238.

41 Cinque, G.M., Szajnman, S.H., Zhong, L., Docampo, R., Schvartzapel, A.J., Rodriguez, J.B., and Gros, E.G. (1998) Structure–activity relationship of new growth inhibitors *Trypanosoma cruzi*. *J. Med. Chem.*, **41**, 1540–1554.

42 Ren, H., Grady, S., Banghart, M., Moulthop, J.S., Kendrick, H., Yardley, V., Croft, S.L., and Moyna, G. (2003) Synthesis and *in vitro* anti-protozoal activity of a series of benzotropolone derivatives incorporating endocyclic hydrazines. *Eur. J. Med. Chem.*, **38**, 949–957.

43 Khabnadideh, S., Pez, D., Musso, A., Brun, R., Luis, M., and Gilbert, I.H. (2005) Design, synthesis and evaluation of 2,4-diaminoquinazolines as inhibitors of trypanosomal and leishmanial dihydrofolate reductase. *Bioorg. Med. Chem. Lett.*, **13**, 2637–2649.

44 Blaney, J.M., Hansch, C., Silipo, C., and Vittoria, A. (1984) Structure–activity relationships of dihydrofolate reductase inhibitors. *Chem. Rev.*, **84**, 333–407.

45 Zuccotto, F., Zvelebil, M., Brun, R., Chowdhury, S.F., Di Lucrezia, R., Leal, I., Maes, L., Ruiz-Perez, L.M., Gonzalez-Pacanowska, D., and Gilbert, I.H. (2001) Novel inhibitors of *Trypanosoma cruzi* dihydrofolate reductase. *Eur. J. Med. Chem.*, **36**, 395–405.

46 Chowdhury, S.F., Di Lucrezia, R., Guerrero, R.H., Brun, R., Goodman, J., Ruiz-Perez, L.M., Pacanowska, D.G., and Gilbert, I.H. (2001) Novel inhibitors of *Leishmanial* dihydrofolate reductase. *Bioorg. Med. Chem. Lett.*, **11**, 977–980.

25
Contribution to New Therapies for Chagas Disease

Patricia S. Doyle and *Juan C. Engel*

Abstract

Chagas disease is a debilitating acute or chronic infection with the kinetoplastid parasite *Trypanosoma cruzi*. An estimated 8–10 million people are infected in South, Central and North America where this endemic disease causes significant morbidity, mortality, and major economic loss. Current therapy with nitrofurans is limited by inadequate efficacy, resistance, and significant toxicity. It is crucial to identify new parasite targets to accomplish parasite eradication in the chronic disease phase. Among new drug targets that are being explored is the parasite cysteine protease cruzain – a clan CA protease expressed in all life cycle stages and implicated in parasite development. Genetic knockout of cruzain is not feasible due to gene redundancy. Instead, this target has been validated using irreversible inhibitors. These inhibitors induce intracellular accumulation of unprocessed cruzain in the Golgi compartment and negligible expression of the protease on the cell membrane of the amastigote form. Cruzain inhibitors also induce activation of host cells harboring amastigotes via the nuclear factor NF-κB P65, which normally is suppressed by cruzain. Finally, cruzain inhibitors rescue animals from lethal *T. cruzi* infection. Cruzain inhibitors that have been reported to have efficacy in animal models of Chagas disease include irreversible aryloxymethyl ketones and covalent-reversible aminoacetonitriles, and K777, an irreversible vinylsulfone-based peptidomimetic inhibitor. Another target of interest for drug development efforts for Chagas disease is the *T. cruzi* C14α-demethylase (CYP51). CYP51 inhibitors induce disruption of sterol metabolism in *T. cruzi*, resulting in parasite death. Both azole and non-azole CYP51 inhibitors have been shown to cure fatal *T. cruzi* infection in experimental animals.

Introduction

Neglected tropical diseases are a health problem of vast proportions worldwide. Among these, Chagas disease is considered the most neglected of all. Chagas is a major health problem throughout Latin America and is now of concern in developed countries. The Centers for Disease Control and Prevention (CDC) currently

* Corresponding Author

Trypanosomatid Diseases: Molecular Routes to Drug Discovery, First edition. Edited by T. Jäger, O. Koch, and L. Flohé.
© 2013 Wiley-VCH Verlag GmbH & Co. KGaA. Published 2013 by Wiley-VCH Verlag GmbH & Co. KGaA.

estimates up to 300 000 infected individuals in the United States and the disease has become prevalent in other developed countries as well, such as Spain.

An estimated 8–10 million people are infected throughout South, Central, and North America with great morbidity and mortality in some areas. Mortality, affecting mostly children and young adults, comprised over 10 000 deaths in 2008 (www.who. int). Estimates of infected patients vary in different endemic geographic regions where triatomid insects maintain the natural cycle of the infectious parasite *Trypanosoma cruzi*. Parasite strains with different biological and genetic character-istics influence the morbidity, mortality, and disease symptomatology. Cardiac manifestations are prevalent in most chagasic patients while megasyndromes are common in Brazil.

Yearly economic loss in Latin America due to this endemic zoonotic infection is enormous. Implementation of medical control (e.g., diagnosis, treatment, clinical surveillance, hospitalization, and organ transplant), epidemiological surveillance, and vector control efforts constitute very significant investments for Latin American governments. Disability and loss of work hours of young adults who are most often afflicted by Chagas disease increase the economic burden.

Current Therapy

High toxicity and low efficacy make current chemotherapy for Chagas disease highly unsatisfactory [1–3]. The two drugs clinically available to treat Chagas disease, nifurtimox and benznidazole, are nitrofurans that cause significant side-effects and require long treatment regimes of 60–120 days. These drugs have been used for almost 50 years with limited success. The pharmaceutical industry has shown little interest in developing new therapy for Chagas disease so far. Moreover, commercial nifurtimox production has been discontinued and benznidazole is at present the only treatment available in Latin America.

Both clinical and experimental evidence indicate that disease progression and pathological cardiac or megasyndrome manifestations are linked to parasite per-sistence in tissues. Ideally, parasite eradication would halt disease progression. However, prolonged treatments are often ineffective, and drug resistance to both nifurtimox and benznidazole has been well documented [4,5]. (Doyle and Engel, unpublished data).

Chemotherapy for Chagas disease was traditionally recommended during the acute and indeterminate stages of infection. By definition, the acute phase of Chagas disease lasts up to 60 days when parasites are usually detected by direct examination of peripheral blood. Acute Chagas disease results in myocarditis in about 60% of patients with an estimated 9% mortality. The indeterminate phase of Chagas disease is defined as the prolonged period of clinically silent infection that follows the phase of acute primary infection. It is considered a stage of host–parasite equilibrium that progresses to the late phase of severe, chronic myocarditis. Both nifurtimox and benznidazole have good efficacy in the treatment of acute cases, with an average index of parasitological cure of around 60% [6–10].

The chronic phase of Chagas disease is considered to begin 3 months post-infection and usually lasts throughout a patient's lifetime. Most chagasic patients die from heart failure associated with cardiomyopathy during the chronic phase. This stage is most resilient to therapy as parasitological cure is only obtained in 10–20% of patients with more than 10 years infection. However, treatment is still recommended as it often decreases pathology progression [11].

Reactivation of Chagas disease leading to meningoencephalitis and/or acute myocarditis occurs in immunosuppressed patients with AIDS, or following organ (e.g., heart, kidney, bone marrow, liver) transplantation and certain cancer treatments. Fatal *T. cruzi* infection was reported in the United States after organ transplantation from chagasic donors [12]. Cardiac transplant in patients with chronic chagasic cardiopathy is now a common procedure, but reactivation of the trypanosomiasis occurs, with clinical manifestations characterized by fever, acute myocarditis, erythematous cutaneous lesions, and abundant *T. cruzi*-infected macrophages. Treatment with nifurtimox or benznidazole can lead to temporary remission and decreased mortality in these patients, although *T. cruzi* infection persists [13]. In addition, both drugs may present with severe side-effects. Benznidazole may induce edema, fever, severe dermatitis, joint and muscle pain, nausea, vomiting, mucosal bleeding, neuropathy, lymphadenopathy, agranulocytosis, sore throat, septicemia, petechiae, and thrombocytopenic purpura. Nifurtimox may trigger weight loss, skin rash, psychosis, nausea and vomiting, leucopenia, neurotoxicity, peripheral neuropathy, and tissue abnormalities documented in adrenal glands, colon, esophagus, testicles, ovaries, and mammary glands [14]. These findings are concerning in particular because Chagas disease often afflicts children and young adults. Both drugs are nevertheless quite well tolerated by children. Until now, pediatric formulations of benznidazole or nifurtimox were not available. Oral administration of benznidazole to children was erratic at best as pills were hand cut by parents or care givers. The Drugs for Neglected Diseases *initiative* (DNDi) is now sponsoring the much-needed development of a benznidazole formulation for pediatric use in endemic countries (http://www.dndi.org/media-centre/press-releases/2008/354-media-centre/press-releases/106-chagas-disease-partnership-will-deliver-safe-easy-to-use-treatment-for-children.html).

New effective drugs are urgently needed to treat Chagas disease. The World Health Organization (www.who.int) and their consultants' indications for new drugs include two key requirements: drugs must be orally effective in the indeterminate and chronic stages of disease, and clinical treatment must be completed in 60 days. Several criteria are required for drug candidates, including low molecular weight, high selectivity, good oral bioavailability, and low toxicity. In addition, drugs with negligible side-effects and good tolerance would decrease the need for medical supervision and increase patient compliance to treatment, both important requirements in rural areas. This in turn may eventually result in reduced rates of infection in endemic areas and decreased drug-resistance of clinical isolates. This chapter summarizes some of the recent contributions to drug discovery for Chagas disease, in particular those made by our team at the University of California, San Francisco.

Targeting the *T. cruzi* Protease Cruzain

Our first approach to developing novel chemotherapy for Chagas disease focused on cruzain (also known as cruzipain, GP51/57), the major cysteine protease of *T. cruzi* [15–17]. Active, mature cruzain consists of a single polypeptide chain folded in two independent domains linked by a polythreonine-rich region [16,17]. Cruzain was first identified as a potential drug target in the 1990s when the efficacy of specific inhibitors of the protease was confirmed [18–20]. The first successful treatment in an acute animal model of Chagas disease with inhibitors designed to inactivate cruzain was with fluoromethyl ketone-derivatized pseudopeptides. The initial optimal scaffold was phenylalanine–homophenylalanine. Among the inhibitors we first tested, morpholine urea-F-hF-fluoromethylketone (Mu-F-hF-FMK), effectively blocked the intracellular cycle of the parasite and resulted in amastigote death *in vitro*. In contrast, mice treated with Z-F-A-FMK that contains natural amino acids had up to 10 000-fold higher parasitemia and survival was significantly decreased.

Peptidomimetics containing at least one non-natural amino acid analog (e.g., hF) do not undergo proteolytic cleavage and bind irreversibly to cruzain [19]. The first effective peptidomimetic was K11002 (i.e., morpholine-urea-F-homo F-vinyl sulfonyl phenyl). To achieve cure of infection, the pseudopeptide scaffold was incorporated into a less toxic vinyl sulfone derivative (i.e., N-methyl-piperazine-F-homo F-vinyl sulfonyl phenyl, K777, K11777) (Figure 25.1). Dr. James Palmer designed K777 while at Khepri Pharmaceuticals. K777 rescued immunocompetent mice from a lethal *T. cruzi* infection, and its efficacy was confirmed in numerous rodent experiments performed subsequently with various dosing and treatment regimes (Doyle and Engel, unpublished data) [19] (http://www.labome.org/grant/r01/ai/k777/ for/k777-for-treatment-of-chagas-disease--ind-enabling-studies-and-ind-submission-7982938.html). K777 was effective even in the background of immunodeficiency and acute *T. cruzi* infection [19]. Rag1 knockout mice constitute a good animal model of human immunodeficiency as they lack functional recombinase leading to defects in recombination of immunoglobulin and T-cell receptor genes. Indeed, Rag1 knockout

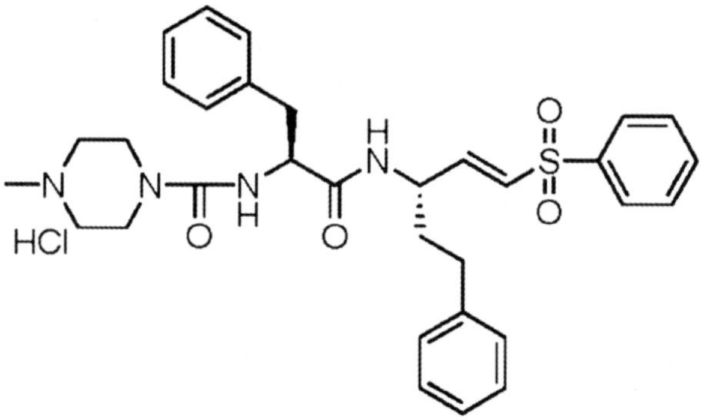

Figure 25.1 Chemical structure of the peptidomimetic K777.

mice were extremely susceptible to *T. cruzi* infection and rapidly died if untreated, while those treated with K777 survived without symptoms of disease [21].

These overall results provided an important proof of concept for the development of cysteine protease inhibitors as chemotherapy for Chagas disease. They clearly demonstrated that animals tolerate irreversible cysteine protease inhibitors at concentrations and dosing schedules that eliminate an intracellular parasite. The absence of any host cell or animal toxicity at therapeutic doses confirmed that parasites are more susceptible to these irreversible cysteine protease inhibitors than mammalian cells, perhaps because of the redundancy of cysteine proteases in the latter [19]. Our findings were then extended to other infectious diseases where cysteine proteases play a key role in pathogenesis, including leishmaniasis, African sleeping sickness, and malaria [22].

Pharmacokinetics of K777 showed adequate and sustained therapeutic levels, and the drug has good oral bioavailability (http://www.labome.org/grant/r01/ai/k777/for/k777-for-treatment-of-chagas-disease--ind-enabling-studies-and-ind-submission-7982938.html). The efficacy and lack of toxicity of cysteine protease inhibitors in treating both acute and chronic *T. cruzi* animal infections support the ongoing development of this lead drug. More potent cysteine protease inhibitors in development are briefly discussed below. Nevertheless, K777 still remains the most extensively characterized inhibitor with studies performed in rodents, dogs and primates. After 15 years of intense experimentation, K777 has passed a pre-IND (Investigational New Drug) meeting with the US Food and Drug Administration and is poised to go into phase I clinical trials. Collaboration between UCSF and DNDi has received funding from the National Institutes of Health to complete primate dosing and pharmacokinetics/pharmacodynamics studies.

Why is Cruzain a Good Drug Target?

The protease is essential for parasite development [19–26]. However, assessment of its biological role has been hampered by genetic redundancy and failure of gene deletion attempts. Cruzain is a reservosomal (lysosomal) cysteine protease in the insect (epimastigote) stage of *T. cruzi*. Its function is vital for epimastigote nutrition and development. The protease also mediates cell remodeling during transformation of epimastigotes to infectious trypomastigotes [17,25]. Trypomastigote infection is facilitated by the cruzain-mediated release of kinin from host cell surfaces and activation of bradykinin receptors [25,27].

Intracellular amastigotes, preferentially infecting muscle cells including myocardiocytes, are responsible for the most common pathological manifestations of Chagas disease. Until recently, the biological role of cruzain in the intracellular amastigote stage and in Chagas disease pathogenesis remained largely unknown. In amastigotes, cruzain localizes mostly to the cell membrane and the flagellar pocket as well as within lysosomes/reservosomes. As intracellular amastigotes divide free within the cytoplasm of the host cell, cruzain is in direct contact with cytoplasmic proteins of the host that may be amenable to proteolytic degradation. Drugs targeting cruzain will preferably have low tropism for lysosomes as the protease is abundantly expressed on the amastigote cell membrane [19].

To investigate the biological role of this vital protease in amastigotes we took two different approaches. First, lethal chemical knockout with cysteine protease inhibitors confirmed the need for cruzain autocatalysis and activation to allow intracellular parasite development. Major morphological alterations in intracellular amastigotes appeared as early as 24 h post-treatment, and host cells were amastigote-free within 20–30 days depending on the inhibitor and treatment regime [19,20]. Cysteine protease inhibitors induced abnormalities in intracellular organelles (i.e., nuclear membrane, endoplasmic reticulum, Golgi complex) due to altered protein trafficking. Abundant double-membrane vacuoles appeared with similar morphology to autophagosomes [20]. Inhibitor treatment significantly reduced cruzain expression both on the cell membrane and within the lysosome consistent with an arrest of cruzain transport in the parasite. A radiolabeled inhibitor was used to confirm access to and specific labeling of the target protease cruzain [20].

Our second approach was to examine the phenotype of cruzain-deficient organisms [28,29]. A K777-resistant and protease-deficient *T. cruzi* retained less than 1% of cruzain activity of the wild-type parental clone. This cruzain-deficient parasite rapidly activated host macrophages via NF-κB P65 and was unable to survive intracellularly. Similarly, infection with wild-type *T. cruzi* followed by treatment with K777 resulted in macrophage activation and parasite death. In contrast, infection with wild-type parasites appeared to induce cruzain-mediated proteolysis of the macrophage nuclear factor NF-κB P65 leading to unresponsiveness of the host macrophage during early infection. Wild-type trypomastigotes rapidly escaped to the cytoplasm of the host cell for transformation and intracellular development. Preventing macrophage activation is crucial for a successful infection. Based on our results, we hypothesize cruzain plays a key role in natural infection. Degradation of NF-κB P65 may hinder activation of innate phagocytes recruited to the bite site. Macrophage unresponsiveness would favor parasite survival in early infection until the onset of the immune response. The cruzain-mediated immune evasion mechanism may be critical for *T. cruzi* survival during the early stages of natural infection with a low number of trypomastigotes [29].

In addition to its enzymatic and immune evasion roles, cruzain is a highly antigenic molecule and anti-cruzain antibodies targeting its glycosylated C-terminal extension are abundant in chagasic sera [30,31]. Human major histocompatibility class I and II epitopes preferentially map to the catalytic domain of cruzain [32–35]. The intensity of inflammatory infiltration in Chagas disease correlates well with the presence of parasites where cruzain is detected immunohistologically [35]. In summary, cruzain has important biological roles in intracellular parasite development and in Chagas disease pathogenesis.

Other Potent Cruzain Inhibitors

K777 and most of other effective trypanocidal inhibitors tested to date act via irreversible covalent modification of the catalytic cysteine residue in the protease

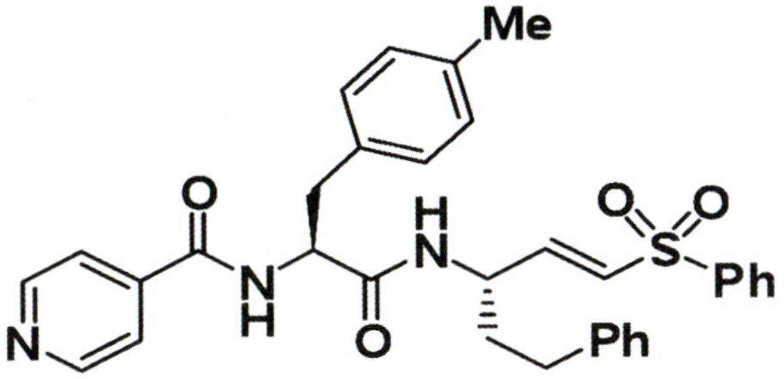

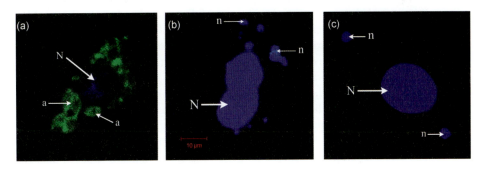

Figure 25.2 Chemical structure of compound **1**, a pyridyl analog of K777.

active site. Chemical scaffolds of current interest include K777 analogs and non-peptidic ketones [36,37]. Replacing the basic piperazine ring in K777 with a less basic pyridine ring produced neutral analogs including compound **1** with 10-fold improved trypanocidal activity (Figures 25.2 and 25.3) [38] (Doyle and Engel, unpublished data). These are among the most potent inhibitors identified to date. Treatment with compound **1** inhibited cruzain expression on the cell surface of the intracellular amastigote similarly to K777.

Among non-peptidic cruzain inhibitors of interest, tetrafluoromethyl ketones were very effective trypanocidal compounds. A 1,2,3-triazole-based tetrafluoro-methyl ketone rescued animals from acute lethal infection at 20 mg/kg weight [39,40]. Promising, albeit quite toxic, ketone derivatives of this compound had high efficacy on *T. cruzi*-infected cells even with short-term treatment regimes (5–10 days) (Doyle and Engel, unpublished data). Further lead optimization may

Figure 25.3 Immunofluorescence microphotographs of bovine muscle skeletal muscle (BESM) cells infected with *T. cruzi* amastigotes. Cruzain was detected using a specific polyclonal antibody followed by an appropriate fluorescent secondary antibody as previously described [20]. Host cell and parasite DNA were stained with 4,6-diamidino-2-phenylindole (DAPI; blue fluorescence). (a) Cruzain (green fluorescence) is abundantly expressed on the cell surface of *T. cruzi* amastigotes within the cytoplasm of an untreated BESM cell. (b) Negligible cruzain expression by intracellular amastigotes treated with 10 μM K777. (c) Negligible cruzain expression by intracellular amastigotes treated with 1 μM compound **1**. N, nucleus of BESM cell; a, amastigote; n, *T. cruzi* DNA.

produce derivatives with better selectivity for the parasite enzyme and less toxicity to the host.

Lack of correlation between biochemical protease inhibition and trypanocidal efficacy was observed with many compounds. Several possibilities may explain these results. (i) Some inhibitor may be sequestered within host cell lysosomes or be degraded by the host. For example, inefficacy of some basic analogs may result from an undesirable accumulation within host cell lysosomes. (ii) Less basic analogs such as pyridyl may reach higher concentrations within the host cell cytoplasm, inducing better inhibition of cruzain expressed on the amastigote cell membrane. The actual amount of inhibitor accessible to cruzain expressed by the intracellular parasite still remains to be quantified. (iii) Compounds with pyridyl rings may also inhibit a second target: the *T. cruzi* sterol C14α-demethylase. This promising drug target discussed below binds small molecules with exposed pyridine rings. Indeed such is the case with compound **1**, a good inhibitor of both enzymatic targets [38] (Doyle and Engel, unpublished data).

To minimize the risk of human toxicity, a clinical drug for Chagas disease should ideally inhibit the protease reversibly. Hundreds of reversible-covalent inhibitors of cruzain were synthesized and tested. Although many of these compounds inhibit the enzyme *in vitro* and some are trypanocidal, we have not yet identified reversible inhibitors as effective as K777 [41] (Doyle and Engel, unpublished data). A possible explanation is that reversible inhibitors may not effectively impair the self-processing of cruzain zymogen in the Golgi necessary for enzymatic activation and proper cellular localization as previously described [20].

Targeting Ergosterol Biosynthesis

Sterol metabolic pathways have been successfully targeted in drug development for fungal diseases. Clinical anti-fungals inhibit the sterol C14α-demethylase (CYP51), which catalyzes the oxidative removal of the 14α-methyl group to produce desaturated intermediates in ergosterol biosynthesis. *T. cruzi* presents similarities to fungi in sterol composition and synthesis. Indeed, CYP51 inhibitors with strong anti-*T. cruzi* activity are in the pipeline for preclinical and clinical development for the treatment of Chagas disease [42–46]. The most potent azole to date is posaconazole (Noxafil®; Merck), which cured infected mice in models of acute and chronic Chagas disease [45]. Posaconazole also parasitologically cured an immunosuppressed patient with concomitant Chagas disease and systemic lupus erythematosus [46]. A clinical trial with this drug is now underway in Barcelona, Spain. The use of posaconazole may be nevertheless restricted by its high cost and by drug-induced hepatotoxicity that requires clinical monitoring during treatment [46]. In addition, DNDi and the Japanese pharmaceutical company Eisai recently signed an agreement for the development of the promising anti-fungal E1224, a ravuconazole pro-drug, to treat Chagas disease. DNDi will coordinate the phase IIA/B clinical trials with E-1224, showing *in vivo* and *in vitro* activity against the pathogen responsible for Chagas disease. Current development of potent azoles has been reviewed in detail by Buckner [47] and Urbina ([45] and Chapter 26 of this volume).

The potential appearance of resistance to azoles is of concern. Although no data on the development of resistance to posaconazole or E1124 resistance in patients with Chagas disease are yet available, azole resistance in fungi is common and mainly due to mutations of the *cyp51* gene. The enzyme region called the posaconazole binding tunnel is prone to mutations. For example, mutations of G54 to R or W in *Aspergillus fumigatus* induce cross-resistance to itraconazole and posaconazole, while mutations in M220 cause resistance to all azole drugs, including posaconazole [48–50]. Similarly, posaconazole-resistant *Candida* is cross-resistant to all azoles [51]. Highlighting this potential problem, Hankins et al. rapidly induced experimental cross-resistance to several azoles in *T. cruzi* [52].

To address some of these concerns, our group explored the development of specific non-azole inhibitors [53,54]. The *N*-[4-pyridyl]-formamide moiety can deliver various chemotypes into the active site of CYP51 enzymes. A first screen identified LP10 with anti-chagasic activity albeit at much higher dose than pos-aconazole. In a mouse model of acute *T. cruzi* infection the cure rate obtained with LP10 was similar to that previously reported with posaconazole [45]. Sterol analyses confirmed that LP10 inhibits the C14α-demethylase, and leads to accumulation of lanosterol and eburicol precursors and reduction of desmethyl sterols in both amastigotes and epimastigotes. The pathogenic intracellular amastigote was more sensitive to treatment than insect epimastigotes. Blockage of 14α-demethylation by both posaconazole and LP10 caused severe ultrastructural and morphological alterations in amastigote membranes, and finally parasite death due to ergosterol deprivation [54]. The inhibitor LP10 served as a starting point for medicinal-chemistry efforts to optimize drug-like properties and develop compounds tailored to specifically inhibit the *T. cruzi* enzyme. It is interesting to note that compound **1** inhibits significantly not only cruzain activity and cell expression, but also CYP51 activity and sterol biosynthesis (Doyle and Engel, unpublished data). Lead compounds with warheads that inhibit specifically the activity of two different enzymatic targets in *T. cruzi* without toxicity to the host have high potential in drug development.

Why Multiple Targets?

T. cruzi strains resistant to current therapy are common. Reported drug resistance to nifurtimox and benznidazole ranges from 0 to 100% [55]. The efficacy of posaconazole and other drugs targeting sterol biosynthesis is unquestionable, although concerns of cost and rapid development of drug resistance remain. On the other hand, the generation of K777 resistance in the laboratory proved to be extremely difficult, and these *T. cruzi* showed significantly lower infectivity and are non-pathogenic for normal mice (Doyle and Engel, unpublished data). To date, the sensitivity of clinical *T. cruzi* isolates to these emerging therapies has not been explored. Given the marked genetic and biological heterogeneity of

T. cruzi, clinical resistance to these drugs may be expected. It then seems prudent to develop therapies targeting various metabolic pathways in *T. cruzi* that may prove useful for future alternative, combinatorial, or synergistic chemotherapy.

Development of Drug Screening Methods

To expedite drug screening for this neglected disease, Buckner *et al.* first developed a rapid quantitative method to test drug sensitivity using β-galactosidase-expressing *T. cruzi* cells. Efficacy was documented by decrease in a colorimetric reaction [56]. Problems with the assay were few and included the possible interference of colored compounds with the final absorbance assay, alterations induced by the β-galactosidase enzyme on some compounds, or inhibition of the activity of the β-galactosidase enzyme by some compounds. Thus effective compounds identified must be retested against untransfected *T. cruzi*.

A second useful method for *in vitro* drug screening utilizes parasites expressing luciferase or the tandem tomato fluorescent protein (tdTomato). The change in fluorescence intensity of tdTomato-expressing lines was measured as an indicator of parasite replication daily for 4 days. This method was used to identify compounds with IC_{50} lower than that of benznidazole [57].

To avoid the problems detailed above with transfected *T. cruzi*, we developed and validated a cell-based, high-throughput assay that can be used with a variety of untransfected *T. cruzi* isolates including clinical parasite isolates and host cells. Our assay simultaneously measures efficacy against the intracellular amastigote stage and toxicity to host cells [58]. Briefly, *T. cruzi*-infected muscle cells are incubated in 96- or 384-well plates with test compounds. Assay plates are automatically imaged and analyzed based on size differences between the DAPI-stained host cell nuclei and parasite kinetoplasts. A reduction in the ratio of *T. cruzi* per host cell provides a quantitative measure of parasite growth inhibition, while a decrease in count of the host nuclei indicates compound toxicity. The assay is now routinely used at UCSF to screen for compounds with trypanocidal efficacy. Automatization has increased drug screening capabilities to 35 000 compounds per week. The flexible assay design allows the use of various parasite strains, including clinical isolates with different biological characteristics such as tissue tropism and drug sensitivity, and a broad range of host cells. Our high-throughput assay now has an important impact on anti-parasitic drug discovery at the Sander Center and has been adapted to screen for anti-parasitic drugs against other human pathogens [59].

To follow up on compound efficacy, we recently developed the minimal trypanocidal assay to determine the minimal trypanocidal concentration (MTC) in 48–96 multiple-well plates infected with Y or CA-I/72 *T. cruzi*. Cultures are treated with decreasing concentrations of drugs or compounds of interest and observed every 48 h by contrast phase microscopy. Following treatment, cultures are incubated for an additional 15 days without drug pressure. In the absence of drug, *T. cruzi* completes its intracellular cycle within 7 days. The MTC is the minimal concentration that results in parasite death and cure of host cells. There is an excellent correlation between efficacy in the MTC assay and efficacy in mouse models of Chagas disease (Doyle and Engel, unpublished data).

In addition to cell-based methods, animal trials are necessary for the final and conclusive evaluation of compound efficacy and for the determination of pharmacokinetic parameters. Experimental models of Chagas disease in several animal species, including mice, rabbits, dogs, and monkeys, are well established and have been extensively used to confirm drug efficacy for over 50 years. Both acute and chronic models in mice are useful for drug screening and a first evaluation of pharmacokinetic properties of compounds. Recently, a number of good *in vivo* testing models became available to assay compound efficacy in mice very rapidly [60].

Conclusions

Endemic Chagas disease is a major health and economic problem in the three American continents affecting millions of people in their prime. Developed countries such as the United States, Spain, France, Japan, and Canada, have already identified Chagas as an important resident infection [61–67]. Adding to the burden of infected chagasic immigrants from Latin American countries, vectors able to transmit *T. cruzi* infection and natural hosts are also found in the US [62,63]. In this era of globalization, Chagas and other neglected tropical diseases have become a worldwide concern. We must address them accordingly by allocating sustained human and financial resources to combat them. Drug discovery is a powerful arm in this equation. In spite of a recent spike in interest on Chagas disease perhaps motivated by the increasing number of infected individuals in developed countries, involvement of established pharmaceutical companies in drug development still remains tenuous. Most efforts to date come from Universities and are sponsored by National Institutes of Health, non-profit organizations, and private donors. Serious challenges encountered in drug development for Chagas disease still remain, and include the lack of adequate financial support, the need for new laboratory methods to evaluate drug efficacy in humans, the identification of markers of cure in patients, and better coordination between basic research and downstream drug development efforts.

Acknowledgements

In memory of James Dvorak (National Institutes of Health) and Robert Smith (Prototek Pharmaceuticals, CA). Thanks to J. Palmer and J.H. McKerrow. The National Institutes of Health (NIAID TDRU AI 35707 and R21 NIH/NINDS NS067590 grants) and the Sandler Family Foundation are gratefully acknowledged for funding our investigations. The authors have no financial affiliations or involvement with any organization or entity with the subject matter or materials discussed in this manuscript. No writing assistance was utilized in this manuscript.

References

1 McKerrow, J.H., Doyle, P.S., Engel, J.C., Podust, L.M., Robertson, S.A., Ferreira, R., Saxton, T., Arkin, M., Kerr, I.D., Brinen, L. S., and Craik, C.S. (2009) Two approaches to discovering and developing new drugs for Chagas disease. *Mem. Inst. Oswaldo Cruz.*, **104**, 263–269.

2 Rassi, A. Jr., Rassi, A., and Marin-Netto, J. A. (2010) Chagas' disease. *Lancet*, **375**, 1388–1402.

3 Urbina, J.A. (2010) Specific chemotherapy for Chagas' disease: relevance, current limitations, and new approaches. *Acta Trop.*, **115**, 55–68.

4 Tsuhako, M.H., Alves, M.J., Colli, W., Filardi, L.S., Brener, Z., and Augusto, O. (1991) Comparative studies of nifurtimox uptake and metabolism by drug-resistant and susceptible strains of *Trypanosoma cruzi. Comp. Biochem. Physiol.*, **99**, 317–321.

5 Filardi, L.S. and Brener, Z. (1987) Susceptibility and natural resistance of *Trypanosoma cruzi* strains to drugs used clinically in Chagas disease. *Trans. R. Soc. Trop. Med. Hyg.*, **81**, 755–759.

6 Sosa Estani, S., Segura, E.L., Ruiz, A.M., Velazquez, E., Porcel, B.M., and Yampotis, C. (1998) Efficacy of chemotherapy with benznidazole in children in the indeterminate phase of Chagas' disease. *Am. J. Trop. Med. Hyg.*, **59**, 526–529.

7 Sosa Estani, S. and Segura, E.L. (1999) Treatment of *Trypanosoma cruzi* infection in the undetermined phase. Experience and current guidelines of treatment in Argentina. *Mem. Inst. Oswaldo Cruz.*, **94**, 363–365.

8 Rodriques Coura, J. and de Castro, S.L. (2002) A critical review on Chagas disease chemotherapy. *Mem. Inst. Oswaldo Cruz*, **97**, 3–24.

9 Gallerano, R.R. and Sosa, R.R. (2000) Interventional study in the natural evolution of Chagas disease. Evaluation of specific antiparasitic treatment. Retrospective-prospective study of antiparasitic therapy. *Rev. Fac. Cien. Med. Univ. Nac. Cordoba*, **57**, 135–162.

10 Jannin, J. and Villa, L. (2007) An overview of Chagas disease treatment. *Mem. Inst. Oswaldo Cruz.*, **102**, 95–97.

11 Fabbro, D.L., Streiger, M.L., Arias, E.D., Bizai, M.L., del Barco, M., and Amicone, N. A. (2007) Trypanocide treatment among adults with chronic Chagas' disease living in Santa Fe city (Argentina), over a mean follow-up of 21 years: parasitological, serological and clinical evolution. *Rev. Soc. Bras. Med. Trop.*, **40**, 1–10.

12 Centers for Disease Control and Prevention (2002) Chagas' disease after organ transplantation – United States. *MMWR Morb. Mortal. Wkly. Rep.*, **51**, 210–212.

13 Ferreira, M.S. (1999) Chagas' disease and immunosuppression. *Mem. Inst. Oswaldo Cruz*, **94**, 325–327.

14 Castro, J.A. and Diaz de Toranzo, E.G. (1988) Toxic effects of nifurtimox and benznidazole, two drugs used against American trypanosomiasis (Chagas' disease). *Biomed. Environ. Sci.*, **1**, 19–33.

15 Bontempi, E., Martinez, J., and Cazzulo, J. J. (1989) Subcellular localization of a cysteine proteinase from *Trypanosoma cruzi. Mol. Biochem. Parasitol.*, **33**, 43–47.

16 Murta, A.C., Persechini, P.M., Padron, T., de, S., de Souza, W., and Guimarães, J.A. (1990) Structural and functional identification of GP57/51 antigen of *Trypanosoma cruzi* as a cysteine proteinase. *Mol. Biochem. Parasitol.*, **43**, 27–38.

17 Eakin, A.E., Mills, A.A., Harth, G., McKerrow, J.H., and Craik, C.S. (1992) The sequence, organization, and expression of the major cysteine protease (cruzain) from *Trypanosoma cruzi. J. Biol. Chem.*, **267**, 7411–7420.

18 Meirelles, M.N., Juliano, L., Carmona, E., Silva, S.G., Costa, E.M., Murta, A.C., and Scharfstein, J. (1992) Inhibitors of the major cysteinyl proteinase (GP57/51) impair host cell invasion and arrest the intracellular development of *Trypanosoma cruzi in vitro. Mol. Biochem. Parasitol.*, **52**, 175–184.

19 Engel, J.C., Doyle, P.S., Hsieh, I., and McKerrow, J.H. (1998) Cysteine protease inhibitors cure an experimental *Trypanosoma cruzi* infection. *J. Exp. Med.*, **188**, 725–734.

20 Engel, J.C., Doyle, P.S., Palmer, J., Hsieh, I., Bainton, D.F., and McKerrow, J.H. (1998) Cysteine protease inhibitors alter Golgi complex ultrastructure and function in *Trypanosoma cruzi*. *J. Cell Sci.*, **111**, 597–606.

21 Doyle, P.S., Zhou, Y.M., Engel, J.C., and McKerrow, J.H. (2007) A cysteine protease inhibitor cures Chagas' disease in an immunodeficient-mouse model of infection. *Antimicrob. Agents Chemother.*, **51**, 3932–3939.

22 Caffrey, C.R., Lima, A.P., and Steverding D. (2011) Cysteine peptidases of kinetoplastid parasites. *Adv. Exp. Med. Biol.*, **712**, 84–99.

23 Doyle, P.S., Sajid, M., O'Brien, T., Dubois, K., Engel, J.C., Mackey, Z.B., and Reed, S. (2008) Drugs targeting parasite lysosomes. *Curr. Pharm. Des.*, **14**, 889–900.

24 Alvarez, V.E., Niemirowicz, G.T., and Cazzulo, J.J. (2012) The peptidases of *Trypanosoma cruzi*: digestive enzymes, virulence factors, and mediators of autophagy and programmed cell death. *Biochem. Biophys. Acta*, **1824**, 195–206.

25 Dos Santos Andrade, D., Serra, R.R., Svensjö, E., de Araújo Lima, A.P., Junior, E. S., da Silva de Azevedo Fortes, F., de Faria Morandini, A.C., Morandi, V., Soeiro, M., de, N., Tanowitz, H.B., and Scharfstein, J. (2012) *Trypanosoma cruzi* invades host cells through the activation of endothelin and bradykinin receptors: a converging pathway leading to chagasic vasculopathy. *Br. J. Pharmacol.*, **165**, 1333–1347.

26 Tomas, A.M., Miles, M.A., and Kelly, J.M. (1997) Overexpression of cruzipain, the major cysteine proteinase of *Trypanosoma cruzi*, is associated with enhanced metacyclogenesis. *Eur. J. Biochem.*, **244**, 596–603.

27 Scharfstein, J., Schmitz., V., Morandi, V., Capella, M.M., Lima, A.P., Morrot, A., Juliano, L., and Müller-Esterl, W. (2000) Host cell invasion by *Trypanosoma cruzi* is potentiated by activation of bradykinin B_2 receptors. *J. Exp. Med.*, **192**, 1289–1300.

28 Engel, J.C., Torres, C., Hsieh, I., Doyle, P. S., and McKerrow, J.H. (2000) Upregulation of the secretory pathway in cysteine protease inhibitor-resistant *Trypanosoma cruzi*. *J. Cell Sci.*, **113**, 1345–1354.

29 Doyle, P.S., Zhou, Y.M., Hsieh, I., Greenbaum, D.C., McKerrow, J.H., and Engel, J.C. (2011) The *Trypanosoma cruzi* protease cruzain mediates immune evasion. *PLoS Pathog.*, **7**, e1002139.

30 Aslund, L., Henriksson, J., Campetella, O., Frasch, A.C., Pettersson, U., and Cazzulo, J.J. (1991) The C-terminal extension of the major cysteine proteinase (cruzipain) from *Trypanosoma cruzi*. *Mol. Biochem. Parasitol.*, **45**, 345–347.

31 Scharfstein, J., Rodrigues, M.M., Alves, C. A., de Souza, W., Previato, J.O., and Mendonça-Previato, L. (1983) *Trypanosoma cruzi*: description of a highly purified surface antigen defined by human antibodies. *J. Immunol.*, **131**, 972–976.

32 Scharfstein, J. (2006) Parasite cysteine proteinase interactions with alpha 2-macroglobulin or kininogens: differential pathways modulating inflammation and innate immunity in infection by pathogenic trypanosomatids. *Immunobiology*, **211**, 117–125.

33 Arnholdt, A.C., Piuvezam, M.R., Russo, D. M., Lima, A.P., Pedrosa, R.C., Reed, S.G., and Scharfstein, J. (1993) Analysis and partial epitope mapping of human T cell responses to *Trypanosoma cruzi* cysteinyl proteinase. *J. Immunol.*, **151**, 3171–3179.

34 Fonseca, S.G., Moins-Teisserenc, H., Clave, E., Ianni, B., Nunes, V.L., Mady, C., Iwai, L.K., Sette, A., Sidney, J., Marin, M.L., Goldberg, A.C., Guilherme., L., Charron, D., Toubert, A., Kalil, J., and Cunha-Neto, E. (2005) Identification of multiple HLA-A*0201-restricted cruzipain and FL-160 CD8$^+$ epitopes recognized by T cells from chronically *Trypanosoma cruzi*-infected patients. *Microbes Infect.*, **7**, 688–697.

35 Morrot, A., Strickland, D.K., Higuchi, M., de, L., Reis, M., Pedrosa, R., and Scharfstein, J. (1997) Human T cell responses against the major cysteine proteinase (cruzipain) of *Trypanosoma cruzi*: role of the multifunctional alpha 2-macroglobulin receptor in antigen presentation by monocytes. *Int. Immunol.*, **9**, 825–834.

36 Jaishankar, P., Hansell, E., Zhao, D.M., Doyle, P.S., McKerrow, J.H., and Renslo, A.R. (2008) Potency and selectivity of P2/P3-modified inhibitors of cysteine proteases from trypanosomes. *Bioorg. Med. Chem. Lett.*, **18**, 624–628.

37 Chen, Y.T., Brinen, L.S., Kerr, I.D., Hansell, E., Doyle, P.S., McKerrow, J.H., and Roush, W.R. (2010) *In vitro* and *in vivo* studies of the trypanocidal properties of WRR-483 against *Trypanosoma cruzi*. *PLoS Negl. Trop. Dis.*, **14**, pii: e825.

38 Robertson, S.A. and Renslo, A.R. (2011) Drug discovery for neglected tropical diseases at the Sandler Center. *Future Med. Chem.*, **3**, 1279–1288.

39 Brak, K., Kerr, I.D., Barrett, K.T., Fuchi, N., Debnath, M., Ang, K., Engel, J.C., McKerrow, J.H., Doyle, P.S., Brinen, L.S., and Ellman, J.A. (2010) Nonpeptidic tetrafluorophenoxymethyl ketone cruzain inhibitors as promising new leads for Chagas disease chemotherapy. *J. Med. Chem.*, **53**, 52–60.

40 Brak, K., Doyle, P.S., McKerrow, J.H., and Ellman, J.A. (2008) Identification of a new class of nonpeptidic inhibitors of cruzain. *J. Am. Chem. Soc.*, **130**, 6404–6410.

41 Mott, B.T., Ferreira, R.S., Simeonov, A., Jadhav, A., Ang, K.K., Leister, W., Shen, M., Silveira, J.T., Doyle, P.S., Arkin, M.R., McKerrow, J.H., Inglese, J., Austin, C.P., Thomas, C.J., Shoichet, B.K., and Maloney, D.J. (2010) Identification and optimization of inhibitors of Trypanosomal cysteine proteases: cruzain, rhodesain, and TbCatB. *J. Med. Chem.*, **53**, 52–60.

42 Buckner, F.S. (2008) Sterol 14 alpha-demethylase inhibitors for *Trypanosoma cruzi* infection. *Adv. Exp. Med. Biol.*, **625**, 61–80.

43 Buckner, F.S. and Navabi, N. (2010) Advances in Chagas' disease drug development: 2009–2010. *Cur. Opin. Infect. Dis.*, **23**, 609–616.

44 Buckner, F.S., Wilson, A.J., White, T.C., and Van Voorhis, W.C. (1998) Induction of resistance to azole drugs in *Trypanosoma cruzi*. *Antimicrob. Agents Chemother.*, **42**, 3245–3250.

45 Urbina, J.A. (2009) Ergosterol biosynthesis and drug development for Chagas disease. *Mem. Inst. Oswaldo Cruz*, **104**, 311–318.

46 Pinazo, M.J., Espinosa, G., Gallego, M., López-Chejade, P.L., Urbina, J.A., and Gascón, J. (2010) Successful treatment with posaconazole of a patient with chronic Chagas disease and systemic lupus erythematosus. *Am. J. Trop. Med. Hyg.*, **82**, 583–587.

47 Buckner, F.S. (2011) Experimental chemotherapy and approaches to drug discovery for *Trypanosoma cruzi* infection. *Adv. Parasitol.*, **75**, 89–119.

48 Mann, P.A., Parmegiani, R.M., Wei, S.Q., Mendrick, C.A., Li, X., Loebenberg, D., DiDomenico, B., Hare, R.S., Walker, S.S., and McNicholas, P.M. (2003) Mutations in *Aspergillus fumigatus* resulting in reduced susceptibility to posaconazole appear to be restricted to a single amino acid in the cytochrome P450 14alpha-demethylase. *Antimicrob. Agents Chemother.*, **47**, 577–581.

49 Mellado, E., Garcia-Effron, G., Alcazar-Fuoli, L., Cuenca-Estrella, M., and Rodriguez-Tudela, J.L. (2004) Substitutions at methionine 220 in the 14alpha-sterol demethylase (Cyp51A) of *Aspergillus fumigatus* are responsible for resistance *in vitro* to azole antifungal drugs. *Antimicrob. Agents Chemother.*, **48**, 2747–2750.

50 Rodriguez-Tudela, J.L., Alcazar-Fuoli, L., Mellado, E., Alastruey-Izquierdo, A., Monzon, A., and Cuenca-Estrella, M. (2008) Epidemiological cutoffs and cross-resistance to azole drugs in *Aspergillus fumigatus*. *Antimicrob. Agents Chemother.*, **52**, 2468–2472.

51 Pinto e Silva, A.T., Costa-de-Oliveira, S., Silva-Dias, A., Pina-Vaz, C., and Rodrigues, A.G. (2009) Dynamics of *in vitro* acquisition of resistance by *Candida parapsilosis* to different azoles. *FEMS Yeast Res.*, **9**, 626–630.

52 Hankins, E.G., Gillespie, J.R., Aikenhead, K., and Buckner, F.S. (2005) Upregulation of sterol C14-demethylase expression in *Trypanosoma cruzi* treated with sterol biosynthesis inhibitors. *Mol. Biochem. Parasitol.*, **144**, 68–75.

53 Chen, C.K., Doyle, P.S., Yermalitskaya, L. V., Mackey, Z.B., Ang, K.K.H., McKerrow, J.H., and Podust, L.M. (2009) *Trypanosoma cruzi* CYP51 inhibitor derived from a *Mycobacterium tuberculosis* screen hit. *PLoS Negl. Trop. Dis.*, **3**, e372.

54 Doyle, P.S., Chen, C.K., Johnston, J.B., Hopkins, S.D., Leung, S.F., Jacobson, M. P., Engel, J.C., McKerrow, J.H., and

Podust, L.M. (2010) A nonazole CYP51 inhibitor cures Chagas' disease in a mouse model of acute infection. *Antimicrobial Agents Chemother.*, **54**, 2480–2488.

55 Filardi, L.S. and Brener, Z. (1987) Susceptibility and natural resistance of *Trypanosoma cruzi* strains to drugs used clinically in Chagas disease. *Trans. R. Soc. Trop. Med. Hyg.*, **81**, 755–759.

56 Buckner, F.S., Verlinde, C.L., La Flamme, A.C., and Van Voorhis, W.C. (1996) Efficient technique for screening drugs for activity against *Trypanosoma cruzi* using parasites expressing beta-galactosidase. *Antimicrob. Agents Chemother.*, **40**, 2592–2607.

57 Canavaci, A.M., Bustamante, J.M., Padilla, A.M., Perez Brandan, C.M., Simpson, L.J., Xu, D., Boehlke, C.L., and Tarleton, R.L. (2010) *In vitro* and *in vivo* high-throughput assays for the testing of anti-*Trypanosoma cruzi* compounds. *PLoS Negl. Trop. Dis.*, **4**, e740.

58 Engel, J.C., Ang, K.K., Chen, S., Arkin, M.R., McKerrow, J.H., and Doyle, P.S. (2010) Image-based high-throughput drug screening targeting the intracellular stage of *Trypanosoma cruzi*, the agent of Chagas' disease. *Antimicrob. Agents Chemother.*, **54**, 3326–3334.

59 De Muylder, G., Ang, K.K., Chen, S., Arkin, M.R., Engel, J.C., and McKerrow, J.H. (2011) A screen against Leishmania intracellular amastigotes: comparison to a promastigote screen and identification of a host cell-specific hit. *PLoS Negl. Trop. Dis.*, **5**, e1253.

60 Bustamante, J.M. and Tarleton, R.L. (2011) Methodological advances in drug discovery for Chagas disease. *Expert Opin. Drug Discov.*, **6**, 653–661.

61 Kirchhoff, L.V. and Pearson, R.D. (2007) The emergence of Chagas disease in the United States and Canada. *Curr. Infect. Dis. Rep.*, **9**, 347–350.

62 Herwaldt, B.L., Grijalva, M.J., Newsome, A.L., McGhee, C.R., Powell, M.R., Nemec, D.G., Steurer, F.J., and Eberhard, M.L. (2000) Use of polymerase chain reaction to diagnose the fifth reported US case of autochthonous transmission of *Trypanosoma cruzi*, in Tennessee, 1998. *J. Infect. Dis.*, **181**, 395–399.

63 Reisenman, C.E., Lawrence, G., Guerenstein, P.G., Gregory, T., Dotson, E., and Hildebrand, J.G. (2010) Infection of kissing bugs with *Trypanosoma cruzi*, Tucson, Arizona, USA. *Emerg. Infect. Dis.*, **16**, 400–405.

64 Ramos, J.M., Milla, A., Rodríguez, J.C., López-Chejade, P., Flóres, M., Rodríguez, J.M., and Gutiérrez, F. (2011) Chagas disease in Latin American pregnant immigrants: experience in a non-endemic country. *Arch. Gynecol. Obstet.*, **285**, 919–92.

65 Gascon, J., Bern, C., and Pinazo, M.J. (2010) Chagas disease in Spain, the United States and other non-endemic countries. *Acta Trop.*, **115**, 22–27.

66 Ueno, Y., Nakamura, Y., Takahashi, M., Inoue, T., Endo, S., Kinoshita, M., and Takeuchi, T. (1995) A highly suspected case of chronic Chagas' heart disease diagnosed in Japan. *Jpn. Circ. J.*, **59**, 219–223.

67 Lescure, F.X., Paris, L., Elghouzzi, M.H., Le Loup, G., Develoux, M., Touafek, F., Mazier, D., and Pialoux, G. (2009) [Experience of targeted screening of Chagas disease in Ile-de-France]. *Bull. Soc. Pathol. Exot.*, **102**, 295–299.

26
Ergosterol Biosynthesis for the Specific Treatment of Chagas Disease: From Basic Science to Clinical Trials

Julio A. Urbina*

Abstract

This chapter reviews the current status and new perspectives on the chemotherapy of Chagas disease, a chronic parasitosis caused by the kinetoplastid protozoon *Trypanosoma cruzi*, which is responsible for the largest parasitic disease burden in the American continent. The activity and limitations of currently available drugs (the nitroheterocyclic compounds nifurtimox and benznidazole) are discussed, as well as potential alternatives, focusing on ergosterol biosynthesis inhibitors (EBIs) – the most advanced candidates for new anti-*T. cruzi* treatments. Such compounds block the *de novo* production of 24-alkyl-sterols, which are essential for parasite survival. Among EBIs, the most promising compounds are new anti-fungal triazole derivatives that inhibit the parasite's sterol C14α-demethylase (CYP51): they have curative activity in animal models of acute and chronic Chagas disease, and are active against nifurtimox- and benznidazole-resistant *T. cruzi* strains, even if the hosts are immunosuppressed. The CYP51 inhibitors posaconazole and ravuconazole have recently entered phase II clinical trials in chronic Chagas disease. Other EBIs with potent and specific anti-*T. cruzi* activity include inhibitors of squalene synthase, lanosterol synthase, 24-methenyl transferase, and squalene epoxidase, as well as compounds with dual mechanisms of action (ergosterol biosynthesis inhibition and free radical generation), but their development is less advanced. The main potential advantages of EBIs over current therapies comprise higher potency in both acute and chronic infections, selectivity and improved safety profile. If safety and efficacy of this class of compounds are confirmed in clinical trials, a new era for the specific treatment of this long-neglected disease is expected.

Introduction

American Trypanosomiasis, or Chagas disease (in honor of Carlos Chagas, a Brazilian physician who described it a century ago [1]), is a chronic parasitosis caused by the kinetoplastid parasite *Trypanosoma* cruzi that has afflicted humanity since its earliest presence in the New World [2] and is still the largest parasitic

* Corresponding Author

Trypanosomatid Diseases: Molecular Routes to Drug Discovery, First edition. Edited by T. Jäger, O. Koch, and L. Flohé.
© 2013 Wiley-VCH Verlag GmbH & Co. KGaA. Published 2013 by Wiley-VCH Verlag GmbH & Co. KGaA.

disease burden of the American continent [3–5], but remains one of the most neglected diseases in the world [6]. The disease is technically a zoonosis, as the natural reservoirs of *T. cruzi* are a large variety of marsupial and placental mammals autochthonous to the American continent, and the parasite is naturally transmitted by hematophagous reduviid insects [5,7,8]. Human disease results from the invasion of natural ecotopes as well as from the establishment of the vectors in human dwellings due to the poor socioeconomic conditions of most rural human populations from Mexico to Argentina, where the disease is endemic [5,7,8]. The parasite can also be transmitted by transfusion of contaminated blood and congenitally from infected mothers to newborns, and these routes of transmission, together with intense international migrations in the last 15 years, have led to the spread of the disease to non-endemic areas, such as the United States and Western Europe [9–12].

Given its zoonotic character, Chagas disease is not eradicable [13]; however, significant advances have taken place in the control of the vectorial and transfusional transmission of the disease in some parts of the continent, particularly by the Southern Cone initiative, which led to a significant drop in the prevalence (from 18–20 million for early 1990s to about 10 million for 2006) and the population at risk (from 100 to 40 million in the same period) [4,14]. Nevertheless, the disease is far from being controlled, due to the uneven extent and quality of control programs in the continent, and limitations of both diagnostic methods and currently available specific treatments [5,13,15–19].

Currently Available Drugs for the Specific Treatment of Chagas Disease: Limitations and Controversies on their Application

Chagas disease is a complex condition resulting from the invasion and successful establishment of *T. cruzi*, an intracellular parasite, in key tissues of its mammalian hosts. In humans, the initial acute phase has a low (less than 10%) mortality and generally mild and unspecific symptoms; macrophages, interferon-γ, $CD4^+$ and $CD8^+$ T 1 lymphocytes are the key elements controlling parasite replication [20–22]. This acute phase is followed by a life-long chronic condition, where the cellular immune response limits the parasite's proliferation but is unable to eradicate the infection, leading to a sustained inflammatory response that underlies the development of one or more of the symptomatic chronic forms of the disease in 30–40% of patients, including chronic Chagas cardiomyopathy (CCC), digestive problems, and neuropathies [21,23,24]. The most severe of these manifestations is CCC, which typically appears decades after the initial infection, and may result in cardiac arrhythmias, ventricular aneurysm, congestive heart failure, thromboembolism, and sudden cardiac death; this condition is the leading cause of cardiac disease and cardiac death in poor rural and rural-originated urban populations in Latin America [15,23,25].

The compounds currently available for the specific treatment of this parasitosis are nifurtimox (Lampit®, Bayer; 5-nitrofuran (3-methyl-4-(5′-nitrofurfurylideneamine) tetrahydro-4H-1,4-tiazine-1,1-dioxide) and benznidazole (Rochagan®, Radanil®,

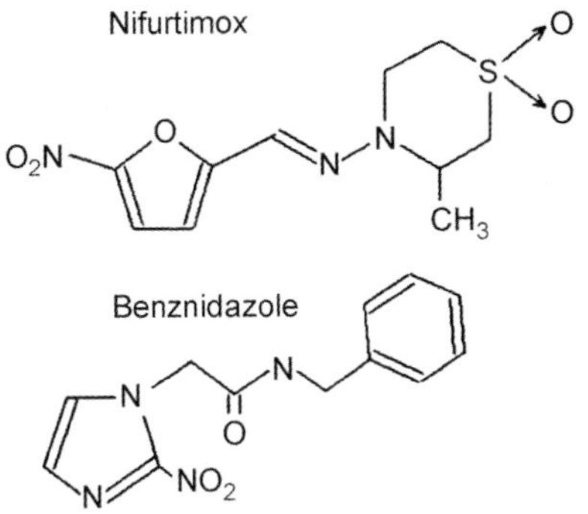

Figure 26.1 Chemical structure of the drugs currently available for the specific treatment of Chagas disease: nifurtimox (a 5-nitrofuran) and benznidazole (a 2-nitroimidazole).

Roche; *N*-benzyl-2-nitroimidazole acetamide), a 2-nitromidazole, which were developed empirically and registered in the late 1960s and early 1970s, originally to treat acute *T. cruzi* infections (Figure 26.1).

Numerous clinical studies, have shown that both drugs have significant activity in congenital and adult acute infections (greater than 95 and 60–80% of parasitological cures, respectively), as defined by negativization of all parasitological and conventional serological tests [26–28], but their efficacy varies according to the geographical area, probably due to differences in drug susceptibility among different *T. cruzi* strains [29–32]. It has been shown, both in experimental animals' and human infections, that the interleukin-12/interferon-γ axis of the immune system plays an essential role in the drug-induced parasitological cure [33,34]. Moreover, it has been reported in the last 15 years that benznidazole has also significant curative activity in early chronic infections, with 60–70% radical parasitological cures observed among children up to 16 years old in Brazil and Argentina [35–37], although other studies on patients of the same age range were unable to detect these high cure rates [32,38,39]. However, the major limitation of these drugs is their lower anti-parasitic activity in the established chronic form of the disease, which is the most prevalent presentation, as 80% or more of treated patients are not parasitologically cured according to the classical criteria indicated above for acute infections [26–28]; these results have now been confirmed using polymerase chain reaction-based and special serological methods in both humans and experimental animals [40–49]. The reasons for the marked difference in the anti-parasitic efficacy of nitroheterocyclic compounds in the acute and chronic stages of the disease are unclear [26], but they may be related to unfavorable pharmacokinetic properties, such as relatively short terminal half-life and limited tissue penetration [16], which will limit their activity in the chronic stage when the parasites are mostly confined to deep tissues and undergo slow replication [16,50]. Nevertheless, several observational clinical studies have shown that chronic patients subjected to anti-parasitic treatment with benznidazole, although not parasitologically cured, have a significant reduction in the occurrence of electrocardiographic changes and a lower frequency of deterioration of their clinical condition [37,51–53], although other studies do not confirm these findings [37,44]. Additionally, both drugs have unwanted side-effects that can lead to treatment discontinuation and are related to their mechanism of action (generation of nitro-reduction intermediates that lead to oxidative stress for nifurtimox or reductive stress for benznidazole [19,54]). In the case of nifurtimox these include anorexia, nausea, and vomiting causing severe weight loss, insomnia, irritability and, less commonly, peripheral polyneuropathy, while for benznidazole the most common adverse effects are allergic dermopathy and gastrointestinal syndromes, and less frequently depression of bone marrow, thrombocytopenic purpura and agranulocytosis, polyneuropathy, paresthesia, and polyneuritis of peripheral nerves [28]. The incidence of such side-effects is variable depending on the age of the patient (less frequent and less severe in younger patients), geographic region, and the quality of the clinical supervision of the treatment [28,32,55].

On the other hand, long-held ideas on the pathogenesis of the disease have discouraged the specific treatment of chronic patients who, as indicated above, are by far the majority of the infected population. Thus, although the role of *T. cruzi* in the pathology of acute phase of Chagas disease and the importance of etiological treatment in that stage are widely accepted [21,28], the participation of the parasite in the pathogenesis of chronic Chagas disease has for decades been the subject of controversies [16,23,56–58]. Several studies implicated autoimmune phenomena as a primary factor leading to the persistent inflammation associated with chronic Chagas disease pathological manifestations, including CCC [59,60]. This hypothesis was based on the apparent absence of parasites in the characteristic inflammatory lesions of the heart and gastrointestinal tract associated with symptomatic chronic Chagas disease and the presence of "anti-self" antibody responses in Chagas disease patients, the latter postulated to result from molecular mimicry between parasite antigens and the host's cellular components [59,60]. According to such hypothesis, after the parasite triggers the autoimmune response in the host, its persistence should not play a pivotal role in the pathogenesis of the disease and even a successful anti-parasitic treatment may not lead to an improvement of the clinical outcome of the patients. In fact, the autoimmune hypothesis of chronic Chagas disease pathogenesis stalled for decades the development of new specific chemotherapeutic approaches for this disease, as anti-parasitic treatment was considered irrelevant for the chronic stage [16,61,62]. This notion, together with the limited efficacy of currently available drugs in long-term chronic infections, have been the main factors responsible for the low treatment coverage as, based on it, the national control programs have traditionally excluded adult chronic patients from their treatment guidelines [5].

However, the autoimmune hypothesis has been strongly challenged by the results of many studies in the last 15 years, which have consistently concluded that the persistence of parasites, coupled with an unbalanced immune response in some individuals, leads to the sustained inflammatory responses that underlie the characteristic lesions of chronic Chagas disease [5,19,23]. This new paradigm indicates, in contrast to previous notions, that eradication of *T. cruzi* may be a prerequisite to arrest the evolution of Chagas disease and avert its irreversible long-term consequences, and implies that this condition must be treated primarily as an infectious, not autoimmune, condition [5,15,16,23,63]. Seen from this new perspective, the positive effect of current specific treatments on the patient's clinical evolution, despite their inability to eradicate the parasite, has been explained by a drug-induced reduction of the parasite load in infected tissues, which presumably should reduce the severity of the associated inflammatory processes [5,51,52,63].

In 1998, based on the clinical experience and the level of understanding of the pathogenesis of the disease at the date, the consensus for the specific treatment of Chagas disease with benznidazole and nifurtimox was summarized by a group of experts as a set of guidelines (Pan-American Health Organization/World Health Organization, document OPS/HCP/HCT140/99), where treatment was recommended for acute cases and recent chronic infections, such as those of seropositive children up to 14 years old, while the treatment of adult chronic patients, with or without cardiac or gastrointestinal involvement, was considered optional. Currently a new consensus is emerging, based on the parasite persistence hypothesis, where etiological treatment is indicated for all seropositive patients (including chronically infected adults, as long as no advanced heart disease is present), aiming to reduce or eliminate their parasite loads [9,15,51,64]. However, many physicians have still strong reservations concerning the use of nifurtimox and benznidazole in chronic patients, due to their questionable risk/benefit ratio. Aiming to clarify this issue, a large-scale, randomized and placebo-controlled clinical trial is currently underway to assess the effects of etiologic treatment with benznidazole in chronic Chagas patients (BENEFIT trial) [65].

Based on the limitations of the currently drugs available anti-*T. cruzi* drugs, particularly for the treatment of chronic infections, new approaches have been pursued in the last 25 years [16,57], among which ergosterol biosynthesis inhibitors (EBIs) are the most promising ones. This strategy will be described in detail in the remaining sections of this chapter.

EBIs as Potential New Therapeutic Agents for Chagas Disease

Structure and Function of Sterols in *T. cruzi*

Sterols are essential lipid molecules in eukaryotes where they act as regulators of membrane physical properties, such as permeability and fluidity, but also have essential roles in aerobic metabolism, regulation of cell cycle, sterol uptake, and sterol transport [66]. The initial steps in cholesterol biosynthesis also lead to the synthesis of other important molecules, including dolichol, ubiquinone, isopentyladenine, heme A, and prenylated proteins. The final products of sterol biosynthesis vary among eukaryotes, with mammals producing cholesterol, while fungi plants and protozoa produce 24-alkyl sterols, with distinct modifications of both the steroid nucleus and the alkyl side-chain for each phylogenetic group. *T. cruzi* is most similar to fungi in its sterol composition, with ergosterol (24-methyl-cholesta-5,7,22-trien-3β-ol) and its 24-ethyl analog (24-ethyl-cholesta-5,7,22-trien-3β-ol) being the major mature sterols in the extracellular epimastigote stages [67–69], while for the intracellular

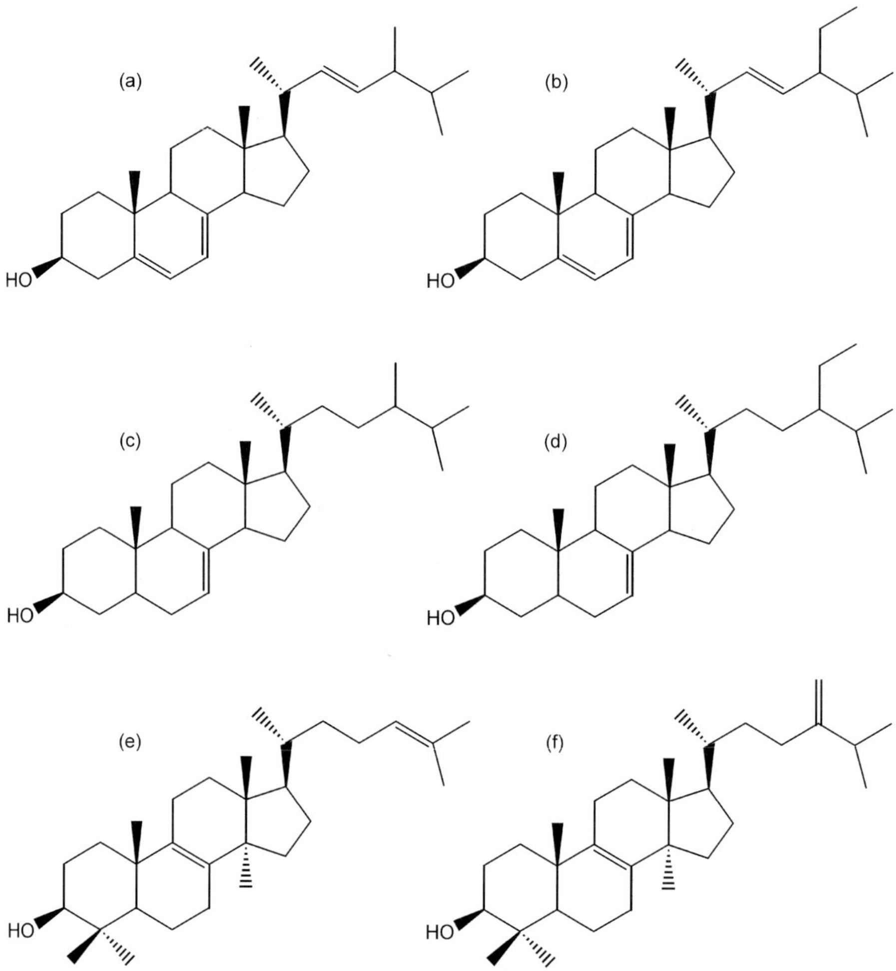

Figure 26.2 Main sterols of *T. cruzi* extracellular epimastigotes, ergosterol (a) and its 24-ethyl analog (b); intracellular amastigotes, fungisterol (c) and its 24-ethyl analog (d); the preferred substrate of mammalian and fungal CYP5, lanosterol (e); the preferred substrate of *T. cruzi* CYP51, eburicol (f).

amastigotes the corresponding compounds are fungisterol (ergosta-7-en-3β-ol) and its 24-ethyl analog (24-ethyl-cholesta-7-en-3β-ol) [70] (Figure 26.2). Although *T. cruzi* incorporates the mammalian hosts' sterol (cholesterol) into its membranes, it has an essential requirement for *de novo* sterol synthesis of 24-alkyl sterols for survival in all stages of its life cycle [69,70] and this biosynthetic pathway has been chemically validated as a drug target in this organism at several different steps (reviewed in [16,57,71]). Biophysical and biochemical studies, using both plasma membranes isolated from *T. cruzi* epimastigotes [72,73] and artificial model membranes [74–76], characterized in detail the far-reaching effects on the physical properties of the lipid bilayer and associated enzymatic activities (including those involved in phospholipid biosynthesis) resulting from changes in the membranes' sterol composition. Other studies revealed the profound alterations in the structure and function of internal organelles resulting from any blockade of the *de novo* sterol synthesis [77,78], particularly in the single giant mitochondrion characteristic of trypanosomatids, which is highly enriched in endogenous sterols [79].

Sterol C14α-Demethylase (CYP51) Inhibitors

Despite the *in vitro* chemical validation of the sterol biosynthesis pathway as a drug target in *T. cruzi*, several subsequent studies showed that commercially available EBIs, which are highly successful in the treatment of fungal diseases (such as ketoconazole, itraconazole, or terbinafine), have suppressive but not curative effects against *T. cruzi* infections in humans or experimental animals and are unable stop the progression of the disease[16,71]. In contrast, in the past 15 years new triazole derivatives (Figure 26.3), potent and selective inhibitors of fungal and protozoan cytochrome P450-dependent sterol C14α-demethylase (CYP51), such as D0870 (Zeneca Pharmaceuticals) and posaconazole (SCH 56592; Schering Plough Research Institute, now Merck), were found to be capable of inducing radical parasitological cure in murine models of acute and chronic Chagas disease [16,71]. These were the first compounds reported to display curative activity in both forms of the disease [80,81]. Furthermore, such compounds were able to eradicate nitrofuran- and nitroimidazole-resistant *T. cruzi* strains from infected mice, even if the hosts were immunosuppressed [16,71].

CYP51 catalyzes an essential step in the *de novo* synthesis of sterols in all eukaryotic organisms; in mammals and yeast, where the substrate is lanosterol (Figure 26.1e), the enzyme is frequently called lanosterol 14α-demethylase. In *T. cruzi*, new data suggests that the preferred substrate is not lanosterol, but rather eburicol (24-methylene-dihydrolanosterol) [82] (Figure 26.1f). CYP51 specifically catalyzes the removal of the C14α methyl group from the sterol scaffold through three successive oxidations resulting in decarboxylation, releasing formic acid [83]. During catalysis, the active-site heme iron is reduced by a P450-reductase enzyme utilizing NADPH from the resting ferric (Fe^{3+}) state to active ferrous (Fe^{2+}) state; the resting state is regenerated in each cycle by the transfer of electrons to oxygen and the incorporation of this atom in the C14α substituent of the sterol substrate [84]. Inhibition of cytochrome P450 enzymes by azole drugs results from coordination of the azole nitrogen to the heme iron, with the lipophilic ligand attached to the azole occupying the binding site for the substrate. These inhibitors prevent both binding of the substrate and oxygen activation [85]. In the last few years crystal structures of trypanosomal CYP51 bound to inhibitors have been described [84,86,87] and, most recently, that of *T. brucei* CYP51 bound to a substrate analog that acts as a mechanism-based (suicide) inhibitor of the *T. cruzi* enzyme [88], which have provided insights into the details of the catalytic site of this enzyme. It was

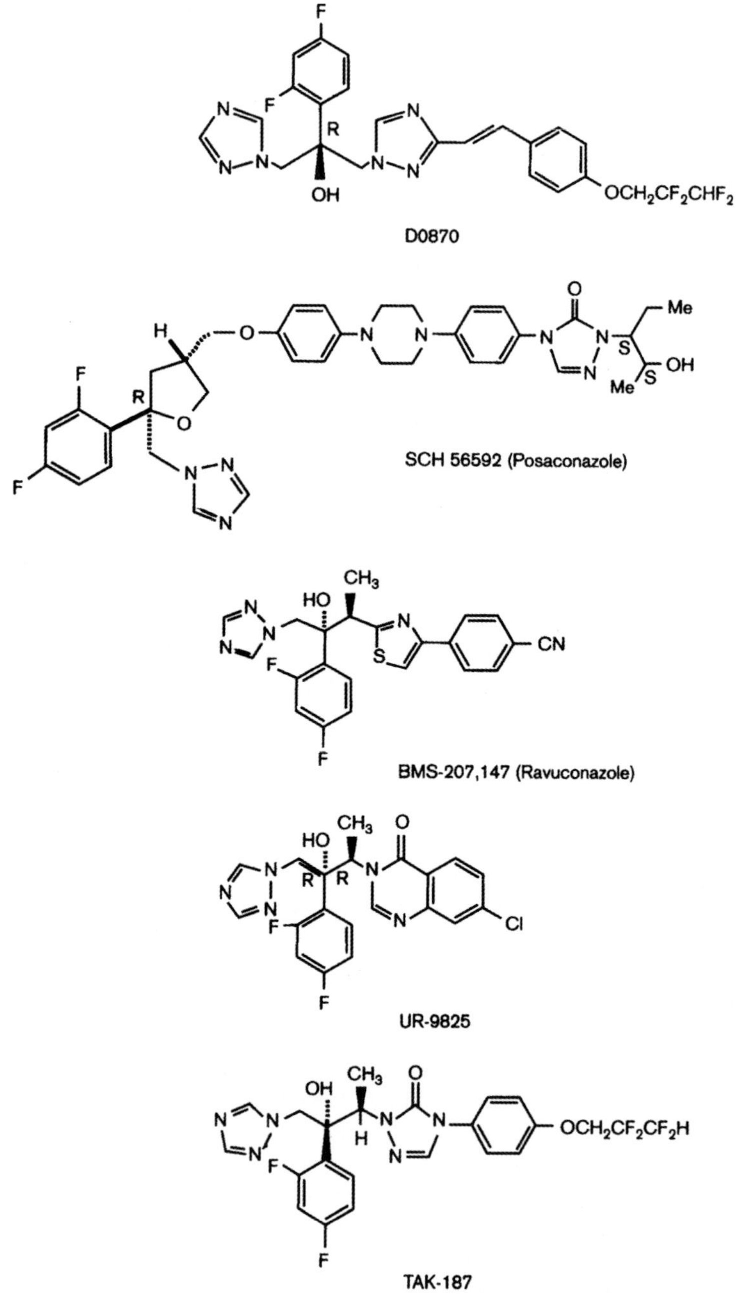

Figure 26.3 Chemical structures of novel triazole derivatives, specific inhibitors of fungal and protozoan sterol C14α-demethylase (CYP51), which have curative activity in animal models of acute and chronic Chagas disease. Posaconazole (Noxafil®; Merck) and ravuconazole (Eisai) are currently the most advanced candidates for a new anti-*T. cruzi* drug, and are in phase II clinical trials for the specific treatment of chronic Chagas disease.

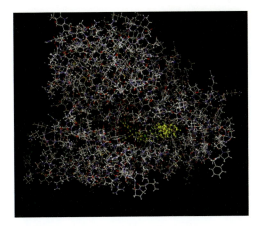

Figure 26.4 Crystal structure of *T. cruzi* CYP51 complexed with posaconazole, seen along the substrate access channel. Protein in displayed gray, posaconazole in bright green, heme in red. Figure prepared with Molegro Molecular Viewer using coordinates from Protein Data Bank ID: 3K1O [86].

found that posaconazole, one of the most potent new triazole derivatives, binds very tightly to *T. cruzi* CYP51, through direct interactions with 13 amino acid side-chains in the active site and 12 in the hydrophobic substrate access channel, which, in fact, have an stabilizing effect on the tertiary structure of the protein [84,86,87] (Figure 26.4).

The remarkable *in vivo* anti-parasitic activities of these triazole derivatives probably result from a combination of their potent and selective intrinsic anti-*T. cruzi* activity (minimal growth inhibitory concentrations against intracellular amastigotes *in vitro* are in the nanomolar to subnanomolar range; in the case of posaconazole, this could be linked to its high binding affinity for *T. cruzi* CYP51, see above) with special pharmacokinetic properties, such as large volumes of distribution (indicating extensive penetration in internal organs) and long terminal half-life [16,89,90]. Furthermore, it has recently been demonstrated that posaconazole and other lipophilic drugs accumulate in the membranes of cells; as a result, the effective local concentrations of these drugs that interact with their membrane-bound CYP51 targets are in fact much higher than their overall cell or tissue levels [91].

Recent studies with posaconazole, which is a structural analog of itraconazole, have shown that this compound can eradicate the intracellular amastigote forms from cultured cardiomyocytes, and at the same time allow the full reassembly of the host cells cytoskeleton and contractile apparatus [92]. Other studies have demonstrated that the anti-*T. cruzi* activity of posaconazole in a murine model of acute Chagas disease is much less dependent on interferon-γ than that of benznidazole [93]. It has also been shown that ablation of TCD4$^+$, TCD8$^+$, and B lymphocytes have distinct effects on posaconazole and benznidazole activity in the same experimental model [94]. posaconazole efficacy was particularly dependent on the presence of functional TCD8$^+$ cells but relatively insensitive to the absence of LB cells, while the reverse was true for benznidazole; the activity of both drugs was markedly reduced in the absence of TCD4$^+$ cells [94]. These results were interpreted in terms of the different parasite stages preferentially targeted by the two drugs (intracellular amastigotes by posaconazole, extracellular trypomastigotes by benznidazole) and distinct cooperation patterns with the host immune system [94]. An independent study in a similar experimental model found that posaconazole was more effective than benznidazole in preventing heart damage and promoting a trypanocidal immune response [95]. Finally, a recent case report from Spain described the successful use of posaconazole to treat a patient with chronic *T. cruzi* infection, compounded by immuno-suppressive treatment required to control a lupus erythematosus condition, who had failed benznidazole chemotherapy [96].

Posaconazole was registered in 2005 in the European Union and Australia for treatment and in 2006 in the United States for the prophylaxis of invasive fungal infections (IFI) as well as for the treatment azole-resistant candidiasis; the drug is currently one of the mainstays for the treatments of IFI due to its potent, broad spectrum, anti-fungal activity and excellent safety profile [97,98]. Based on these antecedents and the results of the preclinical studies as anti-*T. cruzi* agent described above, two proof-of-concept phase II clinical studies with posaconazole for the specific treatment of Chagas disease are under way: the first was launched in October 2010 at the Vall d'Hebron Hospital in Barcelona, Spain (http://clinicaltrials.gov/ct2/show/NCT01162967?term=posaconazole,+Chagas+disease&rank=1) and a second one, sponsored by Merck & Co (http://clinicaltrials.gov/ct2/show/NCT01377480?term=Chagas&rank=1), began recruiting patients in Argentina in the third quarter of 2011. Such studies will take us a big step closer to defining the role of this drug for treating Chagas disease. Unfortunately, posaconazole is an extremely expensive drug, so even if it is shown to be efficacious in humans, there is looming concern that it may be difficult to get it to patients living in resource-limited settings [56], but this issue could potentially be approached through differential pricing, which have been used for other on-patent pharmaceuticals in separate markets [99], or through drug combinations that could lower the dose and/or the length of treatments, thus decreasing their cost (see Section "Combination Therapies").

Other triazoles (Figure 26.3), such as TAK-187 (Takeda Chemical Company) [100,101], UR-9825 (Uriach & Company) [102,103], and ravuconazole (ER-30346, Eisai; BMS 207,147, Bristol-Myers Squibb) [104,105], have also been shown to have trypanocidal activity, both *in vitro* and *in vivo*. TAK-187 is a long-lasting triazole derivative with broad-spectrum anti-fungal activity, which has also very potent anti-*T. cruzi* activity *in vitro*, and is capable of curing both acute and chronic infections in murine hosts even when the infecting strain is nitrofuran- and nitroimidazole-resistant [101]; more recent work has shown than this compound is superior to benznidazole in preventing cardiac damage in a murine model of Chagas disease [100]. UR-9825 is another potent fungal and protozoan CYP51 inhibitor with remarkable *in vitro* anti-*T. cruzi* activity [102]; although its very short half-life in the mouse (less than 0.5 h) precluded *in vivo* studies in this animal model, work in a canine model have demonstrated that the compound has curative activity in established infections of the virulent Y strain of *T. cruzi* with very low toxicity, although drug resistance was encountered with the Berenice-78 strain [103]. Finally, ravuconazole has also been shown to be very active against *T. cruzi in vitro* (comparable to that of posaconazole) but its *in vivo* activity in mice was limited, probably due to inadequate pharmacokinetic properties in this animal model (terminal half-life of 4.5 h) [104]. Similarly, the activity of ravuconazole in a canine model of acute Chagas disease was found to be suppressive, not curative, a result that was again attributed to the relatively short half-life of the compound in dogs (8.8 h)[105]. However, these results do not necessarily rule out the potential usefulness of this compound in the treatment of human *T. cruzi* infections, as the minimal inhibitory concentration against intracellular amastigotes (1 nM) is 1000 to 5000 times lower than the levels attainable in human plasma with multiple oral dosing (which in turn are much lower that the tissue levels, due the large volume of distribution) and its terminal half-life in man is 120 h or more [106,107]. Ravuconazole is currently in phase II clinical trials for the treatment of systemic fungal infections, where is has shown potent activity and very good tolerability [108]. Based on these findings, the Drugs for Neglected Diseases *initiative* (DNDi) announced that it has reached an agreement with Eisai for the clinical development of E1224, a water-soluble pro-drug (mono-lysine derivative) of ravuconazole, for the treatment of chronic human Chagas disease (http://www.dndi.org/press-releases/ 532-eisai-and-dndi-enter-into-a-collaboration.html); the first clinical study was launched in Bolivia in July 2011.

A different type of azole-based CYP51 inhibitors, with potent anti-*T. cruzi* activity *in vitro* and *in vivo*, was serendipitously discovered in the course of a research program to identify parasite-specific inhibitors of protein farnesyltransferase (PFT), based on the structure of the anti-cancer drug tipifarnib [50,109–111]. Since the inhibitory activity on PFT was unnecessary for the anti-*T. cruzi* activity, analogs of tipifarnib were designed to minimize the anti-PFT activity (which could lead to deleterious side-effects) while improving CYP51 inhibitory activity. The current lead compound (Figure 26.5) combines the excellent pharmacokinetic properties of tipifarnib (i.e., oral bioavailability and good metabolic stability) with minimal PFT activity and subnanomolar potency on intracellular *T. cruzi* amastigotes [112]. Working with the same strategic aim, the group led by Lepesheva and Waterman investigated a large variety of compounds as potential CYP51 inhibitors using a high-throughput screening spectroscopic assay that evaluates type II spectral responses to detect strong binders to the sixth coordination position of the heme iron [113,114]. However, it was found than in many cases the apparent binding parameters determined by spectral titration did not correlate with the inhibitory effects of the compounds on the reconstituted enzyme activity; thus, the spectral hits had to be confirmed using the biochemical assay [113,114]. The best results of this approach have been those resulting from a screen of a collection of azole derivatives of the Novartis Research Institute (Vienna, Austria), which led to the identification of two potent β-phenyl imidazoles, VNF (SDZ285604) and VNI (Figure 26.5) [113]. These compounds produce a functionally irreversible inhibition of *T. cruzi* and

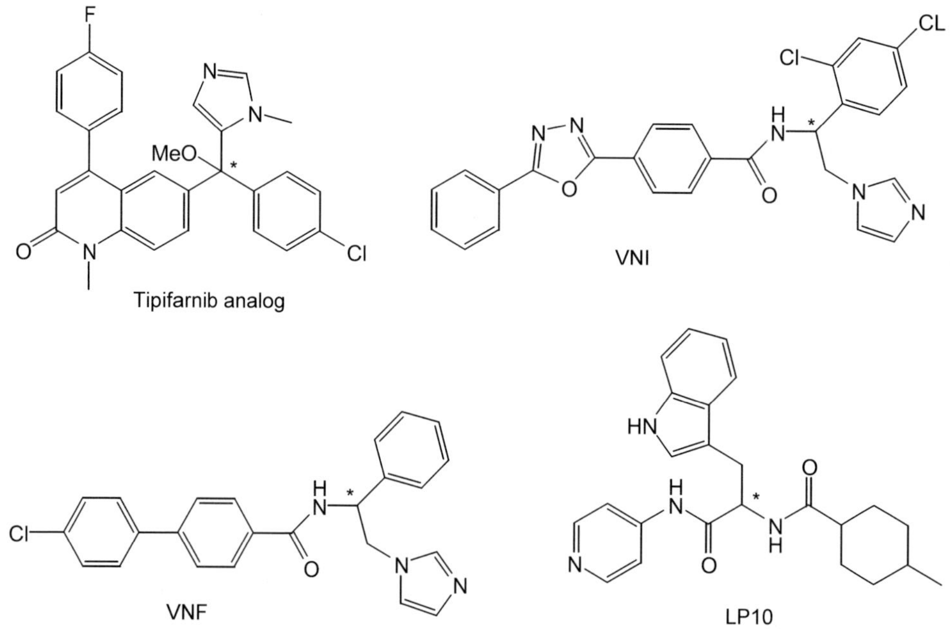

Figure 26.5 Structures of novel *T. cruzi* CYP51 inhibitors discussed in the text: the most active tipifarnib analog; the β-phenyl imidazoles VNI and VNF; the pyridine-indomethacin amide derivative LP-10.

T. brucei CYP51s at a 1:1 inhibitor ratio, and are remarkably selective for the trypanosomatid enzymes (the human enzyme is only slightly affected by a 100-fold excess of the inhibitors [113]). VNF can eradicate *T. cruzi*'s amastigote infection from cultured murine cardiomyocytes at 1 μM [86]. Although such selective activity is promising, it is still 1000-fold less potent that the anti-fungal triazoles discussed above. Interestingly, it was found that VNI binds to *T. brucei* CYP51 in a pose very similar to that of posaconazole bound to *T. cruzi* CYP51, although with less extensive interactions with the substrate access channel [86,115]; such findings may provide insights on how to increase the potency of this class of compounds, while preserving their selectivity. No *in vivo* studies of VNF or VNI have been reported. Another approach by the same team led to the identification of a novel class of non-azole *T. cruzi* CYP51 inhibitors, based on the pyridine–indomethacin amide scaffold [113,116]. However, the most potent compound of this series was only able to fully eradicate amastigotes from infected cardiomyocytes at 20 μM. Remarkably, one of the compounds of that series (ChemDiv-3124-01167, not the most potent one) was independently identified by the team of Podust and McKerrow, from a screen against *Mycobacterium tuberculosis* CYP51, as a potent inhibitor of *T. cruzi* CYP51 [84,117]. The compound, now known as LP-10 (Figure 26.5), was found to bind selectively to *T. cruzi* CYP51 (the authors report no binding to the *T. brucei* enzyme [117], but in the original report by Lepesheva *et al.* [113] binding constants to the two enzymes were comparable) and to eradicate *T. cruzi* amastigotes from infected mouse (J774) macrophages at 10 µM, with no toxicity for the host cells. In a subsequent study [118], the same team reported that LP-10 inhibits the synthesis of endogenous sterol in *T. cruzi* epimastigotes and is curative in about 60% of animals in a murine model of acute Chagas disease. If the ADME/Tox (absorption, distribution, metabolism, elimination, and toxicity) profile of this compound or subsequent derivatives proves to be appropriate for human use it could become an alternative to the proprietary anti-fungal azoles described above, which are the current leading candidates.

Oxidosqualene Cyclase (Lanosterol Synthase) Inhibitors – Amiodarone as an Anti-Parasitic Agent

Another advance in the area of EBIs as anti-parasitic agents is the validation of oxidosqualene cyclase (OSC, lanosterol synthase) as a chemotherapeutic target in *T. cruzi* and related parasites [119–121]. Buckner *et al.* have demonstrated the potent and selective *in vitro* anti-parasitic activities of OSC inhibitors [119,122] and a patent by the same authors claims the use of OSC inhibitors as chemotherapeutic agents for the specific treatment of parasitic infections, including Chagas disease (US Patent WO0076316 [123]). However, no *in vivo* activity of this class of compounds has been reported. In a related development, it was recently discovered that amiodarone (2-butyl-1-benzofuran-3-yl)-[4-(2-diethylaminoethoxy)-3,5-diiodo-phenyl]methanone; Figure 26.6), the anti-arrhythmic drug most frequently used in chronic Chagas disease patients with cardiac compromise [15,25,124], has also

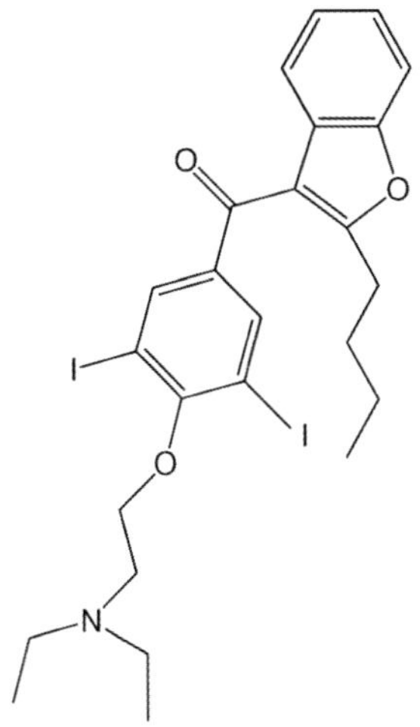

Figure 26.6 Chemical structure of amiodarone, the anti-arrhythmic drug most frequently used in chronic Chagas disease patients with cardiac compromise, now known to have also potent and selective anti-*T. cruzi* activity, *in vitro* and *in vivo*.

intrinsic anti-*T. cruzi* activity *in vitro* and *in vivo*, which is mediated by a blockade of *de novo* ergosterol biosynthesis at the level of OSC and disruption of Ca^{2+} homeostasis [125]. Such mechanism of action explained the additional observation that the combined action of amiodarone and the CYP51 inhibitor posaconazole on *T. cruzi* had synergistic effects, *in vitro* and *in vivo* [125]. Additional studies on the effects of amiodarone on primary cultures of murine cardiomyocytes infected with *T. cruzi* showed that, at concentrations below those required for its anti-arrhythmic action, the drug was able to eradicate the intracellular amastigotes while allowing full recovery of the cytoskeleton, contractile apparatus, and spontaneous contractility of the host cells [126]. The results suggest that Chagas disease patients under treatment with amiodarone to control their arrhythmias may have the added benefit of a reduction of their parasite burden and enhancement of the effects of anti-parasitic treatment. This prediction was recently confirmed by a report of a patient with chronic Chagas disease and advanced cardiac compromise who was treated with a combination of amiodarone and itraconazole, which lead to a marked improvement of his clinical condition as well as to parasitological cure, verified by the disappearance of anti-*T. cruzi* lytic antibodies [48,127]. Subsequent work found very similar effects against *Leishmania mexicana*, *in vitro* and *in vivo*, including a human patient [128–130], indicating a broad anti-parasitic action. New clinical studies on the anti-parasitic activity of this drug, alone or in combinations are expected in the near future.

Squalene Synthase Inhibitors

A different group of promising *T. cruzi* agents among EBIs is that of squalene synthase (SQS) inhibitors. SQS is the first committed step in sterol biosynthesis, and had been the subject of intense study by both academic and industrial groups as it is an attractive target for cholesterol-lowering agents, with potential significant advantages over currently available statins [131–134]. This enzyme has been recently chemically validated as a chemotherapeutic target in *T. cruzi* and *L. mexicana* [135]. Further studies led to the discovery that E5700 and ER-119884, two novel quinuclidine SQS inhibitors that were being developed as cholesterol and triglyceride lowering agents in humans by Eisai (Figure 26.7), have very potent anti-*T. cruzi* activity *in vitro* and one of them (E5700) was able to provide full protection against death and completely arrested development of parasitemia in a murine model of acute disease when given orally [136]; this was the first report of an orally active SQS inhibitor as an anti-infective agent. Although these compounds and other aryl-quinuclidines are also potent inhibitors of mammalian SQS [137–140], their selective anti-parasitic activity *in vitro* and *in vivo* is probably explained by the capacity of the host's cells to compensate for the blockade of *de novo* cholesterol synthesis by upregulating the expression of low-density lipoprotein receptors and taking this sterol from the growth medium or serum [141]; in contrast, there is no way for the parasite to compensate in this manner for the quinuclidine-induced blockade of ergosterol biosynthesis, as there are no appreciable amounts of

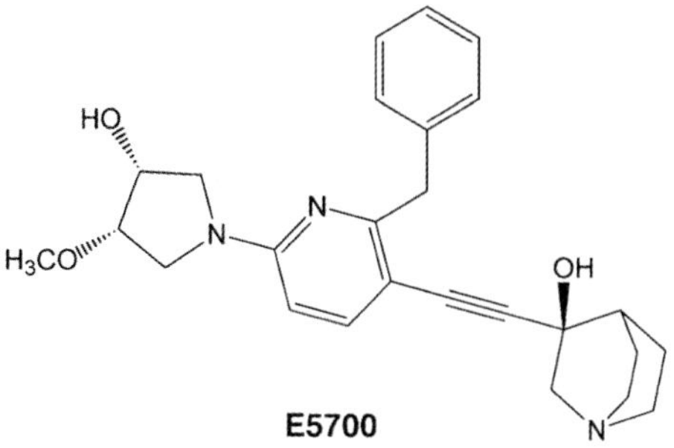

Figure 26.7 Chemical structures of novel aryl-quinuclidine derivatives with potent *in vitro* and *in vivo* (oral) activity against *T. cruzi*.

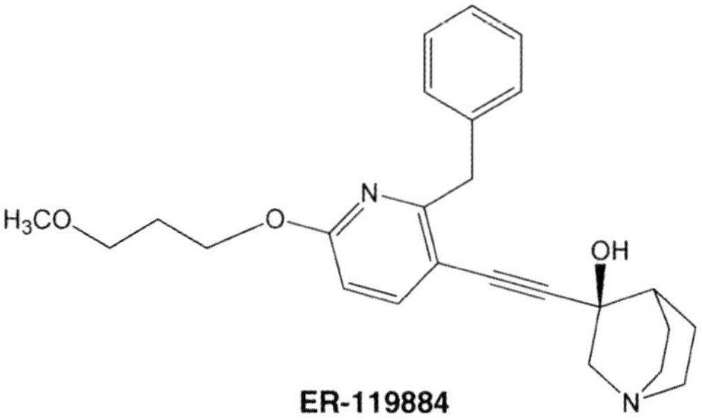

ergosterol in the host cells or growth media [135,136]. However, the requirement of some key organs (such as testis) of an elevated *endogenous* cholesterol supply could pose a significant limitation for the prolonged use of these SQS inhibitors: in fact, sustained use (30 days or longer) of selective SQS inhibitors (and statins) has been associated with testicular atrophy in experimental animals (Eisai, data on file). Thus, the use of this class of compounds as anti-parasitic agents will probably require parasite-specific SQS inhibitors, in much the same way that current anti-fungal azoles are specific for fungal and parasite CYP51s, being much less potent against the mammalian ortholog. Recent work has demonstrated progress towards this goal, as the gene coding *T. cruzi* SQS has been cloned and expressed in *Escherichia coli*, allowing the production of a soluble, fully active, recombinant enzyme, which has been used to identify parasite-specific SQS inhibitors [142,143]. Finally, it has also been shown that aryloxyethyl thiocyanates such as WC-9 (4-phenoxyphenoxye-thylthiocyanate), a new class of potent and selective anti-*T. cruzi* agents [144,145], act by selective inhibition of the parasite's SQS [146].

Hybrid Compounds with a Dual Mechanism of Action

An interesting development in this area is a recent report on the synthesis and chemical/biological characterization of a class of compounds with a dual mechanism of action, resulting from the presence in the same molecule of two pharmacophores: a nitrofuran moiety that leads to free radical generation and redox cycling (see above), and a hetero-allyl moiety that inhibits squalene epoxidase, a key enzyme in sterol biosynthesis [147]. These hetero-allyl-containing 5-nitrofuran compounds were very active against both the extracellular and intracellular forms of the parasite *in vitro* and more potent than nifurtimox and terbinafine, a commercial squalene epoxidase inhibitor with anti-fungal activity. The potential of this new class of compounds is underscored by previous studies [148] that showed that combination therapy with benznidazole and the EBI ketoconazole had synergistic effects in a murine model of acute Chagas disease (see below).

Combination Therapies

Combined anti-infective therapies have several objectives: (i) to reduce the dose and/ or duration of the treatment, with the concomitant reduction in side-effects and costs, as well as improvement in the patient's compliance, (ii) to exploit potential synergic effects of concomitant treatments, and (iii) to forestall the development of drug resistance by the etiological agent. Such combinations have been used for decades in anti-fungal, anti-parasitic, and anti-viral therapy, as well as in the treatment of fastidious bacterial infections such as tuberculosis, but this concept has not yet been incorporated in the specific chemotherapeutic management of human Chagas disease, despite the limitations of currently available drugs and the long (30–60 days) treatments involved.

The emergence of EBI as potential anti-*T. cruzi* agents led from the beginning to interest in the study of combinations of compounds acting at different steps of the pathway, since their combined action was predicted to have synergic effects [90]. Several studies confirmed this hypothesis, demonstrating strong synergism in the anti-*T. cruzi* action of ketoconazole (another CYP51 inhibitor but with suppressive, but not curative, anti-*T. cruzi* activity *in vivo*) combined with terbinafine (squalene epoxidase inhibitor) *in vitro* [77,149] or with mevinolin (lovastatin, an inhibitor of 3-hydroxy-3-methyl-glutaryl-CoA reductase), both *in vitro* and *in vivo* [150]. Furthermore, it was shown that combinations of 22,26-azasterol or 24 (*R,S*),25-epiminolanosterol, inhibitors of sterol 24-methenyl transferase (an essential enzyme in ergosterol biosynthesis, not present in mammals), with ketonazole had strong synergic effects against *T. cruzi*, *in vitro* and *in vivo* [151]. Another study found that combinations of ketoconazole with alkyl-lysophospholipid analogs (inhibitors of the *T. cruzi*'s phosphatidylcholine biosynthesis) had synergic anti-proliferative effects against the parasite *in vitro* [152].

On the other hand, an independent study found that combinations of benznidazole with ketoconazole had synergic effects in a murine model of acute Chagas disease [148] and, as described in Section "Oxidosqualene Cyclase (Lanosterol Synthase) Inhibitors – Amiodarone as an Anti-Parasitic Agent", it is now known that the anti-arrhythmic drug amiodarone also has anti-*T. cruzi* activity and acts synergistically with posaconazole *in vitro* and *in vivo* [125].

Based on these antecedents, drug combinations are being considered for evaluation of their efficacy in both experimental and human Chagas disease:

i)   Combinations of nifurtimox or benznidazole with EBIs such as posaconazole or ravuconazole.
ii) Combinations of amiodarone with benznidazole or nifurtimox, and amiodarone with CYP51 inhibitors (itraconazole, posaconazole, or ravuconazole).
iii) Combinations of EBIs acting at different steps of the pathway such as CYP51 inhibitors (itraconazole, posaconazole, or ravuconazole) with 3-hydroxy-3-methyl-glutaryl-CoA reductase inhibitors (statins) or SQS inhibitors [133,136,153,154].

A recent report [155] described potent synergic effects for combinations of benznidazole or nifurtimox with posaconazole in a murine model of acute Chagas disease. Similar combinations could be incorporated in the initial clinical trials of posaconazole and ravuconazole referred to above.

Conclusions

EBIs are currently the most advanced candidates for new specific treatments for Chagas disease and two of them (posaconazole and ravuconazole) are already under-going phase II, proof-of-concept, clinical trials. After the discovery of the essential requirement of endogenous sterols for the survival and proliferation of *T. cruzi*, the key insight was that, to be effective *in vivo*, the pharmacokinetic properties of the EBIs had to be congruent with the intracellular character and relatively slow growth rate (generation times of 24–30 h) of the clinically relevant amastigote stage of the parasite, necessitating deep tissue penetration (large volumes of distribution) and long terminal half-life [90]. Congruent with this hypothesis, the results of a series of studies with this class of compounds demonstrated that only when an EBI combined nanomolar to subnanomolar activity against intracellular *T. cruzi* amastigotes *in vitro* with the pharmacokinetic profile described above, was curative activity observed in animal models of both acute and chronic of Chagas disease [16,57]; these findings should be kept in mind in future anti-*T. cruzi* drug development efforts, with EBIs or otherwise. The main potential advantages of EBIs over currently available therapies include their higher potency in both acute and chronic infections, activity against nifurtimox- and benznidazole-resistant *T. cruzi* strains, and much better tolerability and safety profile, which results from their selective mechanism of action. Limitations may include complexity and cost of manufacture of the new compounds, and the uneven advancement of different candidates in the drug development process, but there are several options in the pipeline than can address such issues. As for any new drug, such compounds will require extensive clinical testing before being introduced for clinical use. These studies, particularly in chronic patients, will be compounded by the current limitations in the verification of true parasitological cures for *T. cruzi* infections [56], although there are also promising new developments in this area [156–158]. Despite these limiting factors, EBIs are today the best hope for millions of patients currently living with this insidious, silent killer.

References

1 Chagas, C. (1911) Nova entidade morbida do homen. Resumo greal dos estudos etiológicos e clínicos. *Mem. Inst. Oswaldo Cruz*, **3**, 219–275.

2 Aufderheide, A.C., Salo, W., Madden, M., Streitz, J., Buikstra, J., Guhl, F., Arriaza, B. *et al.* (2004) A 9,000-year record of Chagas' disease. *Proc. Natl. Acad Sci. USA*, **101**, 2034–2039.

3 Hotez, P.J., Bottazzi, M.E., Franco-Paredes, C., Ault, S.K., and Periago, M.R. (2008) The neglected tropical diseases of Latin America and the Caribbean: a review of disease burden and distribution and a roadmap for control and elimination. *PLoS Negl. Trop. Dis.*, **2**, e300.

4 Schofield, C.J., Jannin, J., and Salvatella, R. (2006) The future of Chagas disease control. *Trends Parasitol.*, **22**, 583–588.

5 Tarleton, R.L., Reithinger, R., Urbina, J.A., Kitron, U., and Gurtler, R.E. (2007) The challenges of Chagas disease– grim outlook or glimmer of hope. *PLoS Med.*, **4**, e332.

6 Franco-Paredes, C., Bottazzi, M.E., and Hotez, P.J. (2009) The unfinished public health agenda of Chagas disease in the era of globalization. *PLoS Negl. Trop. Dis.*, **3**, e470.

7 Gurtler, R.E., Diotaiuti, L., and Kitron, U. (2008) Commentary: Chagas disease: 100 years since discovery and lessons for the future. *Int. J. Epidemiol.*, **37**, 698–701.

8 Pinto Dias, J.C. (1999) Epidemiologia, in *Trypanosoma cruzi e doença de Chagas* (eds Z. BrenerZ. Andrade, and C. Barral-Netto), Guanabara Koogan, Rio de Janeiro, pp. 48–74.

9 Bern, C., Montgomery, S.P., Herwaldt, B. L., Rassi, A.Jr., Marin-Neto, J.A., Dantas, R.O., Maguire, J.H. *et al.* (2007) Evaluation and treatment of Chagas disease in the United States: a systematic review. *JAMA*, **298**, 2171–2181.

10 Diaz, J.H. (2007) Chagas disease in the United States: a cause for concern in Louisiana? *J. La. State Med. Soc.*, **159** (21–3), 25–29.

11 Piron, M., Verges, M., Munoz, J., Casamitjana, N., Sanz, S., Maymo, R.M., Hernandez, J.M. *et al.* (2008)

Seroprevalence of *Trypanosoma cruzi* infection in at-risk blood donors in Catalonia (Spain). *Transfusion*, **48**, 1862– L 1868.

12 Gascon, J., Albajar, P., Canas, E., Flores, M., Gomez i Prat, J., Herrera, R.N., Lafuente, C.A. *et al.* (2007) Diagnosis, management and treatment of chronic Chagas' heart disease in areas where *Trypanosoma cruzi* infection is not endemic. *Rev. Esp. Cardiol.*, **60**, 285–293.

13 Reithinger, R., Tarleton, R.L., Urbina, J.A., Kitron, U., and Gurtler, R.E. (2009) Eliminating Chagas disease: challenges and a roadmap. *BMJ*, **338**, b1283.

14 Dias, J.C., Silveira, A.C., and Schofield, C. J. (2002) The impact of Chagas disease control in Latin America: a review. *Mem. Inst. Oswaldo Cruz*, **97**, 603–612.

15 Rassi, A.Jr., Dias, J.C., Marin-Neto, J.A., and Rassi, A. (2009) Challenges and opportunities for primary, secondary, and tertiary prevention of Chagas disease. *Heart.*, **95**, 524–534.

16 Urbina, J.A. and Docampo, R. (2003) Specific chemotherapy of Chagas disease: controversies and advances. *Trends Parasitol.*, **19**, 495–501.

17 Pinto Dias, J.C. (2006) The treatment of Chagas disease (South American trypanosomiasis). *Ann. Intern. Med.*, **144**, 772–774.

18 Ribeiro, I., Sevcsik, A.M., Alves, F., Diap, G., Don, R., Harhay, M.O., Chang, S. *et al.* (2009) New, improved treatments for Chagas disease: from the r&d pipeline to the patients. *PLoS Negl. Trop. Dis.*, **3**, e484.

19 Urbina, J.A. (2009) Specific chemotherapy of Chagas disease: relevance, current limitations and new approaches. *Acta Trop.*, **115**, 55–68.

20 Gutierrez, F.R., Guedes, P.M., Gazzinelli, R.T., and Silva, J.S. (2009) The role of parasite persistence in pathogenesis of Chagas heart disease. *Parasite Immunol.*, **31**, 673–685.

21 Brener, Z. and Gazzinelli, R.T. (1997) Immunological control of *Trypanosoma cruzi* infection and pathogenesis of Chagas' disease. *Int. Arch. Allergy Immunol.*, **114**, 103–110.

22 Padilla, A.M., Bustamante, J.M., and Tarleton, R.L. (2009) CD8$^+$ T cells in *Trypanosoma cruzi* infection. *Curr. Opin. Immunol.*, **21**, 385–390.

23 Marin-Neto, J.A., Cunha-Neto, E., Maciel, B.C., and Simoes, M.V. (2007) Pathogenesis of chronic Chagas heart disease. *Circulation*, **115**, 1109–1123.

24 Albareda, M.C., Laucella, S.A., Alvarez, M.G., Armenti, A.H., Bertochi, G., Tarleton, R.L., and Postan, M. (2006) *Trypanosoma cruzi* modulates the profile of memory CD8$^+$ T cells in chronic Chagas' disease patients. *Int. Immunol.*, **18**, 465–471.

25 Rassi, A.Jr., Rassi, A., and Little, W.C. (2000) Chagas' heart disease. *Clin. Cardiol.*, **23**, 883–889.

26 Cançado, J.R. (2002) Long term evaluation of etiological treatment of Chagas disease with benznidazole. *Rev. Inst. Med. Trop. Sao Paulo*, **44**, 29–37.

27 Cançado, J.R. (1999) Criteria of Chagas disease cure. *Mem. Inst. Oswaldo Cruz*, **94** (Suppl. 1), 331–336.

28 Rassi, A.Jr., Dias, J.C., Marin-Neto, J.A., and Rassi, A. (2009) Challenges and opportunities for primary, secondary, and tertiary prevention of Chagas' disease. *Heart*, **95**, 524–534.

29 Kirchhoff, L.V. (1999) Chagas' disease (American Trypanosomiasis): a tropical disease now emerging in the United States, in *Emerging Infections 3* (eds W.M. ScheldW.A. Craig, and J.M. Hughes), ASM Press, Washington, DC, pp. 111–134.

30 Filardi, L.S. and Brener, Z. (1987) Susceptibility and natural resistance of *Trypanosoma cruzi* strains to drugs used clinically in Chagas disease. *Trans. R. Soc. Trop. Med. Hyg.*, **81**, 755–759.

31 Murta, S.M., Gazzinelli, R.T., Brener, Z., and Romanha, A.J. (1998) Molecular characterization of susceptible and naturally resistant strains of *Trypanosoma cruzi* to benznidazole and nifurtimox. *Mol. Biochem. Parasitol.*, **93**, 203–214.

32 Yun, O., Lima, M.A., Ellman, T., Chambi, W., Castillo, S., Flevaud, L., Roddy, P. *et al.* (2009) Feasibility, drug safety, and effectiveness of etiological treatment programs for Chagas disease in Honduras, Guatemala, and Bolivia: 10-year experience of Medecins sans Frontieres. *PLoS. Negl. Trop. Dis.*, **3**, e488.

33 Romanha, A.J., Alves, R.O., Murta, S.M., Silva, J.S., Ropert, C., and Gazzinelli, R.T. (2002) Experimental chemotherapy against *Trypanosoma cruzi* infection: essential role of endogenous interferon-gamma in mediating parasitologic cure. *J. Infect. Dis.*, **186**, 823–828.

34 Bahia-Oliveira, L.M., Gomes, J.A., Cancado, J.R., Ferrari, T.C., Lemos, E.M., Luz, Z.M., Moreira, M.C. *et al.* (2000) Immunological and clinical evaluation of chagasic patients subjected to chemotherapy during the acute phase of *Trypanosoma cruzi* infection 14-30 years ago. *J. Infect. Dis.*, **182**, 634–638.

35 Andrade, A.L., Martelli, C.M., Oliveira, R.M., Silva, S.A., Aires, A.I., Soussumi, L.M., Covas, D.T. *et al.* (2004) Short report: benznidazole efficacy among *Trypanosoma cruzi*-infected adolescents after a six-year follow-up. *Am. J. Trop. Med. Hyg.*, **71**, 594–597.

36 de Andrade, A.L., Zicker, F., de Oliveira, R.M., Almeida Silva, S., Luquetti, A., Travassos, L.R., Almeida, I.C. *et al.* (1996) Randomised trial of efficacy of benznidazole in treatment of early *Trypanosoma cruzi* infection. *Lancet*, **348**, 1407–1413.

37 Sosa-Estani, S. and Segura, E.L. (2006) Etiological treatment in patients infected by *Trypanosoma cruzi*: experiences in Argentina. *Curr. Opin. Infect. Dis.*, **19**, 583–587.

38 Silveira, C.A., Castillo, E., and Castro, C. (2000) Evaluation of an specific treatment for *Trypanosoma cruzi* in children, in the evolution of the indeterminate phase. *Rev. Soc. Bras. Med. Trop.*, **33**, 191–196.

39 Solari, A., Ortiz, S., Soto, A., Arancibia, C., Campillay, R., Contreras, M., Salinas, P. *et al.* (2001) Treatment of *Trypanosoma cruzi*-infected children with nifurtimox: a 3 year follow-up by PCR. *J. Antimicrob. Chemother.*, **48**, 515–519.

40 Martins, H.R., Figueiredo, L.M., Valamiel-Silva, J.C., Carneiro, C.M., Machado-Coelho, G.L., Vitelli-Avelar, D.M., Bahia, M.T. *et al.* (2008) Persistence of PCR-positive tissue in benznidazole-treated

mice with negative blood parasitological and serological tests in dual infections with *Trypanosoma cruzi* stocks from different genotypes. *J. Antimicrob. Chemother.*, **61**, 1319–1327.

41 Anez, N., Carrasco, H., Parada, H., Crisante, G., Rojas, A., Fuenmayor, C., Gonzalez, N. *et al.* (1999) Myocardial parasite persistence in chronic chagasic patients. *Am. J. Trop. Med. Hyg.*, **60**, 726–732.

42 Britto, C., Silveira, C., Cardoso, M.A., Marques, P., Luquetti, A., Macedo, V., and Fernandes, O. (2001) Parasite persistence in treated chagasic patients revealed by xenodiagnosis and polymerase chain reaction. *Mem. Inst. Oswaldo Cruz*, **96**, 823–826.

43 Braga, M.S., Lauria-Pires, L., Arganaraz, E.R., Nascimento, R.J., and Teixeira, A.R. (2000) Persistent infections in chronic Chagas' disease patients treated with anti-*Trypanosoma cruzi* nitroderivatives. *Rev. Inst. Med. Trop. Sao Paulo*, **42**, 157–161.

44 Lauria-Pires, L., Braga, M.S., Vexenat, A. C., Nitz, N., Simoes-Barbosa, A., Tinoco, D.L., and Teixeira, A.R. (2000) Progressive chronic Chagas heart disease ten years after treatment with anti-*Trypanosoma cruzi* nitroderivatives. *Am. J. Trop. Med. Hyg.*, **63**, 111–118.

45 Garcia, S., Ramos, C.O., Senra, J.F., Vilas-Boas, F., Rodrigues, M.M., Campos-de-Carvalho, A.C., Ribeiro-Dos-Santos, R. *et al.* (2005) Treatment with benznidazole during the chronic phase of experimental Chagas' disease decreases cardiac alterations. *Antimicrob. Agents Chemother.*, **49**, 1521–1528.

46 Fernandes, C.D., Tiecher, F.M., Balbinot, M.M., Liarte, D.B., Scholl, D., Steindel, M., and Romanha, A. (2009) Efficacy of benznidazol treatment for asymptomatic chagasic patients from state of Rio Grande do Sul evaluated during a three years follow-up. *Mem. Inst. Oswaldo Cruz*, **104**, 27–32.

47 Krautz, G.M., Kissinger, J.C., and Krettli, A.U. (2000) The targets of the lytic antibody response against *Trypanosoma cruzi*. *Parasitol. Today*, **16**, 31–34.

48 Krautz, G.M., Galvao, L.M., Cancado, J.R., Guevara-Espinoza, A., Ouaissi, A., and Krettli, A.U. (1995) Use of a 24-kilodalton *Trypanosoma cruzi* recombinant protein to monitor cure of human Chagas' disease. *J. Clin. Microbiol.*, **33**, 2086–2090.

49 Pereira-Chioccola, V.L., Fragata-Filho, A. A., Levy, A.M., Rodrigues, M.M., and Schenkman, S. (2003) Enzyme-linked immunoassay using recombinant trans-sialidase of *Trypanosoma cruzi* can be employed for monitoring of patients with Chagas' disease after drug treatment. *Clin. Diagn. Lab. Immunol.*, **10**, 826–830.

50 Buckner, F.S. (2008) Sterol 14-demethylase inhibitors for *Trypanosoma cruzi* infections. *Adv. Exp. Med. Biol.*, **625**, 61–80.

51 Viotti, R. and Vigliano, C. (2007) Etiological treatment of chronic Chagas disease: neglected 'evidence' by evidence-based medicine. *Expert Rev. Anti Infect. Ther.*, **5**, 717–726.

52 Viotti, R., Vigliano, C., Lococo, B., Bertocchi, G., Petti, M., Alvarez, M.G., Postan, M. *et al.* (2006) Long-term cardiac outcomes of treating chronic Chagas disease with benznidazole versus no treatment: a nonrandomized trial. *Ann. Intern. Med.*, **144**, 724–734.

53 Viotti, R., Vigliano, C., Alvarez, M.G., Lococo, B., Petti, M., Bertocchi, G., Armenti, A. *et al.* (2011) Impact of aetiological treatment on conventional and multiplex serology in chronic Chagas disease. *PLoS Negl. Trop. Dis.*, **5**, e1314.

54 Docampo, R. (1990) Sensitivity of parasites to free radical damage by antiparasitic drugs. *Chem. Biol. Interact.*, **73**, 1–27.

55 Pinazo, M.J., Munoz, J., Posada, E., Lopez-Chejade, P., Gallego, M., Ayala, E., Del Cacho, E. *et al.* (2010) Tolerance of benznidazole in the treatment of Chagas disease in adults. *Antimicrob. Agents Chemother.*, **54**, 4896–4899.

56 Urbina, J.A. (2010) New insights in Chagas' disease treatment. *Drugs Future*, **35**, 409–419.

57 Urbina, J.A. (2010) Specific chemotherapy of Chagas disease: relevance, current limitations and new approaches. *Acta Trop.*, **115**, 55–68.

58 Rassi, A.Jr., Rassi, A., and Marin-Neto, J. A. (2009) Chagas heart disease:

pathophysiologic mechanisms, prognostic factors and risk stratification. *Mem. Inst. Oswaldo Cruz*, **104** (Suppl. 1), 152–158.

59 Kalil, J. and Cunha-Neto, E. (1996) Autoimmunity in Chagas disease cardiomyopathy: fullfilling the criteria at last? *Parasitol. Today*, **12**, 396–399.

60 Cunha-Neto, E., Duranti, M., Gruber, A., Zingales, B., De Messias, I., Stolf, N., Bellotti, G. *et al.* (1995) Autoinmunity in Chagas disease cardiopathy: biological relevance of a cardiac myosin-specific epitope crossreactive to an inmunodominant *Trypanosoma cruzi* antigen. *Proc. Natl. Acad. Sci. USA*, **92**, 3541–3545.

61 Urbina, J.A. (1999) Parasitological cure of Chagas disease: is it possible?, Is it relevant? *Mem. Inst. Oswaldo Cruz*, **94** (Suppl. 1), 349–355.

62 Croft, S.L., Barrett, M.P., and Urbina, J.A. (2005) Chemotherapy of trypanosomiases and leishmaniasis. *Trends Parasitol.*, **21**, 508–512.

63 Tarleton, R.L. (2001) Parasite persistence in the aetiology of Chagas disease. *Int. J. Parasitol.*, **31**, 550–554.

64 Apt, W., Heitmann, I., Jercic, L., Jofré, L., Muñoz, P., Noemí, I., San Martin, A.M. *et al.* (2008) Tratamiento antiparasitario de la enfremedad de Chagas. *Rev. Chil. Infect.*, **25**, 384–389.

65 Marin-Neto, J.A., Rassi, A.Jr., Morillo, C. A., Avezum, A., Connolly, S.J., Sosa-Estani, S., Rosas, F. *et al.* (2008) Rationale and design of a randomized placebo-controlled trial assessing the effects of etiologic treatment in Chagas' cardiomyopathy: the BENznidazole Evaluation For Interrupting Trypanosomiasis (BENEFIT). *Am. Heart J.*, **156**, 37–43.

66 Daum, G., Lees, N.D., Bard, M., and Dickson, R. (1998) Biochemistry, cell biology and molecular biology of lipids of Saccharomyces cerevisiae. *Yeast*, **14**, 1471–1510.

67 Furlong, S.T. (1989) Sterols of parasitic protozoa and helminths. *Exp. Parasitol.*, **68**, 482–485.

68 Korn, E.D., Von Brand, T., and Tobie, E.J. (1969) The sterols of *Trypanosoma cruzi* and *Crithidia fasciculata*. *Comp. Biochem. Physiol.*, **30**, 601–610.

69 Liendo, A., Lazardi, K., and Urbina, J.A. (1998) In-vitro antiproliferative effects and mechanism of action of the bis-triazole D0870 and its $S(-)$ enantiomer against *Trypanosoma cruzi*. *J. Antimicrob. Chemother.*, **41**, 197–205.

70 Liendo, A., Visbal, G., Piras, M.M., Piras, R., and Urbina, J.A. (1999) Sterol composition and biosynthesis in *Trypanosoma cruzi* amastigotes. *Mol. Biochem. Parasitol.*, **104**, 81–91.

71 Urbina, J.A. (2009) Ergosterol biosynthesis and drug development for Chagas disease. *Mem. Inst. Oswaldo Cruz*, **104** (Suppl. 1), 311–318.

72 Urbina, J.A., Vivas, J., Ramos, H., Larralde, G., Aguilar, Z., and Avilan, L. (1988) Alteration of lipid order profile and permeability of plasma membranes from *Trypanosoma cruzi* epimastigotes grown in the presence of ketoconazole. *Mol. Biochem. Parasitol.*, **30**, 185–195.

73 Contreras, L.M., Vivas, J., and Urbina, J.A. (1997) Altered lipid composition and enzyme activities of plasma membranes from *Trypanosoma (Schizotrypanum) cruzi* epimastigotes grown in the presence of sterol biosynthesis inhibitors. *Biochem. Pharmacol.*, **53**, 697–704.

74 Montez, B., Oldfield, E., Urbina, J.A., Pekerar, S., Husted, C., and Patterson, J. (1993) Editing ^{13}C-NMR spectra of membranes. *Biochim. Biophys. Acta*, **1152**, 314–318.

75 Urbina, J.A., Pekerar, S., Le, H.B., Patterson, J., Montez, B., and Oldfield, E. (1995) Molecular order and dynamics of phosphatidylcholine bilayer membranes in the presence of cholesterol, ergosterol and lanosterol: a comparative study using ^{2}H-, ^{13}C- and ^{31}P-NMR spectroscopy. *Biochim. Biophys. Acta*, **1238**, 163–176.

76 Urbina, J.A., Moreno, B., Arnold, W., Taron, C.H., Orlean, P., and Oldfield, E. (1998) A carbon-13 nuclear magnetic resonance spectroscopic study of inter-proton pair order parameters: a new approach to study order and dynamics in phospholipid membrane systems. *Biophys. J.*, **75**, 1372–1383.

77 Lazardi, K., Urbina, J.A., and de Souza, W. (1990) Ultrastructural alterations induced by two ergosterol biosynthesis inhibitors, ketoconazole and terbinafine, on epimastigotes and amastigotes of *Trypanosoma (Schizotrypanum) cruzi. Antimicrob. Agents Chemother.*, **34**, 2097–2105.

78 Lazardi, K., Urbina, J.A., and de Souza, W. (1991) Ultrastructural alterations induced by ICI 195,739, a bis-triazole derivative with strong antiproliferative action against *Trypanosoma (Schizotrypanum) cruzi. Antimicrob. Agents Chemother.*, **35**, 736–740.

79 Rodrigues, C.O., Catisti, R., Uyemura, S. A., Vercesi, A.E., Lira, R., Rodriguez, C., Urbina, J.A. *et al.* (2001) The sterol composition of *Trypanosoma cruzi* changes after growth in different culture media and results in different sensitivity to digitonin-permeabilization. *J. Eukaryot. Microbiol.*, **48**, 588–594.

80 Urbina, J.A., Payares, G., Molina, J., Sanoja, C., Liendo, A., Lazardi, K., Piras, M.M. *et al.* (1996) Cure of short- and long-term experimental Chagas' disease using D0870. *Science*, **273**, 969–971.

81 Urbina, J.A., Payares, G., Contreras, L.M., Liendo, A., Sanoja, C., Molina, J., Piras, M. *et al.* (1998) Antiproliferative effects and mechanism of action of SCH 56592 against *Trypanosoma (Schizotrypanum) cruzi: in vitro* and *in vivo* studies. *Antimicrob. Agents Chemother.*, **42**, 1771–1777.

82 Lepesheva, G.I., Zaitseva, N.G., Nes, W. D., Zhou, W., Arase, M., Liu, J., Hill, G.C. *et al.* (2006) CYP51 from *Trypanosoma cruzi*: a phyla-specific residue in the B′ helix defines substrate preferences of sterol 14alpha-demethylase. *J. Biol. Chem.*, **281**, 3577–3585.

83 Fischer, R.T., Stam, S.H., Johnson, P.R., Ko, S.S., Magolda, R.L., Gaylor, J.L., and Trzaskos, J.M. (1989) Mechanistic studies of lanosterol 14 alpha-methyl demethylase: substrate requirements for the component reactions catalyzed by a single cytochrome P-450 isozyme. *J. Lipid. Res.*, **30**, 1621–1632.

84 Lepesheva, G.I., Villalta, F., and Waterman, M.R. (2011) Targeting *Trypanosoma cruzi* sterol 14alpha-demethylase (CYP51). *Adv. Parasitol.*, **75**, 65–87.

85 Walker, K.A., Kertesz, D.J., Rotstein, D. M., Swinney, D.C., Berry, P.W., So, O.Y., Webb, A.S. *et al.* (1993) Selective inhibition of mammalian lanosterol 14 alpha-demethylase: a possible strategy for cholesterol lowering. *J. Med. Chem.*, **36**, 2235–2237.

86 Lepesheva, G.I., Hargrove, T.Y., Anderson, S., Kleshchenko, Y., Furtak, V., Wawrzak, Z., Villalta, F. *et al.* (2010) Structural insights into inhibition of sterol 14alpha-demethylase in the human pathogen *Trypanosoma cruzi. J. Biol. Chem.*, **285**, 25582–25590.

87 Chen, C.K., Leung, S.S., Guilbert, C., Jacobson, M.P., McKerrow, J.H., and Podust, L.M. (2010) Structural characterization of CYP51 from *Trypanosoma cruzi* and *Trypanosoma brucei* bound to the antifungal drugs posaconazole and fluconazole. *PLoS Negl. Trop. Dis.*, **4**, e651.

88 Hargrove, T.Y., Wawrzak, Z., Liu, J., Waterman, M.R., Nes, W.D., and Lepesheva, G.I. (2012) Structural complex of sterol 14alpha-demethylase (CYP51) with 14alpha-methylenecyclopropyl-{delta}7-24,25-dihydrolanosterol. *J. Lipid. Res.*, **52**, 311–320.

89 Urbina, J.A. (2002) Chemotherapy of Chagas disease. *Curr. Pharm. Design*, **8**, 287–295.

90 Urbina, J.A. (1999) Chemotherapy of Chagas' disease: the how and the why. *J. Mol. Med.*, **77**, 332–338.

91 Campoli, P., Al Abdallah, Q., Robitaille, R., Solis, N.V., Fielhaber, J.A., Kristof, A. S., Laverdiere, M. *et al.* (2011) Concentration of antifungal agents within host cell membranes: a new paradigm governing the efficacy of prophylaxis. *Antimicrob. Agents Chemother.*, **55**, 5732–5739.

92 Silva, D.T., de Meirelles Mde, N., Almeida, D., Urbina, J.A., and Pereira, M. C. (2006) Cytoskeleton reassembly in cardiomyocytes infected by *Trypanosoma cruzi* is triggered by treatment with ergosterol biosynthesis inhibitors. *Int. J. Antimicrob. Agents*, **27**, 530–537.

93 Ferraz, M.L., Gazzinelli, R.T., Alves, R.O., Urbina, J.A., and Romanha, A.J. (2007) The anti-*Trypanosoma cruzi* activity of posaconazole in a murine model of acute Chagas' disease is less dependent on gamma interferon than that of benznidazole. *Antimicrob. Agents Chemother.*, **51**, 1359–1364.

94 Ferraz, M.L., Gazzinelli, R.T., Alves, R.O., Urbina, J.A., and Romanha, A.J. (2009) Absence of CD4$^+$ T lymphocytes, CD8$^+$ T lymphocytes, or B lymphocytes has different effects on the efficacy of posaconazole and benznidazole in treatment of experimental acute *Trypanosoma cruzi* infection. *Antimicrob. Agents Chemother.*, **53**, 174–179.

95 Olivieri, B.P., Molina, J.T., de Castro, S.L., Pereira, M.C., Calvet, C.M., Urbina, J.A., and Araujo-Jorge, T.C. (2010) A comparative study of posaconazole and benznidazole in the prevention of heart damage and promotion of trypanocidal immune response in a murine model of Chagas disease. *Int. J. Antimicrob. Agents*, **36**, 79–83.

96 Pinazo, M.J., Espinosa, G., Gallego, M., Lopez-Chejade, P.L., Urbina, J.A., and Gascon, J. (2010) Successful treatment with posaconazole of a patient with chronic Chagas disease and systemic lupus erythematosus. *Am. J. Trop. Med. Hyg.*, **82**, 583–587.

97 Lyseng-Williamson, K.A. (2011) Posaconazole: a pharmacoeconomic review of its use in the prophylaxis of invasive fungal disease in immunocompromised hosts. *Pharmacoeconomics*, **29**, 251–268.

98 Morris, M.I. (2009) Posaconazole: a new oral antifungal agent with an expanded spectrum of activity. *Am. J. Health Syst. Pharm.*, **66**, 225–236.

99 Danzon, P.M. (2007) At what price? *Nature*, **449**, 176–179.

100 Corrales, M., Cardozo, R., Segura, M.A., Urbina, J.A., and Basombrio, M.A. (2005) Comparative efficacies of TAK-187, a long-lasting ergosterol biosynthesis inhibitor, and benznidazole in preventing cardiac damage in a murine model of Chagas' disease. *Antimicrob. Agents Chemother.*, **49**, 1556–1560.

101 Urbina, J.A., Payares, G., Sanoja, C., Molina, J., Lira, R., Brener, Z., and Romanha, A.J. (2003) Parasitological cure of acute and chronic experimental Chagas disease using the long-acting experimental triazole TAK-187. Activity against drug-resistant *Trypanosoma cruzi* strains. *Int. J. Antimicrob. Agents*, **21**, 39–48.

102 Urbina, J.A., Lira, R., Visbal, G., and Bartrolí, J. (2000) In Vitro Antiproliferative Effects and Mechanism of Action of the New Triazole Derivative UR-9825 Against the Protozoan Parasite *Trypanosoma (Schizotrypanum) cruzi*. *Antimicrob. Agents Chemother.*, **44**, 2498–2502.

103 Guedes, P.M., Urbina, J.A., de Lana, M., Afonso, L.C., Veloso, V.M., Tafuri, W.L., Machado-Coelho, G.L. *et al.* (2004) Activity of the new triazole derivative albaconazole against *Trypanosoma (Schizotrypanum) cruzi* in dog hosts. *Antimicrob. Agents Chemother.*, **48**, 4286–4292.

104 Urbina, J.A., Payares, G., Sanoja, C., Lira, R., and Romanha, A.J. (2003) *In vitro* and *in vivo* activities of ravuconazole on *Trypanosoma cruzi*, the causative agent of Chagas disease. *Intern. J. Antimicrob. Agents*, **21**, 27–38.

105 Diniz Lde, F., Caldas, I.S., Guedes, P.M., Crepalde, G., de Lana, M., Carneiro, C.M., Talvani, A. *et al.* (2010) Effects of ravuconazole treatment on parasite load and immune response in dogs experimentally infected with *Trypanosoma cruzi*. *Antimicrob. Agents Chemother.*, **54**, 2979–2986.

106 Andes, D., Marchillo, K., Stamstad, T., and Conklin, R. (2003) *In vivo* pharmacodynamics of a new triazole, ravuconazole, in a murine candidiasis model. *Antimicrob. Agents Chemother.*, **47**, 1193–1199.

107 Mikamo, H., Yin, X.H., Hayasaki, Y., Shimamura, Y., Uesugi, K., Fukayama, N., Satoh, M. *et al.* (2002) Penetration of ravuconazole, a new triazole antifungal, into rat tissues. *Chemotherapy*, **48**, 7–9.

108 Pasqualotto, A.C. and Denning, D.W. (2008) New and emerging treatments for

fungal infections. *J. Antimicrob. Chemother.*, **61** (Suppl. 1), 19–30.

109 Kraus, J.M., Verlinde, C.L., Karimi, M., Lepesheva, G.I., Gelb, M.H., and Buckner, F.S. (2009) Rational modification of a candidate cancer drug for use against Chagas disease. *J. Med. Chem.*, **52**, 1639–1647.

110 Hucke, O., Gelb, M.H., Verlinde, C.L., and Buckner, F.S. (2005) The protein farnesyltransferase inhibitor tipifarnib as a new lead for the development of drugs against Chagas disease. *J. Med. Chem.*, **48**, 5415–5418.

111 Buckner, F., Yokoyama, K., Lockman, J., Aikenhead, K., Ohkanda, J., Sadilek, M., Sebti, S. *et al.* (2003) A class of sterol 14-demethylase inhibitors as anti-*Trypanosoma cruzi* agents. *Proc. Natl. Acad. Sci. USA*, **100**, 15149–15153.

112 Kraus, J.M., Tatipaka, H.B., McGuffin, S. A., Chennamaneni, N.K., Karimi, M., Arif, J., Verlinde, C.L. *et al.* (2010) Second generation analogues of the cancer drug clinical candidate tipifarnib for anti-Chagas disease drug discovery. *J. Med. Chem.*, **53**, 3887–3898.

113 Lepesheva, G.I., Hargrove, T.Y., Kleshchenko, Y., Nes, W.D., Villalta, F., and Waterman, M.R. (2008) CYP51: a major drug target in the cytochrome P450 superfamily. *Lipids*, **43**, 1117–1125.

114 Lepesheva, G.I., Ott, R.D., Hargrove, T.Y., Kleshchenko, Y.Y., Schuster, I., Nes, W.D., Hill, G.C. *et al.* (2007) Sterol 14alpha-demethylase as a potential target for antitrypanosomal therapy: enzyme inhibition and parasite cell growth. *Chem. Biol.*, **14**, 1283–1293.

115 Lepesheva, G.I., Park, H.W., Hargrove, T. Y., Vanhollebeke, B., Wawrzak, Z., Harp, J.M., Sundaramoorthy, M. *et al.* (2010) Crystal structures of *Trypanosoma brucei* sterol 14alpha-demethylase and implications for selective treatment of human infections. *J. Biol. Chem.*, **285**, 1773–1780.

116 Konkle, M.E., Hargrove, T.Y., Kleshchenko, Y.Y., von Kries, J.P., Ridenour, W., Uddin, M.J., Caprioli, R.M. *et al.* (2009) Indomethacin amides as a novel molecular scaffold for targeting *Trypanosoma cruzi* sterol 14alpha-demethylase. *J. Med. Chem.*, **52**, 2846–2853.

117 Chen, C.K., Doyle, P.S., Yermalitskaya, L. V., Mackey, Z.B., Ang, K.K., McKerrow, J. H., and Podust, L.M. (2009) *Trypanosoma cruzi* CYP51 inhibitor derived from a *Mycobacterium tuberculosis* screen hit. *PLoS Negl. Trop. Dis.*, **3**, e372.

118 Doyle, P.S., Chen, C.K., Johnston, J.B., Hopkins, S.D., Leung, S.S., Jacobson, M. P., Engel, J.C. *et al.* (2010) A non-azole CYP51 inhibitor cures chagas disease in a mouse model of acute infection. *Antimicrob. Agents Chemother.*, **54**, 2480–2488.

119 Buckner, F.S., Griffin, J.H., Wilson, A.J., and Van Voorhis, W.C. (2001) Potent anti-*Trypanosma cruzi* activities of oxidosqualene cyclase inhibitors. *Antimicrob. Agents Chemother.*, **45**, 1210–1215.

120 Buckner, F.S., Nguyen, L.N., Joubert, B. M., and Matsuda, S.P. (2000) Cloning and expression of the *Trypanosoma brucei* lanosterol synthase gene. *Mol. Biochem. Parasitol.*, **110**, 399–403.

121 Joubert, B.M., Buckner, F.S., and Matsuda, S.P. (2001) Trypanosome and animal lanosterol synthases use different catalytic motifs. *Org. Lett.*, **14**, 1957–1960.

122 Hinshaw, J.C., Suh, D.Y., Garnier, P., Buckner, F.S., Eastman, R.T., Matsuda, S. P., Joubert, B.M. *et al.* (2003) Oxidosqualene cyclase inhibitors as antimicrobial agents. *J. Med. Chem.*, **46**, 4240–4243.

123 Urbina, J.A. (2003) New chemotherapeutic approaches for the treatment of Chagas disease (American Trypanosomiasis). *Expert Opin. Ther. Pat*, **13**, 661–669.

124 Rosenbaum, M.B., Chiale, P.A., Haedo, A., Lazzari, J.O., and Elizari, M.V. (1983) Ten years of experience with amiodarone. *Am. Heart J.*, **106**, 957–964.

125 Benaim, G., Sanders, J.M., Garcia-Marchan, Y., Colina, C., Lira, R., Caldera, A.R., Payares, G. *et al.* (2006) Amiodarone has intrinsic anti-*Trypanosoma cruzi* activity and acts synergistically with posaconazole. *J. Med. Chem.*, **49**, 892–899.

126 Adesse, D., Azzam, E.M., Meirelles Mde, N., Urbina, J.A., and Garzoni, L.R. (2011)

Amiodarone inhibits *Trypanosoma cruzi* infection and promotes cardiac cell recovery with gap junction and cytoskeleton reassembly *in vitro*. *Antimicrob. Agents Chemother.*, **55**, 203–210.

127 Paniz-Mondolfi, A.E., Perez-Alvarez, A. M., Lanza, G., Marquez, E., and Concepcion, J.L. (2009) Amiodarone and itraconazole: a rational therapeutic approach for the treatment of chronic Chagas' disease. *Chemotherapy*, **55**, 228–233.

128 Serrano-Martin, X., Garcia-Marchan, Y., Fernandez, A., Rodriguez, N., Rojas, H., Visbal, G., and Benaim, G. (2009) Amiodarone destabilizes intracellular Ca^{2+} homeostasis and biosynthesis of sterols in *Leishmania mexicana*. *Antimicrob. Agents Chemother.*, **53**, 1403–1410.

129 Serrano-Martin, X., Payares, G., De Lucca, M., Martinez, J.C., Mendoza-Leon, A., and Benaim, G. (2009) Amiodarone and miltefosine act synergistically against *Leishmania mexicana* and can induce parasitological cure in a murine model of cutaneous leishmaniasis. *Antimicrob. Agents Chemother.*, **53**, 5108–5113.

130 Paniz-Mondolfi, A.E., Perez-Alvarez, A. M., Reyes-Jaimes, O., Socorro, G., Zerpa, O., Slova, D., and Concepcion, J.L. (2008) Concurrent Chagas' disease and borderline disseminated cutaneous leishmaniasis: the role of amiodarone as an antitrypanosomatidae drug. *Ther. Clin. Risk Manag.*, **4**, 659–663.

131 Tansey, T.R. and Shechter, I. (2001) Squalene synthase: structure and regulation. *Prog. Nucleic Acid Res. Mol. Biol.*, **65**, 157–195.

132 Menys, V.C. and Durrington, P.N. (2003) Squalene synthase inhibitors. *Br. J. Pharmacol.*, **139**, 881–882.

133 Charlton-Menys, V. and Durrington, P.N. (2007) Squalene synthase inhibitors: clinical pharmacology and cholesterol-lowering potential. *Drugs*, **67**, 11–16.

134 Suckling, K.E. (2006) The return of two old targets? *Expert Opin. Ther. Targets*, **10**, 785–788.

135 Urbina, J.A., Concepcion, J.L., Rangel, S., Visbal, G., and Lira, R. (2002) Squalene synthase as a chemotherapeutic target in *Trypanosoma cruzi* and *Leishmania mexicana*. *Mol. Biochem. Parasitol.*, **125**, 35–45.

136 Urbina, J.A., Concepcion, J.L., Caldera, A., Payares, G., Sanoja, C., Otomo, T., and Hiyoshi, H. (2004) In vitro and *in vivo* activities of E5700 and ER-119884, two novel orally active squalene synthase inhibitors, against *Trypanosoma cruzi*. *Antimicrob. Agents Chemother.*, **48**, 2379–2387.

137 McTaggart, F., Brown, G.R., Davidson, R. G., Freeman, S., Holdgate, G.A., Mallion, K.B., Mirrlees, D.J. *et al.* (1996) Inhibition of squalene synthase of rat liver by novel 3′ substituted quinuclidines. *Biochem. Pharmacol.*, **51**, 1477–1487.

138 Ward, W.H.J., Holdgate, G.A., Freeman, S., McTaggart, F., Girdwood, P.A., Davidson, R.G., Mallion, K.B. *et al.* (1996) Inhibition of squalene synthase *in vitro* by 3-(biphenyl-4-yl)-quinuclidine. *Biochem. Pharmacol.*, **51**, 1489–1501.

139 Ishihara, T., Kakuta, H., Moritani, H., Ugawa, T., Sakamoto, S., Tsukamoto, S., and Yanagisawa, I. (2003) Syntheses and biological evaluation of novel quinuclidine derivatives as squalene synthase inhibitors. *Bioorg. Med. Chem.*, **11**, 2403–2414.

140 Ishihara, T., Kakuta, H., Moritani, H., Ugawa, T., and Yanagisawa, I. (2004) Synthesis and biological evaluation of quinuclidine derivatives incorporating phenothiazine moieties as squalene synthase inhibitors. *Chem. Pharm. Bull. (Tokyo)*, **52**, 1204–1209.

141 Goldstein, J.L. and Brown, M.S. (2001) The cholesterol quartet. *Science*, **292**, 1310–1312.

142 Orenes Lorente, S., Gomez, R., Jimenez, C., Cammerer, S., Yardley, V., de Luca-Fradley, K., Croft, S.L. *et al.* (2005) Biphenylquinuclidines as inhibitors of squalene synthase and growth of parasitic protozoa. *Bioorg. Med. Chem.*, **13**, 3519–3529.

143 Sealey-Cardona, M., Cammerer, S., Jones, S., Ruiz-Perez, L.M., Brun, R., Gilbert, I. H., Urbina, J.A. *et al.* (2007) Kinetic characterization of squalene synthase from *Trypanosoma cruzi*: Selective

inhibition by quinuclidine derivatives. *Antimicrob. Agents Chemother.*, **51**, 2123–2129.

144 Elhalem, E., Bailey, B.N., Docampo, R., Ujvary, I., Szajnman, S.H., and Rodriguez, J.B. (2002) Design, synthesis, and biological evaluation of aryloxyethyl thiocyanate derivatives against *Trypanosoma cruzi. J. Med. Chem.*, **45**, 3984–3999.

145 Szajnman, S.H., Yan, W., Bailey, B.N., Docampo, R., Elhalem, E., and Rodriguez, J.B. (2000) Design and synthesis of aryloxyethyl thiocyanate derivatives as potent inhibitors of *Trypanosoma cruzi* proliferation. *J. Med. Chem.*, **43**, 1826–1840.

146 Urbina, J.A., Concepcion, J.L., Montalvetti, A., Rodriguez, J.B., and Docampo, R. (2003) Mechanism of action of 4-phenoxyphenoxyethyl thiocyanate (WC-9) against *Trypanosoma cruzi*, the causative agent of Chagas' disease. *Antimicrob. Agents Chemother.*, **47**, 2047–2050.

147 Gerpe, A., Odreman-Nunez, I., Draper, P., Boiani, L., Urbina, J.A., Gonzalez, M., and Cerecetto, H. (2008) Heteroallyl-containing 5-nitrofuranes as new anti-*Trypanosoma cruzi* agents with a dual mechanism of action. *Bioorg. Med. Chem.*, **16**, 569–577.

148 Araujo, M.S., Martins-Filho, O.A., Pereira, M.E., and Brener, Z. (2000) A combination of benznidazole and ketoconazole enhances efficacy of chemotherapy of experimental Chagas' disease. *J. Antimicrob. Chemother.*, **45**, 819–824.

149 Urbina, J.A., Lazardi, K., Aguirre, T., Piras, M.M., and Piras, R. (1988) Antiproliferative synergism of the allylamine SF 86-327 and ketoconazole on epimastigotes and amastigotes of *Trypanosoma (Schizotrypanum) cruzi. Antimicrob. Agents Chemother.*, **32**, 1237–1242.

150 Urbina, J.A., Lazardi, K., Marchan, E., Visbal, G., Aguirre, T., Piras, M.M., Piras, R. *et al.* (1993) Mevinolin (lovastatin)

potentiates the antiproliferative effects of ketoconazole and terbinafine against *Trypanosoma (Schizotrypanum) cruzi*: in vitro and *in vivo* studies. *Antimicrob. Agents Chemother.*, **37**, 580–591.

151 Urbina, J.A., Vivas, J., Lazardi, K., Molina, J., Payares, G., Piras, M.M., and Piras, R. (1996) Antiproliferative effects of delta 24(25) sterol methyl transferase inhibitors on *Trypanosoma (Schizotrypanum) cruzi*: in vitro and *in vivo* studies. *Chemotherapy*, **42**, 294–307.

152 Santa-Rita, R.M., Lira, R., Barbosa, H.S., Urbina, J.A., and de Castro, S.L. (2005) Anti-proliferative synergy of lysophospholipid analogues and ketoconazole against *Trypanosoma cruzi* (Kinetoplastida: Trypanosomatidae): cellular and ultrastructural analysis. *J. Antimicrob. Chemother.*, **55**, 780–784.

153 Davidson, M.H. (2007) Squalene synthase inhibition: a novel target for the management of dyslipidemia. *Curr. Atheroscler. Rep.*, **9**, 78–80.

154 Burnett, J.R. (2006) Drug evaluation: TAK-475–an oral inhibitor of squalene synthase for hyperlipidemia. *Curr. Opin. Investig. Drugs*, **7**, 850–856.

155 Bahia, M.T. (2011) *Evaluation of combined therapies for the treatment of Chagas disease (in portuguese)*, presented at *27th Reunião Anual de Pesquisa Aplicada de Doença de Chagas*, Uberaba, Minas Gerais.

156 Laucella, S.A., Mazliah, D.P., Bertocchi, G., Alvarez, M.G., Cooley, G., Viotti, R., Albareda, M.C. *et al.* (2009) Changes in *Trypanosoma cruzi*-specific immune responses after treatment: surrogate markers of treatment efficacy. *Clin. Infect. Dis.*, **49**, 1675–1684.

157 Cooley, G., Etheridge, R.D., Boehlke, C., Bundy, B., Weatherly, D.B., Minning, T., Haney, M. *et al.* (2008) High throughput selection of effective serodiagnostics for *Trypanosoma cruzi* infection. *PLoS Negl. Trop. Dis.*, **2**, e316.

158 Urbina, J.A. (2009) New advances in the management of a long-neglected disease. *Clin. Infect. Dis.*, **49**, 1685–1687.

27
New Developments in the Treatment of Late-Stage Human African Trypanosomiasis

*Cyrus J. Bacchi, Robert T. Jacobs, and Nigel Yarlett**

Abstract

Human African trypanosomiasis (African sleeping sickness) is a disease caused by various subspecies of the parasite *Trypanosoma brucei* and spread through an insect vector, the tsetse fly, in sub-Saharan Africa. Although only relatively small numbers of patients (estimated by the World Health Organization to be approximately 10 000 per annum) are diagnosed each year, all victims of this disease will progress to a second-stage central nervous system disease that is 100% fatal if untreated. Current treatment options for HAT are limited to old, toxic, and ineffective drugs that are difficult to administer in the disease endemic area, particularly for the second-stage disease. Consequently, there is an urgent need for the discovery and development of new agents to treat Stage 2 HAT. This chapter reviews some recent efforts in this area, in particular the discovery and development of a new class of novel boron-containing compounds, the benzoxaboroles.

Introduction

African trypanosomiasis, human African trypanosomiasis (HAT), and animal trypanosomiasis (Ngana) go back to reports at the beginning of recorded African history. European explorers prior to the nineteenth century describe a disease which could only have been HAT. Later, explorers such as Livingstone, Speke, Stanley, Burton, Bruce, and others began noticing dramatic loss of livestock to a wasting disease that disrupted their intended destination (e.g., the head waters of the Nile, Lake Victoria). Soon human disease, resembling the animal wasting disease, began plaguing members of these expeditions, with usually fatal results. Very often porters and other expedition members would come down with fever, chills, and an extended wasting disease, always after being bitten by a large fly with the hatchet-shaped venations in its wings – the tsetse fly [1].

Epidemics of huge proportions were frequent in preclinical Africa with reports of entire villages being wiped out. By 1900, the disease had been attributed to a microscopic blood flagellate, *Trypanosoma brucei*, with different subspecies proposed

---

* Corresponding Author

Trypanosomatid Diseases: Molecular Routes to Drug Discovery, First edition. Edited by T. Jäger, O. Koch, and L. Flohé.
© 2013 Wiley-VCH Verlag GmbH & Co. KGaA. Published 2013 by Wiley-VCH Verlag GmbH & Co. KGaA.

as agents for the human diseases in West Africa (*T. b. gambiense*), East Africa (*T. b. rhodesiense*), and domestic and wild animals (*T. b., rhodesiense* and *T. b. brucei*). The veterinary trypanosomes prevented large-scale cattle ranching and remain a constant menace for farmers who own livestock [1].

Life Cycle of *T. b. brucei*

The agent of HAT, the trypanosome, is transmitted by the tsetse fly, and has a cyclical life cycle (Figure 27.1) in which it changes morphologically and biochemically between vector insect and human (or veterinary) hosts. After a blood meal from an infected host, bloodstream trypanosomes migrate to the stomach of the fly, undergo transformation (procyclic trypomastigotes), and migrate to the salivary glands where they undergo another transformation (epimastigotes). In the salivary glands of the tsetse they become infectious in the saliva. When the fly bites, these forms (metacyclic trypomastigotes) are transmitted, multiplying at the bite site, and then progressively invading the bloodstream and lymphatics of the new host. The cycle in the fly takes 25–50 days depending on environmental conditions. The fly injects up to 40 000 metacyclic forms when it feeds.

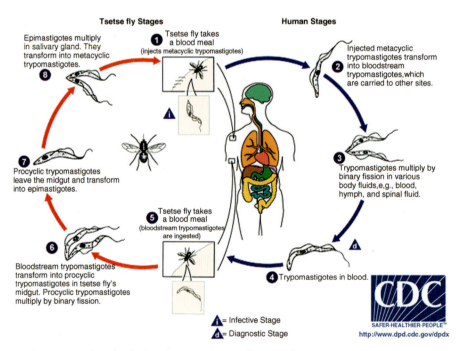

Figure 27.1 Life cycle of *T. brucei*, causative agent of human African trypanosomiasis. (Reproduced from: http://dpd.cdc.gov/dpdx/HTML/ImageLibrary/TrypanosomiasisAfrican_il. htm).

HAT is endemic over 10 million square kilometers of sub-Saharan Africa, threatening 60 million people [2] and all livestock. The human disease is always fatal if untreated. In humans, two types of human disease are recognized, West African sleeping sickness (*T. b. gambiense*) and East African disease (*T. b. rhodesiense*). Of the two diseases, East African HAT is the more rapid developing disease, lasting less than 6 months from initiation of symptoms to death. In West African disease progression is slower with death coming in 1–5 years. Progression of the disease is identical in both cases, with an abscess (chancre) forming at the site of the bite, then trypanosomes migrating to the lymph nodes and eventually to the bloodstream. The organisms then migrate to internal organs and then to the central nervous system (CNS) and brain. Symptoms include fever, convulsions, and later behavioral changes, blindness, coma, and death.

The entire trypanosome surface is covered by a coat – the variant surface glycopeptide (VSG). During infection of mammalian hosts, the VSG genes rapidly switch on and off expression, resulting in variation of the surface coat, which constantly evades the host immune system. There are about 900 genes for VSGs, which prevent practical development of a vaccine [2]. Aside from vector (tsetse fly) control, drug treatment is the only way to control the disease.

Development of chemotherapy has been limited, with few drugs available and only one new drug available clinically since 1947. Early treatment centered on inorganic arsenic administered as H_3AsO_4. After extreme toxicity of this compound was recognized, the scene was ready for a synthetic chemical approach. Paul Ehrlich began synthesizing organic arsenicals in 1905. His early efforts resulted in "Salvarsan 606", the "Magic Bullet" which killed trypanosomes *in vitro* and was later used successfully against syphilis. His work also involved compounds being developed by the German dye industry, which later led to the synthesis of suramin, now used for early-stage disease [1].

Current Chemotherapy

Melarsoprol

In the mid-1940s Ernst Freidheim, working at the Rockefeller University in New York, began chemical synthesis of organic arsenicals based on the early work of Ehrlich. In 1947 he synthesized melarsoprol, a melanophenyl-based arsenical (Figure 27.2). Freidheim traveled to Africa and successfully treated patients with late-stage West African disease using melarsoprol [1,3].

Until recently, melarsoprol was the only available agent for late-stage CNS disease; however, there are serious considerations concerning its use. Melarsoprol causes a post-treatment reactive encephalopathy (PTRE) in about 20% of all patients. About 5% of all patients receiving melarsoprol die from complications of PTRE. Melarsoprol is not water soluble and is soluble only in propylene glycol. Intravenous administration of melarsoprol is painful, and vein thrombophlebitis and atrophy is common [4]. Dose regimens are usually once a day for 10 days, followed by 7 days

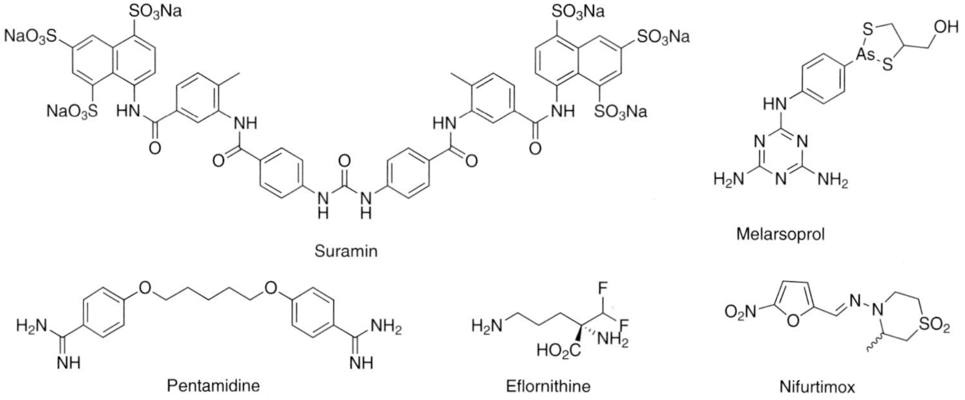

Figure 27.2 Current chemotherapeutic agents for HAT.

rest and an additional 10-day treatment [5]. Recently, failure rates up to 30% have been reported at several clinical locations [6], and in the highly endemic foci of Southern Sudan, Democratic Republic of Congo, Uganda, and Angola [7].

Suramin

This "colorless dye" is used only for early-stage HAT. Suramin (Figure 27.2), first synthesized as part of the German dye industry, was based on the work of Ehrlich using the naphthalene dyes Trypan red and blue. It was first synthesized by Jacobs and Heidelberg at the Rockefeller University in 1919. Suramin has been used for early-stage *T. b. gambiense* and *T. b. rhodesiense* infections since 1940. It is a highly charged molecule and binds to blood proteins, resulting in a long half-life and prophylactic activity. Since it does not penetrate the blood–brain barrier (BBB) it is not used where late-stage disease is suspect [8]. It is given as a series of five intravenous infusions every 3–7 days. Side-effects include neuropathy, rash, fatigue, and renal insufficiency. Resistance to suramin is rare in human disease. The highly charged nature of suramin promotes binding to serum proteins which extends its half-life but prevent BBB penetration [8].

Pentamidine

This diamidine (Figure 27.2) arose from work on synthalin, an agent used to control blood sugar levels in the 1930s [9]. Pentamidine has been in use since the early 1940s, and is used primarily for early-stage *T. b. gambiense* and given as intramuscular injections over 7–10 days [8]. Common side-effects (10% of patients) include reduction of serum glucose, hypotension, and pain at the injection site. Owing to its extensive use, long serum half-life, and multiple uptake transporters in the trypanosome, resistance to pentamidine is not common [7]. It is currently used to treat early-stage HAT infections, primarily *T. b. gambiense*. As it is a highly charged molecule, it does not penetrate the BBB and is not used for late-stage disease [8].

There is no solid evidence for clinical resistance with most failures attributed to incorrect dosing or the presence of low level CNS disease. Uptake of pentamidine has been attributed to three adenine/adenosine-type transporters [10,11] and it is unlikely that resistance due to uptake would arise.

Eflornithine (Ornidyl, Difluoromethylornithine)

Eflornithine (Figure 27.2), an inhibitor of ornithine decarboxylase was developed as an anti-tumor agent that failed in extensive clinical trials. This agent was found to cure early-stage acute *T. b. brucei* laboratory infection [12], and later found to cure a late-stage *T. b. brucei* model infection both alone and in combination with other agents [13,14]. In 1990 eflornithine was licensed for clinical use for late-stage *T. b. gambiense* infection, the first new anti-trypanosomal agent in over 40 years [7]. Although it has no serious side-effects, it must be given in four intravenous doses (total 400 mg), 6 h apart for 2 weeks. This is a serious undertaking in rural clinics resulting in frequent bloodstream infections. Recently, dosing has been reduced to two intravenous doses per day at 12 h intervals for 1 week [6]. In general, eflornithine has been around 90% curative in late-stage *T. b. gambiense* infections [15]. It is not used in *T. b. rhodesiense* infections. Eflornithine is expensive and its synthesis is difficult – a major drawback to widespread use.

Nifurtimox–Eflornithine Combination Therapy

Recent clinical observations with eflornithine and nifurtimox, a nitroimidazole (Figure 27.2) used in single-drug compassionate therapy for relapsed diseases [5], led to the development of an eflornithine-nifurtimox combination regimen [16]. This consists of eflornithine 400 mg/kg/day, intravenously every 12 h for 1 week accompanied by nifurtimox 15 mg/kg/day orally every 8 h for 10 days. This regimen is 96% curative with low adverse effects and is now the standard clinical regimen. Particularly important in the nifurtimox–eflornithine combination therapy (NECT) regimen is the reduction of eflornithine infusions from four per day for 2 weeks to two per day for 1 week [16].

Need for New Chemotherapy

As evident in the preceding discussion, the major problems with current chemotherapy for HAT are drug resistance, toxicity, and inability to penetrate the BBB. Consequently, continued research is needed for new agents that can be given orally in a short-term regimen, and are both non-toxic and effective against Stage 2 CNS disease. This need has been recognized, and there has been a resurgence in research in neglected tropical diseases, including HAT, over the past decade [8]. Numerous reasons for this renewed interest are at play, including the establishment of private–public partnerships such as the Drugs for Neglected Diseases *initiative* (DNDi) and increased philanthropic support from foundations such as the Bill and Melinda Gates Foundation.

Recent Approaches to New Trypanocidal Agents

Nitroimidazoles

Nitroimidazoles (Figure 27.3) are an important class of anti-bacterial and anti-protozoal agents. They include the anti-trichomonad metronidazole, the related tinidazole, the anti-trypanosomal megazole, and the anti-Chagas agent benznidazole. Although metronidazole (trichomoniasis) and benznidazole (Chagas disease) have been in use for many years, these compounds are perceived to be mutagenic because of the nitroaromatic group. More extensive examination of the mechanism of action of nitroheterocycles has suggested that concerns regarding mutagenicity of this class may be less than initially suspected and hence a renewed interest in this class has emerged [17,18].

Fexinidazole

This 5-nitroimidazole (Figure 27.3) is a member of a class of compounds known to have anti-trypanosomal activity [19,20], but was abandoned because of mutagenicity concerns [21]. Following a comprehensive review and *in vitro* assessment of hundreds of nitroheterocycles by the DNDi, recent studies with fexinidazole have demonstrated *in vivo* activity in murine models of both acute and CNS infections [22]. Following extensive characterization of fexinidazole's pharmacokinetics, coupled with no evidence for toxicity or mutagenicity, this compound was progressed to phase I clinical trials in 2010 [22].

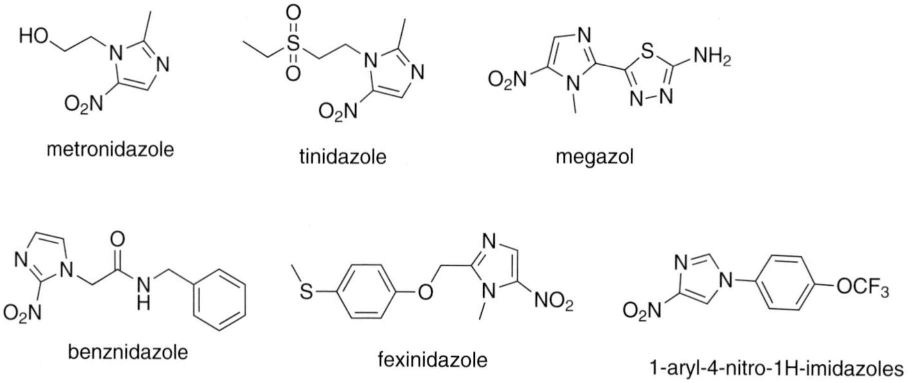

metronidazole

tinidazole

megazol

benznidazole

fexinidazole

1-aryl-4-nitro-1H-imidazoles

Figure 27.3 Nitroheterocycles for HAT.

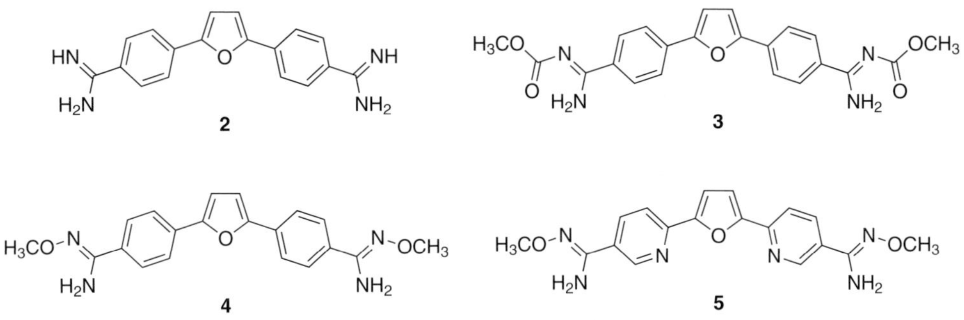

Figure 27.4 Diamidines for HAT.

Aryl-4-nitroimidazoles

In part based on the successful preclinical characterization of fexinidazole, additional nitroimidazoles have been considered as potential candidates for optimization. For example, recent developments in chemistry have allowed synthesis of a series of 1-aryl-4-nitro-1H-imidazoles (Figure 27.3), several of which have been found to be curative in murine models of acute and CNS infections of *T. b. rhodesiense* and *T. b. brucei* [23]. Dosing was orally twice daily for 4 or 5 days. These compounds were not substrates of mammalian nitro-reductases and not genotoxic in mammalian cells. This series needs further investigation to progress to clinical trials as orally administered trypanocides.

Diamidines

Given the clinical utility of pentamidine for treatment of Stage 1 HAT, exploration of the diamidine class has been an active area of research for the Consortium for Parasitic Drug Development (http://www.unc.edu/~jonessk/). Initially focused on exploration of conformationally constrained analogs of pentamidine as potential anti-malarials, the trypanocidal activity of the 2,5-bis(4-guanylphenyl)furan (structure 2, Figure 27.4) was noted [24,25]. These early diamidine analogs were more potent than pentamidine in animal models, but were active only when dosed parenterally. A key advance in the diamidine class occurred when it was discovered that carbamate analogs (structure 3, Figure 27.4) could serve as orally bioavailable prodrugs, initially in anti-microbial models [26]. The prodrug strategy was extended to include amidoximes, resulting in the discovery of DB289 (structure 4, Figure 27.4) as an orally available diamidine analog efficacious in mouse [27–29] and monkey [30] models of Stage 1 HAT. DB289 was not curative in Stage 2 models of HAT [31], presumably due to poor transport across the BBB. DB289 progressed to clinical trials for Stage 1 HAT, where it was found to be effective following a 10-day course of treatment [32]. Unfortunately, further development of DB289 was suspended due to liver and kidney toxicities [32]. More recent research efforts on the diamidine class have identified aza analogs of DB289 (structure 5, Figure 27.4) as having significantly improved efficacy in a murine Stage 2 HAT model [33].

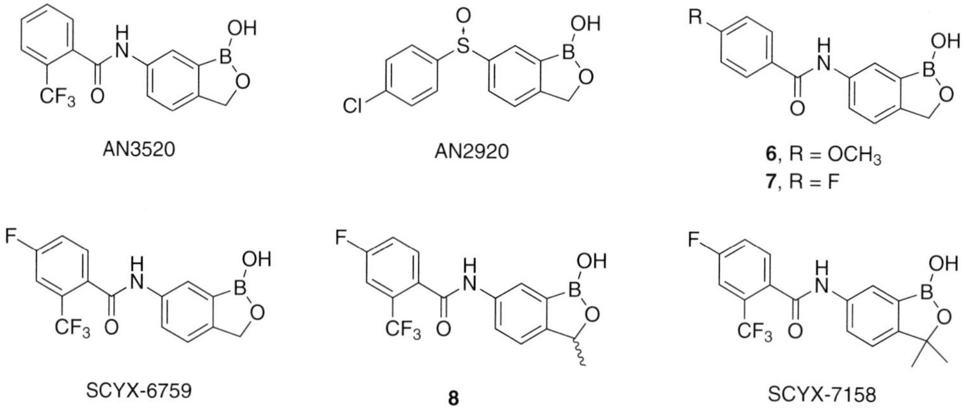

Figure 27.5 Benzoxaboroles for HAT.

Benzoxaboroles

Very recently, a novel series of boron-containing drug candidates, the benzoxaboroles (Figure 27.5), have emerged as a potential treatment for both Stage 1 and Stage 2 sleeping sickness. Initially explored by Anacor Pharmaceuticals as anti-fungal, anti-bacterial, and anti-inflammatory agents [34–36], the benzoxaboroles were found to have anti-parasitic efficacy through screening against *T. brucei* at the Sandler Center of Drug Discovery, UCSF [37]. From approximately 400 benzoxaboroles screened in this early work, two classes of compounds, the 6-carboxamides (represented by AN3520, Figure 27.5) and the 6-sulfoxides (represented by AN2920, Figure 27.5), were determined to have interesting activity and potential for optimization [38]. In addition to the *in vitro* screening conducted by the UCSF group, evaluation of AN2920 in a mouse model of Stage 1 HAT demonstrated that this compound was able to cure mice of the parasitic infection, albeit at a reasonably high dose of 50 mg/kg (i.p. × 5 days). Encouraged by these results, Anacor approached the DNDi to further explore and granted the DNDi a license to develop this series for HAT, leishmaniasis, and Chagas disease. The DNDi had already engaged the biotechnology company Scynexis, in collaboration with the Haskins Laboratories at Pace University, to conduct a lead optimization drug discovery program for HAT and the benzoxaboroles were introduced into the program in early 2008. Following confirmation of the activity of the lead benzoxaboroles in a high throughput *in vitro* assay at Scynexis [39], AN2920 and AN3520 and several close analogs were progressed to a range of *in vitro* ADME (absorption, distribution, metabolism, and elimination) and physicochemical property assays. The profile exhibited by these compounds in these assays suggested that the benzoxaboroles were indeed an attractive series for lead optimization.

Described in detail elsewhere [40,41], it was determined that instability to metabolizing enzymes was one of the primary limitations of the early lead compounds. This liability was confirmed in an *in vivo* pharmacokinetic study, in which relatively rapid disappearance of compounds from the plasma of mice was

Table 27.1 Efficacy of benzoxaboroles in a murine Stage 1 HAT model [13,42].

Compound	Dose (mg/kg)	Route and frequency	Duration (days)	Relapses	Number cured
AN2920	20	i.p., b.i.d.	4	—	3/3
	20	p.o., b.i.d.	4	1-d10, 1-d11	1/3
AN3520	20	i.p., b.i.d.	4	—	3/3
	20	p.o., b.i.d.	4	—	3/3
	10	p.o., b.i.d.	4	1-d11	2/3
<u>6</u>	20	p.o., b.i.d.	4	3-d10	0/3
<u>7</u>	20	p.o., b.i.d.	4	—	3/3
	10	p.o., b.i.d.	4	1-d7	2/3
SCYX-6759	10	p.o., b.i.d.	4	—	5/5
	10	p.o., q.d.	4	—	5/5
	5	p.o., q.d.	4	—	5/5
	2.5	p.o., q.d.	4	—	5/5
	1.25	p.o., q.d.	4	4-d4, 1-d5	0/5
SCYX-7158	10	p.o., q.d.	4	—	5/5
	5	p.o., q.d.	4	—	5/5
	2.5	p.o., q.d.	4	1-d5, 1-d7, 3-d10	0/5

i.p., intraperitoneally; p.o., per os; b.i.d., twice daily; q.d., once daily.

observed after either intraperitoneal or oral dosing. In this study, both AN2920 and AN3520 were found to provide exposure sufficient to suggest that they should be active in a mouse model of Stage 1 HAT. This relationship between pharmacokinetics and pharmacodynamics was confirmed in the Stage 1 mouse model (Table 27.1), where both compounds were found to be active when dosed i.p. at 20 mg/kg (b.i.d. × 4 days) [37,41]. When evaluated in the same model following oral administration at 20 mg/kg (b.i.d. × 4 days), AN2920 was found to be inactive, whereas AN3520 was found to be active. Lower doses of AN3520 were found to be variably active by either route of administration. Analogs of AN3520 were also active following intraperitoneal administration, but exhibited variable efficacy when dosed orally. For example, the 4-methoxybenzamide (structure 6, Figure 27.5) was inactive following a 20 mg/kg (b.i.d. × 4 days) oral dose (Table 27.1). In contrast, the 4-fluorobenzamide (structure 7, Figure 27.5) exhibited full efficacy at 20 mg/kg and partial efficacy at 10 mg/kg (Table 27.1). This structure–activity relationship trend was broadly reflective of metabolic stability, as **6** was less stable in several *in vitro* assays, and the *in vivo* pharmacokinetics of **6** in mice suggested this compound was removed from the bloodstream much more rapidly than either AN3520 or **7** (Wring, unpublished data). Consequently, the focus of the lead optimization program was to improve the metabolic stability of the benzoxaborole 6-carboxamide series.

Of several approaches taken, one of the most straightforward and effective was to simply add a fluorine atom to the 4-position of benzamide region of AN3520,

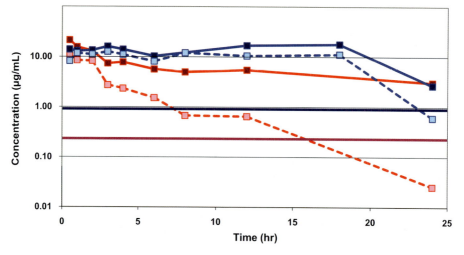

Figure 27.6 Pharmacokinetic profiles for SCYX-6759 (red symbols) and SCYX-7158 (blue symbols) in plasma (solid lines) and brain (dashed lines) of mice.

resulting in SCYX-6759 (Figure 27.5). This compound was also found to be very potent in the *T. b. brucei in vitro* assay, and had good physicochemical and ADME properties [40]. Furthermore, when dosed orally to mice at doses as low as 6.25 mg/kg, plasma levels of SCYX-6759 were found to remain at concentrations at or above the *in vitro* IC$_{50}$ for at least 12 h, suggesting that this compound would exhibit improved efficacy in the *in vivo* mouse model. This was confirmed, as SCYX-6759 was fully efficacious when dosed orally at 2.5 mg/kg (b.i.d. × 4 days). In the pharmacokinetics experiment, brain levels of SCYX-6759 were also measured; this data suggested that concentrations of compound in the brain were maintained at or above the *in vitro* IC$_{50}$ for at least 12 h following a dose of 50 mg/kg (Figure 27.6). Consequently, SCYX-6759 was progressed to a mouse model of Stage 2 HAT [40], where it was found to be curative following a dosing regimen of 50 mg/kg (b.i.d., i. p. × 14 days). While encouraged by this result, it was clear that further improvements in either efficacy and/or brain exposure were required for the benzoxaboroles to be viable as once-daily oral treatments for Stage 2 HAT, which was the Target Product Profile defined by the DNDi at the outset of the project.

As described above, the *in vitro* ADME profiles of SCYX-6759 and related compounds were very good, and it was difficult to identify reasons for the apparent disconnect between plasma and brain exposure. For example, permeability across the BBB, as predicted by an *in vitro* assay using an MDCK-MDRI cell monolayer, was uniformly high for all of the benzoxaborole 6-carboxamides examined, with no evidence of efflux liability by P-glycoprotein [43]. It was hypothesized that other transporters could be at least in part responsible for efflux of the weakly acidic benzoxaboroles from the brain. Therefore, modifications to SCYX-6759 were pursued in an effort to electronically and/or sterically limit access to the acidic

B-OH moiety. Of several approaches pursued, it was found that introduction of substituents at C(3) of the benzoxaborole nucleus were particularly successful, albeit with some limitations [41]. More specifically, introduction of a single methyl group, such as in structure 8 (Figure 27.5), afforded compounds that were more cytotoxic to mammalian cells relative to the C(3)-unsubstituted analogs. From a pharmacokinetic perspective, these analogs did not exhibit the improvements required in terms of brain exposure. More sterically demanding C(3) substituents were found to significantly erode *in vitro* potency versus *T. brucei*. In contrast, the 3,3-dimethyl analogs exemplified by SCYX-7158 (Figure 27.5) were found to not exhibit mammalian cell cytotoxicity, and maintained sufficient *in vitro* potency to progress to *in vivo* efficacy and pharmacokinetic studies.

When evaluated in both the Stage 1 and Stage 2 HAT models, SCYX-7158 exhibited impressive efficacy [44]. In particular, it was observed that complete cure of mice infected with the TREU667 strain in the Stage 2 model could be achieved following a 25 mg/kg (q.d. $\times$ 7 days) oral dosing paradigm. Partial cure (80%) was observed following a 12.5 mg/kg (q.d. $\times$ 7 days) oral dose schedule. *In vivo* pharmacokinetic characterization of SCYX-7158 was consistent with these observations, as it was observed that brain concentrations of SCYX-7158 were maintained at therapeutically relevant levels for close to 24 h after a 25 mg/kg dose and that a 12.5 mg/kg dose provided brain levels slightly below the *in vitro* IC_{50} and/or minimum inhibitory concentration. The relationship between brain concentration and observed efficacy in the Stage 2 HAT model has formed the basis for development of a pharmacokinetics/pharmacodynamics model (Wring, personal communication). SCYX-7158 was thoroughly evaluated in the mouse Stage 2 HAT model as shown in Table 27.2.

Interestingly, while most studies were performed using a standardized 7-day dosing protocol, it was found that cures could be obtained with SCYX-7158 with as little as 3 days of dosing at 50 mg/kg. Reduction of the dosing period from 7 days (to 5 or 3 days) at 25 mg/kg resulted in partial efficacy. Coupled with the extensive pharmacokinetic data generated for SCYX-7158 allowed one to conclude that activity in the mouse model of Stage 2 HAT was both time- and concentration-dependent.

Table 27.2 Efficacy of SCYX-7158 in Stage 2 HAT model [13,45].

Dose (mg/kg)	Route/frequency	Duration (days)	Relapses	Number cured
6.25	p.o., q.d.	7	6-d34, 1-d41, 3-d48	0/10
12.5	p.o., q.d.	7	1-d34, 1-d48	8/10
25	p.o., q.d.	7		10/10
25	p.o., q.d.	5	1-d35, 1-d42, 1-d63	7/10
25	p.o., q.d.	3	2-d35, 1-d42	6/9
50	p.o., q.d.	7		32/32
50	p.o., q.d.	5		14/14
50	p.o., q.d.	3		14/14
50	p.o.	1	1-d22, 4-d28	0/5

p.o., per os; q.d., once daily.

Based on these properties, SCYX-7158 was selected for progression to preclinical development activities [44]. When evaluated in a broad array (greater than 100) of *in vitro* receptor binding, enzyme inhibition, and ion channel inhibition assays, SCYX-7158 showed no significant activity (defined as greater than 50% inhibition at $10\,\mu M$) against any of these mammalian targets. In addition, the compound was found to be functionally inactive against the hERG ion channel [46] and was not mutagenic in an *in vitro* bacterial reverse mutation assay [47].

SCYX-7158 has also been evaluated in a number of *in vivo* safety pharmacology and toxicology studies in rodents and dogs, including single-dose, 7- and 28-day multiple-dose toxicology studies, rat CNS safety pharmacology, dog cardiovascular safety pharmacology, rat respiratory safety pharmacology, and rat gastrointestinal motility. In these studies, no significant safety or toxicity issues were identified. In the toxicology studies, pharmacokinetics were also further evaluated, and it was observed that plasma exposure to SCYX-7158 was well in excess of that required for efficacy in the mouse models, allowing adequate safety margins to be predicted based on these studies. Based on these efforts, SCYX-7158 was progressed to phase I clinical trials following regulatory approval from the European Medicines Association (http://clinicaltrials.gov/show/NCT01533961).

Conclusion

Based on the above compilation of results, it is evident that oxaboroles hold much promise as effective human trypanocides. The results of ongoing clinical trials are keenly awaited and we maintain hope for the emergence of an effective, non-toxic, orally available agent for HAT. This research has shown the rapid progression of a drug lead to clinical candidate through mining of compound data, collaboration of pharmaceutical resources, academic research, and effective private–public partnership and philanthropic foundation support. There is, however, another issue closely linked to HAT: the continuing poverty and malnutrition found in the tsetse belt. Cure of HAT is only part of the answer. The rest of the solution lies in the emergence of a veterinary trypanocide that will allow effective farming and cattle ranching in tsetse-infected areas. Only then will the "curse of flies" be lifted from Africa [1].

References

1 McKelvey, J.J.Jr. (1973) *Man Against Tsetse: Struggle for Africa*, Cornell University Press, Ithaca, NY.

2 Kennedy, P.G.E. (2008) The continuing problem of Human African trypanosomiasis (sleeping sickness). *Ann. Neurol.*, **64**, 116–127.

3 Apted, F.I.C. (1970) Treatment of African trypanosomiasis, in *The African Trypanosomiases* (ed. H.W. Mulligan), George Allen & Unwin, London, pp 152–156.

4 Van Nieuwenhove, S., Schechter, P.J., Declercq, J., Bone, G., Burke, J., and Sjoerdsma, A. (1985) Treatment of gambiense sleeping sickness in the Sudan with oral DFMO (DL-alpha-difluoromethylornithine), an inhibitor of

ornithine decarboxylase; first field trial. *Trans. R. Soc. Trop. Med. Hyg.*, **79**, 692–698.

5 Van Nieuwenhove, S. (1992) Advances in sleeping sickness therapy. *Ann. Soc. Belg. Med. Trop.*, **72** (Suppl. 1), 39–51.

6 Priotto, G., Pinogcs, L., Fursa, I.B., Burke, B., Nicolay, N., Grillet, G., Hewison, C., and Balasegaram, M. (2008) Safety and effectiveness of first line eflornithine for *Trypanosoma brucei gambiense* sleeping sickness in Sudan: cohort study. *BMJ*, **336**, 705–708.

7 Delespaux, V. and de Koning, H.P. (2007) Drugs and drug resistance in African trypanosomiasis. *Drug Resist. Updat.*, **10**, 30–50.

8 Barrett, M.P., Boykin, D.W., Brun, R., and Tidwell, R.R. (2007) Human African trypanosomiasis: pharmacological re-engagement with a neglected disease. *Br. J. Pharmacol.*, **152**, 1155–1171.

9 Barrett, M.P. and Fairlamb, A.H. (1999) The biochemical basis of arsenical-diamidine crossresistance in African trypanosomes. *Parasitol. Today*, **15**, 136–140.

10 de Koning, H.P. (2001) Transporters in African trypanosomes: role in drug action and resistance. *Int. J. Parasitol.*, **31**, 512–522.

11 De Koning, H.P. (2001) Uptake of pentamidine in *Trypanosoma brucei brucei* is mediated by three distinct transporters: implications for cross-resistance with arsenicals. *Mol. Pharmacol.*, **59**, 586–592.

12 Bacchi, C.J., Nathan, H.C., Hutner, S.H., McCann, P.P., and Sjoerdsma, A. (1980) Polyamine metabolism: a potential therapeutic target in trypanosomes. *Science*, **210**, 332–334.

13 Bacchi, C.J., Nathan, H.C., Clarkson, A.B. Jr., Bienen, E.J., Bitonti, A.J., McCann, P.P., and Sjoerdsma, A. (1987) Effects of the ornithine decarboxylase inhibitors DL-alpha-difluoromethylornithine and alpha-monofluoromethyldehydroornithine methyl ester alone and in combination with suramin against *Trypanosoma brucei brucei* central nervous system models. *Am. J. Trop. Med. Hyg.*, **36**, 46–52.

14 Clarkson, A.B.Jr., Bienen, E.J., Bacchi, C.J., McCann, P.P., Nathan, H.C., Hutner, S.H., and Sjoerdsma, A. (1984) New drug combination for experimental late-stage African trypanosomiasis: DL-alpha-difluoromethylornithine (DFMO) with suramin. *Am. J. Trop. Med. Hyg.*, **33**, 1073–1077.

15 Priotto, G., Kasparian, S., Ngouama, D., Ghorashian, S., Arnold, U., Ghabri, S., and Karunakara, U. (2007) Nifurtimox-eflornithine combination therapy for second-stage *Trypanosoma brucei gambiense* sleeping sickness: a randomized clinical trial in Congo. *Clin. Infect. Dis.*, **45**, 1435–1442.

16 Priotto, G., Kasparian, S., Mutombo, W., Ngouama, D., Ghorashian, S., Arnold, U., Ghabri, S., Baudin, E., Buard, V., Kazadi-Kyanza, S., Ilunga, M., Mutangala, W., Pohlig, G., Schmid, C., Karunakara, U., Torreele, E., and Kande, V. (2009) Nifurtimox-eflornithine combination therapy for second-stage African *Trypanosoma brucei gambiense* trypanosomiasis: a multicentre, randomised, phase III, non-inferiority trial. *Lancet*, **374**, 56–64.

17 Bendesky, A., Menéndez, D., and Ostrosky-Wegman, P. (2002) Is metronidazole carcinogenic? *Mutat. Res.*, **511**, 133–144.

18 Buschini, A., Giordani, F., de Albuquerque, C.N., Pellacani, C., Pelosi, G., Rossi, C., Zucchi, T.M., and Poli, P. (2007) Trypanocidal nitroimidazole derivatives: relationships among chemical structure and genotoxic activity. *Biochem. Pharmacol.*, **73**, 1537–1547.

19 Winkelmann, E., Raether, W., Gebert, U., and Sinharay, A. (1977) Chemotherapeutically active nitro compounds. 4. 5-Nitroimidazoles (Part I). *Arzneimittelforschung*, **27**, 2251–2263.

20 Jennings, F.W. and Urquhart, G.M. (1983) The use of the 2 substituted 5-nitroimidazole, Fexinidazole (Hoe 239) in the treatment of chronic *T. brucei* infections in mice. *Z. Parasitenkd.*, **69**, 577–581.

21 Voogd, C.E. (1981) On the mutagenicity of nitroimidazoles. *Mutat. Res.*, **86**, 243–277.

22 Torreele, E., Bourdin Trunz, B., Tweats, D., Kaiser, M., Brun, R., Mazue, G., Bray, M.A., and Pecoul, B. (2010) Fexinidazole – a new oral nitroimidazole drug candidate entering clinical development for the

treatment of sleeping sickness. *PLoS Negl. Trop. Dis.*, **4**, e923.

23 Trunz, B.B., Jedrysiak, R., Tweats, D., Brun, R., Kaiser, M., Suwinski, J., and Torreele, E. (2011) 1-Aryl-4-nitro-1H-imidazoles, a new promising series for the treatment of human African trypanosomiasis. *Eur. J. Med. Chem.*, **46**, 1524–1535.

24 Das, B.P. and Boykin, D.W. (1977) Synthesis and antiprotozoal activity of 2,5-bis(4-guanylphenyl)furans. *J. Med. Chem.*, **20**, 531–536.

25 Steck, E.A., Kinnamon, K.E., Davidson, D. E.Jr., Duxbury, R.E., Johnson, A.J., and Masters, R.E. (1982) *Trypanosoma rhodesiense*: evaluation of the antitrypanosomal action of 2,5-bis(4-guanylphenyl)furan dihydrochloride. *Exp. Parasitol.*, **53**, 133–144.

26 Rahmathullah, S.M., Hall, J.E., Bender, B.C., McCurdy, D.R., Tidwell, R.R., and Boykin, D.W. (1999) Prodrugs for amidines: synthesis and anti-*Pneumocystis carinii* activity of carbamates of 2,5-bis(4-amidinophenyl)furan. *J. Med. Chem.*, **42**, 3994–4000.

27 Zhou, L., Lee, K., Thakker, D.R., Boykin, D.W., Tidwell, R.R., and Hall, J.E. (2002) Enhanced permeability of the antimicrobial agent 2,5-bis(4-amidinophenyl)furan across Caco-2 cell monolayers via its methylamidoidme prodrug. *Pharm. Res.*, **19**, 1689–1695.

28 Ansede, J.H., Anbazhagan, M., Brun, R., Easterbrook, J.D., Hall, J.E., and Boykin, D. W. (2004) *O*-alkoxyamidine prodrugs of furamidine: *in vitro* transport and microsomal metabolism as indicators of *in vivo* efficacy in a mouse model of *Trypanosoma brucei rhodesiense* infection. *J. Med. Chem.*, **47**, 4335–4338.

29 Sturk, L.M., Brock, J.L., Bagnell, C.R., Hall, J.E., and Tidwell, R.R. (2004) Distribution and quantitation of the anti-trypanosomal diamidine 2,5-bis(4-amidinophenyl)furan (DB75) and its *N*-methoxy prodrug DB289 in murine brain tissue. *Acta Trop.*, **91**, 131–143.

30 Mdachi, R.E., Thuita, J.K., Kagira, J.M., Ngotho, J.M., Murilla, G.A., Ndung'u, J.M., Tidwell, R.R., Hall, J.E., and Brun, R. (2009) Efficacy of the novel diamidine

compound 2,5-bis(4-amidinophenyl)-furan-bis-*O*-methlylamidoxime (Pafuramidine, DB289) against *Trypanosoma brucei rhodesiense* infection in vervet monkeys after oral administration. *Antimicrob. Agents Chemother.*, **53**, 953–957.

31 Ansede, J.H., Voyksner, R.D., Ismail, M.A., Boykin, D.W., Tidwell, R.R., and Hall, J.E. (2005) *In vitro* metabolism of an orally active *O*-methyl amidoxime prodrug for the treatment of CNS trypanosomiasis. *Xenobiotica*, **35**, 211–226.

32 Paine, M.F., Wang, M.Z., Generaux, C.N., Boykin, D.W., Wilson, W.D., De Koning, H.P., Olson, C.A., Pohlig, G., Burri, C., Brun, R., Murilla, G.A., Thuita, J.K., Barrett, M.P., and Tidwell, R.R. (2010) Diamidines for human African trypanosomiasis. *Curr. Opin. Investig. Drugs.*, **11**, 876–883.

33 Wenzler, T., Boykin, D.W., Ismail, M.A., Hall, J.E., Tidwell, R.R., and Brun, R. (2009) New treatment option for second-stage African sleeping sickness: *in vitro* and *in vivo* efficacy of aza analogs of DB289. *Antimicrob. Agents Chemother.*, **53**, 4185–4192.

34 Baker, S.J., Akama, T., Zhang, Y.K., Sauro, V., Pandit, C., Singh, R., Kully, M., Khan, J., Plattner, J.J., Benkovic, S.J., Lee, V., and Maples, K.R. (2006) Identification of a novel boron-containing antibacterial agent (AN0128) with anti-inflammatory activity, for the potential treatment of cutaneous diseases. *Bioorg. Med. Chem. Lett.*, **16**, 5963–5967.

35 Baker, S.J., Zhang, Y.K., Akama, T., Lau, A., Zhou, H., Hernandez, V., Mao, W., Alley, M.R., Sanders, V., and Plattner, J.J. (2006) Discovery of a new boron-containing antifungal agent, 5-fluoro-1,3-dihydro-1-hydroxy-2,1- benzoxaborole (AN2690), for the potential treatment of onychomycosis. *J. Med. Chem.*, **49**, 4447–4450.

36 Akama, T., Baker, S.J., Zhang, Y.K., Hernandez, V., Zhou, H., Sanders, V., Freund, Y., Kimura, R., Maples, K.R., and Plattner, J.J. (2009) Discovery and structure–activity study of a novel benzoxaborole anti-inflammatory agent (AN2728) for the potential topical treatment of psoriasis and atopic dermatitis. *Bioorg. Med. Chem. Lett.*, **19**, 2129–2132.

37 Ding, D., Zhao, Y., Meng, Q., Xie, D., Nare, B., Chen, D., Bacchi, C.J., Yarlett, N., Zhang, Y.-K., Hernandez, V., Xia, Y., Freund, Y., Abdulla, M., Ang, K.-H., Ratnam, J., McKerrow, J.H., Jacobs, R.T., Zhou, H., and Plattner, J.J. (2010) Discovery of novel benzoxaborole-based potent antitrypanosomal agents. *ACS Med. Chem. Lett.*, **1**, 165–169.

38 Ding, C.Z., Zhang, Y.K., Li, X., Liu, Y., Zhang, S., Zhou, Y., Plattner, J.J., Baker, S.J., Liu, L., Duan, M., Jarvest, R.L., Ji, J., Kazmierski, W.M., Tallant, M.D., Wright, L.L., Smith, G.K., Crosby, R.M., Wang, A. A., Ni, Z.J., Zou, W., and Wright, J. (2010) Synthesis and biological evaluations of P4-benzoxaborole-substituted macrocyclic inhibitors of HCV NS3 protease. *Bioorg. Med. Chem. Lett.*, **20**, 7317–7322.

39 Bowling, T., Mercer, L., Don, R., Jacobs, R., and Nare, B. (2012) Application of a resazurin-based high-throughput screening assay for the identification and progression of new treatments for human African trypanosomiasis. *Int. J. Parasitol.*, **2**, 262–270.

40 Nare, B., Wring, S., Bacchi, C., Beaudet, B., Bowling, T., Brun, R., Chen, D., Ding, C., Freund, Y., Gaukel, E., Hussain, A., Jarnagin, K., Jenks, M., Kaiser, M., Mercer, L., Mejia, E., Noe, A., Orr, M., Parham, R., Plattner, J., Randolph, R., Rattendi, D., Rewerts, C., Sligar, J., Yarlett, N., Don, R., and Jacobs, R. (2010) Discovery of novel orally bioavailable oxaborole 6-carboxamides that demonstrate cure in a murine model of late-stage central nervous system African trypanosomiasis. *Antimicrob. Agents Chemother.*, **54**, 4379–4388.

41 Jacobs, R.T., Plattner, J.J., Nare, B., Wring, S.A., Chen, D., Freund, Y., Gaukel, E.G., Orr, M.D., Perales, J.B., Jenks, M., Noe, R. A., Sligar, J.M., Zhang, Y.-K., Bacchi, C.J., Yarlett, N., and Don, R. (2011) Benzoxaboroles: a new class of potential drugs for human African trypanosomiasis. *Future Med. Chem.*, **3**, 1259–1278.

42 Bacchi, C.J., Brun, R., Croft, S.L., Alicea, K., and Buhler, Y. (1996) In vivo trypanocidal activities of new S-adenosylmethionine decarboxylase inhibitors. *Antimicrob. Agents Chemother.*, **40**, 1448–1453.

43 Mahar Doan, K.M., Humphreys, J.E., Webster, L.O., Wring, S.A., Shampine, L.J., Serabjit-Singh, C.J., Adkison, K.K., and Polli, J.W. (2002) Passive permeability and P-glycoprotein-mediated efflux differentiate central nervous system (CNS) and non-CNS marketed drugs. *J. Pharmacol. Exp. Ther.*, **303**, 1029–1037.

44 Jacobs, R.T., Nare, B., Wring, S.A., Orr, M.D., Chen, D., Sligar, J.M., Jenks, M.X., Noe, R.A., Bowling, T.S., Mercer, L.T., Rewerts, C., Gaukel, E., Owens, J., Parham, R., Randolph, R., Beaudet, B., Bacchi, C.J., Yarlett, N., Plattner, J.J., Freund, Y., Ding, C., Akama, T., Zhang, Y.K., Brun, R., Kaiser, M., Scandale, I., and Don, R. (2011) SCYX-7158, an orally-active benzoxaborole for the treatment of Stage 2 human African trypanosomiasis. *PLoS Negl. Trop. Dis.*, **5**, e1151.

45 Bacchi, C.J., Nathan, H.C., Yarlett, N., Goldberg, B., McCann, P.P., Sjoerdsma, A., Saric, M., and Clarkson, A.B.Jr. (1994) Combination chemotherapy of drug-resistant *Trypanosoma brucei rhodesiense* infections in mice using DL-alpha-difluoromethylornithine and standard trypanocides. *Antimicrob. Agents Chemother.*, **38**, 563–569.

46 Zhou, Z., Gong, Q., Ye, B., Fan, Z., Makielski, J.C., Robertson, G.A., and January, C.T. (1998) Properties of HERG channels stably expressed in HEK 293 cells studied at physiological temperature. *Biophys. J.*, **74**, 230–241.

47 Ames, B.N., McCann, J., and Yamasaki, E. (1975) Methods for detecting carcinogens and mutagens with the *Salmonella*/mammalian-microsome mutagenicity test. *Mutat. Res.*, **31**, 347–364.

Index

a

acidocalcisomes 266
activated protein-1 (AP-1)
– component 109
active ligands 59
active-site cysteine residue 183
active small molecules, chemical structure 57
adenosine ribose 139
α-difluoromethylornithine (eflornithine) 292
AdoMetDC inhibitors 175
ADP-ribosylation factor-like protein
   (ARL-1) 288
AEP-1 247
African sleeping sickness 57, 58, 405.
   See also Chagas disease
African trypanosomes 43, 184. See also
   human African trypanosomiasis (HAT)
– both TORC1 and TORC2 265
– GLO2-encoding gene 157
– human pathogenic stage 122
– infective form 300, 301
– lacking GLO1 161
– necrosis, after H_2O_2 treatment 262
– potential drug target 301
– synthesis and reduction of
   trypanothione 388
– treatments for 70
– type IA DNA topoisomerases in 253
alanine aminotransferase 39
alanine dehydrogenase (ADH) 127
aldose reductase activity 161
alkylphosphocholine miltefosine 387
allopurinol 9, 22, 23, 141
allopurinol (4-hydroxypyrazolo(3,4-d)
   pyrimidine) 141
alternative oxidase (AO) 123
amastigotes 106
aminobenzimidazole derivative 70
aminoglycoside antibiotic paromomycin 18

aminosidin. See paromomycin
amino sugars catabolism 131
amiodarone, as anti-parasitic agent 501, 502
2-ammino-thiadiazole 466
amphotericin B 9, 18, 387
– deoxycholate 4
– formulations 25
– leishmanicidal properties 25
– monomeric form 24
– side-effect 25
AM1 theory 63
amyloidotic-type neurodegenerative
   diseases 154
animal leishmaniases 19
animal trypanosomiasis (Ngana) 515
anti-Chagas therapy 290
anti-fungal azoles 27
anti-kinetoplastida drug design 59–61
anti-kinetoplastid agents 292
anti-Leishmania antibody 20
anti-leishmanial compounds 27
antimonials, in combined therapy 26
antimony-resistant Indian visceral
   leishmaniasis parasites 5
antioxidant 356, 406
– mechanisms 216
– network 226
anti-parasitic drugs 336
anti-protozoan drugs 81
anti-sleeping sickness drugs 366
anti-trypanosomal compounds
– chemical structure, and biological
   activity 64
anti-trypanosomal drugs 38, 387
anti-trypanosomal hit/lead compounds
   58, 59
anti-trypanosomal N-phenylpyrazole
   benzylidene-carbohydrazides 64
apicoplast 336

Trypanosomatid Diseases: Molecular Routes to Drug Discovery, First edition. Edited by T. Jäger, O. Koch, and L. Flohé.
© 2013 Wiley-VCH Verlag GmbH & Co. KGaA. Published 2013 by Wiley-VCH Verlag GmbH & Co. KGaA.

apoptosis 268–273, 357
– in protozoan parasites 268–273
– in trypanosomes 269, 270
apoptosis-inducing factor (AIF) 269
aquaglyceroporin (AQP2) 45
arabinonolactone oxidase 132
arginine decarboxylase (ADC) 175
aromatic amino-methylene bisphosphonate
    derivatives 139
aryl-quinuclidine derivatives 503
ascorbate peroxidase 226
ASINEX database 72
Aspergillus fumigatus 481
atazanavir 288
*ATG*genes 265
ATG8 genes 267
ATG8-lipidation pathway 267, 355
Atg8 pathway 267
ATP-competitive kinase inhibitors 291
ATP-dependent DNA helicase 250
auranofin 239, 240
AutoDock4 program 72
autophagic pathway in *Leishmania* spp
    109, 354
– ATG4 regulation 355, 356
autophagolysosomal degradation 109
autophagolysosomes 265, 268
autophagosomes 267, 268, 352
– ATG12–ATG5 conjugation pathway, role in
    biogenesis and 358
– biogenesis, molecular machinery for
    352, 355
– degradation 355
autophagy 135, 263, 352
– Atg18–Atg2 complex 264, 265
– autophagic pathway in *Leishmania* spp 354
– autophagosome formation 264, 265
– *Leishmania*'s cathepsins role in
    regulation 356–358
– regulation of induction 264, 265
– in *T. brucei* 266
– TORC complexes 265
– vesicle nucleation 264
autophagy-related proteins (Atg) 134, 265
azoles 480
– resistance 481

b

Bacille Calmette-Guerin (BCG) 9
Bayesian models 89, 90
Baylis–Hillman chemistry 466
B-cells 263
Bcr–Abl kinase 291
benznidazole 387, 467

binding pocket prediction 75
bioinformatics 267
biomarkers 49
N^1,N^8-bis(glutathionyl)spermidine.
    See trypanothione
1,3-bisphosphoglycerate (1,3-PGA) 122
bisphosphonates 140
blood–brain barrier (BBB) 45, 273
blood–CSF barrier 271, 273
B lymphocytes 497
β-phenyl imidazoles 499
6-bromo-5-methylindirubin-3′-oxime 291
buparvaquone 27
L-buthionine-*S*,*R*-sulfoximine (BSO) 173
2-[*trans*(4-*t*-butylcyclohexyl)-methyl]-3-hydroxy-
    1,4-naphthoquinone 27

c

calpains 359
Candida albicans 287
candidate drug targets 141
canine leishmaniasis, and chemotherapy
    19–27
– alkylphosphocholine 23, 24
– allopurinol 22, 23
– aminosidine 26, 27
– amphotericin B 24, 25
– – drug delivery systems, use 25, 26
– – pentamidine 26, 27
– anti-leishmanial drugs, exploration 27, 28
– by *Leishmania* infantum 19, 20
– pentavalent antimonials 20–22
cardiomyocytes 219
caspases 358
catalase 387
cathepsin K inhibitors 288
cathepsins 289, 290, 355
– Kinetoplastid parasites producing 289
– and virulence 356–358
CDD Database 83, 86
– relevant trypanosomal disease screening
    datasets in 87
– screenshot showing data mining
    facilities 89
CD8$^+$ T cells 112
cell antioxidant capacity 209
cell death 261, 283
central nervous system (CNS) 37
central processing units (CPUs) 59
cerebrospinal fluid (CSF) 269, 273
Chagas disease 57, 69, 81, 83, 122, 140, 141,
    215, 226, 386, 474, 476, 480, 490, 492, 501,
    505, 520. *See also* cruzain
– benznidazole 57

– Centers for Disease Control and Prevention (CDC) estimation for   473, 474
– current therapy   474, 475
– – targeting *T. cruzi* protease cruzain   476, 477
– CYP51 inhibitors   480
– cysteine protease inhibitors, as chemotherapy for   477
– drugs, for specific treatment   490–493
– EBIs as potential new therapeutic agents   493–504
– megasyndromes prevalence   474
– mortality   474
– new therapies for   473
– nifurtimox   57
– pharmacokinetics of K777   477
– – clinical trials and studies   477
channel-forming proteins   142
chemical ionization (CI)   41
chemical libraries   61, 66, 68
cheminformatics methods   83
chemotherapeutic agents   18
chinifur   419
chloroquine resistance   343
chloro-quinoline scaffold   64
collaborative drug discovery (CDD) database   81, 86, 87
– capability   88
– screenshot showing data mining facilities   89, 90
Combination therapies   5, 504, 505
– aminosidine   26
– benznidazole with ketoconazole   504
– evaluation of efficacy   505
– ketoconazole with alkyl-lysophospholipid analogs   504
– nifurtimox–eflornithine combination therapy   519
– synergic effects   504
compound libraries   143
computational approaches, used for drug discovery   84, 85
computational machine learning models   89
computational protocol   74
computer-aided drug design   58, 59
contraception method   18
Crithidia fasciculata   44, 181, 205, 243, 430
cruzain   289
– as good drug target   477, 478
– potent inhibitors   478–480
– – lack of correlation, protease inhibition and trypanocidal efficacy   480
– – non-peptidic cruzain inhibitors   479
– – pyridyl analog of K777   479

– – toxicity   480
cruzipaine   68
cryptic infections   20
CxxC-containing oxidoreductases   204
CxxC-containing proteins   207
cyclin-dependent kinases (CDKs)   291
cyclodextrin-based formulations   46
cycloguanil   467
CYP51 activity, and sterol biosynthesis   481
2-Cysperoxiredoxins (2-Cys-Prxs)   388
Cys-protease motif   176
2-Cys PRXs, mechanism of action   202, 203
cysteine peptidases   352
– downregulation in *Leishmania* spp.   352
– inhibitors: opportunities and challenges   359, 360
– – dipeptidyl α-fluorovinyl   359
– – α-ketoheterocyclics   359
– – metal-based inhibitors   359
– – vinyl sulfone inhibitor, K11777   359
cysteine proteases   268
– inhibitors   28, 288
cysteines, overoxidation   180
cytokines   7, 108, 215, 217, 266, 285, 325, 374
cytokinesis   265
cytosolic tryparedoxin peroxidase (cTXNPx)   217
cytosolic TXN, downregulation   207
cytotoxicity   62, 217, 374, 463, 465, 525

d
data analysis   42–44
data mapping   88
DDD85646 selectivity   288
deglutathionylate proteins   180
dehydroepiandrosterone (DHEA)   305
dendritic cells (DCs)   106, 111, 112
– dermal DCs   111
– ICAM-3-grabbing non-integrin (DC-SIGN)   112
– myeloid DCs (mDCs)   111
– plasmacytoid DCs (pDCs)   111
de novo synthesis
– compounds linking BTCP with diaryl sulfide-based inhibitors   392
– of Spd   173, 175
– of sterols   495
– of trypanothione   407
density functional theory (DFT) level   63
deoxyribonucleotides synthesis   181
2′-deoxythymidine-5′-monophosphate (dTMP)   446
2,4-diaminopyrimidines   467
2,4-diaminoquinazolines   468

diaryl sulfides   420
1-(3,4-dichloro-benzyl)-2-amino-
  benzimidazole   467
2,7-dichlorodihydrofluorescein diacetate
  (DCFH₂)   217
diffusion   337–339
difluoromethylornithine (DFMO)   174, 387
D,L-difluoromethyl ornithine (DFMO). *See*
  eflornithine
dihydrofolate reductase (DHFR)   46, 343,
  445, 446
– crystallographic structures
– – available from PDB   454
– – of *Tc*DHFR-TS   454
– folate analogs acting as DHFR
  inhibitors   446
– inhibition of   467, 468
– pathways involving   447
– structural studies   453–455
– x-ray crystal structures   446
dihydropteroate synthetase   343
dihydroxyacetone phosphate (DHAP)   154
diminazene aceturate resistance   343
dinitrosyl-iron complex (DNIC)   178
dipyridamole   283
"direct-squirt" method   39
5,5'-dithiobis(2-nitrobenzamide)
  (DTNBA)   407
DNA-binding protein   247
DNA degradation   269
DNA fragments   45
DNA helicases   246, 250, 251
DNA polymerases   246, 249, 250, 257
DNA primases   246, 248, 249
DNA synthesis   182
DNA TopoII_{mt}   250
DNA topoisomerases   244, 252, 253
docking analysis   73
docking-based binding mode   74
– analysis   73
dolichol-phosphate mannose synthase
  (DPMS)   318, 326, 327
domperidone   27
*Dpn*II-PCR-RFLP   343, 344
drug delivery systems, development   111
drug design, and screening
– computer-aided drug design   58, 59
– ligand-based approaches, against
  trypanosoma parasites   61–65
– molecular modeling, and anti-kinetoplastida
  drug design   59–61
– protein druggability, in silico
  prediction   74–76
– *in silico* approaches   57–76

– structure-based drug design and
  screening   65–67
– – workflow   65–67
– supercomputers and other technical
  resources   59
– virtual screening approaches against
  trypanosome proteins   67–74
drug discovery program   89
druggability of target protein   74
drug incubation *Glossina* infectivity test
  (DIGIT)   342
drug incubation infectivity test (DIIT)   342
drug mechanisms, biochemical
  investigation   48
drug resistance   179, 180
drug screening, for neglected disease   482
– high-throughput assay   482
– MTC assay and efficacy   483
– quantitative method to test drug
  sensitivity   482
– targeting ergosterol biosynthesis   480
– *in vitro* drug screening   482
drugs for neglected diseases initiative
  (DNDi)   475, 480, 499, 522
drugs, for specific treatment of chagas
  disease   490. *See also* chagas disease
– benznidazole   490, 492, 493
– ergosterol biosynthesis inhibitors
  (EBIs)   493
– guidelines   493
– limitations   490–493
– nifurtimox   490, 492, 493
– 2-nitromidazole   490

e
eflornithine   47, 48, 387, 519
eflornithine (D,L-difluoromethyl ornithine
  (DFMO))   47
electronic descriptors   60
Embden–Meyerhof pathway   298
endocytic pathway   111
endocytosis   45, 266, 268, 288, 357
endonuclease G   269
endoplasmic reticulum (ER)   128, 316
enolase (ENO)   122
Entamoeba invadens   352
enzyme-linked immunosorbent assay   19
enzyme-mediated actions   179
enzyme-selective inhibitors   141
enzyme substitution mechanism   202
epiandrosterone (EA)   305
epimastigotes   128
ergosterol biosynthesis inhibitors (EBIs)
  489, 493

Ergosterol synthesis 285
Escherichia coli 41
Euglena 405
eukaryotic elongation factor 1B (eEF1B) 179
exocytosis 266
exponential-phase promastigotes 161

f
Fansidar 343
Farnesylation 285
Fcγ receptor-mediated phagocytosis 111
fingerprint for ligands and proteins (FLAP) 76
FK-binding protein 12, 264
flavin-disulfide oxidoreductases 405
flavoenzyme TR 387
5-formyl-6-hydroxy-2-naphthyl di-sodium phosphate 139
Fourier transform ion cyclotron resonance (FT-ICR) mass spectrometers 41
FRED program 72
fructose-1,6-bisphosphatase (FBPase) 131
fructose-6-phosphate 138, 317
fumarate hydratase (FH) 127
functional genomics projects 143

g
GDP-mannose, biosynthesis and consumption 316
GDP mannose dehydratase (GMD) 138
GDP-mannose-dependent mannosyltransferases 316, 327
GDP-mannose pyrophosphorylase (GDP-MP) 125, 317
GDP-mannose transporter (LPG2) 327, 328
gene expression profiles 157
γ-glutamylcysteine synthetase (GSH1) 387
GLO1-encoding gene 155
GLO1–green fluorescent protein construct 158
glomerular filtration rate 23
glucantime 21
gluconeogenesis 130, 298
gluconeogenic enzymes 131
glucosamine-6-phosphate *N*-acetyltransferase (GNA) 138
glucose
– based metabolism, of trypanosomatids 39, 298
– consumption 271
glucose-6-phosphate (G6P) 130, 298
glucose-6-phosphate dehydrogenase (G6PDH) 46, 125, 178, 298
glucose transporter 124, 125

γ-glutamylcysteine synthetase (GshA) 46, 173
glutaredoxins 388
glutathione (GSH) 336, 429
– functional replacement 153
glutathione peroxidase (GPX) 201, 225, 254
glutathione reductase (GR) 387
– protein backbone for human GR(hGR) 410
glutathione synthetase 173, 388
glutathionylspermidines 406
glutathionyl spermidine synthetase (GspS) 175, 430
glyceraldehyde-3-phosphate (Gly3P) 154, 298
glyceraldehyde-3-phosphate dehydrogenase (GAPDH) 122
glycerol kinase (GK) 124
glycerol-3-phosphate/DHAP shuttle 158
glycerol-3-phosphate oxidase (GPO) system 123
glycine 267, 355
glycoconjugates 316
– mannosylation 317
glycogen synthase kinase-3 (GSK-3) 291
glycolipids 315
glycolysis 21, 43, 128, 141, 262, 298
– in trypanosomes 263
glycolytic enzymes 127, 262
– in cell-free assays 46
glycolytic flux 125, 133, 160
glycolytic pathway 130, 298
glycosomal enzymes 141
– kinetic properties 127
glycosomal membrane 133
– controlled communication across 132–134
glycosomal NADH-dependent glycerol-3-phosphate dehydrogenase (G3PDH) 123
glycosomal solute transporters 142
glycosomal targeting signal 204
glycosomes 121, 262, 298
– inhibitors of glycosomal enzymes/processes 138–141
– integration of glycosomal metabolism
–– relation to life cycle differentiation 134, 135
– potential drug targets 136, 137
– target characterization, achievements 135, 138
glycosylation, eukaryotic 315
glycosylinositolphospholipids (GIPLs) 317
glycosylphosphatidylinositol (GPI) 315
glyoxalase enzymes
– glyoxalase I 155–157
– glyoxalase II 157, 158
– glyoxalase pathway 153–155

– – regulation 158–160
– – as therapeutic target 160–162
– in trypanosomatids 153–163
glyoxalase pathway 153–155, 161
– regulation 158–160
– as therapeutic target 160–162
glyoxalase system, in trypanosomatids 154
GOLD docking program 72
GPXs three-dimensional structure 206
GPx-type peroxidases 182, 184, 185
graphic processing units (GPUs) 59
graphic user interface (GUI) 87
GRID force field parameterization 76
GTPase Ras-related protein (Rab) 112
guanosine-diphospho-D-mannose
    pyrophosphorylase (GDP-MP) 325, 326
guide RNA (gRNA) molecules 244

h

HAT. *See* human African trypanosomiasis
    (HAT)
HeLa cells 184
helper T (T_h) cells 216
hemolymphatic system 37
hetero-oligomers 139
hexadecylphosphocholine 23
hexokinase 122, 317, 322, 323
– crystallographic analysis 322
– inhibitors 139, 322
– isozymes 322
hexose transporter 130, 318, 322
HGPRT ligands 141
high-affinity pentamidine transporter
    (HAPT1) 44
high-throughput screening (HTS)
    technologies 67, 82, 138, 177, 184
histone H1-like proteins 248
H_2O_2-induced programmed cell death 208
homeostasis 352
homologous protein 60
homology modeling docking crystal structure
– of *Tb*Atg8 to Atg4 from rat 267
homolysis 219
host cells, of *Leishmania* 106–111
host-nitrated proteins 219
host's defense mechanisms 167
host's oxidative defense 135
HTS Data for machine learning models
    89–98
HTS repurposing molecules, for trypanosomal
    diseases 82
human African trypanosomiasis (HAT) 37,
    365, 515
– current chemotherapeutic agents for 518

– – eflornithine (ornidyl,
        difluoromethylornithine) 519
– – melarsoprol 517, 518
– – nifurtimox–eflornithine combination
        therapy 519
– – pentamidine 518, 519
– – philanthropic support from
        foundations 520
– – suramin 518
– DFMO treatment 174
– life cycle of trypanosome 516, 517
– new trypanocidal agents 520
– – benzoxaboroles 522–526
– – diamidines 521
– – fexinidazole 520, 521
– – nitroimidazoles 520
human glutathione reductase (hGR) 71
human leishmaniasis 17
human parasitic trypanosomatid species,
    glycosomal enzymes 142
Hybrid compounds, with a dual mechanism
    of action 503, 504
hydrogen bond 224, 336, 337, 393, 448,
    452, 465
hydrolytic enzymes 352
hydroperoxide metabolism 181, 182
hydroperoxide-reducing enzymes 201, 207
hydroperoxides
– broad spectrum 201
– TXN/TXN dependent Prx (TXNPx)-mediated
    removal 179
hydrophilic interaction chromatography
    (HILIC) 41
hydrophobic interaction 466
1-(3-(4-hydroxybutoxy)-4-methoxyphenyl)-3-
    methylbutan-1-one 283
hypoglycemic shock 262
hypoxanthine 22
hypoxanthine-guanine
    phosphoribosyltransferase (HGPRT) 129

i

IDN-6556 288
IFATtest 23
immune evasion strategies 112
immunomodulating molecules 106
immuno-stimulated macrophages 217
indirect fluorescent antibody test (IFAT) 19
inducible nitric oxide synthase (iNOS)
    108, 215
inhibitors targeting, conserved proteins 284
inorganic pyrophosphate (PPi) 127, 129
in silico structure-based approaches 58,
    60, 70

in silico two-dimensional (2-D) bond based linear indices   62
in silico virtual screening approaches   71
intellectual property (IP) arrangements   83
inter alia proteins   184
interferon (IFN)-γ   8, 217
interferon (IFN)-γ–inducible protein (IP)-10   107
interleukin-2   263
intraglycosomal inorganic pyrophosphate (PPi)   129
in vitro fluorimetric assays   69
iron–sulfur cluster (ISC) metabolism   168, 178, 179
isoprenoids   129
itraconazole   481

j
Janus kinase/signal transducer and activator of transcription (JAK/STAT)   108

k
kala-azar   25, 386, 405
KAP3 and KAP4 proteins   248
kDNA chain elongation   249
kDNA repair enzymes   251
kDNA replication   244, 249, 251
– genes, periodic expression   254, 255
– machinery as an anti-trypanosomal drug target   256, 257
– machinery, components   247
– model   245
– proteins   253
– regulation   253, 255
–– replication initiation   253, 254
–– role of mitochondrial HslVU protease   255
– replication proteins, and complexes   247
– role of DNA topoisomerases   252
– topological reactions during   252
kinases   290–292
– inhibitors   292
kinetoplast-associated proteins (KAPs)   243
kinetoplast DNA (kDNA)   243
kinetoplast DNA helicases   250
kinetoplastida   238, 266
– drug targets   74
kinetoplastid selenoproteome   238, 239
kinetoplasts   248
Krebs cycle   21
Kyoto Encyclopedia of Genes and Genomes (KEGG)   43

l
lactaldehyde dehydrogenase system   158
S-ᴅ-lactoyltrypanothione   155
Langerhans cells (LCs)   111
Laplacian-corrected Bayesian classifier models   89
Leishmania amastigotes   130, 135
Leishmania amazonensis   108, 109
– MAPK/ERK pathway in   112
Leishmania braziliensis   107, 208
Leishmania chagasi   17, 19, 207
Leishmania chemotactic factor (LCF)   107
Leishmania donovani   3, 18, 107, 405, 430
– proliferation   177
Leishmania–host cell relationships   105
Leishmania infantum   3, 18, 19, 153, 205, 430
– detoxification enzymes   160
– glyoxalase II, trypanothione specificity in   159
– infections by   19
– methylglyoxal metabolism in   161
– progressive reduction   24
– resistant strains   26
Leishmania-infected macrophages   108
Leishmania major   282, 317, 352, 430
– GDP-mannose   317
– glucokinases   323
– TryS crystal structure   176
Leishmania mexicana   18, 327, 352
– Δ*lpg2* mutants   327
Leishmania parasites
– dendritic cells (DCs)   111, 112
– glycosomes   130–132
– host cells   106–111
– interaction with host cells functional consequences   105–113
– life cycle   105, 106
– macrophages   107–111
– neutrophils   106, 107
– non-essential enzyme in   208
– promastigotes
–– phagocytosis   110, 111
– TXNPx   180
leishmaniasis   297, 351
– chemotherapy   17–28, 386
–– canine leishmaniasis   19–27
–– status   17, 18
– muco-cutaneous leishmaniasis (espundia)   386
– visceral leishmaniasis   386
Leishmania tarentolae   243
Leishmania tropica   405
leishmanicidal compounds   110

ligand-based approaches   60, 61, 63
– against trypanosoma parasites   61–65
ligand binding sites   76
ligand–protein interactions   67
ligand similarity filter   71
LIG kα protein   252
LIG kβ expression   *252*
linear discriminant analysis (LDA)   61
Lipinski's rule   69
lipoamide dehydrogenase (LipDH)   406, 409
lipophilic hydroperoxides   201
lipophilic pockets   75
lipophosphoglycans (LPGs)   111, 317
liposomal amphotericin B   4, 8
– single-dose treatment   5
low-affinity pentamidine transporter (LAPT1)   44
low-cost drug delivery system   26
lowest unoccupied molecular orbital (LUMO)   64
LP10 inhibitor   481
lysosomal hydrolases   111, 265
lysosomes   336, 352
lysosomotropism   289

m
machine learning models   99
macroautophagy   352
macromolecules synthesis   174
macrophage inflammatory protein (MIP)-1β   107
macrophages   107–111, 218, 356
– functions, manipulation   107–110
– parasitophorous vacuoles in   110, 111
major histocompatibility complex (MHC) class II   108
malate dehydrogenase (MDH)   127
mammalian target of rapamycin (mTOR)   108
– proteolytical cleavage   109
mammals *vs* kinetoplastids
– enzymes and transporters involved in mannosylation   318–322
– – dolichol-phosphate mannose synthase (DPMS)   326, 327
– – GDP-mannose-dependent mannosyltransferases   327
– – GDP-mannose transporter   327, 328
– – guanosine-diphospho-D-mannose pyrophosphorylase (GDP-MP)   325, 326
– – hexokinase   322, 323
– – hexose transporter   318, 322
– – mannosyl phosphate transferases (MPTs)   328
– – phosphoglucose isomerase (PGI)   323, 324

– – phosphomannomutase (PMM)   324, 325
– – phosphomannose isomerase (PMI)   324
– mannosylation pathways   317, 318
mannogen synthesis   131
mannose-1-phosphate (M1P)   317
mannose-6-phosphate (M6P)   317
mannosylation pathways
– mammals vs kinetoplastids   317, 318
mannosyl phosphate transferases (MPTs)   318, 328
matrix proteins   134
meglumine antimoniate   20, 22, 387
melarsen oxide–trypanothione conjugate (MelT)   46
melarsen–trypanothione adduct (MelT)   47
melarsoprol   46, 47, 387, 517, 518
melarsoprol–DFMO combined therapy   174
metabolite translocation   134
metabolomics   37, 407
– new technologies applied to Trypanosomes   38–44
– – data analysis   42–44
– – MS-based metabolomics   40–42
– – NMR-based metabolomics   39, 40
– – sample preparation   38
– potential role   49
metacaspases (MCAs)   269, 357
metacyclic promastigotes   106
methemoglobinemia   418
methionine sulfoxide reductase (MSR)   183, 388
– nucleophilic cysteine   183
methylene blue   418
– redox cycles   419
methylglyoxal   179
– catabolizing enzymes   160
– formation system   158
– metabolism   160
– pathway   153
– steady-state concentration   161
methylglyoxal (MG) metabolism
– sensitivity analysis   162
methylthioadenosine phosphorylase   184
mevalonate kinase (MK)   131
Microsoft Excel-based application   43
MIF-like proteins   110
migration inhibitory factor (MIF)-like proteins   110
miltefosine   9, 23, 24, 358
– dog leishmaniasis treatment   23
– limitation   24
– pharmacokinetic profile   5
– in visceral leishmaniasis treatment   3
mitochondrial DNA ligases   251, 252

mitochondrial DNA primases   255
mitochondrial DNA replication   183
mitochondrial DNA TopoII$_{mt}$ 246
mitochondrial HslVU protease   255
mitochondrial outer membrane
   permeabilization (MOMP)   357
mitogen-activated protein kinase (MAPK)
   pathways   108
MM-GBSA approaches   66
molecular mechanics (MM) methods   58
molecular modeling   59–61
mononuclear phagocytic cells   107
mononuclear phagocytic system   19
MS-based metabolomics   40–42
– GC-MS-based metabolomics   40, 41
– LC-MS-based metabolomics   41, 42
multidrug treatment regimens, advantage   7
multiple reaction monitoring (MRM)
   approaches   42
mutations   343
– indicative G→A point mutation   343
– *PfCRT1*   343
– point mutation in *TcoAT1*   343
– resistance-associated ("mutated") *TcoAT1*
   allele   343

n
N-acetylcysteine   356
NAD-dependent fumarate reductase
   (FRD)   127
NAD(P)-dependent lactaldehyde
   dehydrogenase   179
NADPH-dependent aldose reductase   160
NADPH-dependent disulfide reductases   406
NADPH-dependent flavoenzyme TR, in
   kinetoplastid parasites   406
NADPH-dependent glutathione/GR
   system   406
NADPH-dependent methylglyoxal
   reductase   158
NADPH-dependent trypanothione
   reductase   167
NADPH oxidase   215
Nagana cattle disease   405
naphthoquinone (NQ) derivative   27, 409
– derived from menadione, plumbagin, and
   juglone, structures   412
– 1,4-NQs as trypanocidal agents   409–413
– oxidoreduction   409
– structures of trypanocidal 1,4-NQs
– – acting as subversive substrates   411
natural killer (NK) cells   107, 216
necrosis   261

neglected diseases   105
neglected tropical diseases (NTDs)   3, 386
network-based representations   43
neutrophils   106, 107
new anti-leishmanial drugs, exploration
   of   27, 28
new chemical entity (NCE)   10
N-glycosylated proteins   315
Ni^{2+}-dependent proteins   156
nifurtimox   48, 61, 387, 413
nifurtimox–eflornithine combination therapy
   (NECT)   44, 48, 387
nifurtimox-resistant   289
nitric oxide ($^{•}$NO)   178, 216
nitrofurans   413, 473
– anti-trypanosomal drugs
– – development events   413
– – nitrofurazone   416
– – prodrug NFOH-121   416
– – recently developed, with anti-parasitic
   activity   416
– – synthesis of hydroxymethylnitrofurazone
   from   416
– derivative   409
– parasitic targets, and mechanism
   of action   414, 415
– redox cycle in presence of molecular
   oxygen   415
– toxicity   413
nitrofurazone   416
nitroimidazoles   413
NMR-based metabolomics   39, 40
N-myristoyltransferase (NMT)   287, 288
– inhibition and trypanocidal activity   288
non-folate-related DHFR inhibitors   468
non-homologous enzymes   135
non-ionic surfactant vesicles   22
NOS isoforms   218
Noxafil$^{®}$ 480, 496
nsGPXs, mechanism of action   202, 203
nuclear factor "kappa light chain enhancer" of
   activated B cells (NF-κB)   110
nuclear magnetic resonance (NMR)   38, 60
– Bringaud's systematic application   40
nucleic acids, as chemical building blocks   38
nucleoprotein complex   254

o
odanacatib   288
ODC expression   47
Okazaki fragments   245, 252
oligosaccharide mannogen   131
open-access chemistry databases   83

Oriental sore   405
origin recognition complexes (ORCs)   253
ornithine decarboxylase (ODC)   46, 47, 174, 292, 387
orotidine-5'-monophosphate decarboxylase   132
orphan drug   18
osteoporosis   288
oxidative stress   407
oxidoreductase tryparedoxin (TXN)   168
oxidosqualene cyclase (lanosterol synthase) inhibitors   501, 502
2-oxoaldehyde   153
oxygen metabolites   106

p
parallel artificial membrane permeation assay (PAMPA)   337
parasitemia   271
parasite persistence mechanisms   8
parasite's redox homeostasis   177
parasite target-oriented compounds   18
parasitophorous vacuoles (PVs)   105, 106
paromomycin   18, 26, 27, 387
– non-inferiority   5
– in visceral leishmaniasis treatment   3
part fatal diseases   17
pathogen–host cell interactions   113
PC-based database systems   86
PDSP dataset   88
pentamidine   44, 45, 518, 519
pentamidine dimetasulfonate   27
pentamidine isethionate   26
pentavalent antimonials   20
pentose-phosphate pathways (PPP)   122, 128, 135, 298, 300, 301
– enzymes, from trypanosomatids   125, 129, 303–305
– inhibitor discovery against enzymes   305–308
pentose phosphate shunt   178
PEP carboxykinase (PEPCK)   127
peptidases   352
– Clan CA peptidases, with roles in ubiquitination   358
– mitochondrion ubiquitin-like peptidase (MUP)   359
– potential peptidase targets in *Leishmania* spp.   353
peptide-based drugs, drawbacks   290
peptidic substrate   184
peptidomimetic K777   476
peroxidases   217
– as drug targets   184, 185

peroxidatic cysteine   202, 205
peroxins (PEXs)   121, 134
peroxiredoxin (PRX)   201
peroxisomal enzymes   122
peroxisomal membranes   133
peroxisome-targeting signal (PTS)   128
peroxynitrite anion (ONOO⁻)   216
peroxynitrite detoxification systems   222–226
peroxynitrite diffusion   219–222
peroxynitrite formation
– in immuno-stimulated-infected macrophages   218
– during *T. cruzi*–mammalian host cell interaction   216
peroxynitrite reactivity with *T. cruzi* targets   219–222
peroxynitrite reduction kinetics   225
peroxynitrous acid (ONOOH)   216
PEX proteins   142
P38 gene   248
PGK reaction   124
phagophore   263, 355
4-phenoxyphenoxyethylthiocyanate (WC-9)   140
1-phenyl-4-glycosyl-dihydropyridines   465
phosphatidylethanolamine (PE)   265, 355
phosphatidylinositol-3 kinase (PI3K) pathway   108
phosphatidylinositol-3-phosphate   265
5-phosphoarabinonohydroxamic acid (5PAH)   324
phosphodiesterases (PDEs)   282
– inhibitors   282, 283
phosphoenolpyruvate (PEP)   127
phosphofructokinase (PFK) reactions   122
6-phosphogluconate dehydrogenase (6PGDH)   125, 298
6-phosphogluconolactonase (6PGL)   298
phosphoglucose isomerase (PGI)   317, 323, 324
– expression products encoded by   323
6-phosphoglunocolactone dehydrogenase   178
3-phosphoglycerate (3-PGA)   122
phosphoglycerate kinase (PGK)   44, 122
phosphoglycerate mutase (PGAM)   122
phosphoinositide 3-kinase (PI3K)   291
phospholipid bilaminar complexes   25
phospholipids   352
phosphomannomutase (PMM)   317, 324, 325
phosphomannose isomerase (PMI)   317, 324
– deficiency   324
– leishmanial and trypanosomal   324
phosphorylated hexoses   128

phosphoseryl-tRNA kinase (PSTK)   239
piperidine derivative   71
plant peroxisomes   133
plasma membrane hexose transporter   128
Plasmodium falciparum   156, 182, 392, 405
– glutathione reductase (GR) schematic
   presentation   407
pleiotropism   185
Pneumocystis carinii   26
PocketPicker   75
polar replication model   247
polyamines   47, 48, 388
– deficient media   174
– production   174
polycyclic compound   71
polymerase chain reaction (PCR)   19
posaconazole   286, 480, 481, 496–498
– efficacy   481
post-kala-azar dermal leishmaniasis
   (PKDL)   3, 4, 8–10
– *Leishmania donovani*   8
– *Leishmania infantum*   8
– pathology and immunopathology   8, 9
– susceptibility   9
– treatment options for   9, 10
potential resistance mechanisms   49
PPi-susceptible glycosomal enzymes   140
PPP enzymes   125, 140
pre-autophagosomal structure (PAS)   263
PRI1 gene   249
procyclic-form trypanosomes   125
procyclic promastigotes   106
procyclic trypanosomes   39
pro-inflammatory cytokines   109
prolactin production   27
proof-of-concept   7
– study   49
propidium iodide   261
prostaglandin (PG) D_2 (PGD$_2$)   269
– applications   269
proteases   288
– cellular functions   370
–– proteasome   373
–– *Tb*CALPs   371
–– *Tb*CATB and *Tb*CATL   370
–– *Tb*GPI8   372
–– *Tb*MCA2, *Tb*MCA3, and *Tb*MCA5   371, 372
–– *Tb*MSP-B   373
–– *Tb*OPB and *Tb*POP   372
– as drug targets   373
–– proteasome   377, 378
–– *Tb*CALPs   374
–– *Tb*CATB and *Tb*CATL   373, 374

–– *Tb*GPI8   374, 375
–– *Tb*MCAs   374
–– *Tb*MSP-B   377
–– *Tb*OPB and *Tb*POP   375, 376
– inhibitors   288
Protein Data Bank   393
Protein Data Bank (PDB)   60, 393
protein druggability, in silico prediction
   74–76
protein farnesyltransferase (PFT)   285, 499
protein–ligand complexes   66, 399
protein–protein interactions   76
protein structures, x-ray resolution   67
protein tyrosine phosphatase (PTP)   108
proteolytical modification, of transcription
   factors   109
proteomic analysis   47
proteophosphoglycans (PPGs)   317
protozoan parasites   282
protozoan transporters, selective uptake
   by   339–341
Pseudomonas aeruginosa   156
Pseudomonas putida   156
pteridine reductase (PTR1)   445, 446
– crystallographic structures, available in
   PDB   450
– from DHFR to PTR1 Inhibitors   465, 466
–– docking studies on compounds   465
– discovery and development of
   inhibitors   455
–– chemical structures and activity
   values   456–464
–– compounds with similar structures   455
–– 5-deazapteridines   455
–– diaminopteridines   455
–– pteridine-like compounds   455, 465
–– quinazolines   455
– *Lm*PTR1 structure   451
– non-pteridine-like PTR1 inhibitors   466, 467
– pathways involving   447
– promising drug targe   446
– residues forming *Lm*PTR1 active site   451
– structural studies   446, 448, 451–453
– in trypanosomatidic parasites
–– alignment of PTR1 sequences   449
–– identity (and similarity) among PTR1
   sequences   448
– x-ray crystal structures   446
purine metabolism   23
purine salvage   298
PYK isoenzymes   138
pyridine-indomethacin amide derivative
   LP-10   500

pyrimidine biogenesis   298
pyruvate kinase (PYK)   122
pyruvate phosphate dikinase (PPDK)   127

q
QM methods   63
QM simulations   58
quantitative statistical models   74
quantitative structure–activity relationship
   (QSAR)   61, 62, 64, 83
quantum mechanics (QM) methods   58
quinols   423, 424
– proposed mode of action   424
quinones   409

r
Radanil®   387
rapamycin   263, 264, 267
rapid filtration method   39
ravuconazole   286
reactive oxygen species (ROS)   271
receiver operating characteristic (ROC)
   value   90
recombinant enzyme   140
recombinant proteins   183
recombinant *Tb*PIF5 DNA helicase   250
recombinant *Tb*PIF1 protein   250
redoxin and DNA synthesis   182, 183, 184
redoxin-dependent enzymes   183
redoxin-dependent functions   180, 181
redoxin-independent functions   178
redoxins   184
– as drug targets   184, 185
redox metabolism   182
redox sensors   168
relacatib   288
ribonucleotide reductase (RnR)   182, 388
ribose-5-phosphate (R5P)   298
ribose-5-phosphate isomerase (RPI)   298
– from trypanosomatids   304
ribosomes   265
ribulose-5-phosphate epimerase (RPE)   298
RITSeq approach   45, 47, 48
RNA interference (RNAi)   124, 168, 207, 281
– analysis   247
– drug targets by   135
– mediated downregulation   173
– pathway   45
roflumilast   283

s
Saccharomyces cerevisiae   156
S-adenosylmethionine decarboxylase
   (SAMDC)   44

salicylhydroxamic acid (SHAM)   124
sample preparation   38, 39
saquinavir   288
Schizosaccharomyces pombe   183
scoring function   66
screening approaches towards TR   391
– combined *in vitro*/*in silico* screening
   campaign   393
– – workflow   394
– consensus pharmacophore building
   398, 399
– – by docking and clustering
   experiments   399
– – Drugscore^Maps approach   398
– – kinetic analysis   398
– current state of the art   391–393
– second *in vitro* screen   397, 398
– *in silico* screening   396, 397
– TR assay adaptation   395
– *in vitro* screening   395, 396
Sec insertion sequence (SECIS) element   238
SECISearch   238
SecS genes   239, 240
selenocysteine (Sec)   237
selenocysteine-containing glutathione
   peroxidases (GPXs)   181, 387
selenoproteome   239, 240
– default pattern of SECISearch   238
– dispensable   239, 240
– of kinetoplastids   239
– relevant for long-term protection   240
short-coursemultidrug treatment regimes   5
signal-to-noise ratios   82
single-dose liposomal amphotericin B plus
   miltefosine   7
site-directed mutagenesis   202
sleeping sickness   272, 365, 385, 386
– chemotherapy   366
sodium stibogluconate   4, 21, 387
spermidine   48, 387, 388, 430
spermidine-interacting residues   158
spermidine synthase (SpdS)   175, 388
squalene synthase (SQS)   129, 140
squalene synthase inhibitors   502, 503
Sterol C14α-demethylase (CYP51)   489
– inhibitors   495–501
sterols   493
stoichiometry-based models   43
Streptomyces hygroscopicus   263
Streptomyces nodosus   24
structure–activity relationship (SAR)
   analysis   62, 83, 135
structure-based approaches   66, 68
– requirement for   65

structure-based docking 73
structure-based drug design, and
    screening 65–67
structure-based pharmacophore models 66,
    72, 75
structure-based virtual screening 65, 71
structure-specific endonuclease 1 (SSE1) 246
substrate-binding pocket 185
sugar nucleotides 125
supercomputers 59
superoxide radical 215
suramin 45, 46, 518

t

TAC proteins p166 247
target of rapamycin (TOR) 291
target protein 74
target receptor 60, 75
– 3-D structure 59
Tau protein 418
TbGPXA2
– crystal structure 206
*Tb*HslVU protease 250
TbPDEB1 inhibitor 283
TbPIF5 allele 250
– overexpression 251
*Tb*PIF1 and *Tb*PIF2 DNA helicase 250
TB project 86
TCA cycle 127
T-cell receptor genes 476
T-cells 263
TcoAT1 resistance allele 344
teratogenicity 351
tetrafluoromethyl ketones 479
tetrahydrophthalazinone 283
thiol-dependent reactions 167
thiol–disulfide exchange 202
thiol/disulfide oxidoreductases 180
thiol group 352
thiol peroxidases
– function in trypanosomatids 207–209
– mechanism of reaction 202–204
– thiol-dependent peroxidases in
    trypanosomatids 201, 202
– trypanosomatid GPXs 205–207
– trypanosomatid PRXs 204, 205
– of trypanosomatids 201–209
thioredoxin homolog "tryparedoxin"
    (TXN) 429
thioredoxin recognition 207
thioredoxin reductase (TrxR) 387
thioredoxins 204, 388
thioredoxin/TrxR system 406

thymidylate synthase (TS) 445, 446
time-of-flight (TOF) 41
tipifarnib 499
– analog 500
α-tocopherol
– water-soluble version 182
TOF detectors 42
topological molecular computer design
    (TOMOCOMD) approach 61–63
TORC complexes 265
TOR complex 1 (TORC1) 264
TOR kinases 265
TOR-like proteins 265
Toxoplasma gondii 185, 352
track sugar nucleotide 42
transaldolase (TAL) 298
transcription factor 183
transferrin 268
transforming growth factor (TGF)-β 107
transketolase 298
transporters
– protozoan transporters, selective uptake
    by 339–341
– role of efflux transporters 341, 342
1,2,3-triazole-based tetrafluoromethyl
    ketone 479
triazole derivatives, chemical structures 496
– ravuconazole 496, 498
– TAK-187 496, 498
– UR-9825 496, 498
tricarboxylic acid (TCA) cycle 40
– enzymes 122
Trichomonas vaginalis 336
tricyclic system 72
trimethoprim 467
2,2,4-trimethyl-1,2-dihydroquinolines
    (THQs) 417, 418
– with anti-trypanosomal activities 417
– anti-trypanosomal mechanism of 418
– *in vitro* anti-trypanosomal structure–activity
    relationship 417
TR inhibitors 72
triosephosphate isomerase (TPI) 124
triostam 387
tripartite attachment complex (TAC) 247
triple-quadrupole mass spectrometers 42
TriTryp genomes 173
trypanocidal drugs
– mode of action 38
trypanocidal drugs, metabolic affects
    44–48
– eflornithine 47, 48
– melarsoprol 46, 47

– NECT   48
– pentamidine   44, 45
– suramin   45, 46
Trypanosoma brucei   37, 81, 122, 153, 157, 336, 352, 429
– cathepsins   290
– cell density regulation in   272
– cellular functions of proteases   370–373
– classes of proteases   366
–– calpain-like proteins   368
–– cathepsin B- and L-like proteases   366
–– cysteine peptidases   366
–– GPI : protein transamidase   368, 369
–– metacaspases   368
–– metalloproteases   369, 370
–– serine peptidases   369
–– threonine proteases   370
– etiological agent of HAT   365
– genome   43
– GLO1 enzyme in   161
– glycosomes   122–125
– hexokinases   323
– infection   40
– lipidomic analysis   42
– PDEBs as drug targets   284
– PEX proteins   134
– 6PGDH   304
– procyclic forms   39
– proteases, as drug targets   373–378
– pteridine reductase 1 (PTR1)   69, 70
– resistance against diamidine compounds   343
– statistics on X-ray resolution of protein structures   67
– subspecies, disease patterns caused by   365
–– *gambiense*   365
–– *rhodesiense*   365
– UCSF dataset   95–98
Trypanosoma brucei gambiense   41, 405
– life cycle   516, 517
– polyamine biosynthesis in   48
Trypanosoma brucei pteridine reductase 1 (PTR1)   69, 70
Trypanosoma brucei rhodesiense   37, 405
Trypanosoma brucei St Jude's dataset   91–94
Trypanosoma congolense   405
Trypanosoma cruzi   215, 352, 405, 430
– antioxidant enzymes, as virulence mediators   226–228
– antioxidant network   226
– chemical structure and biological activity   62, 64
–– discovered by using the *in silico*-based technique   62

– competitive inhibitors   68
– cruzain activity   478
– cruzain identified by means of virtual screening   68
– crystal structure of CYP51 complexed with posaconazole   497
– dihydrofolate reductase (DHFR)   69
–– chemical structure and inhibitory activity   70
–– function   70
– DNA primase 1 (*Tb*PRI1)   216
– epimastigote forms   61
– glucokinases   322, 323
– glycosomes   125–130
– inhibitory activity of *Tc*TS inhibitor   69
– killing by intraphagosomal peroxynitrite and   227
– lead compounds, inhibiting enzymatic targets   481
– mammalian host cell interaction   216–219
– nitrofurazone, reduced by LipDH   416
– peroxynitrite formation during mammalian host cell interaction   216
– PIF1-like proteins   251
– *PRI1* gene   255
– resistant to current therapy   481, 482
– SPS2   240
– statistics on the X-ray resolution of protein structures   67
– sterols   494
–– structure and function of   493–495
– TR inhibitor
–– chemical structure and inhibitory activity   72
– trypanothione reductase (TR)   70–74
–– protein backbone   410
–– schematic presentation   407
Trypanosoma cruzi trans-sialidase (TcTS)
– chemical structure and inhibitory activity   69
Trypanosoma evansi   44
trypanosomal diseases   99
– CDD database   83–89
– computational approaches and collaborative drug discovery   81–99
– drug discovery, computational approaches for   84, 85
– HTS repurposing molecules for   82
– machine learning models, using HTS data for   89–98
– screening datasets   87
trypanosomal proteasome   370, 373, 378
trypanosomatids   141, 246
– carbonyl and redox stresses in   163

– Chagas disease (*See* Chagas disease)
– function of thiol peroxidases 207–209
– glyoxalase enzymes 153–163
– – connection between carbonyl and redox
   stresses 163
– – glyoxalase I 155–157
– – glyoxalase II 157, 158
– – glyoxalase pathway 153–155
– – glyoxalase pathway as a therapeutic
   target 160–162
– – glyoxalase pathway regulation 158–160
– glyoxalases
– – X-ray crystallographic structures 156
– glyoxylase system 178
– GPXs 205–207
– hydroperoxide elimination in 201
– hydroperoxide-reducing enzymes 209
– major metabolic pathways/parts of pathways
   found in 123
– mechanism of reaction of thiol
   peroxidases 202–204
– metabolism
– – controlled communication essentiality
   across glycosomal membrane 132–134
– – correct integration essentiality of
   glycosomal metabolism in 134, 135
– – glycosomal enzymes/processes, inhibitors
   development 138–141
– – glycosomal metabolism pathway, diagram
   presenting enzymes 123
– – glycosomes function and glycosomal
   proteins as drug targets 121–143
– – *Leishmania* spp., glycosomes 130–132
– – metabolic processes, enzymes presents
   in 126
– – target characterization 135–138
– – *T. brucei*, glycosomes 122–125
– – *T. cruzi*, glycosomes 125–130
– Nagana (Surra) cattle disease 386
– nsGPXs 206
– oxoaldehyde metabolism 179
– parasitic diseases caused by 385, 386
– pathogenic 121
– potential drug targets in glycosomes 136, 137
– PRXs 204, 205
– *T. b. rhodesiense* 386
– *T. brucei gambiense* 385
– thiol-dependent peroxidases 201, 202
– thiol-dependent redox system 168
– thiol redox metabolism 167–173, 387, 388
– trypanothione-based redox
   metabolism 167–186
– – thiol redox metabolism 167–173

Trypanosoma vivax 405
trypanosome PEX amino acid sequences 135
trypanosome-specific 18S-PCR-RFLP
   343, 344
trypanosomes, pharmacological
   metabolomics 37–49
– data analysis 42–44
– eflornithine 47, 48
– melarsoprol 46, 47
– MS-based metabolomics 40–42
– new technologies applied to 38–44
– nifurtimox in combination therapy
   (NECT) 48
– NMR-based metabolomics 39, 40
– pentamidine 44, 45
– sample preparation 38, 39
– suramin 45, 46
– trypanocidal drugs, metabolic affects 44–48
trypanosomiasis 297
– cerebral 338
– chemotherapy 386
– human African trypanosomiasis
– – life cycle of *T. brucei*, causative agent 516
– melarsoprol-refractory 413
– as neglected tropical diseases (NTDs) 386
trypanothione 167, 336, 406
– in African trypanosomes 388
– – synthesis and reduction 388
– Ellman's-reagent-mediated
   regeneration 408
trypanothione (bis(glutathionyl)
   spermidine 387
trypanothione-based redox metabolism
– of trypanosomatids 167–186
– – thiol redox metabolism 167–173
– trypanothione biosynthesis 173–177
– trypanothione recycling 177, 178
– trypanothione utilization 178–185
– – hydroperoxide metabolism 181, 182
– – redoxin and DNA synthesis 182, 183, 184
– – redoxin-dependent functions 180, 181
– – redoxin-independent functions 178
– – redoxins and peroxidases as drug
   targets 184, 185
– – trypanothione-dependent detoxification
   reactions and drug resistance 179, 180
– – trypanothione-dependent ligation of iron,
   NO complexes and ISCs 178, 179
trypanothione biosynthesis 173–177
– glutathione synthesis 173
– polyamine synthesis, salvage, and
   uptake 173, 175
– trypanothione synthesis 175–177

trypanothione-dependent detoxification
reactions   177, 179, 180
trypanothione-dependent glyoxalase
pathway   154
trypanothione-dependent hydroperoxide
metabolism   183
trypanothione metabolism   21, 169
trypanothione-reactive agents   420
– reaction mechanisms
– – for modification of protein thiols
(RSH)   421
– – for polymer formation and
fragmentation   422
– unsaturated mannich bases as dithiol-
alkylating agents   420, 423
trypanothione recycling   177, 178
trypanothione reductase (TR)   70, 254, 387
– active site of *T. cruzi* TR   390
– as drug target molecule   407, 408
– inhibitors   63, 140
– screening approaches (*See* screening
approaches towards TR)
– turncoat inhibitors (subversive substrates/
redox cyclers)   408, 409
– as validated drug target   389
– *vs.* human glutathione reductase (GR)
389, 391
trypanothione-related pathways
– components   170–172
trypanothione-related protein   70
trypanothione synthetase (TryS)   175, 226,
387, 429, 430
– functional and structural
characteristics   430–436
– – alternative routes of T(SH)$_2$
biosynthesis   431
– – ATP-grasp fold loop   434
– – *Lm*TryS model structure   435
– – spermidine and glutathione analogs as
substrates in T(SH)2 biosynthesis   433
– – TryS-amidase X-ray structure   432
– GSH analogs with inhibitory activity   437
– Gsp analogs mimic transition state during
Gsp formation   438
– inhibitor design   436–440
– natural product with inhibitory activity   440
– N^5-substituted paullone inhibiting *Cf*
TryS   438
– TryS inhibitors derived from random
screening   439
trypanothione system   185, 388
trypanothione utilization   178–185
– hydroperoxide metabolism   181, 182
– redoxin and DNA synthesis   182, 183, 184

– redoxin-dependent functions   180, 181
– redoxin-independent functions   178
– redoxins and peroxidases as drug
targets   184, 185
– trypanothione-dependent
– – detoxification reactions and drug
resistance   179, 180
– – ligation of iron, NO complexes and
ISCs   178, 179
tryparedoxin (Tpx)   204, 388
T(SH)$_2$-dependent enzymes   429
T(SH)$_2$ synthesis   176
tumor necrosis factor (TNF)-α   8, 108, 217
TUNEL test   269
TXN-dependent peroxidase activity   204
type IA DNA topoisomerases   253
type II DNA topoisomerase   253

u

ubiquitin-activating enzyme   184
UDP-*N*-acetylglucosamine pyrophosphorylase
(UAP)   138
UDP-glucose-4′-epimerase (UGE)   138
UDP-glucose pyrophosphorylase (UGP)
138
UMS-binding protein (UMSBP)   247, 253
– DNA-binding activity and its redox
state   253, 254
– surface plasmon resonance (SPR)
analysis   254
UMSBP gene   247
universal mini circle sequence binding
protein   183
uridine-5-monophosphate (UMP)
synthase   132

v

variant surface glycoprotein (VSG)   269,
270, 271
– coat   288
– VSG-specific antibodies   271, 272
vinylsulfone K11777   289
virtual screening approaches   65, 72
– against trypanosome proteins   67–74
virulence   352
– factors   228
visceral leishmaniasis
– anti-leishmanial drugs and treatment
options   4–8
– available drugs   4, 5
– clinical drug efficacy, regional differences
in   7, 8
– clinical features   3
– drugs and treatment regimes   6

– drugs, pharmacokinetic/pharmacodynamic
   profiles   7
– open questions and needs   10
– PKDL   8–10
– treatments and needs   3–10

w
World Health Organization   18
– guidelines   493
– key requirements, for drugs   475
– 17 NTDs   386
– screening program supported by   417

x
xanthine phosphoribosyltransferase
   (XPRT)   132
xanthine urolithiasis   23
X-ray crystallography   67, 68, 69
X-ray *Trypanosoma*'s protein structures
– statistics   60

z
Z-DNA region   248
zinc-dependent protease (MSP-B)   273
zoonosis   386, 490